NUTRITION AND DIET RESEARCH PROGRESS

PLANT FLAVONOIDS AFFECT CANCER CHEMOTHERAPEUTIC EFFICACY

A HANDBOOK FOR DOCTORS AND PATIENTS

NUTRITION AND DIET RESEARCH PROGRESS

Additional books and e-books in this series can be found
on Nova's website under the Series tab.

NUTRITION AND DIET RESEARCH PROGRESS

PLANT FLAVONOIDS AFFECT CANCER CHEMOTHERAPEUTIC EFFICACY

A HANDBOOK FOR DOCTORS AND PATIENTS

KATRIN SAK

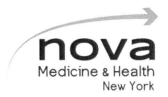

Copyright © 2019 by Nova Science Publishers, Inc.

All rights reserved. No part of this book may be reproduced, stored in a retrieval system or transmitted in any form or by any means: electronic, electrostatic, magnetic, tape, mechanical photocopying, recording or otherwise without the written permission of the Publisher.

We have partnered with Copyright Clearance Center to make it easy for you to obtain permissions to reuse content from this publication. Simply navigate to this publication's page on Nova's website and locate the "Get Permission" button below the title description. This button is linked directly to the title's permission page on copyright.com. Alternatively, you can visit copyright.com and search by title, ISBN, or ISSN.

For further questions about using the service on copyright.com, please contact:
Copyright Clearance Center
Phone: +1-(978) 750-8400   Fax: +1-(978) 750-4470   E-mail: info@copyright.com.

NOTICE TO THE READER

The Publisher has taken reasonable care in the preparation of this book, but makes no expressed or implied warranty of any kind and assumes no responsibility for any errors or omissions. No liability is assumed for incidental or consequential damages in connection with or arising out of information contained in this book. The Publisher shall not be liable for any special, consequential, or exemplary damages resulting, in whole or in part, from the readers' use of, or reliance upon, this material. Any parts of this book based on government reports are so indicated and copyright is claimed for those parts to the extent applicable to compilations of such works.

Independent verification should be sought for any data, advice or recommendations contained in this book. In addition, no responsibility is assumed by the Publisher for any injury and/or damage to persons or property arising from any methods, products, instructions, ideas or otherwise contained in this publication.

This publication is designed to provide accurate and authoritative information with regard to the subject matter covered herein. It is sold with the clear understanding that the Publisher is not engaged in rendering legal or any other professional services. If legal or any other expert assistance is required, the services of a competent person should be sought. FROM A DECLARATION OF PARTICIPANTS JOINTLY ADOPTED BY A COMMITTEE OF THE AMERICAN BAR ASSOCIATION AND A COMMITTEE OF PUBLISHERS.

Additional color graphics may be available in the e-book version of this book.

Library of Congress Cataloging-in-Publication Data

ISBN: 978-1-53615-957-8

Published by Nova Science Publishers, Inc. † New York

To my ancestors; above all, to my parents.
With gratitude and honor

CONTENTS

Preface		ix
Introduction		xi
Abbreviations		xvii
Chapter 1	Overview of the Most Common Cancer Types	1
Chapter 2	Cancer Development Step by Step	33
Chapter 3	Conventional Chemotherapy and Its Limitations	39
Chapter 4	Complex Mechanisms of Cancer Drug Resistance: Possibilities for Intervention with Natural Compounds	51
Chapter 5	Plant Flavonoids: Their Natural Sources, Bioavailability and Anticancer Properties	89
Chapter 6	Effects of Plant Flavonoids on Chemotherapeutic Efficacy of Cancer Drugs	135
Chapter 7	Conclusion and Further Perspectives to Improve Cancer Therapeutic Outcome	385
About the Author		395
Index of Drugs		397
Index of Flavonoids		399
Related Nova Publications		403

PREFACE

Despite intensive work done in the understanding of molecular mechanisms underlying malignant transformation, progression and metastasis of cancer, but also continuous development of novel drugs and therapeutic regimens against various types of human malignancies, cancer has still often remained an incurable disease, especially in the case of its advanced and metastatic stages. Therefore, with the hope to gain therapeutic advantage or even miracle cure, even more than 50% of cancer patients consume any kind of herbal supplements when undergoing chemotherapeutic treatment with traditional cytotoxic antineoplastic agents. As knowledge about the possible interactions of bioactive natural plant compounds and chemotherapeutic drugs is generally poor, such consumption of plant-derived dietary supplements is mostly injudicious and unreasonable. This book is the first one to systematically compile currently available information about the modulation of chemotherapeutic efficacy by flavonoids as bioactive constituents of plant-based food products and dietary supplements. To date, numerous combinations of these phytochemicals and different conventional cytotoxic anticancer agents have been studied in preclinical settings, i.e., cancer cell lines *in vitro* and xenograft models *in vivo*. As a result, both desired (additive to highly synergistic) as well as undesired (antagonistic) interactions have been demonstrated, meaning that coadministration of flavonoids and chemotherapeutic drugs can lead to both augmentation as well as abolishment of therapeutic efficacy. Cancer patients should be informed about these antagonistic combinations to be able to abstain from products containing contraindicated flavonoids during the active treatment phase with certain chemotherapeutic drugs, with the aim not to impair therapeutic responses. On the other hand, synergistic combinations should be the subject of further therapeutic development, including initiation of clinical trials, to improve the current therapeutic protocols by addition of flavonoids as valuable adjuvant agents. As a consequence, enhanced treatment responses would be achieved at lower drug doses, thereby reducing the extent of severe adverse side effects caused by cytotoxic anticancer agents, altogether leading to better clinical outcome, improved quality of life and prolonged overall survival of patients. Most importantly, patients should be well-informed about different interactions of plant secondary metabolites and chemotherapeutic drugs to be able to make conscious choices in selecting proper plant products during anticancer treatment. This book will hopefully assist them at that, providing contemporary evidence-based information.

INTRODUCTION

Cancer is one of the major public health problems in humans all over the world, whereas both incidence as well as mortality of this devastating disease are rapidly growing. According to the recent report of the International Agency for Research on Cancer (IARC), GLOBOCAN 2018, about 18.1 million cancer cases and 9.6 million cancer deaths were estimated to have occurred in 2018 [1]. By 2030, as many as 13 million people are expected to die from malignant disorders each year [2]. Thus, although being still the second leading cause of mortality, cancer is predicted to surpass cardiovascular diseases in the near future, affecting populations of diverse ethnic, economic and social features [3, 4]. This life-threatening disorder is generally defined as the uncontrolled proliferation and spread of abnormal cells which could occur in any human tissue, whereas its increasing burden is associated with both population aging and growth, adoption of unhealthy lifestyle choices, such as tobacco smoking, alcohol consumption, physical inactivity and obesity, as well as exposure to environmental carcinogens, including radiation. Only 5-10% of all malignant disorders have been related to inherent genetic factors, highlighting the role of lifestyle and environment in the development of disease [5]. Accordingly, it is estimated that almost one-third of new cancer cases would be preventable by minimizing the exposure to known risk factors [1].

Despite intensive studies and several important advances on the comprehension of the mechanisms underlying development, progression and metastasis of malignant disorders, cancer mortality rate continues to rise with only little therapeutic progress made in the past decades [6-8]. As a multifactorial disease, cancer requires also multimodal therapies, including surgery, chemotherapy and radiotherapy. Although chemotherapy has remained one of the most important weapons in the battle against cancer, it self-represents a heavy burden for patients. Indeed, most chemotherapeutic drugs effectively target not only rapidly-dividing malignant cells, but damage also fast-growing normal cells, leading to serious adverse side effects and remarkably impairing quality of life of patients. In addition, a major factor causing the failure of chemotherapy is the resistance to antineoplastic drugs. Whereas on the one hand over the half of cancer patients receive chemotherapeutic treatments [9], on the other hand, nearly 50% of human tumors are either intrinsically resistant to chemotherapy or respond only transiently to conventional anticancer agents and acquire resistance in the course of the repeated treatment regimens [10]. Therefore, faced with the troubles of adverse reactions and drug resistance, but mainly due to the feelings of helplessness and fear in their situation, many cancer patients decide to alter their diet markedly increasing the proportion of plant-based foods and to use, on a voluntary basis, different herbal supplements. Indeed, many plant-derived preparations are widely utilized as complementary medication by cancer patients who are undergoing the treatment with conventional chemotherapeutic drugs, with the belief to gain treatment advantage or even miracle cure. Green tea extract, soy-based supplements and milk thistle silymarin are probably just some of the most frequently used herbal products consumed by oncological patients. Based on the recent studies, even as many as 50-60% of cancer patients utilize diverse phytochemicals-based supplements concurrently with their standard anticancer therapies [11, 12].

Flavonoids are the main bioactive components of plant-derived food products, such as fruits and vegetables, but also many herbal supplements. This large group of phytochemicals with over 8000 structurally different compounds constitutes an integral part of human everyday diet, being usually consumed in the amount of approximately 1 g per day. Intake of these plant secondary metabolites has been associated with several health benefits, coming from their antioxidant, antiinflammatory, antibacterial, antiviral, antiangiogenic, antiproliferative and anticancer properties. Intake of these dietary polyphenols as herbal supplements seems to be particularly attractive due to their safety and non-toxic nature, proven through exposure of mankind to flavonoids as constituents of plant-derived food items and medicinal herbs already for millennia [13-15]. However, although interactions between flavonoids and chemotherapeutic drugs are highly possible, available information about the role of these plant secondary metabolites on chemoresistance and chemotherapeutic efficacy of conventional antineoplastic agents is still incomplete, often controversial and also unsystematic, leaving cancer patients alone in the dark.

Therefore, the aim of this book is to compile all the current knowledge on interactions between flavonoids and standard antineoplastic agents and present it systematically by chemotherapeutic drugs. In this way, this book provides a common evidence-based fundament and supporting material for cancer patients who have decided to alter their diet and consume plant-derived dietary supplements, to do it in conscious and well-informed manner for the best therapeutic outcome. This book can be a good assistant also for medical doctors and dietary counselors who are everyday faced with multiple questions of patients about the utility of different herbal supplements, their suitability or contraindication during chemotherapeutic treatment regimens, with the aim not to impair clinical success. Last but not least, as this book highlights the most attractive synergistic combinations of flavonoids and antineoplastic agents in certain types of malignancies described in the preclinical settings so far, it clearly indicates the urgent need to initiate clinical trials by medical researchers and clinical scientists. To be better understandable for patients who are not familiar with cellular physiology and molecular malignant mechanisms, the first five Chapters of this book are devoted to give a short survey about development and progression of cancer, to explain why the current treatment modalities are often ineffective in curing malignant disorders and to demonstrate the possibilities for intervention in these bottlenecks using natural plant-derived flavonoids. In the Chapter 6, all the currently available knowledge about the interactions of flavonoids and chemotherapeutic drugs in certain cancer cells is presented. To be as concise as possible, some limitations were placed in the exposition of these data. First, only the effects of flavonoids on therapeutic efficacy of antineoplastic agents are involved, whereas protection of normal cells against therapy-induced toxic side effects is not the subject of this book. Secondly, only pure natural flavonoids are considered, leaving out herbal extracts in which cases we cannot be sure on the specific bioactive compounds. Also, oligomeric flavonoids, such as proanthocyanidins, and synthetically modified flavonoids or semisynthetic compounds are excluded from this book. As chemotherapeutic drugs, traditional cytotoxic anticancer agents are concerned, i.e., drugs which act on the DNA (alkylating drugs, platinum compounds, topoisomerase inhibitors), antimetabolites and drugs which target microtubules, leaving interactions of flavonoids with hormonal anticancer agents, targeted biological therapeutics and immunomodulating agents for the subject of further discussions. This book explores the modulation of chemotherapeutic efficacy by different flavonoids in both solid tumors as well as hematological malignancies, but it is still important to emphasize that most of the studies have been performed in preclinical settings, i.e., *in vitro* cancer cell lines and *in vivo* tumor xenograft animal models.

Differently from traditional chemotherapeutic drugs which are designed to modulate single cellular pathway to block the growth and survival of malignant cells [16], flavonoids can simultaneously impact multiple molecular targets, affecting thus the therapeutic efficacy of conventional anticancer agents. As demonstrated in this book, such interactions might be desired (additive to highly synergistic) but also undesired (antagonistic). Positive cooperation between flavonoids and chemotherapeutics towards killing cancerous cells certainly requires additional *in vivo* studies and further clinical trials with patients suffering from advanced and resistant tumors. After thorough optimization of concentrations, sequences and schedules, these studies will hopefully lead to improvements of current chemotherapeutic protocols by introducing flavonoids as novel non-toxic adjuvant agents, allowing to reduce the dosage of cytotoxic drugs and thereby decreasing the extent of severe adverse reactions. However, antagonistic interactions of certain flavonoids and chemotherapeutic drugs found in preclinical studies will probably never investigated further in clinical trials due to the ethical principles not to harm the human's health. Therefore, in the case of antagonistic combinations which have demonstrated to decrease or even abolish the therapeutic efficacy resulting in promotion of drug resistance and disease progression, the only possibility is to fully trust the findings of preclinical studies. Hence, this book is unique in its construction summarizing all the current knowledge about both beneficial as well as potentially deleterious interactions between natural dietary flavonoids and traditional cytotoxic antineoplastic agents. To facilitate the use of this book, contraindicated flavonoids during the treatment of certain cancer types with specific chemotherapeutic drugs are separately brought forth in the end of the subsections devoted to these drugs in the Chapter 6. Altogether, if pose a question whether cancer patients should consume herbal supplements during their active treatment phase with chemotherapeutic drugs, the answer is "yes" – consciously chosen flavonoids can act as valuable adjuvant agents potentiating the anticancer action and allowing to achieve enhanced therapeutic responses at lower doses of cytotoxic drugs, thereby improving quality of life and overall survival of patients. But the answer is also "no" – certain flavonoids can suppress the therapeutic efficacy of specific chemotherapeutic drugs leading to a substantial impairment of clinical outcome. Therefore, cancer patients should be well-informed and conscious about these undesired interactions to be able to avoid the exposure to food products and dietary supplements containing contraindicated flavonoids when undergoing treatment with specific chemotherapeutic drugs. If the detailed information is not available, it is probably better to be precautious in coadministering chemotherapeutic drugs and supplements rich in bioactive flavonoids, as the possibility to do more harm than good always remains.

Finally, although numerous previous studies have shown that flavonoids can exert several anticancer activities, these effects usually appear at high micromolar concentrations which are unachievable via oral consumption. However, the modulatory effects of flavonoids on chemotherapeutic action of antineoplastic agents have been shown to occur at remarkably lower doses possibly attainable in physiological conditions after oral administration of products rich in these phytochemicals. Therefore, it can be even supposed that the actual application of flavonoids in the future anticancer therapies is augmentation of chemotherapeutic efficacy in combinational regimens with cytotoxic drugs, rather than development of monotherapeutic strategies. In any case, interactions of flavonoids with traditional antineoplastic agents are probably of high clinical importance, constituting an area that definitely requires further investigations in the near future.

REFERENCES

[1] Bray F, Ferlay J, Soerjomataram I, Siegel RL, Torre LA, Jemal A. Global cancer statistics 2018: GLOBOCAN estimates of incidence and mortality worldwide for 36 cancers in 185 countries. *CA Cancer J Clin* 2018; 68: 394-424.

[2] GLOBOCAN 2018: Counting the toll of cancer. *Lancet* 2018; 392: 985.

[3] Krajnovic T, Kaluderovic GN, Wessjohann LA, Mijatovic S, Maksimovic-Ivanic D. Versatile antitumor potential of isoxanthohumol: Enhancement of paclitaxel activity in vivo. *Pharmacol Res* 2016; 105: 62-73.

[4] de Oliveira Junior RG, Christiane Adrielly AF, da Silva Almeida JRG, Grougnet R, Thiery V, Picot L. Sensitization of tumor cells to chemotherapy by natural products: A systematic review of preclinical data and molecular mechanisms. *Fitoterapia* 2018; 129: 383-400.

[5] Flores-Perez A, Marchat LA, Sanchez LL, Romero-Zamora D, Arechaga-Ocampo E, Ramirez-Torres N, Chavez JD, Carlos-Reyes A, Astudillo-de la Vega H, Ruiz-Garcia E, Gonzales-Perez A, Lopez-Camarillo C. Differential proteomic analysis reveals that EGCG inhibits HDGF and activates apoptosis to increase the sensitivity of non-small cells lung cancer to chemotherapy. *Proteomics Clin Appl* 2016; 10: 172-82.

[6] Lewandowska U, Gorlach S, Owczarek K, Hrabec E, Szewczyk K. Synergistic interactions between anticancer chemotherapeutics and phenolic compounds and anticancer synergy between polyphenols. *Postepy Hig Med Dosw (Online)* 2014; 68: 528-40.

[7] Delmas D, Xiao J. Natural polyphenols properties: chemopreventive and chemosensitizing activities. *Anticancer Agents Med Chem* 2012; 12: 835.

[8] Gao AM, Ke ZP, Wang JN, Yang JY, Chen SY, Chen H. Apigenin sensitizes doxorubicin-resistant hepatocellular carcinoma BEL-7402/ADM cells to doxorubicin via inhibiting PI3K/Akt/Nrf2 pathway. *Carcinogenesis* 2013; 34: 1806-14.

[9] Pashaei-Asl F, Pashaei-Asl R, Khodadadi K, Akbarzadeh A, Ebrahimie E, Pashaiasl M. Enhancement of anticancer activity by silibinin and paclitaxel combination on the ovarian cancer. *Artif Cells Nanomed Biotechnol* 2018; 46: 1483-7.

[10] Mei Y, Wei D, Liu J. Reversal of multidrug resistance in KB cells with tea polyphenol antioxidant capacity. *Cancer Biol Ther* 2005; 4: 468-73.

[11] Abaza MS, Orabi KY, Al-Quattan E, Al-Attiyah RJ. Growth inhibitory and chemo-sensitization effects of naringenin, a natural flavanone purified from Thymus vulgaris, on human breast and colorectal cancer. *Cancer Cell Int* 2015; 15: 46.

[12] Hemalswarya S, Doble M. Potential synergism of natural products in the treatment of cancer. *Phytother Res* 2006; 20: 239-49.

[13] Sak K. Cytotoxicity of dietary flavonoids on different human cancer types. *Pharmacogn Rev* 2014; 8: 122-46.

[14] Sak K. Site-specific anticancer effects of dietary flavonoid quercetin. *Nutr Cancer* 2014; 66: 177-93.

[15] Sak K. Intake of individual flavonoids and risk of carcinogenesis: Overview of epidemiological evidence. *Nutr Cancer* 2017; 69: 1119-50.

[16] Chavoshi H, Vahedian V, Saghaei S, Pirouzpanah MB, Raeisi M, Samadi N. Adjuvant therapy with silibinin improves the efficacy of paclitaxel and cisplatin in MCF-7 breast cancer cells. *Asian Pac J Cancer Prev* 2017; 18: 2243-7.

ABBREVIATIONS

ABC   ATP-binding cassette
Abl   Abelson murine leukemia viral oncogene homolog
ACF   aberrant crypt foci
AIF   apoptosis-inducing factor
AKR   aldo-keto reductase
Akt   protein kinase B
ALCL   anaplastic large cell lymphoma
ALKL   anaplastic lymphoma kinase-positive
ALL   acute lymphoblastic leukemia
AML   acute myelogenous leukemia
AMPK   AMP-activated protein kinase
Ang   angiopoietin
Apaf-1   apoptotic protease activating factor 1
APE1   apurinic/apyrimidinic endonuclease 1
AR   androgen receptor
ARE   antioxidant responsive element
Ask1   apoptosis signal-regulating kinase 1
ATC   anaplastic thyroid cancer
ATG   autophagy-related
ATM   ataxia telangiectasia mutated
ATR   ATM and Rad3-related
AuNP   gold NP
AVO   acidic vesicular organelle
BAD   Bcl-2-associated death promoter
Bak   Bcl-2 homologous antagonist/killer

Abbreviations

Bax	Bcl-2-associated X protein
BBB	blood-brain barrier
Bcl-2	B-cell lymphoma 2
Bcl-xl	B-cell lymphoma-extra large
Bcr	breakpoint cluster region
BCRP	breast cancer resistance protein
BCSC	breast cancer stem cell
BECN	beclin
Bid	BH3 interacting-domain death agonist
Bim	Bcl-2-like protein 11
BIRC5	baculovirus inhibitor of apoptosis repeat-containing 5
BOK	Bcl-2 related ovarian killer
BPL	biotin-modified PEGylated liposomes
BRCA	breast cancer gene
BrdU	bromodeoxyuridine
BTN	biotin
CBR	carbonyl reductase
CDC	cell division cycle
CDK	cyclin-dependent kinase
CDKN1A	cyclin dependent kinase inhibitor 1A
CFU-L	colony forming unit-leukemic
Chk1	checkpoint kinase 1
CHOP	CCAAT/enhancer binding protein homologues protein
CI	combination index
cIAP1	cellular inhibitor of apoptosis protein 1
CLL	chronic lymphocytic leukemia
CML	chronic myeloid leukemia
CNT	carbon nanotubes
COX	cyclooxygenase
CSC	cancer stem cell
CSLC	cancer stem-like cells
CTR1	copper transporter 1
Cx	connexin
CXCR	chemokine receptor
CYP1B1	cytochrome P450 1B1
CYR61	cysteine-rich angiogenic induces 61
cyt c	cytochrome c
d	day
dCdR	deoxycytidine
DCK	deoxycytidine kinase

dCTP	deoxycytidine triphosphate
Dex-CT	dextran-catechin
dFdC	2`,2`-difluoro-2`-deoxycytidine
dFdCDP	5`-diphosphate of dFdC
dFdCMP	5`-monophosphate of dFdC
dFdCTP	5`-triphosphate of dFdC
DHFU	dihydrofluorouracil
DMBA	7,12-dimethylbenz[a] anthracene
DMH	1,2-dimethyl hydrazine
DNMT	DNA methyltransferase
DNROL	daunorubicinol
DPD	dihydropyrimidine dehydrogenase
DR	death receptor
DRSP	drug-resistant sphere
DSB	double-stranded DNA break
dTMP	deoxythymidine monophosphate
dUMP	deoxyuridine monophosphate
dUTP	deoxyuridine triphosphate
E2	estradiol
EAC	Ehrlich ascites carcinoma
EBS	estrogen binding sites
EBV	Epstein-Barr Virus
ECM	extracellular matrix
EGFR	epidermal growth factor receptor
EMT	epithelial-mesenchymal transition
EPR	enhanced permeability and retention effect
ER	estrogen receptor
ERK	extracellular signal-regulated kinase
ERS	endoplasmic reticulum stress
ESCC	esophageal squamous cell carcinoma
f_a	fraction affected
FADD	Fas-associated death domain
FAK	focal adhesion kinase
FANCD2	Fanconi anemia group D2
FasL	Fas ligand
FDG	2-fluorodeoxyglucose
FdUMP	fluorodeoxyuridine monophosphate
FGF	fibroblast growth factor
Fox	forkhead box
FUMP	fluorouridine monophosphate

FUTP	fluorouridine triphosphate
FZD7	frizzled homolog protein 7
GATA3	GATA binding protein 3
GBM	glioblastoma multiforme
GJ	gap junction
GJIC	GJ intercellular communication
GLT	gelatin
GLUT	glucose transporter
GPx	glutathione peroxidase
GRP	glucose-regulated protein
GSH	glutathione
GSK	glycogen synthase kinase
GST	glutathione S-transferase
GTP	guanosine 5`-triphosphate
HA	hyaluronic acid
HCC	hepatocellular carcinoma
HDAC	histone deacetylase
HDGF	hepatoma-derived growth factor
HER2	human epidermal growth factor receptor 2 (erbB2)
HIF-1α	hypoxia-inducible factor 1α
HK2	hexokinase 2
HNC	head and neck cancer
HNSC	head and neck squamous carcinoma
HNSCC	head and neck squamous cell carcinoma
HO-1	heme oxygenase-1
HPV	human papillomavirus
Hsp	heat shock protein
i.d.	intradermically, intradermally
i.g.	intragastrically
i.m.	intramuscularly
i.p.	intraperitoneally
i.v.	intravenously
IAP	inhibitor of apoptosis
IARC	International Agency for Research on Cancer
IC$_{50}$	half-maximal inhibitory concentration
ICAM-1	intercellular adhesion molecule 1
IFP	interstitial fluid pressure
IGF	insulin like growth factor
IGF-1R	IGF 1 receptor
IGFBP	IGF binding protein

Abbreviations xxi

IKK	IκB kinase
IL	interleukin
ILS	increase in the life span
IMP	inosine 5`-monophosphate
IP$_3$	inositol 1, 4, 5-trisphosphate
IκBα	nuclear factor of kappa light polypeptide gene enhancer in B-cells inhibitor, α
JNK	c-Jun N-terminal kinase
Keap1	Kelch-like ECH-associated protein 1
Lam	laminin
LC$_{50}$	50% lethal concentration
LDHA	lactate dehydrogenase A
LDM	low-dose metronomic therapy
LLC	Lewis lung carcinoma
LPN	lipid-polymeric nanocarrier
LRP	lung resistance protein
Luc	luciferase
MAPK	mitogen-activated protein kinase
MARK2	microtubule affinity-regulating kinase 2
Mcl-1	myeloid cell leukemia 1
MDR	multidrug resistance
MET	mesenchymal-epithelial transition
MG-CMB	monochloromonoglutathionyl CMB
MGMT	O^6-methylguanine DNA methyltransferase
miR	microRNA
MMP	matrix metalloproteinase
MMR	mismatch repair
MN	micronuclei
MNC	mononuclear cell
MnSOD	manganese superoxide dismutase
MRP	multidrug resistance-associated protein
MRT	mean residence time
MSI	microsatellite instability
MTHF	5,10-methylenetetrahydrofolate
mTOR	mammalian target of rapamycin
MVD	microvessel density
NE	nanoemulsion
NEAT	nuclear enriched abundant transcript
NF-κB	nuclear factor-κB
NGO	nanographene oxide

NHL	Non-Hodgkin lymphoma
NL	nanoliposome
NLC	nanostructured lipid carrier
NP	nanoparticle
NQO	NAD(P)H:quinone oxidoreductase
Nrf2	nuclear factor (erythroid-derived 2)-like 2
NSCLC	non-small cell lung cancer
NZB mice	New Zealand Black mice
OCSC	oral cancer stem cell
OCTN2	organic cation/carnitine transporter 2
OPG	osteoprotegerin
OSCC	oral squamous cell carcinoma
p.o.	per oral
PARP	poly (ADP-ribose) polymerase
PBMC	peripheral blood mononuclear cell
PCNA	proliferating cell nuclear antigen
PCSC	prostate cancer stem cell
PDGF	platelet-derived growth factor
PDK1	pyruvate dehydrogenase kinase 1
PDT	photodynamic therapy
PEG	polyethylene glycol
PEG-PCD	poly(ethylene glycol)-block-poly(2-methyl-2-carboxyl-propylene carbonate-graft-dodecanol)
PEI	polyethyleneimine
PGE2	prostaglandin E2
P-gp	P-glycoprotein
PGRMC1	progesterone receptor membrane component 1
PI3K	phosphoinositide 3-kinase
PIC	polyion complex
PLGA	poly(lactic-co-glycolic acid)
PMAA	polymethacrylic acid
PN-1	protease nexin-1
PR	progesterone receptor
PSA	prostate-specific antigen
PSi	porous silicon
Pt	platinum
PTEN	phosphatase and tensin homolog
PUMA	p53 upregulated modulator of apoptosis
QoL	quality of life
RANK	receptor activator of nuclear factor-κB

Abbreviations

RANKL	RANK ligand
Rb	retinoblastoma
RCC	renal cell carcinoma
ROS	reactive oxygen species
RR-M2	ribonucleotide reductase M2 subunit
s.c.	subcutaneously
SCLC	small cell lung cancer
SDH	silibinin di-hemisuccinate
SiLN	silica nanoparticle
SIRT1	sirtuin 1
SLN	solid lipid nanoparticle
SOD	superoxide dismutase
Sox2	sex-determining region Y-Box
STAT3	signal transducer and activator of transcription 3
TACE	transarterial chemoembolization
tBid	truncated Bid
TEM	Tie2-expressing monocyte
Tf	transferrin
TGF-β	transforming growth factor β
TKI	tyrosine kinase inhibitor
TLR4	Toll-like receptor 4
TN	triple negative
TNBC	triple negative breast cancer
TNFR	tumor necrosis factor receptor
TNF-α	tumor necrosis factor-α
Topo	topoisomerase
TRAILR	TNF-related apoptosis-inducing ligand receptor
TS	thymidylate synthase
TUNEL	terminal deoxynucleotidyl transferase dUTP nick end labeling
ULK	Unc-51 like autophagy activating kinase
uPA	urokinase-type plasminogen activator
VEGF	vascular endothelial growth factor
VEGF-R	VEGF receptor
w	week
WHO	World Health Organization
wt	wild type
XIAP	X-linked inhibitor of apoptosis protein
YB-1	Y-box binding protein 1
$\Delta\Psi m$	mitochondrial membrane potential

Chapter 1

OVERVIEW OF THE MOST COMMON CANCER TYPES

Cancer incidence and mortality are rapidly growing all over the world so that malignant tumors are expected to rank as the leading cause of death in the 21st century. Indeed, according to the GLOBOCAN 2018 estimates reported by the International Agency for Research on Cancer (IARC), there was an estimated 18.1 million new cancer cases and 9.6 million cancer deaths worldwide in 2018 [1]. Moreover, predictions suggest that by 2030, even 13 million people die from cancer each year [2]. The reasons for these rising trends are complex comprising both aging and growing population in the world but also changes in the prevalence of the main risk factors, including unhealthy lifestyle and exposure to environmental carcinogens (tobacco smoking, alcohol consumption, infection with carcinogenic viruses, obesity, physical inactivity). It is reported that from one-third to two-fifths of new cancer cases would be avoidable by eliminating or minimizing exposure to known risk factors [1]. However, implementation of the means of primary prevention is still not an active international priority. As about 60% of the global population resides in Asia, nearly one-half of the cancer cases and over one-half of the deaths are estimated to occur in this region. However, despite only 9% of the global population residing in Europe, 23.4% of cancer incidence and 20.3% of mortality occur in European countries. America accounts for 21% of the total cancer cases and 14.4% of cancer deaths [1], probably showing the greatest progress in diagnostic and therapeutic strategies in the management of malignant disorders.

The global statistics of incidence and mortality of ten most frequent malignancies in both men and women in 2018 are presented in Figure 1. This diagram is composed by the data of GLOBOCAN 2018 published in [1]. A short overview of the most common cancer types, both solid tumors as well as hematological malignancies, which will be further concerned in this book, is presented as follows.

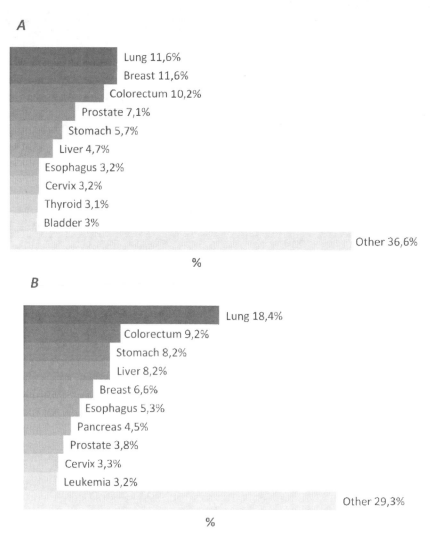

Figure 1.1. Global cancer incidence (A) and mortality (B) in men and women in 2018. The diagram is composed by the data of GLOBOCAN 2018 published in [1].

1.1. SOLID TUMORS

1.1.1. Respiratory Tract

1.1.1.1. Lung Cancer

Lung cancer, also known as pulmonary carcinoma, remains the most commonly diagnosed malignant tumor and the global leading cause of cancer-associated death in both men and women. With continuously increasing incidence, lung cancer represents a serious and life-threatening problem for public health all over the world requiring each year more lives than breast, prostate and colon cancer combined [3-8]. Due to the lack of screening methods, lung cancer is generally diagnosed in relatively advanced stage and despite improvements in staging, integrated application of surgery, radiotherapy and chemotherapy, and discovery of molecular targets the long-term survival is only hardly changed over the past several decades. Thus, about 80-85% of patients experience recurrence and metastasis and the 5-year survival rate is just 17-18% [3, 5-7, 9-11]. On basis of histology, lung cancer can be broadly classified into small cell lung carcinoma (SCLC) originating from neuroendocrine cells and non-small cell lung carcinoma (NSCLC). NSCLC is the most frequent type of lung cancer accounting for about 85% of all cases, further categorized into adenocarcinoma as the most common lung cancer in the Western world, squamous cell carcinoma accounting for about 30% of all lung cancers, and large cell carcinoma, all differing by their cellular origin and morphology [3, 5, 8, 10, 12-14]. At the time of diagnosis, numerous patients with NSCLC already exhibit advanced stage surgically unresectable disease, with the median survival only between 8 and 12 months and the 1-year survival rates ranging from 30% to 50% [3, 8, 15]. For these inoperable NSCLC patients, systemic chemotherapy and radiotherapy remain the mainstay of the treatment. However, despite the availability of different approved chemotherapeutics with platinum-based compounds (cisplatin) as the recommended first-line treatment possibility, the clinical applicability of these drugs is often limited due to emergence of resistance and numerous intolerable adverse effects [3, 5, 6, 7, 10, 11, 16-21]. Therefore, enhancement of chemosensitivity to current drugs and/or development of novel antitumor agents are the major goals to improve the efficacy of lung cancer therapy and prognosis and reduce its high mortality rate.

1.1.1.2. Malignant Mesothelioma

With a very poor prognosis, malignant mesothelioma is an aggressive and highly lethal tumor developing from pleural, peritoneal or pericardial mesothelial cells after a long-term exposure to asbestos and/or erionite. Although cisplatin-based combination therapies are conventionally administrated, this is not successful due to therapeutic resistance. No successful treatment options are currently available for this deadly disease [22, 23].

1.1.1.3. Nasopharyngeal Carcinoma

Nasopharyngeal carcinoma is another respiratory tract malignancy of epithelial origin that represents a distinct geographical distribution being common in Southern China, North Africa and South East Asia. This cancer type is strongly associated with latent infection of the Epstein-Barr virus (EBV) and its standard treatment modalities include radiotherapy with concurrent chemotherapy. However, for patients with locoregionally advanced disease the current treatment has proven mostly unsuccessful [24].

1.1.2. Digestive Tract

1.1.2.1. Oral Cancer

Oral squamous cell carcinoma (OSCC) is one of the most frequent and lethal malignancies of head and neck region [25]. Current treatments are of rather limited efficacy in preventing tumor progression and recurrence and the prognosis of patients with advanced disease is relatively poor. Treatment strategies rely on surgical resection, radiotherapy and chemotherapy; the efficacy of chemotherapy is impeded mainly by drug resistance. Hence, it is crucial to elucidate the mechanisms underlying chemoresistance and develop novel therapeutic strategies for OSCC [25-27].

1.1.2.2. Laryngeal Cancer

Laryngeal cancer is another most common head and neck malignancies. Treatment of advanced stage disease relies on combination of surgery, radiation and chemotherapy; however, the survival has not substantially improved over the last few decades due to emergence of resistance to current drugs [28].

1.1.2.3. Esophageal Cancer

Esophageal cancer is a global health problem being the sixth most frequent cause of cancer mortality worldwide [29, 30]. It is one of the most aggressive malignancies with late presentation, rapid progression and early distant metastasis. At the time of diagnosis, the majority of patients have already developed advanced stage tumor with no possibilities for complete surgical resection [29, 31, 32]. Therefore, systemic chemotherapy is the main therapeutic method to improve survival with 5-fluorouracil (5-FU) as a universal first-line treatment option. However, gradual emergence of drug resistance and toxic side effects besides a poor general medical status of patients limit its clinical application, pointing to an urgent need to identify candidates for enhancement of 5-FU therapeutic efficacy and to find novel therapeutic treatment regimens [29-34].

1.1.2.4. Gastric Cancer

Gastric cancer is the fifth most commonly diagnosed malignant disorder and the third leading cause of cancer death in the world [35-37]. Several factors including infection with *Helicobacter pylori*, tobacco smoking, unhealthy diet and obesity have been linked to the carcinogenesis in stomach [38]. However, progress in clinical management of this highly heterogenous and aggressive disease has been rather limited and prognosis of patients is still disappointing. In fact, due to its high recurrence rate, local invasion and metastasis the estimated overall 5-year survival of gastric cancer patients is only around 20%, with a median survival time of about 24 months [39-42]. Although surgical resection is the most common strategy of treating patients with early stage gastric cancer, even after complete surgical resection of tumors only about 40% of patients remain disease-free [36, 37, 43]. Moreover, the majority of patients are already at advanced stage at diagnosis, contradicting the use of a surgical operation [44]. Therefore, chemotherapy is an important strategy for clinical treatment of most gastric cancer patients. 5-FU has remained the most important standard drug used as single or combined therapy for treatment of gastric cancer. However, the response rate is low, and resistance and unmanageable toxic side effects still represent unresolved problems leading to the failure of gastric cancer chemotherapy [35-37, 39, 40, 44-46]. Hence, more effective and tolerable therapeutic strategies with novel agents and drug combinations are urgently required to improve clinical outcomes of gastric cancer treatment.

1.1.2.5. Colorectal Cancer

Colorectal cancer is ranked the third most common cancer type and a second leading cause of cancer-associated mortality worldwide [47-49]. In 2018, over 1.8 million new cases have been estimated to occur throughout the world resulting in more than 861 000 deaths [1]. Approximately 90% of colorectal cancers arise from benign adenomatous lesions which progress during 5-15 years through complex mechanisms into invasive malignant adenocarcinomas [50, 51]. Despite plenty of information accumulated about the dietary, lifestyle and medical risk factors about carcinogenesis in colorectum, occurrence and mortality of this aggressive tumor type are steadily increasing and its prognosis remains poor [47, 49]. Some progress has been recently made in primary prevention, screening and diagnosis of colorectal cancer as well as in development of therapeutic approaches; however, chemoresistance and short-term tumor recurrence still remain the major challenges to successful clinical management of this malignancy [47, 49, 50]. Colorectal tumors are often diagnosed at advanced stages where chemotherapy is the mainstream of treatment option. Among chemotherapeutics used, 5-FU has been regarded as a drug of choice and the principal component of multidrug regimen applied with topoisomerase inhibitor irinotecan or platinum compound oxaliplatin to improve the overall response rate and prolong the survival of patients. However, advancements in clinical treatment are impeded by the emergence of resistance and serious adverse effects [48, 49, 52-58]. Therefore, it is clear that new therapeutic strategies are highly needed to enhance the efficacy of 5-FU-based regimens and overcome the current bottlenecks in clinical management of colorectal cancer.

1.1.2.6. Liver Cancer

Liver cancer represents a major global health burden. Although its incidence varies geographically, the rate is increasing throughout the world. Hepatocellular carcinoma is the major histological subtype, accounting for 85-90% of all primary liver cancer cases with an incidence in men twice of that in women [59-61]. Hepatocellular carcinoma is the sixth most common cancer type and the fourth leading cause of cancer-related mortality in the world [62, 63]. More than 50% of cases of this highly lethal tumor occur in China and other Asia-Pacific region [64]. Hepatocellular carcinoma is a very aggressive malignancy with a dismal outcome; patients usually survive less than one year after diagnosis and the 5-year survival rate is only about 15% [60, 65, 66]. Moreover, the prognosis has not been significantly changed in the past decades. Although tumor resection, liver transplantation and percutaneous thermal ablation are potentially curative interventions, they are applicable only for patients with early-stage disease, and even among those treated with curative intent, postoperative relapse rates are very high (up to 70%) being a major obstacle for improving prognosis [61, 62, 64, 67-69]. Furthermore, the majority of patients are diagnosed at advanced stages negating surgical operation due to metastatic spread [70]. Low-invasive local therapies such as transarterial chemoembolization (TACE) can be employed on the basis of general hypervascularity of hepatocellular carcinoma when radical therapies are not feasible [71, 72]. However, for those patients with inoperable metastatic disease systemic chemotherapy remains the traditional treatment option. Doxorubicin and 5-FU are commonly utilized drugs for chemotherapy of advanced hepatocellular carcinoma [68, 70, 71, 73, 74]. However, the efficacy of chemotherapeutic drugs in palliative treatment of advanced tumor is low and insufficient, and resistance to treatments also contributes to the poor survival rate [61, 65, 71, 72, 75]. Therefore, developing more efficient treatment strategies for clinical management of hepatocellular carcinoma is urgently needed to increase the survival of patients.

1.1.2.7. Gallbladder Cancer

Gallbladder carcinoma is the most common tumor type of biliary tract. Due to the silent clinical character and late presentation, aggressive biological behavior and low response to conventional therapeutic methods, it is associated with poor prognosis and high mortality rate worldwide [76-78]. The only curative treatment option is complete surgical resection at an early stage of disease but only less than 30% of patients are candidates to benefit from the radical operation because of lack of early diagnosis [77, 79]. For those patients with unresectable tumor, treatment options include radiotherapy and systemic chemotherapy. However, the response rate to drugs such as gemcitabine and 5-FU is not satisfactory, and recurrence occurs in a large proportion of patients who eventually succumb to their disease; the overall survival is only about 8 months [76, 77, 79]. Novel therapeutic strategies are highly needed to improve the response rate and prolong the survival.

1.1.3. Excretory System

1.1.3.1. Renal Cancer
Renal cell carcinoma is the most common malignancy arising in the kidney accounting for 90-95% of renal cancers. It is about twice as common in men than in women, with median age at diagnosis of approximately 60 years [80, 81]. Surgical resection is the preferred treatment method for localized primary tumors; however, a large proportion of patients (25-30%) have metastatic disease at the time of diagnosis and the median survival for those with advanced stage disease is only about 13 months. Available chemotherapeutic drugs alone as monotherapy are rather ineffective and not recommended for use against metastatic renal cell carcinoma [80, 81].

1.1.3.2. Bladder Cancer
Bladder cancer is one of the most commonly diagnosed tumors in genito-urinary system with transitional cell carcinoma accounting for more than 90% of all bladder cancer cases [82]. Stage at diagnosis is a major prognostic factor and surgery remains the mainstream treatment option for localized disease. However, bladder cancer is notorious for its high recurrence rate, whereas the risk of recurrence after resection is reported to be up to 70% [82, 83]. Epirubicin is the traditional first-line chemotherapeutic agent used in patients with bladder cancer to prevent recurrence. Unfortunately, emergence of resistance is a great obstacle for achieving successful treatment outcome, besides adverse effects accompanying high-dose intravesical chemotherapeutic treatment [82]. Development of novel agents behaving as chemosensitizers to current drugs is imperative for improvement of response rate in bladder cancer treatment.

1.1.4. Endocrine System

1.1.4.1. Pancreatic Cancer
Pancreatic cancer (pancreatic ductal adenocarcinoma) is a highly lethal malignancy being the fourth leading cause of cancer-associated mortality in the Western world [84, 85]. It has an extremely poor prognosis with the median survival time only around six months [84, 85]. The 5-year survival rate has remained about 5% for the past few decades and is the lowest for any malignancy. In the case of this devastating disease, the mortality rate almost equals the incidence rate [85-87]. Poor prognosis is due to highly aggressive nature and rapid progression of pancreatic cancer, lack of specific signs and symptoms, making the early diagnosis and curative treatment difficult, but also lack of screening possibilities [86, 88]. The only potentially curative treatment option is surgical resection, pancreatectomy, although relapses are common even in these cases [84]. Moreover, about 80% of patients have locally advanced or metastatic disease at the time of initial

diagnosis making the dismal prognosis inevitable [85, 87, 89]. Currently, there are no effective therapies for pancreatic cancer. The recommended standard treatment is gemcitabine, given alone or in combination with other agents; however, the impact is very modest and limited by chemoresistance [84-86, 90-92]. Therefore, overcoming of drug resistance and identifying of novel therapeutic regimens are critical to improve the clinical outcome and overall survival of patients with pancreatic cancer.

1.1.4.2. Thyroid Cancer

Anaplastic thyroid cancer is an undifferentiated thyroid malignancy. Due to its poor differentiation, this tumor has a tendency to invade to the surrounding tissues, such as trachea being one of the most lethal human cancers. Its treatment strategy depends on the stage and extent of disease, and includes surgical resection, radioactive iodine treatment, hormone therapy, radiation, chemotherapy and targeted therapy, alone or combined [93].

1.1.5. Reproductive System

1.1.5.1. Breast Cancer

Breast cancer is the most frequently diagnosed cancer and the leading cause of cancer-related mortality in women worldwide, accounting for 2.09 million new cases in 2018 (24.2% of the total new cancer cases and 15.0% of cancer deaths among women) [1]. Despite recent improvements in primary prevention, early detection and treatment, the lifetime risk of breast cancer development for women is as high as 1 in 8 in the Western world, the incidence continues to rise and mortality rate has remained high [94-96]. Breast cancer can be characterized and the clinical management is mostly guided by the presence or absence of estrogen receptor, progesterone receptor and human epidermal growth factor receptor 2 (HER2) in tumor cells [97, 98]. Standard treatment methods include surgical resection, radiotherapy, hormonal therapy, chemotherapy and gene-targeting therapy. Antihormonal treatment and HER2 targeted therapeutic modalities have improved the clinical outcome and survival rates of the patients who are responsive to these treatments [98]. However, triple negative breast cancer that fail to express estrogen and progesterone receptors and HER2 progresses typically more aggressively and has a poorer prognosis than other breast cancer subtypes. Treatment options for triple negative breast cancer are restricted to cytotoxic chemotherapy, whereas recurrence risk is still rather high. Overexpression of HER2 oncogene has been observed in about 25-30% of all breast cancer patients and is believed to be associated with increased chemoresistance [97, 99-101]. For breast tumors, chemotherapy is often prescribed at different stages of disease as combination of drugs, based on anthracyclines (doxorubicin), taxanes and platinum compounds. However, because of resistance, the clinical response in the case of advanced disease is mostly temporary, accompanied by

Overview of the Most Common Cancer Types 9

reduced quality of life due to several toxic side effects and relapse remains a major challenge contributing to the treatment failure [94-96, 102-107]. Hence, the need to develop new effective therapeutic strategies and novel agents for clinical management of breast cancer, especially triple negative breast cancer, is ever increasing with the global rise of breast cancer incidence.

1.1.5.2. Ovarian Cancer

Ovarian carcinoma is the most lethal type of gynecological malignancy being responsible for 3.4% of all total new cancer cases and 4.4% of cancer-related deaths in women worldwide. Its incidence continues to grow [1, 108-110]. More than 90% of ovarian cancers arise from epithelial cells [111, 112]. As ovarian cancer typically reveals no early symptoms and is difficult to detect, it is mostly (in more than two-third of cases) diagnosed at advanced clinical stage when the disease has already spread beyond the ovaries. Exfoliation of tumor cells from the ovarian surface and dissemination in peritoneal cavity is therefore common [108, 110, 112-117]. Conventional treatment options typically consist of extensive surgical resection and cytotoxic chemotherapy, whereas chemotherapy mostly represents an indispensable next step following surgical approach [113, 118-120]. Chemotherapy with platinum-based agents (cisplatin) and taxanes (paclitaxel) has been the standard choice for care of ovarian cancer [108, 109, 111, 114, 117, 121]. However, despite successful initial treatment and early clinical remission (about 80% of women are responsive to first-line cisplatin treatment), the majority of patients (nearly 70%) ultimately develop platinum resistance, suffer from tumor recurrence, progress and succumb to their disease [108, 109, 112, 113, 116, 118, 121-124]. Recurrent ovarian cancer is currently only minimally responsive to further treatments; moreover, chemotherapy resistance has been suggested to enhance the malignant degree of tumor and promote metastasis. Thus, the overall 5-year survival rate has remained as low as around 40-45% [108, 110, 111, 116, 122, 125]. As the currently available standard chemotherapeutic drugs have not improved the survival rate of ovarian cancer patients and platinum resistance represents a major challenge in the successful cure, identifying novel effective chemosensitizing agents to overcome resistance is the most important goal for combating the disease and achieving a better clinical outcome. Development of such new modulators has been further complicated by the highly heterogenous nature of ovarian tumor [114, 126].

1.1.5.3. Cervical Cancer

Malignant tumor in cervix uteri is a prevalent gynecologic cancer being the fourth most common cancer type and fourth leading cause of cancer mortality among women throughout the world [1, 127]. Combination of surgery, chemotherapy and radiotherapy is the standard strategy in the clinical management of cervical cancer, whereas cisplatin has been one of the most effective chemotherapeutic drugs used in treatment of advanced stage disease [128-130]. Chemoresistance of tumor cells is still the major reason of unsatisfactory results and therapeutic failure. Hence, more effective and tolerable treatment options are required to improve the clinical outcome.

1.1.5.4. Choriocarcinoma

Choriocarcinoma is the most frequently diagnosed gestational trophoblastic neoplasia. Chemotherapy is an important therapeutic modality after removal of tumor mass to prevent further invasiveness. Although 80% of patients can be successfully treated by methotrexate and dactinomycin regimen, numerous side effects including teratogenicity can limit their use and almost 20% of patients experience recurrence or failure due to resistance [131].

1.1.5.5. Prostate Cancer

Prostate cancer is the second most common type of malignancy and the fifth leading cause of cancer death among men worldwide; its rate is steadily rising [1, 132]. It has been reported that 1 in 3 men has the chance to develop prostatic intraepithelial neoplasia (an early precancerous event of prostatic malignant transformation), and 1 in 6 men develop prostate cancer during their life time, whereas aging and previous family history are the known risk factors [133, 134]. Prostate tumors can be characterized by multifocality and heterogeneity and despite advances in screening and translational research, such molecular complexity renders the prognosis rather poor [134, 135]. The standard treatment options for patients with initial stages or organ confined tumors include surgical resection and radiotherapy, being curative in the majority of patients. Since the growth of prostate and prostate cancer is regulated by androgens, the advanced cases with tumors spread beyond the pelvis are generally first treated with androgen deprivation therapy [136, 137]. However, despite initial response, nearly all patients on hormonal ablation therapy progress within 18-24 months to castration-resistant cancer that has remained a big challenge to treat. Docetaxel is a first-line and cabazitaxel a second-line chemotherapeutic agent for metastatic and androgen-independent prostate cancer; however, the median progression-free survival with docetaxel treatment has remained only around 6 months. Besides serious toxic side effects and reduced quality of life, it has been reported that tumors become even more invasive and aggressive with emergence of taxane resistance. Moreover, skeletal metastasis is a common cause of bone pain and immobility [134-136, 138-140]. Unfortunately, the best treatment for progressive prostate cancer after docetaxel treatment is still not well defined, most patients die of tumor metastasis and the median survival of men with advanced metastatic androgen-independent disease has remained less than 2 years [139, 141-143]. Therefore, it is crucial to develop novel anticancer agents and adjuvants to overcome taxane resistance in prostate cancer to improve the clinical outcome and prolong the survival of patients. Given that prostate cancer afflicts mostly elderly age group of men, these new agents must be better tolerated and safe to administer.

1.1.5.6. Testicular Cancer

The incidence of testicular carcinoma has steadily increased during the last decades becoming one of the most common cancer types in young men. Cisplatin is a conventional drug for treatment of germ cell originating testicular teratocarcinoma and embryonal carcinoma; however, its use is limited by various adverse effects [144].

1.1.6. Brain and Nervous System

1.1.6.1. Gliomas

Primary brain tumors are a heterogenous group of diseases originating from different cells. Due to their location, aggressive metastatic nature and diffuse infiltrative growth between normal cells, brain tumors are often intractable and have remained one of the most challenging diseases to treat [145, 146]. Most of malignant gliomas are classified as high-grade tumors and comprise WHO grade III tumors (anaplastic forms of astrocytoma, oligodendroglioma and oligoastrocytoma) and WHO grade IV tumors (glioblastoma multiforme) [147, 148]. Glioblastoma multiforme occurs mostly in elderly adults (aged 50-70 years) accounting for almost half of all brain tumors [146, 147, 149]. Anaplastic astrocytoma represents about 25% of all primary brain tumors [150]. The conventional treatment strategy consists of maximal surgical resection, followed by radiotherapy and chemotherapy with alkylating agent temozolomide that has the capacity to cross the blood-brain barrier [146, 148, 149, 151, 152]. However, due to diffusive infiltrative growth between normal cells and probable invasion into the life-critical brain structures, complete surgical resection is nearly impossible [147, 150, 153]. Moreover, failure of chemotherapy is another major issue in the treatment of brain tumors due to the insufficient accumulation of drugs in the tumor site and emergence of resistance to temozolomide [145, 154]. Thus, the median survival time of patients with glioblastoma multiforme is only about 10-15 months with no significant improvements reported over the past few decades [146, 147, 152, 153, 155, 156]. Although the growth of anaplastic astrocytomas is somewhat slower, they are also ultimately fatal with survival time of patients for 30-50 months [146, 150]. Hence, there is an urgent need for identifying specific molecular targets and finding novel drug candidates against glioma, but also developing new therapeutic combination regimens with adjuvant agents to augment the efficacy of temozolomide and improve the prognosis of glioma patients.

1.1.6.2. Medulloblastoma

Medulloblastoma is the most common malignant brain tumor in children with a peak incidence around 5 years of age. These highly heterogenic tumors arise from neural precursors of the cerebellum and brainstem [157]. Advancements in multimodal therapy comprising combination of surgical excision, postoperative radiation and polychemotherapy with different drugs have greatly improved the prognosis with overall 5-year survival rate reaching 60-80% [157]. However, the majority of medulloblastoma survivors suffer from life-long adverse effects, both endocrine impairments and neurological disabilities, including motor, cognitive, and/or vision impairments as well as psychosocial dysfunction, all contributing to reduced quality of life [157, 158]. Therefore, novel therapeutic regimens for treatment of medulloblastoma are needed not only to improve clinical response, but also to reduce the life-long adverse effects caused by the current treatment modalities. Moreover, as growth and migration of medulloblastoma has been reported to be stimulated by estrogens and estradiol can increase the resistance to cytotoxic agents, exposure to environmental estrogens should be avoided with the aim not to impair the chemosensitivity of medulloblastoma to drugs [157].

1.1.6.3. Neuroblastoma

Neuroblastoma is the third most commonly diagnosed malignancy in childhood accounting for about 15% of pediatric cancer-related deaths. It is an extracranial neuroendocrine tumor developing most often in one of the adrenal glands, but can also arise in nerve tissues in the chest, neck, abdomen, or pelvis [159-161]. The 5-year survival rate for high-risk neuroblastoma patients treated with multimodal strategy (surgery, radiotherapy, chemotherapy) has remained dismal being around 30% [159, 160]. Moreover, because of toxic adverse effects, neuroblastoma survivors often experience life-long health issues from the chemotherapeutic treatments received in childhood [159].

1.1.7. Musculoskeletal System

1.1.7.1. Sarcomas

Sarcomas are an heterogenous group of mesenchymal neoplasms with more than 50 histological types [162]. Sarcomas are notoriously chemoresistant with an overall 5-year survival rate of 50-60% [162, 163]. Soft tissue sarcomas comprise a rare group of tumors with extremely poor prognosis when diagnosed at metastatic stage [164]. Osteosarcoma is the most common primary malignancy of bone tissue, characterized by histologic heterogeneity, and occurring mainly in children and adolescents [163, 165-167]. Cytotoxic chemotherapy with different agents, such as doxorubicin, cisplatin, cyclophosphamide, methotrexate and etoposide, is regarded as the mainstream clinical approach for treatment of osteosarcomas [165-169]. However, such chemotherapy faces major limitations, including emergence of chemoresistant phenotypes and toxic side effects, resulting in poor prognosis [163, 166, 169, 170]. Interestingly, the incidence rate of osteosarcoma in dogs is estimated to be about 10 times higher than that among humans. Canine osteosarcoma is known by its aggressiveness, rapid progression and easy metastasis to the lungs, all contributing to a poor survival time of only about 243 days [171]. Therefore, it is important to find alternative combination regimens to improve the outcome of clinical management of sarcomas in human patients, but also in the case of treating canine osteosarcoma. Due to the high heterogeneity and complexity of this disease, development of targeted therapies has still been unsuccessful.

1.1.8. Integumentary System

1.1.8.1. Melanoma

Melanoma is the most aggressive form of cutaneous malignancy being often a treatment-refractory and metastasis-prone neoplasm [172-175]. The incidence of melanoma is increasingly raised over the last several decades, whereas the main reason is believed to be increased exposure to ultraviolet radiation from sunlight [172, 176-178]. According to the estimates from IARC, 287 723 new melanoma cases occurred worldwide in 2018 and this is 1.24-fold more than the global melanoma cases estimated in 2012 [1, 179]. Invasiveness, rapid metastasis and the lack of effective therapy make the long-term survival poor for patients with advanced stage disease [172, 174]. The alkylating agent dacarbazine is considered one of the most effective chemotherapies for metastatic melanoma used for decades, but the response rate is low, typically not durable and accompanied by toxic side effects and reduced quality of life [174, 178, 180]. Hence, there is a great clinical interest in identifying novel drugs to be used either in monotherapy or combination therapy for treating patients with unresectable metastatic melanoma.

1.2. HEMATOLOGICAL MALIGNANCIES

1.2.1. Acute Myeloid Leukemia

Acute myeloid leukemia (AML) is characterized by an uncontrolled proliferation and abnormal accumulation of myeloid precursors that interferes with the production and maturation of normal white blood cells in the bone marrow [181, 182]. AML accounts for about 80% of all acute leukemia cases in adults and the number of new cases is stably increasing every year [183, 184]. Despite advances in studies of molecular mechanisms, identification of prognostic factors and modification of treatment protocols, AML has remained a disease which is difficult to treat [183]. Standard therapeutic regimens mostly comprise combination chemotherapies of cytarabine and anthracyclines (daunorubicin, idarubicin), whereas cytarabine has been used for AML treatment for already more than 40 years [181, 182, 184, 185]. Although such treatment usually results in initial remission around 70% of individuals, the disease eventually relapses in the majority of patients. Both the resistance to current drugs as well as treatment-related toxicity are the major drawbacks, especially in the population of elderly individuals [181, 183]. Thus, the mortality rate is high and an average survival for adult AML patients is less than 12 months [181]. Ways to increase the therapeutic response to treat AML by development of novel drugs or alternative combinations are still intensively sought. However, heterogeneity of this disease further complicates the finding of a single molecule to target or single agent to employ in treatment regimens.

1.2.2. Chronic Myeloid Leukemia

Chronic myeloid leukemia (CML) accounts for about 20% of all adult leukemia cases [186]. It is characterized by a rapid growth and accumulation of myeloid cells and their precursors, being associated with the lesion in Bcr-Abl fusion gene and abnormal functions of the respective protein as a constitutively active receptor tyrosine kinase [186, 187]. BCR-ABL specific tyrosine kinase inhibitors have improved the 10-year survival time in 80% of CML patients, but most individuals eventually relapse upon cessation of drug treatment [186-188]. CML usually starts with a chronic phase and over the course of years ultimately progresses to blast crisis, becoming increasingly resistant to any current drugs [186].

1.2.3. Acute Lymphoid Leukemia

Acute lymphoid leukemia (ALL) is the most common form of childhood malignancy, accounting for about 75% of all childhood leukemias [189-191]. Multiagent chemotherapy has remained the mainstay treatment strategy for ALL, combining several anticancer drugs, such as vincristine and methotrexate [189-191]. However, resistance of leukemic cells to these agents is one of the major causes of treatment failure, whereas the further treatment of relapsed patients has remained a major challenge in the clinical management of childhood ALL [189, 191]. Possible treatment option of these individuals includes hematopoietic stem cell transplantation; however, recurrence is still the major impediment to success [191]. Therefore, identifying new molecular targets and developing rationally designed novel drugs are essential to overcome the chemotherapeutic resistance in relapsed ALL patients.

1.2.4. Chronic Lymphoid Leukemia

Chronic lymphoid leukemia (CLL) is the most common leukemia type in adult population constituting 22-30% of all leukemia cases [192, 193]. This disease is characterized by a progressive clonal expansion of mature CD5+ B lymphocytes within lymphoid organs and peripheral blood [193, 194]. About half of all individuals with CLL remain asymptomatic and are diagnosed incidentally by unrelated lymphocytosis [192]. Therefore, treatment strategies also largely depend on the clinical staging. Development of combined chemo-immunotherapy employing antimetabolites like fludarabine with humanized monoclonal antibodies has significantly improved the clinical outcome for CLL patients; current first-line treatment includes combination of fludarabine, cyclophosphamide and monoclonal antibodies [192, 194]. However, this regimen is intolerable for old patients and/or those suffering from several comorbidities. Moreover, a significant subset of treated patients eventually become refractory, develop resistance, relapse and face a poor prognosis; thus, indicating the urgent need for better tolerable and more effective alternative therapies for treatment of this highly heterogenous disease [192, 194].

1.2.5. Multiple Myeloma

Multiple myeloma accounts for 13.4% of all hematological malignancies and is characterized by the accumulation of malignant plasma cells in bone marrow. Chemotherapy with multiple agents is the standard approach to treatment; however, only limited effects have been observed with these regimens and multiple myeloma has still remained an incurable disease [195]. Identifying novel effective drugs is imperative to improve the clinical outcomes of multiple myeloma treatment.

1.2.6. Lymphoma

Non-Hodgkin lymphoma (NHL) is the most prevalent hematological cancer with steadily increased incidence over the past few decades. It represents a heterogenous set of malignancies arising from lymph glands and other lymphoid tissues. Among the subgroups, diffuse large B-cell lymphoma is the most frequently diagnosed type of Non-

Hodgkin lymphoma accounting for about 30-40% of all NHL cases in adults. Chemotherapy is the mainstream treatment option for clinical management of NHL, whereas treatment with cyclophosphamide, vincristine, doxorubicin and prednisolone has remained the standard care for diffuse large B-cell lymphoma. Resistance, toxicity and eventual relapse are the major clinical challenges for lymphoma management showing the need for further development of new and more effective treatment strategies [196].

REFERENCES

[1] Bray F, Ferlay J, Soerjomataram I, Siegel RL, Torre LA, Jemal A. Global cancer statistics 2018: GLOBOCAN estimates of incidence and mortality worldwide for 36 cancers in 185 countries. *CA Cancer J Clin* 2018; 68: 394-424.

[2] GLOBOCAN 2018: Counting the toll of cancer. *Lancet* 2018; 392: 985.

[3] Lu L, Yang LN, Wang XX, Song CL, Qin H, Wu YJ. Synergistic cytotoxicity of ampelopsin sodium and carboplatin in human non-small cell lung cancer cell line SPC-A1 by G1 cell cycle arrested. *Chin J Integr Med* 2017; 23: 125-31.

[4] Kiartivich S, Wei Y, Liu J, Soiampornkul R, Li M, Zhang H, Dong J. Regulation of cytotoxicity and apoptosis-associated pathways contributes to the enhancement of efficacy of cisplatin by baicalein adjuvant in human A549 lung cancer cells. *Oncol Lett* 2017; 13: 2799-804.

[5] Lu C, Wang H, Chen S, Yang R, Li H, Zhang G. Baicalein inhibits cell growth and increases cisplatin sensitivity of A549 and H460 cells via miR-424-3p and targeting PTEN/PI3K/Akt pathway. *J Cell Mol Med* 2018; 22: 2478-87.

[6] Varela-Castillo O, Cordero P, Gutierrez-Iglesias G, Palma I, Rubio-Gayosso I, Meaney E, Ramirez-Sanchez I, Villarreal F, Ceballos G, Najera N. Characterization of the cytotoxic effects of the combination of cisplatin and flavanol (-)-epicatechin on human lung cancer cell line A549. An isobolographic approach. *Exp Oncol* 2018; 40: 19-23.

[7] Yu S, Gong LS, Li NF, Pan YF, Zhang L. Galangin (GG) combined with cisplatin (DDP) to suppress human lung cancer by inhibition of STAT3-regulated NF-κB and Bcl-2/Bax signaling pathways. *Biomed Pharmacother* 2018; 97: 213-24.

[8] Punia R, Raina K, Agarwal R, Singh RP. Acacetin enhances the therapeutic efficacy of doxorubicin in non-small-cell lung carcinoma cells. *PLoS One* 2017; 12: e0182870.

[9] Wu L, Yang W, Zhang SN, Lu JB. Alpinetin inhibits lung cancer progression and elevates sensitization drug-resistant lung cancer cells to cis-diammined dichloridoplatium. *Drug Des Devel Ther* 2015; 9: 6119-27.

[10] Singh VK, Arora D, Satija NK, Khare P, Roy SK, Sharma PK. Intricatinol synergistically enhances the anticancerous activity of cisplatin in human A549 cells via p38 MAPK/p53 signalling. *Apoptosis* 2017; 22: 1273-86.

[11] Wang A, Wang W, Chen Y, Ma F, Wei X, Bi Y. Deguelin induces PUMA-mediated apoptosis and promotes sensitivity of lung cancer cells (LCCs) to doxorubicin (Dox). *Mol Cell Biochem* 2018; 442: 177-86.

[12] Hou X, Bai X, Gou X, Zeng H, Xia C, Zhuang W, Chen X, Zhao Z, Huang M, Jin J. 3`,4`,5`,5,7-pentamethoxyflavone sensitizes Cisplatin-resistant A549 cells to Cisplatin by inhibition of Nrf2 pathway. *Mol Cells* 2015; 38: 396-401.

[13] Sadava D, Kane SE. Silibinin reverses drug resistance in human small-cell lung carcinoma cells. *Cancer Lett* 2013; 339: 102-6.

[14] Zhang BY, Wang YM, Gong H, Zhao H, Lv XY, Yuan GH, Han SR. Isorhamnetin flavonoid synergistically enhances the anticancer activity and apoptosis induction by cis-platin and carboplatin in non-small cell lung carcinoma (NSCLC). *Int J Clin Exp Pathol* 2015; 8: 25-37.

[15] Liu D, Yan L, Wang L, Tai W, Wang W, Yang C. Genistein enhances the effect of cisplatin on the inhibition of non-small cell lung cancer A549 cell growth *in vitro* and *in vivo. Oncol Lett* 2014; 8: 2806-10.

[16] Klimaszewska-Wisniewska A, Halas-Wisniewska M, Tadrowski T, Gagat M, Grzanka D, Grzanka A. Paclitaxel and the dietary flavonoid fisetin: a synergistic combination that induces mitotic catastrophe and autophagic cell death in A549 non-small cell lung cancer cells. *Cancer Cell Int* 2016; 16: 10.

[17] Zhuo W, Zhang L, Zhu Y, Zhu B, Chen Z. Fisetin, a dietary bioflavonoid, reverses acquired Cisplatin-resistance of lung adenocarcinoma cells through MAPK/ Survivin/Caspase pathway. *Am J Transl Res* 2015; 7: 2045-52.

[18] Zhou DH, Wang X, Feng Q. EGCG enhances the efficacy of cisplatin by downregulating hsa-miR-98-5p in NSCLC A549 cells. *Nutr Cancer* 2014; 66: 636-44.

[19] Jiang P, Wu X, Wang X, Huang W, Feng Q. NEAT1 upregulates EGCG-induced CTR1 to enhance cisplatin sensitivity in lung cancer cells. *Oncotarget* 2016; 7: 43337-51.

[20] Xu Z, Mei J, Tan Y. Baicalin attenuates DDP (cisplatin) resistance in lung cancer by downregulating MARK2 and p-Akt. *Int J Oncol* 2017; 50: 93-100.

[21] Yu M, Qi B, Xiaoxiang W, Xu J, Liu X. Baicalein increases cisplatin sensitivity of A549 lung adenocarcinoma cells via PI3K/Akt/NF-κB pathway. *Biomed Pharmacother* 2017; 90: 677-85.

[22] Demiroglu-Zergeroglu A, Basara-Cigerim B, Kilic E, Yanikkaya-Demirel G. The investigation of effects of quercetin and its combination with Cisplatin on malignant mesothelioma cells in vitro. *J Biomed Biotechnol* 2010; 2010: 851589.

[23] Demiroglu-Zergeroglu A, Ergene E, Ayvali N, Kuete V, Sivas H. Quercetin and Cisplatin combined treatment altered cell cycle and mitogen activated protein kinase expressions in malignant mesotelioma cells. *BMC Complement Altern Med* 2016; 16: 281.

[24] Daker M, Ahmad M, Khoo AS. Quercetin-induced inhibition and synergistic activity with cisplatin – a chemotherapeutic strategy for nasopharyngeal carcinoma cells. *Cancer Cell Int* 2012; 12: 34.

[25] Chen SF, Nieh S, Jao SW, Liu CL, Wu CH, Chang YC, Yang CY, Lin YS. Quercetin suppresses drug-resistant spheres via the p38 MAPK-Hsp27 apoptotic pathway in oral cancer cells. *PLoS One* 2012; 7: e49275.

[26] Yang SF, Yang WE, Chang HR, Chu SC, Hsieh YS. Luteolin induces apoptosis in oral squamous cancer cells. *J Dent Res* 2008; 87: 401-6.

[27] Hu FW, Yu CC, Hsieh PL, Liao YW, Lu MY, Chu PM. Targeting oral cancer stemness and chemoresistance by isoliquiritigenin-mediated GRP78 regulation. *Oncotarget* 2017; 8: 93912-23.

[28] Xu YY, Wu TT, Zhou SH, Bao YY, Wang QY, Fan J, Huang YP. Apigenin suppresses GLUT-1 and p-AKT expression to enhance the chemosensitivity to cisplatin of laryngeal carcinoma Hep-2 cells: an in vitro study. *Int J Clin Exp Pathol* 2014; 7: 3938-47.

[29] Wang L, Feng J, Chen X, Guo W, Du Y, Wang Y, Zang W, Zhang S, Zhao G. Myricetin enhance chemosensitivity of 5-fluorouracil on esophageal carcinoma in vitro and in vivo. *Cancer Cell Int* 2014; 14: 71.

[30] Li J, Li B, Xu WW, Chan KW, Guan XY, Qin YR, Lee NP, Chan KT, Law S, Tsao SW, Cheung AL. Role of AMPK signaling in mediating the anticancer effects of silibinin in esophageal squamous cell carcinoma. *Expert Opin Ther Targets* 2016; 20: 7-18.

[31] Wang J, Yang ZR, Guo XF, Song J, Zhang JX, Wang J, Dong WG. Synergistic effects of puerarin combined with 5-fluorouracil on esophageal cancer. *Mol Med Rep* 2014; 10: 2535-41.

[32] Chuang-Xin L, Wen-Yu W, Yao C, Xiao-Yan L, Yun Z. Quercetin enhances the effects of 5-fluorouracil-mediated growth inhibition and apoptosis of esophageal cancer cells by inhibiting NF-κB. *Oncol Lett* 2012; 4: 775-8.

[33] Zhang C, Ma Q, Shi Y, Li X, Wang M, Wang J, Ge J, Chen Z, Wang Z, Jiang H. A novel 5-fluorouracil-resistant human esophageal squamous cell carcinoma cell line Eca-109/5-FU with significant drug resistance-related characteristics. *Oncol Rep* 2017; 37: 2942-54.

[34] Liu L, Ju Y, Wang J, Zhou R. Epigallocatechin-3-gallate promotes apoptosis and reversal of multidrug resistance in esophageal cancer cells. *Pathol Res Pract* 2017; 213: 1242-50.

[35] Lei CS, Hou YC, Pai MH, Lin MT, Yeh SL. Effects of quercetin combined with anticancer drugs on metastasis-associated factors of gastric cancer cells: in vitro and in vivo studies. *J Nutr Biochem* 2018; 51: 105-13.

[36] Hong ZP, Wang LG, Wang HJ, Ye WF, Wang XZ. Wogonin exacerbates the cytotoxic effect of oxaliplatin by inducing nitrosative stress and autophagy in human gastric cancer cells. *Phytomedicine* 2018; 39: 168-75.

[37] Zhang Y, Ge Y, Ping X, Yu M, Lou D, Shi W. Synergistic apoptotic effects of silibinin in enhancing paclitaxel toxicity in human gastric cancer cell lines. *Mol Med Rep* 2018; 18: 1835-41.

[38] Ramachandran L, Manu KA, Shanmugam MK, Li F, Siveen KS, Vali S, Kapoor S, Abbasi T, Surana R, Smoot DT, Ashktorab H, Tan P, Ahn KS, Yap CW, Kumar AP, Sethi G. Isorhamnetin inhibits proliferation and invasion and induces apoptosis through the modulation of peroxisome proliferator-activated receptor γ activation pathway in gastric cancer. *J Biol Chem* 2012; 287: 38028-40.

[39] Fang J, Zhang S, Xue X, Zhu X, Song S, Wang B, Jiang L, Qin M, Liang H, Gao L. Quercetin and doxorubicin co-delivery using mesoporous silica nanoparticles enhance the efficacy of gastric carcinoma chemotherapy. *Int J Nanomedicine* 2018; 13: 5113-26.

[40] Chen F, Zhuang M, Zhong C, Peng J, Wang X, Li J, Chen Z, Huang Y. Baicalein reverses hypoxia-induced 5-FU resistance in gastric cancer AGS cells through suppression of glycolysis and the PTEN/Akt/HIF-1α signaling pathway. *Oncol Rep* 2015; 33: 457-63.

[41] Xu GY, Tang XJ. Troxerutin (TXN) potentiated 5-Fluorouracil (5-Fu) treatment of human gastric cancer through suppressing STAT3/NF-κB and Bcl-2 signaling pathways. *Biomed Pharmacother* 2017; 92: 95-107.

[42] Hyun HB, Moon JY, Cho SK. Quercetin suppresses CYR61-mediated multidrug resistance in human gastric adenocarcinoma AGS cells. *Molecules* 2018; 23: E209.

[43] Zhou L, Wu Y, Guo Y, Li Y, Li N, Yang Y, Qin X. Calycosin enhances some chemotherapeutic drugs inhibition of Akt signaling pathway in gastric cells. *Cancer Invest* 2017; 35: 289-300.

[44] Guo XF, Yang ZR, Wang J, Lei XF, Lv XG, Dong WG. Synergistic antitumor effect of puerarin combined with 5-fluorouracil on gastric carcinoma. *Mol Med Rep* 2015; 11: 2562-8.

[45] Lin X, Tian L, Wang L, Li W, Xu Q, Xiao X. Antitumor effects and the underlying mechanism of licochalcone A combined with 5-fluorouracil in gastric cancer cells. *Oncol Lett* 2017; 13: 1695-701.

[46] Guo XF, Liu JP, Ma SQ, Zhang P, Sun WD. Avicularin reversed multidrug-resistance in human gastric cancer through enhancing Bax and BOK expressions. *Biomed Pharmacother* 2018; 103: 67-74.

[47] Li N, Zhang Z, Jiang G, Sun H, Yu D. Nobiletin sensitizes colorectal cancer cells to oxaliplatin by PI3K/Akt/MTOR pathway. *Front Biosci (Landmark Ed)* 2019; 24: 303-12.

[48] Qu Q, Qu J, Guo Y, Zhou BT, Zhou HH. Luteolin potentiates the sensitivity of colorectal cancer cell lines to oxaliplatin through the PPARγ/OCTN2 pathway. *Anticancer Drugs* 2014; 25: 1016-27.

[49] Shi DB, Li XX, Zheng HT, Li DW, Cai GX, Peng JJ, Gu WL, Guan ZQ, Xu Y, Cai SJ. Icariin-mediated inhibition of NF-κB activity enhances the in vitro and in vivo antitumour effect of 5-fluorouracil in colorectal cancer. *Cell Biochem Biophys* 2014; 69: 523-30.

[50] Wang Z, Sun X, Feng Y, Liu X, Zhou L, Sui H, Ji Q, E Q, Chen J, Wu L, Li Q. Dihydromyricetin reverses MRP2-mediated MDR and enhances anticancer activity induced by oxaliplatin in colorectal cancer cells. *Anticancer Drugs* 2017; 28: 281-8.

[51] Li QC, Liang Y, Hu GR, Tian Y. Enhanced therapeutic efficacy and amelioration of cisplatin-induced nephrotoxicity by quercetin in 1,2-dimethyl hydrazine-induced colon cancer in rats. *Indian J Pharmacol* 2016; 48: 168-71.

[52] Chan JY, Tan BK, Lee SC. Scutellarin sensitizes drug-evoked colon cancer cell apoptosis through enhanced caspase-6 activation. *Anticancer Res* 2009; 29: 3043-7.

[53] Chian S, Li YY, Wang XJ, Tang XW. Luteolin sensitizes two oxaliplatin-resistant colorectal cancer cell lines to chemotherapeutic drugs via inhibition of the Nrf2 pathway. *Asian Pac J Cancer Prev* 2014; 15: 2911-6.

[54] Hu F, Wei F, Wang Y, Wu B, Fang Y, Xiong B. EGCG synergizes the therapeutic effect of cisplatin and oxaliplatin through autophagic pathway in human colorectal cancer cells. *J Pharmacol Sci* 2015; 128: 27-34.

[55] Xavier CP, Lima CF, Rohde M, Pereira-Wilson C. Quercetin enhances 5-fluorouracil-induced apoptosis in MSI colorectal cancer cells through p53 modulation. *Cancer Chemother Pharmacol* 2011; 68: 1449-57.

[56] Samuel T, Fadlalla K, Mosley L, Katkoori V, Turner T, Manne U. Dual-mode interaction between quercetin and DNA-damaging drugs in cancer cells. *Anticancer Res* 2012; 32: 61-71.

[57] Ha J, Zhao L, Zhao Q, Yao J, Zhu BB, Lu N, Ke X, Yang HY, Li Z, You QD, Guo QL. Oroxylin A improves the sensitivity of HT-29 human colon cancer cells to 5-FU through modulation of the COX-2 signaling pathway. *Biochem Cell Biol* 2012; 90: 521-31.

[58] Guo J, Zhou AW, Fu YC, Verma UN, Tripathy D, Frenkel EP, Becerra CR. Efficacy of sequential treatment of HCT116 colon cancer monolayers and xenografts with docetaxel, flavopiridol, and 5-fluorouracil. *Acta Pharmacol Sin* 2006; 27: 1375-81.

[59] Wen Y, Zhao RQ, Zhang YK, Gupta P, Fu LX, Tang AZ, Liu BM, Chen ZS, Yang DH, Liang G. Effect of Y6, an epigallocatechin gallate derivative, on reversing doxorubicin drug resistance in human hepatocellular carcinoma cells. *Oncotarget* 2017; 8: 29760-70.

[60] Liang G, Tang A, Lin X, Li L, Zhang S, Huang Z, Tang H, Li QQ. Green tea catechins augment the antitumor activity of doxorubicin in an in vivo mouse model for chemoresistant liver cancer. *Int J Oncol* 2010; 37: 111-23.

[61] Chen L, Ye HL, Zhang G, Yao WM, Chen XZ, Zhang FC, Liang G. Autophagy inhibition contributes to the synergistic interaction between EGCG and doxorubicin to kill the hepatoma Hep3B cells. *PLoS One* 2014; 9: e85771.

[62] Zhao JL, Zhao J, Jiao HJ. Synergistic growth-suppressive effects of quercetin and cisplatin on HepG2 human hepatocellular carcinoma cells. *Appl Biochem Biotechnol* 2014; 172: 784-91.

[63] Wang G, Zhang J, Liu L, Sharma S, Dong Q. Quercetin potentiates doxorubicin mediated antitumor effects against liver cancer through p53/Bcl-xl. *PLoS One* 2012; 7: e51764.

[64] Jia H, Yang Q, Wang T, Cao Y, Jiang QY, Ma HD, Sun HW, Hou MX, Yang YP, Feng F. Rhamnetin induces sensitization of hepatocellular carcinoma cells to a small molecular kinase inhibitor or chemotherapeutic agents. *Biochim Biophys Acta* 2016; 1860: 1417-30.

[65] Gao AM, Zhang XY, Hu JN, Ke ZP. Apigenin sensitizes hepatocellular carcinoma cells to doxorubic through regulating miR-520b/ATG7 axis. *Chem Biol Interact* 2018; 280: 45-50.

[66] Sun L, Chen W, Qu L, Wu J, Si J. Icaritin reverses multidrug resistance of HepG2/ADR human hepatoma cells via downregulation of MDR1 and P-glycoprotein expression. *Mol Med Rep* 2013; 8: 1883-7.

[67] Chen P, Hu MD, Deng XF, Li B. Genistein reinforces the inhibitory effect of Cisplatin on liver cancer recurrence and metastasis after curative hepatectomy. *Asian Pac J Cancer Prev* 2013; 14: 759-64.

[68] Yurtcu E, Iseri Ö, Sahin F. Genotoxic and cytotoxic effects of doxorubicin and silymarin on human hepatocellular carcinoma cells. *Hum Exp Toxicol* 2014; 33: 1269-76.

[69] Chen Z, Huang C, Ma T, Jiang L, Tang L, Shi T, Zhang S, Zhang L, Zhu P, Li J, Shen A. Reversal effect of quercetin on multidrug resistance via FZD7/β-catenin pathway in hepatocellular carcinoma cells. *Phytomedicine* 2018; 43: 37-45.

[70] Yang XW, Wang XL, Cao LQ, Jiang XF, Peng HP, Lin SM, Xue P, Chen D. Green tea polyphenol epigallocatehin-3-gallate enhances 5-fluorouracil-induced cell growth inhibition of hepatocellular carcinoma cells. *Hepatol Res* 2012; 42: 494-501.

[71] Jung EU, Yoon JH, Lee YJ, Lee JH, Kim BH, Yu SJ, Myung SJ, Kim YJ, Lee HS. Hypoxia and retinoic acid-inducible NDRG1 expression is responsible for doxorubicin and retinoic acid resistance in hepatocellular carcinoma cells. *Cancer Lett* 2010; 298: 9-15.

[72] Kwak MS, Yu SJ, Yoon JH, Lee SH, Lee SM, Lee JH, Kim YJ, Lee HS, Kim CY. Synergistic anti-tumor efficacy of doxorubicin and flavopiridol in an in vivo hepatocellular carcinoma model. *J Cancer Res Clin Oncol* 2015; 141: 2037-45.

[73] Dai W, Gao Q, Qiu J, Yuan J, Wu G, Shen G. Quercetin induces apoptosis and enhances 5-FU therapeutic efficacy in hepatocellular carcinoma. *Tumour Biol* 2016; 37: 6307-13.

[74] Zhao L, Sha YY, Zhao Q, Yao J, Zhu BB, Lu ZJ, You QD, Guo QL. Enhanced 5-fluorouracil cytotoxicity in high COX-2 expressing hepatocellular carcinoma cells by wogonin via the PI3K/Akt pathway. *Biochem Cell Biol* 2013; 91: 221-9.

[75] Yurtcu E, Darcansov Iseri O, Iffet Sahin F. Effects of silymarin and silymarin-doxorubicin applications on telomerase activity of human hepatocellular carcinoma cell line HepG2. *J BUON* 2015; 20: 555-61.

[76] Li Y, Huang X, Huang Z, Feng J. Phenoxodiol enhances the antitumor activity of gemcitabine in gallbladder cancer through suppressing Akt/mTOR pathway. *Cell Biochem Biophys* 2014; 70: 1337-42.

[77] Gao H, Xie J, Peng J, Han Y, Jiang Q, Han M, Wang C. Hispidulin inhibits proliferation and enhances chemosensitivity of gallbladder cancer cells by targeting HIF-1α. *Exp Cell Res* 2015; 332: 236-46.

[78] Mayr C, Wagner A, Neureiter D, Pichler M, Jakab M, Illig R, Berr F, Kiesslich T. The green tea catechin epigallocatechin gallate induces cell cycle arrest and shows potential synergism with cisplatin in biliary tract cancer cells. *BMC Complement Altern Med* 2015; 15: 194.

[79] Zhang DC, Liu JL, Ding YB, Xia JG, Chen GY. Icariin potentiates the antitumor activity of gemcitabine in gallbladder cancer by suppressing NF-κB. *Acta Pharmacol Sin* 2013; 34: 301-8.

[80] Sato A, Sekine M, Kobayashi M, Virgona N, Ota M, Yano T. Induction of the connexin 32 gene by epigallocatechin-3-gallate potentiates vinblastine-induced cytotoxicity in human renal carcinoma cells. *Chemotherapy* 2013; 59: 192-9.

[81] Chang HR, Chen PN, Yang SF, Sun YS, Wu SW, Hung TW, Lian JD, Chu SC, Hsieh YS. Silibinin inhibits the invasion and migration of renal carcinoma 786-O cells in vitro, inhibits the growth of xenografts in vivo and enhances chemosensitivity to 5-fluorouracil and paclitaxel. *Mol Carcinog* 2011; 50: 811-23.

[82] Pan XW, Li L, Huang Y, Huang H, Xu DF, Gao Y, Chen L, Ren JZ, Cao JW, Hong Y, Cui XG. Icaritin acts synergistically with epirubicin to suppress bladder cancer growth through inhibition of autophagy. *Oncol Rep* 2016; 35: 334-42.

[83] Di Lorenzo G, Pagliuca M, Perillo T, Zarrella A, Verde A, De Placido S, Buonerba C. Complete response and fatigue improvement with the combined use of cyclophosphamide and quercetin in a patient with metastatic bladder cancer: A case report. *Medicine (Baltimore)* 2016; 95: e2598.

[84] Kim N, Kang MJ, Lee SH, Son JH, Lee JE, Paik WH, Ryu JK, Kim YT. Fisetin enhances the cytotoxicity of gemcitabine by down-regulating ERK-MYC in MiaPaca-2 human pancreatic cancer cells. *Anticancer Res* 2018; 38: 3527-33.

[85] Löhr JM, Karimi M, Omazic B, Kartalis N, Verbeke CS, Berkenstam A, Frödin JE. A phase I dose escalation trial of AXP107-11, a novel multi-component crystalline form of genistein, in combination with gemcitabine in chemotherapy-naive patients with unresectable pancreatic cancer. *Pancreatology* 2016; 16: 640-5.

[86] Johnson JL, Gonzalez de Mejia E. Interactions between dietary flavonoids apigenin or luteolin and chemotherapeutic drugs to potentiate anti-proliferative effect on human pancreatic cancer cells, in vitro. *Food Chem Toxicol* 2013; 60: 83-91.

[87] Liu P, Feng J, Sun M, Yuan W, Xiao R, Xiong J, Huang X, Xiong M, Chen W, Yu X, Sun Q, Zhao X, Zhang Q, Shao L. Synergistic effects of baicalein with gemcitabine or docetaxel on the proliferation, migration and apoptosis of pancreatic cancer cells. *Int J Oncol* 2017; 51: 1878-86.

[88] Tang SN, Fu J, Shankar S, Srivastava RK. EGCG enhances the therapeutic potential of gemcitabine and CP690550 by inhibiting STAT3 signaling pathway in human pancreatic cancer. *PLoS One* 2012; 7: e31067.

[89] Suzuki R, Kang Y, Li X, Roife D, Zhang R, Fleming JB, Genistein potentiates the antitumor effect of 5-Fluorouracil by inducing apoptosis and autophagy in human pancreatic cancer cells. *Anticancer Res* 2014; 34: 4685-92.

[90] Xu XD, Zhao Y, Zhang M, He RZ, Shi XH, Guo XJ, Shi CJ, Peng F, Wang M, Shen M, Wang X, Li X, Qin RY. Inhibition of autophagy by deguelin sensitizes pancreatic cancer cells to doxorubicin. *Int J Mol Sci* 2017; 18: E370.

[91] Wu W, Xia Q, Luo RJ, Lin ZQ, Xue P. In vitro study of the antagonistic effect of low-dose liquiritigenin on gemcitabine-induced capillary leak syndrome in pancreatic adenocarcinoma via inhibiting ROS-mediated signalling pathways. *Asian Pac J Cancer Prev* 2015; 16: 4369-76.

[92] Johnson JL, Dia VP, Wallig M, Gonzalez de Mejia E. Luteolin and gemcitabine protect against pancreatic cancer in an orthotopic mouse model. *Pancreas* 2015; 44: 144-51.

[93] Park CH, Han SE, Nam-Goong IS, Kim YI, Kim ES. Combined effects of baicalein and docetaxel on apoptosis in 8505c anaplastic thyroid cancer cells via downregulation of the ERK and Akt/mTOR pathways. *Endocrinol Metab (Seoul)* 2018; 33: 121-32.

[94] Kuo CY, Zupko I, Chang FR, Hunyadi A, Wu CC, Weng TS, Wang HC. Dietary flavonoid derivatives enhance chemotherapeutic effect by inhibiting the DNA damage response pathway. *Toxicol Appl Pharmacol* 2016; 311: 99-105.

[95] Sato Y, Sasaki N, Saito M, Endo N, Kugawa F, Ueno A. Luteolin attenuates doxorubicin-induced cytotoxicity to MCF-7 human breast cancer cells. *Biol Pharm Bull* 2015; 38: 703-9.

[96] Zhang J, Luo Y, Zhao X, Li X, Li K, Chen D, Qiao M, Hu H, Zhao X. Co-delivery of doxorubicin and the traditional Chinese medicine quercetin using biotin-PEG2000-DSPE modified liposomes for the treatment of multidrug resistant breast cancer. *RSC Adv* 2016; 6: 113173.

[97] Smith ML, Murphy K, Doucette CD, Greenshields AL, Hoskin DW. The dietary flavonoid fisetin causes cell cycle arrest, caspase-dependent apoptosis, and enhanced cytotoxicity of chemotherapeutic drugs in triple-negative breast cancer cells. *J Cell Biochem* 2016; 117: 1913-25.

[98] Wong MY, Chiu GN. Liposome formulation of co-encapsulated vincristine and quercetin enhanced antitumor activity in a trastuzumab-insensitive breast tumor xenograft model. *Nanomedicine* 2011; 7: 834-40.

[99] Xue JP, Wang G, Zhao ZB, Wang Q, Shi Y. Synergistic cytotoxic effect of genistein and doxorubicin on drug-resistant human breast cancer MCF-7/Adr cells. *Oncol Rep* 2014; 32: 1647-53.

[100] Sharma R, Gatchie L, Williams IS, Jain SK, Vishwakarma RA, Chaudhuri B, Bharate SB. Glycyrrhiza glabra extract and quercetin reverses cisplatin resistance in triple-negative MDA-MB-468 breast cancer cells via inhibition of cytochrome P450 1B1 enzyme. *Bioorg Med Chem Lett* 2017; 27: 5400-3.

[101] Choi EJ, Kim GH. 5-Fluorouracil combined with apigenin enhances anticancer activity through induction of apoptosis in human breast cancer MDA-MB-453 cells. *Oncol Rep* 2009; 22: 1533-7.

[102] Staedler D, Idrizi E, Kenzaoui BH, Juillerat-Jeanneret L. Drug combinations with quercetin: doxorubicin plus quercetin in human breast cancer cells. *Cancer Chemother Pharmacol* 2011; 68: 1161-72.

[103] Li SZ, Qiao SF, Zhang JH, Li K. Quercetin increase the chemosensitivity of breast cancer cells to doxorubicin via PTEN/Akt pathway. *Anticancer Agents Med Chem* 2015; 15: 1185-9.

[104] Fu P, Du F, Liu Y, Hong Y, Yao M, Zheng S. Wogonin increases doxorubicin sensitivity by down-regulation of IGF-1R/AKT signaling pathway in human breast cancer. *Cell Mol Biol (Noisy-le-grand)* 2015; 61: 123-7.

[105] Wang Z, Wang N, Liu P, Chen Q, Situ H, Xie T, Zhang J, Peng C, Lin Y, Chen J. MicroRNA-25 regulates chemoresistance-associated autophagy in breast cancer cells, a process modulated by the natural autophagy inducer isoliquiritigenin. *Oncotarget* 2014; 5: 7013-26.

[106] Tyagi T, Treas JN, Mahalingaiah PK, Singh KP. Potentiation of growth inhibition and epigenetic modulation by combination of green tea polyphenol and 5-aza-2`-deoxycytidine in human breast cancer cells. *Breast Cancer Res Treat* 2015; 149: 655-68.

[107] Chavoshi H, Vahedian V, Saghaei S, Pirouzpanah MB, Raeisi M, Samadi N. Adjuvant therapy with silibinin improves the efficacy of paclitaxel and cisplatin in MCF-7 breast cancer cells. *Asian Pac J Cancer Prev* 2017; 18: 2243-7.

[108] Zheng AW, Chen YQ, Zhao LQ, Feng JG. Myricetin induces apoptosis and enhances chemosensitivity in ovarian cancer cells. *Oncol Lett* 2017; 13: 4974-8.

[109] Dia VP, Pangloli P. Epithelial-to-mesenchymal transition in paclitaxel-resistant ovarian cancer cells is downregulated by luteolin. *J Cell Physiol* 2017; 232: 391-401.

[110] Liu M, Qi Z, Liu B, Ren Y, Li H, Yang G, Zhang Q. RY-2f, an isoflavone analog, overcomes cisplatin resistance to inhibit ovarian tumorigenesis via targeting the PI3K/AKT/mTOR signaling pathway. *Oncotarget* 2015; 6: 25281-94.

[111] Pashaei-Asl F, Pashaei-Asl R, Khodadadi K, Akbarzadeh A, Ebrahimie E, Pashaiasl M. Enhancement of anticancer activity by silibinin and paclitaxel combination on the ovarian cancer. *Artif Cells Nanomed Biotechnol* 2018; 46: 1483-7.

[112] Pan Q, Xue M, Xiao SS, Wan YJ, Xu DB. A combination therapy with baicalein and taxol promotes mitochondria-mediated cell apoptosis: Involving in Akt/β-catenin signaling pathway. *DNA Cell Biol* 2016; 35: 646-56.

[113] Xu Y, Wang S, Chan HF, Lu H, Lin Z, He C, Chen M. Dihydromyricetin induces apoptosis and reverses drug resistance in ovarian cancer cells by p53-mediated downregulation of survivin. *Sci Rep* 2017; 7: 46060.

[114] Mazumder ME, Beale P, Chan C, Yu JQ, Huq F. Epigallocatechin gallate acts synergistically in combination with cisplatin and designed trans-palladiums in ovarian cancer cells. *Anticancer Res* 2012; 32: 4851-60.

[115] Chan MM, Soprano KJ, Weinstein K, Fong D. Epigallocatechin-3-gallate delivers hydrogen peroxide to induce death of ovarian cancer cells and enhances their cisplatin susceptibility. *J Cell Physiol* 2006; 207: 389-96.

[116] Wang H, Luo Y, Qiao T, Wu Z, Huang Z. Luteolin sensitizes the antitumor effect of cisplatin in drug-resistant ovarian cancer via induction of apoptosis and inhibition of cell migration and invasion. *J Ovarian Res* 2018; 11: 93.

[117] Bieg D, Sypniewski D, Nowak E, Bednarek I. Morin decreases galectin-3 expression and sensitizes ovarian cancer cells to cisplatin. *Arch Gynecol Obstet* 2018; 298: 1181-94.

[118] Maciejczyk A, Surowiak P. Quercetin inhibits proliferation and increases sensitivity of ovarian cancer cells to cisplatin and paclitaxel. *Ginekol Pol* 2013; 84: 590-5.

[119] Wang X, Jiang P, Wang P, Yang CS, Wang X, Feng Q. EGCG enhances cisplatin sensitivity by regulating expression of the copper and cisplatin influx transporter CTR1 in ovary cancer. *PLoS One* 2015; 10: e0125402.

[120] Zhu X, Ji M, Han Y, Guo Y, Zhu W, Gao F, Yang X, Zhang C. PGRMC1-dependent autophagy by hyperoside induces apoptosis and sensitizes ovarian cancer cells to cisplatin treatment. *Int J Oncol* 2017; 50: 835-46.

[121] Li J, Wang Y, Lei JC, Hao Y, Yang Y, Yang CX, Yu JQ. Sensitisation of ovarian cancer cells to cisplatin by flavonoids from Scutellaria barbata. *Nat Prod Res* 2014; 28: 683-9.

[122] Bible KC, Peethambaram PP, Oberg AL, Maples W, Groteluschen DL, Boente M, Burton JK, Gomez Dahl LC, Tibodeau JD, Isham CR, Maguire JL, Shridhar V, Kukla AK, Voll KJ, Mauer MJ, Colevas AD, Wright J, Doyle LA, Erlichman C; Mayo Phase 2 Consortium (P2C); North Central Cancer Treatment Group (NCCTG). A phase 2 trial of flavopiridol (Alvocidib) and cisplatin in platin-resistant ovarian and primary peritoneal carcinoma: MC0261. *Gynecol Oncol* 2012; 127: 55-62.

[123] Yellepeddi VK, Vangara KK, Kumar A, Palakurthi S. Comparative evaluation of small-molecule chemosensitizers in reversal of cisplatin resistance in ovarian cancer cells. *Anticancer Res* 2012; 32: 3651-8.

[124] Su YK, Huang WC, Lee WH, Bamodu OA, Zucha MA, Astuti I, Suwito H, Yeh CT, Lin CM. Methoxyphenyl chalcone sensitizes aggressive epithelial cancer to cisplatin through apoptosis induction and cancer stem cell eradication. *Tumour Biol* 2017; 39: 1010428317691689.

[125] Song Y, Xin X, Zhai X, Xia Z, Shen K. Sequential combination of flavopiridol with Taxol synergistically suppresses human ovarian carcinoma growth. *Arch Gynecol Obstet* 2015; 291: 143-50.

[126] Solomon LA, Ali S, Banerjee S, Munkarah AR, Morris RT, Sarkar FH. Sensitization of ovarian cancer cells to cisplatin by genistein: the role of NF-kappaB. *J Ovarian Res* 2008; 1: 9.

[127] Lo YL, Wang W. Formononetin potentiates epirubicin-induced apoptosis via ROS production in HeLa cells in vitro. *Chem Biol Interact* 2013; 205: 188-97.

[128] Zhang L, Yang X, Li X, Li C, Zhao L, Zhou Y, Hou H. Butein sensitizes HeLa cells to cisplatin through the AKT and ERK/p38 MAPK pathways by targeting FoxO3a. *Int J Mol Med* 2015; 36: 957-66.

[129] Singh M, Bhui K, Singh R, Shukla Y. Tea polyphenols enhance cisplatin chemosensitivity in cervical cancer cells via induction of apoptosis. *Life Sci* 2013; 93: 7-16.

[130] Yi JL, Shi S, Shen YL, Wang L, Chen HY, Zhu J, Ding Y. Myricetin and methyl eugenol combination enhances the anticancer activity, cell cycle arrest and

apoptosis induction of cis-platin against HeLa cervical cancer cell lines. *Int J Clin Exp Pathol* 2015; 8: 1116-27.

[131] Telli E, Genc H, Tasa BA, Sinan Özalp S, Tansu Koparal A. In vitro evaluation of combination of EGCG and Erlotinib with classical chemotherapeutics on JAR cells. *In Vitro Cell Dev Biol Anim* 2017; 53: 651-8.

[132] Erdogan S, Turkekul K, Serttas R, Erdogan Z. The natural flavonoid apigenin sensitizes human CD44+ prostate cancer stem cells to cisplatin therapy. *Biomed Pharmacother* 2017; 88: 210-7.

[133] Hörmann V, Kumi-Diaka J, Durity M, Rathinavelu A. Anticancer activities of genistein-topotecan combination in prostate cancer cells. *J Cell Mol Med* 2012; 16: 2631-6.

[134] Nagaprashantha LD. Vatsyayan R, Singhal J, Fast S, Roby R, Awasthi S, Singhal SS. Anti-cancer effects of novel flavonoid vicenin-2 as a single agent and in synergistic combination with docetaxel in prostate cancer. *Biochem Pharmacol* 2011; 82: 1100-9.

[135] Mukhtar E, Adhami VM, Siddiqui IA, Verma AK, Mukhtar H. Fisetin enhances chemotherapeutic effect of cabazitaxel against human prostate cancer cells. *Mol Cancer Ther* 2016; 15: 2863-74.

[136] Flaig TW, Su LJ, Harrison G, Agarwal R, Glode LM. Silibinin synergizes with mitoxantrone to inhibit cell growth and induce apoptosis in human prostate cancer cells. *Int J Cancer* 2007; 120: 2028-33.

[137] Tyagi AK, Singh RP, Agarwal C, Chan DC, Agarwal R. Silibinin strongly synergizes human prostate carcinoma DU145 cells to doxorubicin-induced growth inhibition, G2-M arrest, and apoptosis. *Clin Cancer Res* 2002; 8: 3512-9.

[138] Wang P, Henning SM, Heber D, Vadgama JV. Sensitization of docetaxel in prostate cancer cells by green tea and quercetin. *J Nutr Biochem* 2015; 26: 408-15.

[139] Li B, Jin X, Meng H, Hu B, Zhang T, Yu J, Chen S, Guo X, Wang W, Jiang W, Wang J. Morin promotes prostate cancer cells chemosensitivity to paclitaxel through miR-155/GATA3 axis. *Oncotarget* 2017; 8: 47849-60.

[140] Zhang S, Wang Y, Chen Z, Kim S, Iqbal S, Chi A, Ritenour C, Wang YA, Kucuk O, Wu D. Genistein enhances the efficacy of cabazitaxel chemotherapy in metastatic castration-resistant prostate cancer cells. *Prostate* 2013; 73: 1681-9.

[141] Wang G, Zhang D, Yang S, Wang Y, Tang Z, Fu X. Co-administration of genistein with doxorubicin-loaded polypeptide nanoparticles weakens the metastasis of malignant prostate cancer by amplifying oxidative damage. *Biomater Sci* 2018; 6: 827-35.

[142] Wen D, Peng Y, Lin F, Singh RK, Mahato RI. Micellar delivery of miR-34a modulator rubone and paclitaxel in resistant prostate cancer. *Cancer Res* 2017; 77: 3244-54.

[143] McPherson RA, Galettis PT, de Souza PL. Enhancement of the activity of phenoxodiol by cisplatin in prostate cancer cells. *Br J Cancer* 2009; 100: 649-55.

[144] Tripathi R, Samadder T, Gupta S, Surolia A, Shaha C. Anticancer activity of a combination of cisplatin and fisetin in embryonal carcinoma cells and xenograft tumors. *Mol Cancer Ther* 2011; 10: 255-68.

[145] Hu J, Wang J, Wang G, Yao Z, Dang X. Pharmacokinetics and antitumor efficacy of DSPE-PEG2000 polymeric liposomes loaded with quercetin and temozolomide: Analysis of their effectiveness in enhancing the chemosensitization of drug-resistant glioma cells. *Int J Mol Med* 2016; 37: 690-702.

[146] Elhag R, Mazzio EA, Soliman KF. The effect of silibinin in enhancing toxicity of temozolomide and etoposide in p53 and PTEN-mutated resistant glioma cell lines. *Anticancer Res* 2015; 35: 1263-9.

[147] Jakubowicz-Gil J, Langner E, Wertel I, Piersiak T, Rzeski W. Temozolomide, quercetin and cell death in the MOGGCCM astrocytoma cell line. *Chem Biol Interact* 2010; 188: 190-203.

[148] Jia WZ, Zhao JC, Sun XL, Yao ZG, Wu HL, Xi ZQ. Additive anticancer effects of chrysin and low dose cisplatin in human malignant glioma cell (U87) proliferation and evaluation of the mechanistic pathway. *J BUON* 2015; 20: 1327-36.

[149] Yang L, Wang Y, Guo H, Guo M. Synergistic anti-cancer effects of icariin and temozolomide in glioblastoma. *Cell Biochem Biophys* 2015; 71: 1379-85.

[150] Jakubowicz-Gil J, Langner E, Rzeski W. Kinetic studies of the effects of Temodal and quercetin on astrocytoma cells. *Pharmacol Rep* 2011; 63: 403-16.

[151] Zhang Y, Wang SX, Ma JW, Li HY, Ye JC, Xie SM, Du B, Zhong XY. EGCG inhibits properties of glioma stem-like cells and synergizes with temozolomide through downregulation of P-glycoprotein inhibition. *J Neurooncol* 2015; 121: 41-52.

[152] Wang Y, Liu W, He X, Fei Z. Hispidulin enhances the anti-tumor effects of temozolomide in glioblastoma by activating AMPK. *Cell Biochem Biophys* 2015; 71: 701-6.

[153] Shervington A, Pawar V, Menon S, Thakkar D, Patel R. The sensitization of glioma cells to cisplatin and tamoxifen by the use of catechin. *Mol Biol Rep* 2009; 36: 1181-6.

[154] Hayashi T, Adachi K, Ohba S, Hirose Y. The Cdk inhibitor flavopiridol enhances temozolomide-induced cytotoxicity in human glioma cells. *J Neurooncol* 2013; 115: 169-78.

[155] Jakubowicz-Gil J, Langner E, Badziul D, Wertel I, Rzeski W. Apoptosis induction in human glioblastoma multiforme T98G cells upon temozolomide and quercetin treatment. *Tumour Biol* 2013; 34: 2367-78.

[156] Zhang P, Sun S, Li N, Ho ASW, Kiang KMY, Zhang X, Cheng YS, Poon MW, Lee D, Pu JKS, Leung GKK. Rutin increases the cytotoxicity of temozolomide in glioblastoma via autophagy inhibition. *J Neurooncol* 2017; 132: 393-400.

[157] Belcher SM, Burton CC, Cookman CJ, Kirby M, Miranda GL, Saeed FO, Wray KE. Estrogen and soy isoflavonoids decrease sensitivity of medulloblastoma and central nervous system primitive neuroectodermal tumor cells to chemotherapeutic cytotoxicity. *BMC Pharmacol Toxicol* 2017; 18: 63.

[158] Khoshyomn S, Manske GC, Lew SM, Wald SL, Penar PL. Synergistic action of genistein and cisplatin on growth inhibition and cytotoxicity of human medulloblastoma cells. *Pediatr Neurosurg* 2000; 33: 123-31.

[159] Vittorio O, Le Grand M, Makharza SA, Curcio M, Tucci P, Iemma F, Nicoletta FP, Hampel S, Cirillo G. Doxorubicin synergism and resistance reversal in human neuroblastoma BE(2)C cell lines: An in vitro study with dextran-catechin nanohybrids. *Eur J Pharm Biopharm* 2018; 122: 176-85.

[160] Vittorio O, Brandl M, Cirillo G, Spizzirri UG, Picci N, Kavallaris M, Iemma F, Hampel S. Novel functional cisplatin carrier based on carbon nanotubes-quercetin nanohybrid induces synergistic anticancer activity against neuroblastoma in vitro. *RSC Adv* 2014; 4: 31378.

[161] Zanini C, Giribaldi G, Madili G, Carta F, Crescenzio N, Bisaro B, Doria A, Foglia L, di Montezemolo LC, Timeus F, Turrini F. Inhibition of heat shock proteins (HSP) expression by quercetin and differential doxorubicin sensitization in neuroblastoma and Ewing`s sarcoma cell lines. *J Neurochem* 2007; 103: 1344-54.

[162] Zhang B, Yu X, Xia H. The flavonoid luteolin enhances doxorubicin-induced autophagy in human osteosarcoma U2OS cells. *Int J Clin Exp Med* 2015; 8: 15190-7.

[163] Zhang B, Shi ZL, Liu B, Yan XB, Feng J, Tao HM. Enhanced anticancer effect of gemcitabine by genistein in osteosarcoma: the role of Akt and nuclear factor-kappaB. *Anticancer Drugs* 2010; 21: 288-96.

[164] Jacobs H, Bast A, Peters GJ, van der Vijgh WJ, Haenen GR. The semisynthetic flavonoid monoHER sensitises human soft tissue sarcoma cells to doxorubicin-induced apoptosis via inhibition of nuclear factor-κB. *Br J Cancer* 2011; 104: 437-40.

[165] Wang Z, Yang L, Xia Y, Guo C, Kong L. Icariin enhances cytotoxicity of doxorubicin in human multidrug-resistant osteosarcoma cells by inhibition of ABCB1 and down-regulation of the PI3K/Akt pathway. *Biol Pharm Bull* 2015; 38: 277-84.

[166] Ferreira de Oliveira JMP, Pacheco AR, Coutinho L, Oliveira H, Pinho S, Almeida L, Fernandes E, Santos C. Combination of etoposide and fisetin results in anti-cancer efficiency against osteosarcoma cell models. *Arch Toxicol* 2018; 92: 1205-14.

[167] Zhang X, Guo Q, Chen J, Chen Z. Quercetin enhances cisplatin sensitivity of human osteosarcoma cells by modulating microRNA-217-KRAS axis. *Mol Cells* 2015; 38: 638-42.

[168] Luke JJ, D`Adamo DR, Dickson MA, Keohan ML, Carvajal RD, Maki RG, de Stanchina E, Musi E, Singer S, Schwartz GK. The cyclin-dependent kinase inhibitor flavopiridol potentiates doxorubicin efficacy in advanced sarcomas: preclinical investigations and results of a phase I dose-escalation clinical trial. *Clin Cancer Res* 2012; 18: 2638-47.

[169] Coutinho L, Oliveira H, Pacheco AR, Almeida L, Pimentel F, Santos C, Ferreira de Oliveira JM. Hesperetin-etoposide combinations induce cytotoxicity in U2OS cells: Implications on therapeutic developments for osteosarcoma. *DNA Repair (Amst)* 2017; 50: 36-42.

[170] Xia YZ, Ni K, Guo C, Zhang C, Geng YD, Wang ZD, Yang L, Kong LY. Alopecurone B reverses doxorubicin-resistant human osteosarcoma cell line by inhibiting P-glycoprotein and NF-kappa B signaling. *Phytomedicine* 2015; 22: 344-51.

[171] Ryu S, Park S, Lim W, Song G. Effects of luteolin on canine osteosarcoma: Suppression of cell proliferation and synergy with cisplatin. *J Cell Physiol* 2019; 234: 9504-14.

[172] Liao B, Ying H, Yu C, Fan Z, Zhang W, Shi J, Ying H, Ravichandran N, Xu Y, Yin J, Jiang Y, Du Q. (-)-Epigallocatechin gallate (EGCG)-nanoethosomes as a transdermal delivery system for docetaxel to treat implanted human melanoma cell tumors in mice. *Int J Pharm* 2016; 512: 22-31.

[173] Krajnovic T, Kaluderovic GN, Wessjohann LA, Mijatovic S, Maksimovic-Ivanic D. Versatile antitumor potential of isoxanthohumol: Enhancement of paclitaxel activity in vivo. *Pharmacol Res* 2016; 105: 62-73.

[174] Kluger HM, McCarthy MM, Alvero AB, Sznol M, Ariyan S, Camp RL, Rimm DL, Mor G. The X-linked inhibitor of apoptosis protein (XIAP) is up-regulated in metastatic melanoma, and XIAP cleavage by Phenoxodiol is associated with Carboplatin sensitization. *J Transl Med* 2007; 5: 6.

[175] Shi H, Wu Y, Wang Y, Zhou M, Yan S, Chen Z, Gu D, Cai Y. Liquiritigenin potentiates the inhibitory effects of cisplatin on invasion and metastasis via downregulation of MMP-2/9 and PI3K/AKT signaling pathway in B16F10 melanoma cells and mice model. *Nutr Cancer* 2015; 67: 761-70.

[176] Thangasamy T, Sittadjody S, Limesand KH, Burd R. Tyrosinase overexpression promotes ATM-dependent p53 phosphorylation by quercetin and sensitizes melanoma cells to dacarbazine. *Cell Oncol* 2008; 30: 371-87.

[177] Liu JD, Chen SH, Lin CL, Tsai SH, Liang YC. Inhibition of melanoma growth and metastasis by combination with (-)-epigallocatechin-3-gallate and dacarbazine in mice. *J Cell Biochem* 2001; 83: 631-42.

[178] Thangasamy T, Sittadjody S, Mitchell GC, Mendoza EE, Radhakrishnan VM, Limesand KH, Burd R. Quercetin abrogates chemoresistance in melanoma cells by modulating deltaNp73. *BMC Cancer* 2010; 10: 282.

[179] Ferlay J, Soerjomataram I, Dikshit R, Eser S, Mathers C, Rebelo M, Parkin DM, Forman D, Bray F. Cancer incidence and mortality worldwide: sources, methods and major patterns in GLOBOCAN 2012. *Int J Cancer* 2015; 136: E359-86.

[180] Wu J, Guan M, Wong PF, Yu H, Dong J, Xu J. Icariside II potentiates paclitaxel-induced apoptosis in human melanoma A375 cells by inhibiting TLR4 signaling pathway. *Food Chem Toxicol* 2012; 50: 3019-24.

[181] Lee JJ, Koh KN, Park CJ, Jang S, Im HJ, Kim N. The combination of flavokawain B and daunorubicin induces apoptosis in human myeloid leukemic cells by modifying NF-κB. *Anticancer Res* 2018; 38: 2771-8.

[182] Desai UN, Shah KP, Mirza SH, Panchal DK, Parikh SK, Rawal RM. Enhancement of the cytotoxic effects of cytarabine in synergism with hesperidine and silibinin in acute myeloid leukemia: An in-vitro approach. *J Cancer Res Ther* 2015; 11: 352-7.

[183] Papiez MA, Bukowska-Strakova K, Krzysciak W, Baran J. (-)-Epicatechin enhances etoposide-induced antileukaemic effect in rats with acute myeloid leukaemia. *Anticancer Res* 2012; 32: 2905-13.

[184] Shen J, Tai YC, Zhou J, Stephen Wong CH, Cheang PT, Fred Wong WS, Xie Z, Khan M, Han JH, Chen CS. Synergistic antileukemia effect of genistein and chemotherapy in mouse xenograft model and potential mechanism through MAPK signaling. *Exp Hematol* 2007; 35: 75-83.

[185] Teofili L, Pierelli L, Iovino MS, Leone G, Scambia G, De Vincenzo R, Benedetti-Panici P, Menichella G, Macri E, Piantelli M, Ranelletti FO, Larocca LM. The combination of quercetin and cytosine arabinoside synergistically inhibits leukemic cell growth. *Leuk Res* 1992; 16: 497-503.

[186] Wang Y, Miao H, Li W, Yao J, Sun Y, Li Z, Zhao L, Guo Q. CXCL12/CXCR4 axis confers adriamycin resistance to human chronic myelogenous leukemia and oroxylin A improves the sensitivity of K562/ADM cells. *Biochem Pharmacol* 2014; 90: 212-25.

[187] Davenport A, Frezza M, Shen M, Ge Y, Huo C, Chan TH, Dou QP. Celastrol and an EGCG pro-drug exhibit potent chemosensitizing activity in human leukemia cells. *Int J Mol Med* 2010; 25: 465-70.

[188] Xu X, Zhang X, Zhang Y, Yang L, Liu Y, Huang S, Lu L, Kong L, Li Z, Guo Q, Zhao L. Wogonin reversed resistant human myelogenous leukemia cells via inhibiting Nrf2 signaling by Stat3/NF-κB inactivation. *Sci Rep* 2017; 7: 39950.

[189] Goto H, Yanagimachi M, Goto S, Takeuchi M, Kato H, Yokosuka T, Kajiwara R, Yokota S. Methylated chrysin reduced cell proliferation, but antagonized cytotoxicity of other anticancer drugs in acute lymphoblastic leukemia. *Anticancer Drugs* 2012; 23: 417-25.

[190] Chen YJ, Wu CS, Shieh JJ, Wu JH, Chen HY, Chung TW, Chen YK, Lin CC. Baicalein triggers mitochondria-mediated apoptosis and enhances the antileukemic effect of vincristine in childhood acute lymphoblastic leukemia CCRF-CEM cells. *Evid Based Complement Alternat Med* 2013: 2013: 124747.

[191] Uckun FM, Qazi S, Ozer Z, Garner AL, Pitt J, Ma H, Janda KD. Inducing apoptosis in chemotherapy-resistant B-lineage acute lymphoblastic leukaemia cells by targeting HSPA5, a master regulator of the anti-apoptotic unfolded protein response signalling network. *Br J Haematol* 2011; 153: 741-52.

[192] Russo M, Spagnuolo C, Volpe S, Mupo A, Tedesco I, Russo GL. Quercetin induced apoptosis in association with death receptors and fludarabine in cells isolated from chronic lymphocytic leukaemia patients. *Br J Cancer* 2010; 103: 642-8.

[193] Mansour A, Chang VT, Srinivas S, Harrison J, Raveche E. Correlation of ZAP-70 expression in B cell leukemias to the ex vivo response to a combination of fludarabine/genistein. *Cancer Immunol Immunother* 2007; 56: 501-14.

[194] Rebolleda N, Losada-Fernandez I, Perez-Chacon G, Castejon R, Rosado S, Morado M, Vallejo-Cremades MT, Martinez A, Vargas-Nunez JA, Perez-Aciego P. Synergistic activity of deguelin and fludarabine in cells from chronic lymphocytic leukemia patients and in the New Zealand Black murine model. *PLoS One* 2016; 11: e0154159.

[195] Chen X, Wu Y, Jiang Y, Zhou Y, Wang Y, Yao Y, Yi C, Gou L, Yang J. Isoliquiritigenin inhibits the growth of multiple myeloma via blocking IL-6 signaling. *J Mol Med (Berl)* 2012; 90: 1311-9.

[196] Zhu B, Yu L, Yue Q. Co-delivery of vincristine and quercetin by nanocarriers for lymphoma combination chemotherapy. *Biomed Pharmacother* 2017; 91: 287-94.

Chapter 2

CANCER DEVELOPMENT
STEP BY STEP

Cancer development is a complex multistep process, simplified depicted in Figure 2.1. Exposure to diverse carcinogens (chemicals, radiation, oncogenic viruses) causes mutations in the genes which induce carcinogenesis, whereas transformation of normal cells to cancerous includes different genetic changes, such as activation of oncogenes and loss of tumor suppressors. Besides mutations also epigenetic gene regulation, including DNA methylation, plays a certain role in the etiology of cancer [1]. Initiation, promotion and tumor progression are all associated with alterations in morphological and molecular features of cells, including the loss of normal regulatory signaling pathways involved in cell proliferation, differentiation and apoptosis, leading to unrestricted cellular expansion and growth of tumor mass [2-6]. Thus, the neoplastic growth results not only from uncontrolled sustain proliferation but also reduced cell death (apoptosis) [7].

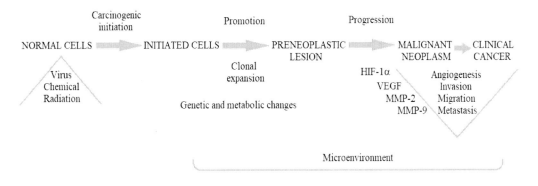

Figure 2.1. Main steps of complex carcinogenesis process (HIF-1α, hypoxia-inducible factor 1α; MMP, matrix metalloproteinase; VEGF, vascular endothelial growth factor).

The aberrant growth of malignant cells and fast expansion of tumor mass are supported by metabolic adaptations that satisfy the energy demand and nutritional requirements for rapidly dividing cells. Metabolic reprogramming to survive and respond to environmental alterations is one of the crucial hallmarks of malignant tumors [8]. The rapid malignant growth usually outpaces new vascular generation, leading to inadequate blood supply in tumor tissue and a hypoxic microenvironment [9]. Hypoxia-inducible factor 1α (HIF-1α) is an important molecule in adaptation with these strict conditions, whereas induction of glycolytic pathway to generate ATP is critical for survival of tumor cells under hypoxic circumstances [9]. Due to mitochondrial injuries, cancer cells exhibit the switch from oxidative phosphorylation to anaerobic glycolysis, even in the presence of oxygen, characterized by the higher glucose uptake and lactate production; this event is known as Warburg effect [8]. Another crucial hallmark of further cancer progression is angiogenesis, i.e., the formation of new intratumoral blood vessels, as malignant cells need nutrients and oxygen supplied by the vascular system [10-13]. Tumor angiogenesis is tightly modulated by proangiogenic mediators, such as vascular endothelial growth factor (VEGF), and antiangiogenic factors. Overexpression of VEGF has been described in a variety of malignant cells being strictly correlated with microvessel density, but also with disease stage and tumor burden [11, 12, 14-18].

Metastasis, a process within primary tumors are spread and transferred from initial site to a regional or distant organ to form secondary tumors, has remained one of the greatest challenges in cancer management and is the major cause of mortality in cancer patients [4, 19-22]. This complicated multifactorial process comprises several sequential events, including detachment of cancer cells from initial tumor, local invasion, intravasation, circulation, extravasation, and formation of new metastatic sites [19, 23]. Capacity of epithelial cells to migrate determines the invasive potential of tumor and therefore, acquisition of epithelial-mesenchymal transition (EMT) is an indispensable process in cancer metastasis and progression. Mesenchymal cells present increased motility and invasiveness owing to decreased cell-cell contact and reduced cell polarity, whereas cadherins as a group of cell-adhesion molecules represent key mediators in this transition [11, 24-26]. In fact, downregulation of epithelial marker E-cadherin and increase in mesenchymal markers, such as N-cadherin and vimentin result in higher metastatic dissemination and tumor recurrence [2, 11, 12, 27]. Indeed, a loss of E-cadherin has been described in several human malignancies, including colorectal, lung, pancreatic, prostate, and breast tumors being correlated with poor prognosis. At that, inflammatory mediators represent one of the negative regulators of E-cadherin expression [27, 28]. Contribution of inflammation to cancer cell proliferation and progression has been suggested already for more than one hundred and fifty years ago (1863), when Virchow observed the origination of tumors from the sites of chronic inflammation [29]. The link between inflammatory reactions and cancer is probably much more complex and multifactorial and still not completely unraveled.

Degradation of extracellular matrix (ECM) is another crucial step in metastasis. ECM forms a natural physical barrier and self-protective microenvironment that can be proteolytically degraded by matrix metalloproteinases (MMPs) [19]. These zinc-binding endopeptidases cleave almost all ECM components and destruct the basal membrane enabling tumor cells to migrate through the matrix and invade surrounding tissues, including blood or lymphatic system [20, 30-32]. Among all MMPs, MMP-2 and MMP-9 are the key regulator enzymes in ECM degradation, whereas their upregulated expression and enhanced activity increase the invasiveness and metastatic ability of tumor cells. Hence, both MMP-2 and MMP-9 levels are considered as markers for evaluation of diagnosis and prognosis of patients and should be downregulated to prevent metastatic spread and improve the clinical outcome [19, 20, 23, 32-34]. In the past decade, control of malignant metastasis and targeting tumor cell migration and invasion have emerged as a promising approach for decreasing cancer mortality. However, there are no effective antimetastatic drugs currently available in clinical application [22].

A comprehensive understanding of the molecular mechanisms underlying cancer development and progression, its biology and behavior may lead to the better therapeutic strategies for clinical application. At that, all the relevant cellular events for complex multistep carcinogenesis process (Figure 2.1) can be considered as potential therapeutic targets. For instance, tumor vasculature is suggested to be an attractive target and angiogenesis inhibitors using VEGF antibodies have been employed. Despite initial halt, tumors are able to develop an adaptive response and progress, even with increased invasiveness [14, 15]. Therefore, the main focus of current treatment regimens has still relied on the suppression of proliferation and subsequent induction of death (apoptosis) of cancer cells, or so-called cytotoxic therapy [22, 35]. However, increasing evidence has exposed that some of such frequently used cytostatic chemotherapeutic drugs, such as paclitaxel, cisplatin or cyclophosphamide, may induce or accelerate metastatic processes [22]. As cancer development and progression is a multistep process, the effective treatment strategy should probably impact all the key events at the same time, i.e., exerting antiproliferative, proapoptotic, antiangiogenic, antiinvasive, antimigratory, antimetastatic and antiinflammatory action. Currently, there is no existing drug or therapy clinically available that would be known to effectively target all these aspects. Therefore, a synergistic approach with carefully chosen agents is probably the most reasonable solution to gain the best outcome in cancer management.

REFERENCES

[1]   Sato A, Sekine M, Kobayashi M, Virgona N, Ota M, Yano T. Induction of the connexin 32 gene by epigallocatechin-3-gallate potentiates vinblastine-induced cytotoxicity in human renal carcinoma cells. *Chemotherapy* 2013; 59: 192-9.

[2] Liu Q, Sun Y, Zheng JM, Yan XL, Chen HM, Chen JK, Huang HQ. Formononetin sensitizes glioma cells to doxorubicin through preventing EMT via inhibition of histone deacetylase 5. *Int J Clin Exp Pathol* 2015; 8: 6434-41.

[3] Mihaila M, Bostan M, Hotnog D, Ferdes M, Brasoveanu LL. Real-time analysis of quercetin, resveratrol and/or doxorubicin effects in MCF-7 cells. *Rom Biotechnol Lett* 2013; 18: 8106-14.

[4] Zhang BY, Wang YM, Gong H, Zhao H, Lv XY, Yuan GH, Han SR. Isorhamnetin flavonoid synergistically enhances the anticancer activity and apoptosis induction by cis-platin and carboplatin in non-small cell lung carcinoma (NSCLC). *Int J Clin Exp Pathol* 2015; 8: 25-37.

[5] Liu L, Ju Y, Wang J, Zhou R. Epigallocatechin-3-gallate promotes apoptosis and reversal of multidrug resistance in esophageal cancer cells. *Pathol Res Pract* 2017; 213: 1242-50.

[6] Kiartivich S, Wei Y, Liu J, Soiampornkul R, Li M, Zhang H, Dong J. Regulation of cytotoxicity and apoptosis-associated pathways contributes to the enhancement of efficacy of cisplatin by baicalein adjuvant in human A549 lung cancer cells. *Oncol Lett* 2017; 13: 2799-804.

[7] Moon JY, Cho M, Ahn KS, Cho SK. Nobiletin induces apoptosis and potentiates the effects of the anticancer drug 5-fluorouracil in p53-mutated SNU-16 human gastric cancer cells. *Nutr Cancer* 2013; 65: 286-95.

[8] Catanzaro D, Gabbia D, Cocetta V, Biagi M, Ragazzi E, Montopoli M, Carrara M. Silybin counteracts doxorubicin resistance by inhibiting GLUT1 expression. *Fitoterapia* 2018; 124: 42-8.

[9] Chen F, Zhuang M, Zhong C, Peng J, Wang X, Li J, Chen Z, Huang Y. Baicalein reverses hypoxia-induced 5-FU resistance in gastric cancer AGS cells through suppression of glycolysis and the PTEN/Akt/HIF-1α signaling pathway. *Oncol Rep* 2015; 33: 457-63.

[10] Garcia-Vilas JA, Quesada AR, Medina MA. Screening of synergistic interactions of epigallocatechin-3-gallate with antiangiogenic and antitumor compounds. *Synergy* 2016; 3: 5-13.

[11] Lei CS, Hou YC, Pai MH, Lin MT, Yeh SL. Effects of quercetin combined with anticancer drugs on metastasis-associated factors of gastric cancer cells: in vitro and in vivo studies. *J Nutr Biochem* 2018; 51: 105-13.

[12] Park CH, Han SE, Nam-Goong IS, Kim YI, Kim ES. Combined effects of baicalein and docetaxel on apoptosis in 8505c anaplastic thyroid cancer cells via downregulation of the ERK and Akt/mTOR pathways. *Endocrinol Metab (Seoul)* 2018; 33: 121-32.

[13] Mukhtar E, Adhami VM, Siddiqui IA, Verma AK, Mukhtar H. Fisetin enhances chemotherapeutic effect of cabazitaxel against human prostate cancer cells. *Mol Cancer Ther* 2016; 15: 2863-74.

[14] Touil YS, Seguin J, Scherman D, Chabot GG. Improved antiangiogenic and antitumour activity of the combination of the natural flavonoid fisetin and cyclophosphamide in Lewis lung carcinoma-bearing mice. *Cancer Chemother Pharmacol* 2011; 68: 445-55.

[15] Mendes LP, Gaeti MP, de Avila PH, de Sousa Vieira M, Dos Santos Rodrigues B, de Avila Marcelino RI, Dos Santos LC, Valadares MC, Lima EM. Multicompartimental nanoparticles for co-encapsulation and multimodal drug delivery to tumor cells and neovasculature. *Pharm Res* 2014; 31: 1106-19.

[16] Wu H, Xin Y, Xu C, Xiao Y. Capecitabine combined with (-)-epigallocatechin-3-gallate inhibits angiogenesis and tumor growth in nude mice with gastric cancer xenografts. *Exp Ther Med* 2012; 3: 650-4.

[17] Wu J, Guan M, Wong PF, Yu H, Dong J, Xu J. Icariside II potentiates paclitaxel-induced apoptosis in human melanoma A375 cells by inhibiting TLR4 signaling pathway. *Food Chem Toxicol* 2012; 50: 3019-24.

[18] Wu H, Xin Y, Xiao Y, Zhao J. Low-dose docetaxel combined with (-)-epigallocatechin-3-gallate inhibits angiogenesis and tumor growth in nude mice with gastric cancer xenografts. *Cancer Biother Radiopharm* 2012; 27: 204-9.

[19] Li J, Zhang J, Wang Y, Liang X, Wusiman Z, Yin Y, Shen Q. Synergistic inhibition of migration and invasion of breast cancer cells by dual docetaxel/quercetin-loaded nanoparticles via Akt/MMP-9 pathway. *Int J Pharm* 2017; 523: 300-9.

[20] Ma L, Wang R, Nan Y, Li W, Wang Q, Jin F. Phloretin exhibits an anticancer effect and enhances the anticancer ability of cisplatin on non-small cell lung cancer cell lines by regulating expression of apoptotic pathways and matrix metalloproteinases. *Int J Oncol* 2016; 48: 843-53.

[21] Ramachandran L, Manu KA, Shanmugam MK, Li F, Siveen KS, Vali S, Kapoor S, Abbasi T, Surana R, Smoot DT, Ashktorab H, Tan P, Ahn KS, Yap CW, Kumar AP, Sethi G. Isorhamnetin inhibits proliferation and invasion and induces apoptosis through the modulation of peroxisome proliferator-activated receptor γ activation pathway in gastric cancer. *J Biol Chem* 2012; 287: 38028-40.

[22] Klimaszewska-Wisniewska A, Halas-Wisniewska M, Grzanka A, Grzanka D. Evaluation of anti-metastatic potential of the combination of fisetin with paclitaxel on A549 non-small cell lung cancer cells. *Int J Mol Sci* 2018; 19: E661.

[23] Shi H, Wu Y, Wang Y, Zhou M, Yan S, Chen Z, Gu D, Cai Y. Liquiritigenin potentiates the inhibitory effects of cisplatin on invasion and metastasis via downregulation of MMP-2/9 and PI3K/AKT signaling pathway in B16F10 melanoma cells and mice model. *Nutr Cancer* 2015; 67: 761-70.

[24] Staedler D, Idrizi E, Kenzaoui BH, Juillerat-Jeanneret L. Drug combinations with quercetin: doxorubicin plus quercetin in human breast cancer cells. *Cancer Chemother Pharmacol* 2011; 68: 1161-72.

[25] Dia VP, Pangloli P. Epithelial-to-mesenchymal transition in paclitaxel-resistant ovarian cancer cells is downregulated by luteolin. *J Cell Physiol* 2017; 232: 391-401.

[26] Hyun HB, Moon JY, Cho SK. Quercetin suppresses CYR61-mediated multidrug resistance in human gastric adenocarcinoma AGS cells. *Molecules* 2018; 23: E209.

[27] Mateen S, Raina K, Agarwal C, Chan D, Agarwal R. Silibinin synergizes with histone deacetylase and DNA methyltransferase inhibitors in upregulating E-cadherin expression together with inhibition of migration and invasion of human non-small cell lung cancer cells. *J Pharmacol Exp Ther* 2013; 345: 206-14.

[28] Nagaprashantha LD. Vatsyayan R, Singhal J, Fast S, Roby R, Awasthi S, Singhal SS. Anti-cancer effects of novel flavonoid vicenin-2 as a single agent and in synergistic combination with docetaxel in prostate cancer. *Biochem Pharmacol* 2011; 82: 1100-9.

[29] Wang HW, Lin CP, Chiu JH, Chow KC, Kuo KT, Lin CS, Wang LS. Reversal of inflammation-associated dihydrodiol dehydrogenases (AKR1C1 and AKR1C2) overexpression and drug resistance in nonsmall cell lung cancer cells by wogonin and chrysin. *Int J Cancer* 2007; 120: 2019-27.

[30] Chen P, Hu MD, Deng XF, Li B. Genistein reinforces the inhibitory effect of Cisplatin on liver cancer recurrence and metastasis after curative hepatectomy. *Asian Pac J Cancer Prev* 2013; 14: 759-64.

[31] Tsai LC, Hsieh HY, Lu KY, Wang SY, Mi FL. EGCG/gelatin-doxorubicin gold nanoparticles enhance therapeutic efficacy of doxorubicin for prostate cancer treatment. *Nanomedicine (Lond)* 2016; 11: 9-30.

[32] Ramadass SK, Anantharaman NV, Subramanian S, Sivasubramanian S, Madhan B. Paclitaxel/epigallocatechin gallate coloaded liposome: a synergistic delivery to control the invasiveness of MDA-MB-231 breast cancer cells. *Colloids Surf B Biointerfaces* 2015; 125: 65-72.

[33] Liu JD, Chen SH, Lin CL, Tsai SH, Liang YC. Inhibition of melanoma growth and metastasis by combination with (-)-epigallocatechin-3-gallate and dacarbazine in mice. *J Cell Biochem* 2001; 83: 631-42.

[34] Ho BY, Lin CH, Apaya MK, Chao WW, Shyur LF. Silibinin and paclitaxel cotreatment significantly suppress the activity and lung metastasis of triple negative 4T1 mammary tumor cell in mice. *J Tradit Complement Med* 2011; 2: 301-11.

[35] Dai W, Gao Q, Qiu J, Yuan J, Wu G, Shen G. Quercetin induces apoptosis and enhances 5-FU therapeutic efficacy in hepatocellular carcinoma. *Tumour Biol* 2016; 37: 6307-13.

Chapter 3

CONVENTIONAL CHEMOTHERAPY AND ITS LIMITATIONS

Current cancer treatment regimens depend largely on the type, stage and location of disease, including surgical resection of tumor mass, radiotherapy, chemotherapy, targeted therapy and immunotherapy, used alone or in different multimodal combinations [1-6]. The main aims with such therapies are to reduce the size and progression of tumor growth, eradicate malignant cells, improve the outcomes, and increase disease-free and overall survival of patients, without affecting the normal healthy tissues [7]. Detection of a tumor at its early developmental stages provides nowadays a rather high chance for curative treatment; however, regionally and/or distantly spread metastatic cancers represent a major challenge to clinical management, whereas an effective cure for advanced tumors has still remained an elusive dream for all mankind [5, 8].

Chemotherapy is a mainstream anticancer treatment approach to induce the death and suppress survival of a wide variety of malignant cells, both of solid tumors as well as hematological malignancies [4, 9-11]. Investigation of chemotherapeutic agents since the early 1940s has resulted in the discovery of more than 50 drugs to date. The first developed and used drugs were nitrogen mustards (chlorambucil, cyclophosphamide) for treatment of non-Hodgkin lymphoma. Afterwards, numerous other anticancer compounds were identified, including antimetabolites and vinca alkaloids. The currently approved chemotherapeutic drugs have different cellular targets and act through diverse molecular mechanisms, based on which these agents are broadly classified into DNA-interfering drugs (alkylating agents, platinum compounds and topoisomerase inhibitors), antimetabolites and microtubules-targeting drugs [5, 12, 13]. A number of different regimens are being used in administration of these chemotherapeutics, including neoadjuvant treatment where drugs are given before surgery or radiation to compress the tumor size for more effective local therapy, adjuvant treatment with continued drug intake after surgical resection to eliminate residual cancer cells and prevent the recurrence risk, and palliative treatment involving drug dosage only to reduce the tumor load and increase life expectancy without any curative goals [12]. Despite benefits achieved with intensive chemotherapeutic treatments, the rate of remission and metastasis is still high and long-term survival poor, reflecting several disadvantages and significant limitations in clinical application of chemotherapeutic drugs [5, 14]. Indeed, there are several obstacles to successful anticancer treatment, including emergence of drug resistance, various deleterious adverse reactions and high cost of conventional chemotherapeutic agents [15-22]. The most critical limitations impeding success of current chemotherapeutic regimens with possible ways of further solutions are depicted in Figure 3.1.

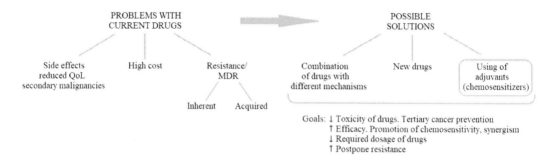

Figure 3.1. Major problems accompanying with chemotherapeutic drugs, possible solutions and principal goals (MDR, multidrug resistance; QoL, quality of life).

While antitumor drugs can successfully obliterate rapidly dividing malignant cells, they exert cytotoxic effects and damage also proliferating normal healthy cells leading to severe side effects and unacceptable organ toxicities, such as immune dysfunction, myelosuppression, fatigue, anorexia, constipation, diarrhea, nausea, vomiting, oral mucositis, alopecia, skin rashes, fever, cardiotoxicity, nephrotoxicity, hepatotoxicity, ototoxicity and neurotoxicity [4, 5, 7, 23-26]. The adverse events caused by specific drugs are described in more detail in the respective subsections of Chapter 6. Such undesirable injury to normal tissues not only involves physical and mental trauma to cancer patients and reduces their quality of life, but also limits the doses of chemotherapeutics applied in clinical practice or even causes discontinuance of treatment, being closely associated with metastasis and unfavorable prognosis. In addition, secondary malignancies are an increasingly recognized late complication after chemo- (but also radio-) therapy [5, 27-30]. Therefore, novel treatment strategies with higher efficacy and selectivity towards cancerous cells protecting at the same time normal healthy tissues from toxic side effects are highly needed.

Another fundamental impediment with the use of antineoplastic drugs leading to treatment failure, tumor recurrence and mortality of patients is chemoresistance, i.e., the lack of complete and long-lasting response to chemotherapy in many human cancers [3, 9, 28, 31-37]. Even with the initial response to chemotherapy treatment, many types of sensitive tumors may become resistant to standard drugs over time. A high degree of molecular genetic heterogeneity facilitates the adaptation of tumors to the usual cytotoxic compounds [1, 6, 11, 38]. Otherwise, the disease can be refractory to chemotherapy already at diagnosis. So, malignant cells may exhibit inherent (primary, intrinsic, natural, de novo) resistance or acquire resistance (secondary) in the course of repeated chemotherapeutic drug regimens [39-44]. Moreover, tumors not only become resistant to the single cytotoxic drugs originally used to treat them, but also to a broad range of chemically and structurally unrelated agents with different molecular targets and intracellular action mechanisms. Such cross-resistance phenomenon is termed multidrug resistance (MDR) and was first described by Kessel et al already in 1968 [41, 42, 44, 45]. At present, MDR is a common clinical problem and one of the major obstacles to successful chemotherapy and long-term regression in management of various cancer types [29, 46-49]. The only way to circumvent the acquired chemoresistance in cancer cells is to increase the drug dosage; however, this can in turn result in higher cytotoxicity and undesirable side effects to normal tissues [32, 44, 50-53]. Thus, tumor cells exhibit drug resistance and potential invasiveness in order to survive chemotherapy, and significant efforts must be made to overcome this chemoresistance and solve MDR to reduce the rate of relapse and metastasis and improve the prognosis of cancer patients.

It is clear that recent treatment regimens have remained suboptimal and development of novel specific strategies for suppressing tumor growth and enhancing chemosensitivity without damaging normal tissues has been the focus of much medical research in the past decades. The most attractive chemotherapeutic schedule involves achievement of higher long-term response rate, minimized systemic toxicity, postponed emergence of drug resistance, but also reduced treatment costs (Figure 3.1). Identification of new potential targets, detailed intracellular mechanisms, and novel more effective and selective anticancer drugs is inevitable for further improving the clinical management of malignant disorders. Thus, numerous *in vitro* and *in vivo* studies are necessary using various cancerous cell lines and human tumor xenografts in nude mice as experimental models. It has been shown that predictions done with these xenografts concerning tumor response, resistance and toxicity level correspond well to the respective estimates obtained for humans in clinical trials [54]. However, promising *in vitro* findings are often followed by much less compelling results *in vivo*, due to very high drug doses needful for therapeutic activity at the site of action [55]. Therefore, research and evaluation of novel more specific cytotoxic anticancer agents with fewer side effects are still justified and must be continued.

In order to overcome above-described limitations and combat multiple survival mechanisms of tumor cells, at present, most cancers are clinically managed by using combinations of various drugs, usually in binary or ternary drug regimens, to obtain synergistic or at least additive effects [15, 19, 56-58]. Compared to single-agent therapies, such multiagent regimens allow to achieve increased therapeutic effects, prolong survival and exhibit lower probability of drug resistance because of the different targets and action mechanisms of applied drugs. Moreover, rational combinations render it possible to employ single chemotherapeutics at lower doses contributing to decreased individual drug-related toxicities [53, 57, 59-62]. However, the reality is that drug combinations bring along some disadvantages, such as added systemic toxicity requiring in turn the dose reduction and leading to poor treatment outcome. In addition, such multiagent chemotherapies are not effective once malignant neoplasms become chemoresistant [40, 63-68]. Also, sequential administrative schedules may have substantial therapeutic implications [69, 70]. Hence, there is still a tremendous need for development of optimal therapeutic strategies for clinical treatment of human cancers, to overcome or delay resistance, prevent recurrence and metastasis, and improve clinical outcome.

A promising approach for future anticancer arsenal comprises identification of non-toxic (chemopreventive) agents preferably from natural sources to sensitize malignant cells toward conventional chemotherapeutic drugs. Such adjuvant combination strategy may produce considerably potentiated response rates and improved therapeutic outcomes, while attenuating the toxic side effects due to reducing the required dosages of traditional cytotoxic agents [56, 71-75]. Previous investigations have shown that suppressing tumor cell defenses against chemotherapeutic agents can inhibit drug-induced chemoresistance and lead to synergistic antitumor effects [76-78]. At that, chemosensitizers act on various molecular targets and affect different intracellular signaling mechanisms. Identification and use of novel effective chemomodulators to improve efficacy, reduce toxicity and reverse multidrug resistance to standard cytotoxic drugs used in the treatment of different human tumor types is an indisputable priority of current cancer research, whereas nature has remained the most important and plentiful source for such attractive compounds [8, 18, 46, 79-81]. Finding and clinical application of such novel adjuvants may be especially beneficial to patients with refractory and/or recurrent disease.

Although combination strategy is devised with the aim to augment the clinical anticancer response of standard drugs, both the chemical structure of combined agents, their molar ratio as well as sequential administration schedule must be carefully chosen. When two agents are administrated together, they can exhibit additivity, synergism or antagonism exerting equal, greater or less than the sum of individual drugs effect, respectively [82]. This means that not all combinations are advantageous and added compound may not only boost the drug action (synergism) but also counteract it (antagonism) leading to smaller total effect than the summary activities of individual agents [83]. The total effect is generally characterized quantitively by combination index (CI) calculated by Chou and Talalay equation (1981), whereas CI value below 1 indicates synergism, CI=1 suggests additive effects and antagonism is defined by CI>1. As farther is the CI value from 1, the stronger is the drug interaction [62, 84-87].

Furthermore, despite potentiating efficacy of administered combinations observed *in vitro* assays, the synergistic ratio of agents might not be maintained *in vivo* conditions due to distinct pharmacokinetic profiles of different compounds and their inconsistent biodistribution [83]. In these cases, co-encapsulation of both agents in fixed molar ratios in an appropriately designed drug delivery system based on nanoparticles platform can assure the simultaneous drug release at the same destination and thus, maximal therapeutic efficacy in fighting against cancer [83, 88, 89]. Thorough preclinical combination studies *in vitro* and *in vivo* conditions using clinically relevant drug concentrations are inevitable to move on with clinical trials [90].

REFERENCES

[1] Kim EH, Jang H, Roh JL. A novel polyphenol conjugate sensitizes cisplatin-resistant head and neck cancer cells to cisplatin via Nrf2 inhibition. *Mol Cancer Ther* 2016; 15: 2620-9.

[2] Varela-Castillo O, Cordero P, Gutierrez-Iglesias G, Palma I, Rubio-Gayosso I, Meaney E, Ramirez-Sanchez I, Villarreal F, Ceballos G, Najera N. Characterization of the cytotoxic effects of the combination of cisplatin and flavanol (-)-epicatechin on human lung cancer cell line A549. An isobolographic approach. *Exp Oncol* 2018; 40: 19-23.

[3] Catanzaro D, Gabbia D, Cocetta V, Biagi M, Ragazzi E, Montopoli M, Carrara M. Silybin counteracts doxorubicin resistance by inhibiting GLUT1 expression. *Fitoterapia* 2018; 124: 42-8.

[4] Abaza MS, Orabi KY, Al-Quattan E, Al-Attiyah RJ. Growth inhibitory and chemo-sensitization effects of naringenin, a natural flavanone purified from Thymus vulgaris, on human breast and colorectal cancer. *Cancer Cell Int* 2015; 15: 46.

[5] Mohan A, Narayanan S, Sethuraman S, Krishnan UM. Combinations of plant polyphenols & anti-cancer molecules: a novel treatment strategy for cancer chemotherapy. *Anticancer Agents Med Chem* 2013; 13: 281-95.

[6] de Oliveira Junior RG, Christiane Adrielly AF, da Silva Almeida JRG, Grougnet R, Thiery V, Picot L. Sensitization of tumor cells to chemotherapy by natural products: A systematic review of preclinical data and molecular mechanisms. *Fitoterapia* 2018; 129: 383-400.

[7] Singh M, Bhui K, Singh R, Shukla Y. Tea polyphenols enhance cisplatin chemosensitivity in cervical cancer cells via induction of apoptosis. *Life Sci* 2013; 93: 7-16.

[8] Maciejczyk A, Surowiak P. Quercetin inhibits proliferation and increases sensitivity of ovarian cancer cells to cisplatin and paclitaxel. *Ginekol Pol* 2013; 84: 590-5.

[9] Sharma R, Gatchie L, Williams IS, Jain SK, Vishwakarma RA, Chaudhuri B, Bharate SB. Glycyrrhiza glabra extract and quercetin reverses cisplatin resistance in triple-negative MDA-MB-468 breast cancer cells via inhibition of cytochrome P450 1B1 enzyme. *Bioorg Med Chem Lett* 2017; 27: 5400-3.

[10] Xu Z, Mei J, Tan Y. Baicalin attenuates DDP (cisplatin) resistance in lung cancer by downregulating MARK2 and p-Akt. *Int J Oncol* 2017; 50: 93-100.

[11] Li N, Zhang Z, Jiang G, Sun H, Yu D. Nobiletin sensitizes colorectal cancer cells to oxaliplatin by PI3K/Akt/MTOR pathway. *Front Biosci (Landmark Ed)* 2019; 24: 303-12.

[12] Raina K, Agarwal R. Combinatorial strategies for cancer eradication by silibinin and cytotoxic agents: efficacy and mechanisms. *Acta Pharmacol Sin* 2007; 28: 1466-75.

[13] Tredaniel J. *Cancer Drugs. A practical approach to drugs available to us.* ESKA Publishing, 2015. 352 pp.

[14] Farzaei MH, Bahramsoltani R, Rahimi R. Phytochemicals as adjunctive with conventional anticancer therapies. *Curr Pharm Des* 2016; 22: 4201-18.

[15] Wang Y, Wang Q, Zhang S, Zhang Y, Tao L. Baicalein increases the cytotoxicity of cisplatin by enhancing gap junction intercellular communication. *Mol Med Rep* 2014; 10: 515-21.

[16] Singh VK, Arora D, Satija NK, Khare P, Roy SK, Sharma PK. Intricatinol synergistically enhances the anticancerous activity of cisplatin in human A549 cells via p38 MAPK/p53 signalling. *Apoptosis* 2017; 22: 1273-86.

[17] Gaballah HH, Gaber RA, Mohamed DA. Apigenin potentiates the antitumor activity of 5-FU on solid Ehrlich carcinoma: Crosstalk between apoptotic and JNK-mediated autophagic cell death platforms. *Toxicol Appl Pharmacol* 2017; 316: 27-35.

[18] Zhang Y, Ge Y, Ping X, Yu M, Lou D, Shi W. Synergistic apoptotic effects of silibinin in enhancing paclitaxel toxicity in human gastric cancer cell lines. *Mol Med Rep* 2018; 18: 1835-41.

[19] Chavoshi H, Vahedian V, Saghaei S, Pirouzpanah MB, Raeisi M, Samadi N. Adjuvant therapy with silibinin improves the efficacy of paclitaxel and cisplatin in MCF-7 breast cancer cells. *Asian Pac J Cancer Prev* 2017; 18: 2243-7.

[20] Guo XF, Liu JP, Ma SQ, Zhang P, Sun WD. Avicularin reversed multidrug-resistance in human gastric cancer through enhancing Bax and BOK expressions. *Biomed Pharmacother* 2018; 103: 67-74.

[21] Brito AF, Ribeiro M, Abrantes AM, Pires AS, Teixo RJ, Tralhao JG, Botelho MF. Quercetin in cancer treatment, alone or in combination with conventional therapeutics? *Curr Med Chem* 2015; 22: 3025-39.

[22] Simoben CV, Ibezim A, Ntie-Kang F, Nwodo JN, Lifongo LL. Exploring cancer therapeutics with natural products from African medicinal plants, Part I: Xanthones, quinones, steroids, coumarins, phenolics and other classes of compounds. *Anticancer Agents Med Chem* 2015; 15: 1092-111.

[23] Hosseinimehr SJ, Jalayer Z, Naghshvar F, Mahmoudzadeh A, Hesperidin inhibits cyclophosphamide-induced tumor growth delay in mice. *Integr Cancer Ther* 2012; 11: 251-6.

[24] Donia TIK, Gerges MN, Mohamed TM. Amelioration effect of Egyptian sweet orange hesperidin on Ehrlich ascites carcinoma (EAC) bearing mice. *Chem Biol Interact* 2018; 285: 76-84.

[25] Johnson JL, Dia VP, Wallig M, Gonzalez de Mejia E. Luteolin and gemcitabine protect against pancreatic cancer in an orthotopic mouse model. *Pancreas* 2015; 44: 144-51.

[26] Tyagi T, Treas JN, Mahalingaiah PK, Singh KP. Potentiation of growth inhibition and epigenetic modulation by combination of green tea polyphenol and 5-aza-2`-deoxycytidine in human breast cancer cells. *Breast Cancer Res Treat* 2015; 149: 655-68.

[27] Zhao H, Yuan X, Li D, Chen H, Jiang J, Wang Z, Sun X, Zheng Q. Isoliquiritigen enhances the antitumour activity and decreases the genotoxic effect of cyclophosphamide. *Molecules* 2013; 18: 8786-98.

[28] Ferreira de Oliveira JMP, Pacheco AR, Coutinho L, Oliveira H, Pinho S, Almeida L, Fernandes E, Santos C. Combination of etoposide and fisetin results in anticancer efficiency against osteosarcoma cell models. *Arch Toxicol* 2018; 92: 1205-14.

[29] Xu GY, Tang XJ. Troxerutin (TXN) potentiated 5-Fluorouracil (5-Fu) treatment of human gastric cancer through suppressing STAT3/NF-κB and Bcl-2 signaling pathways. *Biomed Pharmacother* 2017; 92: 95-107.

[30] Lecumberri E, Dupertuis YM, Miralbell R, Pichard C. Green tea polyphenol epigallocatechin-3-gallate (EGCG) as adjuvant in cancer therapy. *Clin Nutr* 2013; 32: 894-903.

[31] Zhang L, Yang X, Li X, Li C, Zhao L, Zhou Y, Hou H. Butein sensitizes HeLa cells to cisplatin through the AKT and ERK/p38 MAPK pathways by targeting FoxO3a. *Int J Mol Med* 2015; 36: 957-66.

[32] Punia R, Raina K, Agarwal R, Singh RP. Acacetin enhances the therapeutic efficacy of doxorubicin in non-small-cell lung carcinoma cells. *PLoS One* 2017; 12: e0182870.

[33] Gao AM, Zhang XY, Hu JN, Ke ZP. Apigenin sensitizes hepatocellular carcinoma cells to doxorubic through regulating miR-520b/ATG7 axis. *Chem Biol Interact* 2018; 280: 45-50.

[34] Li X, Wan L, Wang F, Pei H, Zheng L, Wu W, Ye H, Wang Y, Chen L. Barbigerone reverses multidrug resistance in breast MCF-7/ADR cells. *Phytother Res* 2018; 32: 733-40.

[35] Vittorio O, Le Grand M, Makharza SA, Curcio M, Tucci P, Iemma F, Nicoletta FP, Hampel S, Cirillo G. Doxorubicin synergism and resistance reversal in human neuroblastoma BE(2)C cell lines: An in vitro study with dextran-catechin nanohybrids. *Eur J Pharm Biopharm* 2018; 122: 176-85.

[36] Li WG, Wang HQ. Inhibitory effects of Silibinin combined with doxorubicin in hepatocellular carcinoma; an in vivo study. *J BUON* 2016; 21: 917-24.

[37] Chen Z, Huang C, Ma T, Jiang L, Tang L, Shi T, Zhang S, Zhang L, Zhu P, Li J, Shen A. Reversal effect of quercetin on multidrug resistance via FZD7/β-catenin pathway in hepatocellular carcinoma cells. *Phytomedicine* 2018; 43: 37-45.

[38] Alvero AB, O`Malley D, Brown D, Kelly G, Garg M, Chen W, Rutherford T, Mor G. Molecular mechanism of phenoxodiol-induced apoptosis in ovarian carcinoma cells. *Cancer* 2006; 106: 599-608.

[39] Hwang JT, Ha J, Park OJ. Combination of 5-fluorouracil and genistein induces apoptosis synergistically in chemo-resistant cancer cells through the modulation of AMPK and COX-2 signaling pathways. *Biochem Biophys Res Commun* 2005; 332: 433-40.

[40] Li Y, Ahmed F, Ali S, Philip PA, Kucuk O, Sarkar FH. Inactivation of nuclear factor kappaB by soy isoflavone genistein contributes to increased apoptosis induced by chemotherapeutic agents in human cancer cells. *Cancer Res* 2005; 65: 6934-42.

[41] Shen M, Chan TH, Dou QP. Targeting tumor ubiquitin-proteasome pathway with polyphenols for chemosensitization. *Anticancer Agents Med Chem* 2012; 12: 891-901.

[42] Bansal T, Jaggi M, Khar RK, Talegaonkar S. Emerging significance of flavonoids as P-glycoprotein inhibitors in cancer chemotherapy. *J Pharm Pharm Sci* 2009; 12: 46-78.

[43] Zhang FY, Du GJ, Zhang L, Zhang CL, Lu WL, Liang W. Naringenin enhances the anti-tumor effect of doxorubicin through selectively inhibiting the activity of multidrug resistance-associated proteins but not P-glycoprotein. *Pharm Res* 2009; 26: 914-25.

[44] Iriti M, Kubina R, Cochis A, Sorrentino R, Varoni EM, Kabala-Dzik A, Azzimonti B, Dziedzic A, Rimondini L, Wojtyczka RD. Rutin, a quercetin glycoside, restores chemosensitivity in human breast cancer cells. *Phytother Res* 2017; 31: 1529-38.

[45] Borska S, Sopel M, Chmielewska M, Zabel M, Dziegiel P. Quercetin as a potential modulator of P-glycoprotein expression and function in cells of human pancreatic carcinoma line resistant to daunorubicin. *Molecules* 2010; 15: 857-70.

[46] Yu S, Gong LS, Li NF, Pan YF, Zhang L. Galangin (GG) combined with cisplatin (DDP) to suppress human lung cancer by inhibition of STAT3-regulated NF-κB and Bcl-2/Bax signaling pathways. *Biomed Pharmacother* 2018; 97: 213-24.

[47] Wen Y, Zhao RQ, Zhang YK, Gupta P, Fu LX, Tang AZ, Liu BM, Chen ZS, Yang DH, Liang G. Effect of Y6, an epigallocatechin gallate derivative, on reversing doxorubicin drug resistance in human hepatocellular carcinoma cells. *Oncotarget* 2017; 8: 29760-70.

[48] Wang ZD, Wang RZ, Xia YZ, Kong LY, Yang L. Reversal of multidrug resistance by icaritin in doxorubicin-resistant human osteosarcoma cells. *Chin J Nat Med* 2018; 16: 20-8.

[49] Yuan Z, Wang H, Hu Z, Huang Y, Yao F, Sun S, Wu B. Quercetin inhibits proliferation and drug resistance in KB/VCR oral cancer cells and enhances its sensitivity to vincristine. *Nutr Cancer* 2015; 67: 126-36.

[50] Luo H, Daddysman MK, Rankin GO, Jiang BH, Chen YC. Kaempferol enhances cisplatin`s effect on ovarian cancer cells through promoting apoptosis caused by down regulation of cMyc. *Cancer Cell Int* 2010; 10: 16.

[51] Arafa el-SA, Zhu Q, Barakat BM, Wani G, Zhao Q, El-Mahdy MA, Wani AA. Tangeretin sensitizes cisplatin-resistant human ovarian cancer cells through downregulation of phosphoinositide 3-kinase/Akt signaling pathway. *Cancer Res* 2009; 69: 8910-7.

[52] Liang G, Tang A, Lin X, Li L, Zhang S, Huang Z, Tang H, Li QQ. Green tea catechins augment the antitumor activity of doxorubicin in an in vivo mouse model for chemoresistant liver cancer. *Int J Oncol* 2010; 37: 111-23.

[53] Yang YI, Lee KT, Park HJ, Kim TJ, Choi YS, Shih IeM, Choi JH. Tectorigenin sensitizes paclitaxel-resistant human ovarian cancer cells through downregulation of the Akt and NFκB pathway. *Carcinogenesis* 2012; 33: 2488-98.

[54] Hofmann J, Fiebig HH, Winterhalter BR, Berger DP, Grunicke H. Enhancement of the antiproliferative activity of cis-diamminedichloroplatinum(II) by quercetin. *Int J Cancer* 1990; 45: 536-9.

[55] Liao B, Ying H, Yu C, Fan Z, Zhang W, Shi J, Ying H, Ravichandran N, Xu Y, Yin J, Jiang Y, Du Q. (-)-Epigallocatechin gallate (EGCG)-nanoethosomes as a transdermal delivery system for docetaxel to treat implanted human melanoma cell tumors in mice. *Int J Pharm* 2016; 512: 22-31.

[56] Jia WZ, Zhao JC, Sun XL, Yao ZG, Wu HL, Xi ZQ. Additive anticancer effects of chrysin and low dose cisplatin in human malignant glioma cell (U87) proliferation and evaluation of the mechanistic pathway. *J BUON* 2015; 20: 1327-36.

[57] Li S, Wang L, Li N, Liu Y, Su H. Combination lung cancer chemotherapy: Design of a pH-sensitive transferrin-PEG-Hz-lipid conjugate for the co-delivery of docetaxel and baicalin. *Biomed Pharmacother* 2017; 95: 548-55.

[58] Mukhtar E, Adhami VM, Siddiqui IA, Verma AK, Mukhtar H. Fisetin enhances chemotherapeutic effect of cabazitaxel against human prostate cancer cells. *Mol Cancer Ther* 2016; 15: 2863-74.

[59] Desai UN, Shah KP, Mirza SH, Panchal DK, Parikh SK, Rawal RM. Enhancement of the cytotoxic effects of cytarabine in synergism with hesperidine and silibinin in acute myeloid leukemia: An in-vitro approach. *J Cancer Res Ther* 2015; 11: 352-7.

[60] Fang J, Zhang S, Xue X, Zhu X, Song S, Wang B, Jiang L, Qin M, Liang H, Gao L. Quercetin and doxorubicin co-delivery using mesoporous silica nanoparticles enhance the efficacy of gastric carcinoma chemotherapy. *Int J Nanomedicine* 2018; 13: 5113-26.

[61] Xu H, Yang T, Liu X, Tian Y, Chen X, Yuan R, Su S, Lin X, Du G. Luteolin synergizes the antitumor effects of 5-fluorouracil against human hepatocellular carcinoma cells through apoptosis induction and metabolism. *Life Sci* 2016; 144: 138-47.

[62] Wang W, Xi M, Duan X, Wang Y, Kong F. Delivery of baicalein and paclitaxel using self-assembled nanoparticles: synergistic antitumor effect in vitro and in vivo. *Int J Nanomedicine* 2015; 10: 3737-50.

[63] Silasi DA, Alvero AB, Rutherford TJ, Brown D, Mor G. Phenoxodiol: pharmacology and clinical experience in cancer monotherapy and in combination with chemotherapeutic drugs. *Expert Opin Pharmacother* 2009; 10: 1059-67.

[64] Wang P, Henning SM, Heber D, Vadgama JV. Sensitization of docetaxel in prostate cancer cells by green tea and quercetin. *J Nutr Biochem* 2015; 26: 408-15.

[65] Kuhar M, Sen S, Singh N. Role of mitochondria in quercetin-enhanced chemotherapeutic response in human non-small cell lung carcinoma H-520 cells. *Anticancer Res* 2006; 26: 1297-303.

[66] Lin X, Tian L, Wang L, Li W, Xu Q, Xiao X. Antitumor effects and the underlying mechanism of licochalcone A combined with 5-fluorouracil in gastric cancer cells. *Oncol Lett* 2017; 13: 1695-701.

[67] Wang T, Gao J, Yu J, Shen L. Synergistic inhibitory effect of wogonin and low-dose paclitaxel on gastric cancer cells and tumor xenografts. *Chin J Cancer Res* 2013; 25: 505-13.

[68] Lee SH, Ryu JK, Lee KY, Woo SM, Park JK, Yoo JW, Kim YT, Yoon YB. Enhanced anti-tumor effect of combination therapy with gemcitabine and apigenin in pancreatic cancer. *Cancer Lett* 2008; 259: 39-49.

[69] Guo J, Zhou AW, Fu YC, Verma UN, Tripathy D, Frenkel EP, Becerra CR. Efficacy of sequential treatment of HCT116 colon cancer monolayers and

xenografts with docetaxel, flavopiridol, and 5-fluorouracil. *Acta Pharmacol Sin* 2006; 27: 1375-81.

[70] Park S, Kim JH, Hwang YI, Jung KS, Jang YS, Jang SH. Schedule-dependent effect of epigallocatechin-3-gallate (EGCG) with paclitaxel on H460 cells. *Tuberc Respir Dis (Seoul)* 2014; 76: 114-9.

[71] Yi JL, Shi S, Shen YL, Wang L, Chen HY, Zhu J, Ding Y. Myricetin and methyl eugenol combination enhances the anticancer activity, cell cycle arrest and apoptosis induction of cis-platin against HeLa cervical cancer cell lines. *Int J Clin Exp Pathol* 2015; 8: 1116-27.

[72] Luo T, Wang J, Yin Y, Hua H, Jing J, Sun X, Li M, Zhang Y, Jiang Y. (-)-Epigallocatechin gallate sensitizes breast cancer cells to paclitaxel in a murine model of breast carcinoma. *Breast Cancer Res* 2010; 12: R8.

[73] Ho BY, Lin CH, Apaya MK, Chao WW, Shyur LF. Silibinin and paclitaxel cotreatment significantly suppress the activity and lung metastasis of triple negative 4T1 mammary tumor cell in mice. *J Tradit Complement Med* 2011; 2: 301-11.

[74] Telli E, Genc H, Tasa BA, Sinan Özalp S, Tansu Koparal A. In vitro evaluation of combination of EGCG and Erlotinib with classical chemotherapeutics on JAR cells. *In Vitro Cell Dev Biol Anim* 2017; 53: 651-8.

[75] Zhang BY, Wang YM, Gong H, Zhao H, Lv XY, Yuan GH, Han SR. Isorhamnetin flavonoid synergistically enhances the anticancer activity and apoptosis induction by cis-platin and carboplatin in non-small cell lung carcinoma (NSCLC). *Int J Clin Exp Pathol* 2015; 8: 25-37.

[76] Kachadourian R, Leitner HM, Day BJ. Selected flavonoids potentiate the toxicity of cisplatin in human lung adenocarcinoma cells: a role for glutathione depletion. *Int J Oncol* 2007; 31: 161-8.

[77] Lv L, Liu C, Chen C, Yu X, Chen G, Shi Y, Qin F, Qu J, Qiu K, Li G. Quercetin and doxorubicin co-encapsulated biotin receptor-targeting nanoparticles for minimizing drug resistance in breast cancer. *Oncotarget* 2016; 7: 32184-99.

[78] Khan M, Maryam A, Mehmood T, Zhang Y, Ma T. Enhancing activity of anticancer drugs in multidrug resistant tumors by modulating P-glycoprotein through dietary nutraceuticals. *Asian Pac J Cancer Prev* 2015; 16: 6831-9.

[79] Huang HY, Niu JL, Lu YH. Multidrug resistance reversal effect of DMC derived from buds of Cleistocalyx operculatus in human hepatocellular tumor xenograft model. *J Sci Food Agric* 2012; 92: 135-40.

[80] Hu XY, Liang JY, Guo XJ, Liu L, Guo YB. 5-Fluorouracil combined with apigenin enhances anticancer activity through mitochondrial membrane potential ($\Delta\Psi$m)-mediated apoptosis in hepatocellular carcinoma. *Clin Exp Pharmacol Physiol* 2015; 42: 146-53.

[81] Huang HY, Niu JL, Zhao LM, Lu YH. Reversal effect of 2`,4`-dihydroxy-6`-methoxy-3`,5`-dimethylchalcone on multi-drug resistance in resistant human hepatocellular carcinoma cell line BEL-7402/5-FU. *Phytomedicine* 2011; 18: 1086-92.

[82] Chen P, Hu MD, Deng XF, Li B. Genistein reinforces the inhibitory effect of Cisplatin on liver cancer recurrence and metastasis after curative hepatectomy. *Asian Pac J Cancer Prev* 2013; 14: 759-64.

[83] Wong MY, Chiu GN. Simultaneous liposomal delivery of quercetin and vincristine for enhanced estrogen-receptor-negative breast cancer treatment. *Anticancer Drugs* 2010; 21: 401-10.

[84] Hofmann J, Doppler W, Jakob A, Maly K, Posch L, Uberall F, Grunicke HH. Enhancement of the antiproliferative effect of cis-diamminedichloroplatinum(II) and nitrogen mustard by inhibitors of protein kinase C. *Int J Cancer* 1988; 42: 382-8.

[85] Su YK, Huang WC, Lee WH, Bamodu OA, Zucha MA, Astuti I, Suwito H, Yeh CT, Lin CM. Methoxyphenyl chalcone sensitizes aggressive epithelial cancer to cisplatin through apoptosis induction and cancer stem cell eradication. *Tumour Biol* 2017; 39: 1010428317691689.

[86] Brechbuhl HM, Kachadourian R, Min E, Chan D, Day BJ. Chrysin enhances doxorubicin-induced cytotoxicity in human lung epithelial cancer cell lines: the role of glutathione. *Toxicol Appl Pharmacol* 2012; 258: 1-9.

[87] Hyun HB, Moon JY, Cho SK. Quercetin suppresses CYR61-mediated multidrug resistance in human gastric adenocarcinoma AGS cells. *Molecules* 2018; 23: E209.

[88] Cheng T, Liu J, Ren J, Huang F, Ou H, Ding Y, Zhang Y, Ma R, An Y, Liu J, Shi L. Green tea catechin-based complex micelles combined with doxorubicin to overcome cardiotoxicity and multidrug resistance. *Theranostics* 2016; 6: 1277-92.

[89] Wong MY, Chiu GN. Liposome formulation of co-encapsulated vincristine and quercetin enhanced antitumor activity in a trastuzumab-insensitive breast tumor xenograft model. *Nanomedicine* 2011; 7: 834-40.

[90] Klimaszewska-Wisniewska A, Halas-Wisniewska M, Tadrowski T, Gagat M, Grzanka D, Grzanka A. Paclitaxel and the dietary flavonoid fisetin: a synergistic combination that induces mitotic catastrophe and autophagic cell death in A549 non-small cell lung cancer cells. *Cancer Cell Int* 2016; 16: 10.

Chapter 4

COMPLEX MECHANISMS OF CANCER DRUG RESISTANCE: POSSIBILITIES FOR INTERVENTION WITH NATURAL COMPOUNDS

Resistance to chemotherapy is a serious clinical problem and one of the major challenges in treating different types of human malignancies, eventually leading to treatment failure, adverse side effects, recurrence, metastasis and poor therapeutic outcome [1-3]. Drug resistance as a multifactorial phenomenon is attributed to various causes including (but not limited to) alteration in drug metabolism (drug inhibition and degradation), increased rates of drug efflux and/or decreased uptake resulting in reduced accumulation of anticancer drugs in tumor cells, enhanced DNA repair capacity, abnormalities of drug targets, altered cell cycle regulation, escape of cells from death pathways, and dysregulation of survival signaling, including increase in expression of nuclear factor-kappa B (NF-κB), upregulation of protein kinase B (Akt) and cyclooxygenase-2 (COX-2) etc. [4-12]. All these complex mechanisms can act independently or in diverse combinations comprising numerous signaling pathways and complicating the possible modulation. Our current understanding about the molecular targets and multiple processes responsible for chemotherapy resistance as well as possibilities to overcome it are still rather limited. In principle, specific non-toxic agents and approaches that intervene in these cancer-specific deregulated events and (re-)sensitize tumor cells to conventional drugs may allow for development of novel clinical therapies enhancing the effects of standard chemotherapeutics [13-16]. Such agents are called multidrug resistance (MDR) modulators or chemosensitizers and their identification, preferably from natural sources, could be pivotal to improve quality of life and survival of patients suffering from different tumors. The major mechanisms contributing to chemoresistance are presented in Figure 4.1 and described in more detail in following subsections.

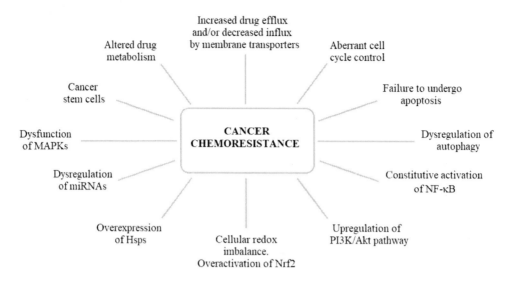

Figure 4.1. Major cellular mechanisms contributing to cancer drug resistance (Akt, protein kinase B; Hsp, heat shock protein; MAPK, mitogen-activated protein kinase; miRNA, microRNA; NF-κB, nuclear factor-κB; Nrf2, nuclear factor (erythroid-derived 2)-like 2; PI3K, phosphoinositide 3-kinase).

4.1. Overexpression and -Activity of Membrane Transporters: P-gp, MRP1/2 and BCRP

Multidrug resistance (MDR) is a phenomenon that comprises various adaptations of malignant cells to escape the killing activities of standard chemotherapeutic drugs contributing to progression of cancer [17]. The major cause of MDR is attributed to the family of efflux pumps that are identified as ATP binding cassette (ABC) plasma membrane transporters, including at least 48 members described in humans so far, characterized by their homologous ATP binding domains and using ATP hydrolysis as the energetic source. The ABC transporters family is generally divided into seven subfamilies (ABCA-ABCG), whereas transporters that are most relevant in malignancies are P-glycoprotein (P-gp, ABCB1), multidrug resistance-associated proteins (MRPs) 1 (ABCC1) and 2 (ABCC2), and breast cancer resistance protein (BCRP, ABCG2) [9, 17-29]. The physiological role of ABC transporters in normal cells is to decrease the body load of potentially harmful compounds, i.e., metabolic waste and xenobiotics, such as environmental toxins and carcinogens [30, 31]. However, overexpression of efflux pumps in tumors strongly promotes the transport of clinically administered antineoplastic agents through the cell membrane outside the cells reducing the intracellular bioavailability and accumulation of drugs [22, 32-35]. Thus, many-fold higher expression of drug transporters in cancer cells compared to normal tissue prevents the achievement of effective doses and reduces cytotoxicity of various structurally different chemotherapeutics in target cells, leading to MDR phenomenon in a number of tumors

[17, 30, 33]. To achieve cellular therapeutic concentrations, increasingly higher dosages of drugs are needed, which in turn may cause severe toxicity to normal healthy tissues [34]. At that, distribution of transporters can widely vary among different cancer types [23].

One of the most extensively studied and best understood classical MDR phenotypes is characterized by the rapid extrusion of numerous structurally and functionally unrelated cytotoxic drugs from target cancer cells due to overexpression of P-gp, a 170 kDa transmembranous efflux pump encoded by MDR1 gene in humans [9, 18, 19, 21, 36-43]. P-gp protein was the first identified MDR transporter (discovered in 1976 in Chinese hamster ovary cells) and hypoxia plays a certain role in its expression, in a hypoxia inducible factor 1α (HIF-1α) dependent manner [9, 44-46]. P-gp could expel a wide variety of substrate drugs, including mitomycin C, etoposide, doxorubicin, daunorubicin, dactinomycin, methotrexate, vinblastine, vincristine, paclitaxel and docetaxel, whereas overexpression of P-gp has been correlated with unsatisfactory chemotherapeutic response, poor survival and prognosis for many human cancers [18, 20, 36, 41, 45-62]. This drug transporter is expressed in about half of all human malignancies at the levels which are sufficient to confer MDR phenotype and treatment failure [63]. For instance, about 40% of breast tumors express P-gp being approximately three times less sensitive to doxorubicin chemotherapy compared to tumors with no P-gp expression [36]. Also, overexpression of P-gp has been found in nearly 80% of renal cell carcinomas [54]. Therefore, overcoming such P-gp mediated chemotherapy resistance is a challenge in treatment of various malignancies.

The inhibitor specificities of P-gp are highly overlapping with those of MRPs and BCRP [17]. MRP1 can efflux diverse cytotoxic drugs, such as topotecan, etoposide, doxorubicin, methotrexate and vincristine, and thus confers MDR phenotype [26, 28, 61]. The level of this 190 kDa membrane protein has become an effective marker for the chemotherapeutic efficacy and overall survival rate of non-small cell lung cancer [22, 64, 65]. Increased expression of MRP2 in tumor cells has been demonstrated to strengthen the resistance to cisplatin, oxaliplatin, etoposide and vincristine [61, 66], whereas overexpression of MRP5 confers resistance to cisplatin, 5-fluorouracil, gemcitabine and methotrexate [67]. BCRP is another member of ABC transporter family (72.1 kDa) with expression profile not limited to breast cancer cells. Overexpression of BCRP has been associated with poor response to clinical treatment of structurally distinct drugs, including SN-38 (active metabolite of irinotecan), topotecan, etoposide, doxorubicin, mitoxantrone and methotrexate [25, 64, 68-70]. Lung resistance protein (LRP) is a transport protein that localizes in the nuclear membrane and its overexpression is believed to induce MDR by altering the endonuclear distribution of chemotherapeutics [40, 64]. The simplified representation of cancer-related MDR transporters with respective substrate drugs is depicted in Figure 4.2.

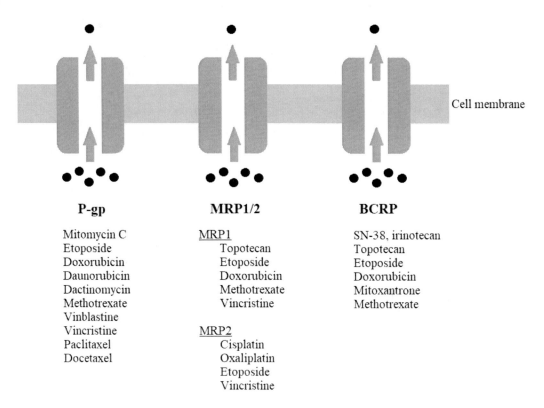

Figure 4.2. Membrane pumps expelling anticancer drugs out of cells (BCRP, breast cancer resistance protein; MRP, multidrug resistance-associated protein; P-gp, P-glycoprotein) [18, 20, 22, 25, 26, 28, 36, 40, 41, 45-48, 50-62, 64, 66-70].

Active export of anticancer drugs from malignant cells is one of the major mechanisms of drug resistance. Therefore, much effort has been directed for finding compounds which could act to reverse MDR by recovering sensitivity of cancer cells to different chemotherapeutic drugs. These agents are called MDR modulators, MDR inhibitors, chemosensitizers or reversal agents. Although downregulation or inhibition of ATP-dependent efflux pumps may be an important strategy to improve the transport of chemotherapeutic agents across the cell membrane inside the cells leading to increase in intracellular bioavailability and concentration of drugs and amelioration of the state of MDR, the results of clinical trials have still been disappointing and no MDR modulators are in clinical use today [10, 32, 36, 40, 71]. This failure may be partly due to redundancy of efflux pumps in resistant neoplasms, but also to several other transport-independent mechanisms being involved in MDR. Besides, more than one mechanism may occur in concert in the resistant cancer cells [17, 45]. The potential chemosensitizers are able either to bind to ABC transporters and directly block their efflux function, or downregulate the membrane expression level of respective proteins [19, 38, 45, 55, 72]. In addition, considering the importance of optimal ATPase activity in functioning of MDR transporters, influencing ATPase activity may have essential implications [47, 51, 73]. Moreover, as anticancer drugs are often expelled from tumor cells in the form of glutathione (GSH) conjugates formed in the reaction catalyzed by glutathione S-transferase (GST), depleting high cellular GSH content and GST activity in cancer cells might also limit the development of MDR [26, 39, 74]. Since the 1980s, the first three generations of pharmaceutical MDR inhibitors have been examined, co-administered with drugs, both in cell cultures, animal models and clinical studies [27, 52, 72]. These tested chemosensitizers have included cyclosporines, calmodulin antagonists, indole alkaloids, coronary vasodilators, quinolines, hormones and calcium channel blockers, whereas verapamil and cyclosporin A are the classical first-generation modulators [9, 17, 20, 37, 73]. However, the clinical use of MDR modifiers has been limited by unfavorable changes in pharmacokinetics and low affinity requiring the use of high doses of modulators associated with unacceptable toxic reactions in normal tissues, including cardiotoxic or immunosuppressive effects [9, 18, 21, 22, 36, 37, 40, 75-77]. Because most MDR transporters have important functions also in normal tissues, inhibition of these proteins may implicate serious consequences on common metabolic processes and increased sensitivity to xenobiotic exposure [27, 30]. Therefore, newer strategies and novel safe and potent compounds with fewer side effects and lower toxicity are currently being investigated to reverse MDR in patients suffering from different types of cancer, with traditional herbs and medicinal plants receiving considerable attention [9, 10, 32, 36, 39, 40]. Due to the clinical failure of the first three generation inhibitors, development of fourth generation MDR modulators from natural products has drawn very high expectations [27, 31].

4.2. EVASION OF DRUG-INDUCED APOPTOSIS

Apoptosis, also known as type I programmed cell death (PCD), is one of the key mechanisms by which various chemotherapeutic drugs destroy and eliminate tumor cells [78-82]. It is active and highly organized physiological process to eradicate damaged or abnormal mutated cells [83-85]. In response to stress stimuli, including cytotoxic drugs or radiation, cell division checkpoints are alerted and cell cycle blocked to initiate DNA repair. However, if the damage is beyond cellular capability to be repaired, apoptosis is normally induced [86]. The progression of cell cycle is strictly regulated by a set of cyclins, cyclin-dependent kinases (CDKs) and CDK inhibitors (CDKIs), whereas strong evidence supports that sensitivity of cancer cells to neoplastic agents-induced apoptosis is highest at the G2/M phase arrest of cell cycle [33, 87-92]. However, malignant cells trigger multiple pathways to escape from apoptotic cascade, and allow tumor cells to survive and progress [78, 93]. Programmed cell death is frequently dysregulated in carcinogenesis exhibiting numerous alterations in signaling pathways that control this process, making resistance to apoptosis a hallmark of cancer [3, 16, 66, 93]. Moreover, defective and dysfunctional apoptosis represents one of the principal mechanisms responsible for multidrug resistance of tumors to conventional cytotoxic chemotherapeutic drugs and accounts for numerous treatment failures [14, 94-99]. Thus, suppression of apoptotic cell death constitutes a major barrier to effective treatment and strategies to sensitize malignant cells to undergo drug-induced apoptosis are highly needed to overcome resistance and improve clinical outcome in management of different cancer types [11, 77, 100, 101].

Multiple morphological changes, including cell shrinkage, membrane blebbing, nuclear condensation, DNA fragmentation and formation of apoptotic bodies are characteristic indicators of cells dying by apoptosis [82, 102-104]. At that, the molecular mechanisms leading to apoptotic death are complex and involve a number of cellular pathways [94]. Apoptosis may occur via two signaling processes: death receptor-mediated (extrinsic) and mitochondrial (intrinsic) pathways [65, 105-108]. The mitochondrial pathway is triggered by various apoptotic stress stimuli, including cytotoxic chemotherapeutic drugs or radiation, and is mediated by B-cell lymphoma 2 (Bcl-2) family proteins. There are two main groups of these proteins: antiapoptotic (Bcl-2, Bcl-xl, Mcl-1) and proapoptotic proteins (Bax, Bak, Bad, Bid, Bim, Bok) [94, 106, 109-112]. Bcl-2 functions as an inhibitor of intrinsic apoptosis by binding to Bax and forming heterodimers. The balance between these proteins, i.e., Bax/Bcl-2 ratio, is a crucial factor indicating whether apoptotic response is initiated and thus, determines the fate of tumor cell. Therefore, overexpression of Bcl-2 and/or downregulation of Bax can contribute to multidrug resistance phenotype and poor therapeutic prognosis [14, 77, 81, 93-95, 98, 106, 109, 113-115]. In fact, suppression of Bax has been related to acquired resistance to cisplatin and 5-fluorouracil in clinical settings [81]. Insertion of proapoptotic Bcl-2 proteins (Bax) in the mitochondrial membrane induces disruption of mitochondrial membrane potential ($\Delta\Psi$m) and subsequent release of cytochrome c from mitochondria to cytoplasm [105, 106, 116, 117]. Cytosolic cytochrome c then combines with apoptotic protease activating factor 1 (Apaf-1) and procaspase-9 to form apoptosome, which further leads to caspase-9 activation and eventually, cleavage of downstream executive caspase-3 [65, 93, 107, 118, 119].

The extrinsic apoptotic pathway is triggered through activation of death receptors on the cell surface, i.e., tumor necrosis factor receptor (TNFR) and Fas. Once activated, they recruit Fas-associated death domain (FADD) and procaspase-8 to form death-inducing signaling complex (DISC), further leading to caspase-8 activation [105, 106, 108, 112, 113, 120]. Both intrinsic and extrinsic routes converge to a final common pathway correlated with processing of caspase-3 [105, 112]. Otherwise, activated caspase-8 can lead to Bid truncation that further translocates into mitochondrial membrane, induces its permeabilization and release of cytochrome c [106]. Caspase-3 activation causes the cleavage of DNA repair enzyme poly(ADP-ribose)polymerase (PARP) and ultimately, elimination of damaged cell by apoptotic death [121-123]. Thus, the family of cysteine-requiring aspartate proteases, known as caspases, plays a pivotal role in both intrinsic and extrinsic apoptosis, and is divided into initiator caspases (caspases-8 and -9) and effector caspases (caspase-3) [93, 94, 124, 125]. Loss of caspase-3 is often detected in a number of solid tumors, such as colon and breast cancers, being associated with resistance to standard chemotherapeutic drugs and poor survival of patients [81]. The simplified scheme of extrinsic and intrinsic apoptotic pathways is depicted in Figure 4.3.

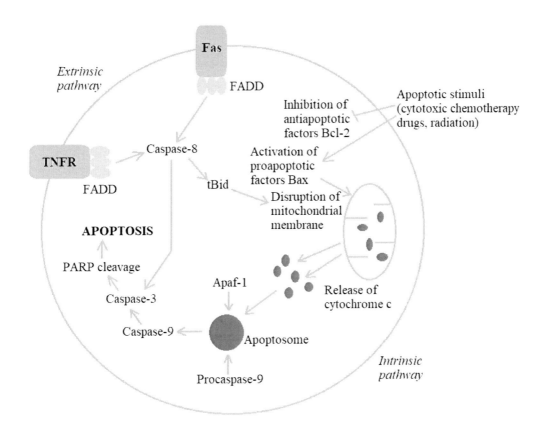

Figure 4.3. Simplified scheme of extrinsic and intrinsic apoptotic pathways (Apaf-1, apoptotic protease activating factor 1; Bax, Bcl-2-associated X protein; Bcl-2, B-cell lymphoma 2; Bid, BH3 interacting-domain death agonist; FADD, Fas-associated death domain; PARP, poly(ADP-ribose)polymerase; tBid, truncated Bid; TNFR, tumor necrosis factor receptor).

Both intrinsic and extrinsic apoptotic pathways can be suppressed by a group of proteins called inhibitors of apoptosis (IAP) [82, 126]. Among them, X-linked inhibitor of apoptosis protein (XIAP) is a key member that selectively binds and directly inhibits caspases-3 and -7, suppresses apoptosome-mediated activation of caspase-9 and thereby blocks apoptosis [86, 112, 126-128]. Increased expression of XIAP has been related to aggressive behavior and metastatic progression of a variety of malignancies, including breast cancer, prostate cancer, lung cancer, renal cell carcinoma, leukemia and lymphoma. In the case of melanoma, significantly higher levels of this protein have been detected compared to benign nevi, whereas expression in metastatic lesions exceeds that of primary tumors [126-128]. Moreover, upregulation of XIAP has been correlated with resistance of tumor cells to chemotherapeutic drugs and radiotherapy. In fact, resistance of melanoma cells to carboplatin and epithelial ovarian cancer cells to cisplatin and docetaxel has been associated with XIAP overexpression [82, 126, 128, 129]. Therefore, development of XIAP-targeting therapies downregulating its expression by non-toxic natural agents can be a useful and attractive approach to sensitize tumor cells to standard cytotoxic drugs and thus overcome chemoresistance. Another important member of the IAP proteins family is survivin that also contributes to evasion of cancer cells from apoptotic death [130]. Overexpression of survivin has been observed in most of the human malignancies and is related to disease progression, drug resistance, recurrences and unfavorable prognosis [59, 109, 131, 132]. At that, it is only scarcely detected in normal cells and healthy tissues [132]. Finding of possibilities to reduce survivin expression or function and thereby promote efficacy of drugs in apoptosis induction may lead to sensitization of tumors to chemotherapy and thus, provides an essential complement in our current anticancer arsenal.

Among the regulators of apoptosis, tumor suppressor protein p53 represents a crucial molecule that participates in apoptosis in a very complex way, both through controlling the cell cycle progression as well as transactivation of proapoptotic proteins [116, 120, 133, 134]. Under normal unstressed conditions, p53 is maintained at low levels in cytoplasm; however, in response to different stress stimuli (including cytotoxic drugs), p53 is activated and stabilized by phosphorylation and acetylation, and translocated to nucleus to induce apoptotic cascade [113, 120, 135]. In general, p53 mediates apoptosis in both transcription-dependent and -independent manners [113]. The transcription-dependent processes involve direct regulation of expression of p53 downstream genes that impact the sensitivity to apoptosis, such as Bax, Bid, p53 upregulated modulator of apoptosis (PUMA) and certain death-related receptors [113, 118, 120]. Besides, p53 can also move out of nucleus and directly interact with mitochondrial proteins, including Bcl-2 and Bcl-xl, acting as an important negative regulator for these antiapoptotic proteins in a transcription-independent manner [113, 118, 120, 136]. Loss of the functional p53 is a characteristic feature to a wide variety of tumors and has been associated with resistance to several cytotoxic drugs, including doxorubicin and 5-fluorouracil. Indeed, more than 50% of human cancers from different tissue origins have been estimated to carry mutated p53 [85, 133, 135, 137-143].

Altogether, there are apparently several potential ways to enhance susceptibility of cancer cells to drug-induced apoptosis and thereby overcome multidrug resistance, using potential chemosensitizing agents. For instance, upregulation of proapoptotic and downregulation of antiapoptotic Bcl-2 family proteins, promotion of caspase-3 level, inhibition of expression and function of XIAP and survivin, and activation of tumor suppressor protein p53 [81, 98, 106, 125, 128, 136, 144, 145]. Bcl-2 was the first discovered death regulator and its suppression has been shown to promote apoptosis to several anticancer drugs [14, 146]. Also, mitochondria may be a relevant target for novel therapeutic agents designed to modulate apoptosis [147, 148]. Therefore, identification of potent non-toxic compounds, preferably from natural sources, involved in augmentation of complex apoptotic cascade is one of the most important challenges for cancer researchers to improve the clinical outcome of oncotherapy in the future.

4.3. DYSREGULATION OF AUTOPHAGY

Increasing evidence suggests that response of tumor cells to chemotherapeutic drugs is not only confined to apoptosis, but involves also other modes of cell death [80]. Autophagy is an evolutionarily well-conserved dynamic intracellular process by which damaged or long-lived organelles and unnecessary cytoplasmic proteins are sequestered by autophagosome and eliminated via lysosomal degradation to maintain homeostasis [78, 149-154]. The series of biochemical steps of autophagy is characterized by changes in several proteins, whereas conversion of LC3-I to LC3-II is the hallmark of autophagy [149, 150, 153-156].

However, the role of autophagy in tumor formation and chemotherapy has remained ambiguous and controversial. Autophagy can play a dual role in cancer therapy, exerting either pro-survival (cytoprotective) or pro-death (cytotoxic) mechanism depending on the context and stimuli [78, 149, 152, 155, 157, 158]. On one hand, it exerts a protective mechanism that enables malignant cells to survive under stressful conditions caused by cytotoxic drugs or radiation [155, 157]. Autophagy can provide recycled metabolic substrates which help meet increased energetic demands of tumor cells to survive, adapt to adverse environment and progress [78, 150, 159]. Indeed, autophagy is activated in malignant cells compared to normal healthy cells, whereas enhanced autophagy has been generally observed in advanced stages of carcinogenesis [150, 155, 160]. Such cytoprotective autophagy contributes to chemoresistance and treatment failure, whereas its inhibition sensitizes cancer cells to drug-induced apoptosis and promotes tumor regression [78, 133, 150, 155, 157]. Therefore, finding novel non-toxic autophagy inhibitors is an attractive strategy to overcome resistance to anticancer drugs and improve therapeutic outcome.

On the other hand, autophagy may also constitute a cell death mechanism, known as type II programmed cell death (PCD), by degrading essential cellular components and excessive self-digestion [149, 151, 153, 157, 161]. In this case, autophagy induction may be therapeutically beneficial, as it mediates cytotoxic effects of antineoplastic agents leading to death of tumor cells [78, 156, 157, 162]. Moreover, autophagy and apoptosis may function independently in parallel pathways or influence each other and act in complex collaboration [78, 149, 157].

As autophagy can be considered a double-edged sword in cancer formation, from therapeutical view, it is highly needed first to determine whether the induction of autophagy involves sensitization or increase in resistance to standard cytotoxic treatment [155, 157, 160]. Appropriate modulation of autophagy with novel natural compounds in favor to inhibit its cytoprotective effects and induce autophagic cell death might be a promising novel strategy to overcome resistance of various human cancer types to conventional chemotherapeutic drugs [157, 160, 163].

4.4. CONSTITUTIVE ACTIVATION OF NUCLEAR FACTOR-κB

Nuclear factor-κB (NF-κB) is an essential transcription factor that plays a central role in chemoresistance of cancer cells to cytotoxic therapy, both in solid tumors as well as hematological malignancies [74, 164-167]. This transcription factor was first identified in murine B lymphocytes in 1986 and since then, its action in normal and tumor cells has been extensively studied [168]. Among various stressful stimuli, activation of NF-κB is induced by treatment with different chemotherapeutic drugs, including cisplatin, camptothecin, etoposide, doxorubicin, daunorubicin, 5-fluorouracil, gemcitabine, vinblastine, vincristine, paclitaxel and docetaxel [57, 74, 97, 98, 110, 116, 169-172]. Under non-stimulating conditions, NF-κB is primarily retained in the cytoplasm as an inactive complex through direct binding to its endogenous inhibitor IκB. After exposure to neoplastic agents, IκB protein is phosphorylated by IκB kinase and degraded, allowing NF-κB to translocate to the nucleus where it binds to DNA and activates transcription of a wide variety of its downstream target genes [97, 98, 166, 169, 170, 173, 174]. As a result, NF-κB plays important roles in proliferation of malignant cells, their invasion and migration through extracellular matrix, angiogenesis, metastasis, inflammatory responses, overexpression of P-gp drug efflux pump, and defective apoptotic pathways by initiating expression of antiapoptotic proteins like Bcl-2, Bcl-xl, survivin and XIAP [12, 18, 57, 99, 106, 121, 132, 168, 169, 172, 174-177]. The major targets of NF-κB in promotion of cancer progression and chemoresistance are depicted in Figure 4.4.

Constitutive activation of NF-κB has been observed in a wide variety of malignant cells contributing essentially to chemoresistant phenotype of different human cancer types and treatment failure [18, 97, 106, 117, 137, 168, 175, 177, 178]. Indeed, high levels of NF-κB have been correlated with poor disease prognosis and even used as a prognostic marker for grade IV gastric cancer [116, 177]. Accumulating evidence also suggests that inhibition of NF-κB potentiates cytotoxic efficacy of standard chemotherapeutics in various tumor cells, contributing to their elimination via apoptosis induction, and thereby improves therapeutic outcome [97, 116, 117, 172, 179, 180]. Therefore, NF-κB might be considered as an attractive target candidate for novel natural non-toxic compounds to sensitize cancer cells to chemotherapeutic drugs by suppression of this transcription factor.

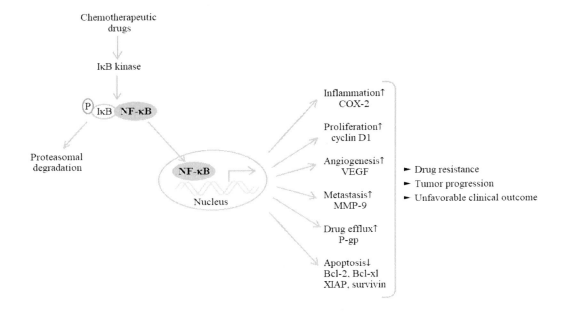

Figure 4.4. Activation and targets of nuclear factor-κB (NF-κB) in promoting tumor progression and chemoresistance (Bcl-2, B-cell lymphoma 2; Bcl-xl, B-cell lymphoma-extra large; COX-2, cyclooxygenase 2; MMP-9, matrix metalloproteinase 9; P-gp, P-glycoprotein; VEGF, vascular endothelial growth factor; XIAP, X-linked inhibitor of apoptosis protein).

4.5. UPREGULATION OF PROTEIN KINASE B PATHWAY

The protein kinase B or Akt pathway is one of the most prevalently overactivated signaling pathways in human cancers being a critical determinant of biological aggressiveness and chemoresistance for both solid tumors as well as hematological malignancies [13, 32, 116, 181-184]. Akt is a downstream target of phosphoinositide 3-kinase (PI3K) which is activated as a result of the ligand-dependent activation of epidermal growth factor receptors (EGFRs), including human epidermal growth factor receptor 2 (HER2 or ErbB2) [185, 186]. Overexpression of EGFR has been observed in a wide variety of human malignancies, being correlated with chemoresistance, reduced survival and adverse clinical prognosis in patients suffering from non-small cell lung cancer [187, 188] or head and neck squamous cell carcinoma [141]. Once activated, PI3K phosphorylates and activates Akt that functions as an oncogene and regulates several cellular downstream components, including NF-κB and mammalian target of rapamycin (mTOR) (Figure 4.5), thereby mediating numerous molecular events associated with cancer progression, invasion, metastasis and treatment resistance [6, 169, 189-191].

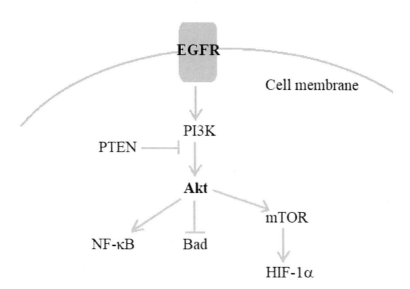

Figure 4.5. Protein kinase B (Akt) as an essential nodal point in signaling cascade implicated in chemoresistance (Bad, Bcl-2-associated death promoter; EGFR, epidermal growth factor receptor; HIF-1α, hypoxia-inducible factor 1α; mTOR, mammalian target of rapamycin; NF-κB, nuclear factor-κB; PI3K, phosphoinositide 3-kinase; PTEN, phosphatase and tensin homolog).

PI3K/Akt/NF-κB pathway mediates epithelial-mesenchymal transition (EMT) of cancer cells by downregulating the epithelial marker E-cadherin, and thereby contributes to chemoresistance phenotype. During EMT, malignant cells lose their polarity and cell-cell contacts leading to increase in invasive and migratory behavior. Chemotherapy-induced EMT is considered one of the mechanisms of tumor resistance, molecularly well characterized for paclitaxel resistance in ovarian cancer cells [190, 192]. In addition, PI3K/Akt/NF-κB pathway also mediates inflammatory responses via regulation of cyclooxygenase-2 (COX-2) activity, participating in the development of chemoresistant phenotype [174, 193, 194]. Increased expression of this inflammatory enzyme and its biosynthetic product prostaglandin E2 (PGE2) has been observed in several malignant tissues, including hepatocellular carcinoma, breast, colon, lung and pancreatic neoplasms [193, 195]. In the case of colorectal carcinoma, overexpression of COX-2 has been associated with resistance to 5-fluorouracil [195]. In chronic lymphocytic leukemia (CLL) cells, overactivation of PI3K/Akt/NF-κB pathway has been associated with acquisition of resistance to fludarabine [196].

Another important downstream target of PI3K/Akt pathway, mTOR, is also involved in a number of aspects of tumorigenesis, regulating cellular proliferation and growth, but is also involved in development of hypoxic environment within a cancerous tissue, mediated by hypoxia-inducible factor 1α (HIF-1α) [6, 197, 198]. Hypoxia has been recognized as one of the key factors rendering tumor cells insensitive to cancer treatment, whereas high rate of glycolysis under hypoxic conditions and poor vascularization of hypoxic tissue can essentially contribute to chemoresistance to most of the conventional drugs [9, 44, 198, 199]. Indeed, overexpression of HIF-1α has been observed in a number of tumors, including gastric cancer, enhancing the resistance of gastric cancer patients to 5-fluorouracil-based chemotherapy [198]. Also, decrease in sensitivity to doxorubicin treatment has been reported in hypoxic hepatocellular carcinoma cells [199]. In addition, overactivation of PI3K/Akt/mTOR pathway has been described in development of resistance to platinum compounds in ovarian cancer cells [191], whereas inhibition of this pathway has been shown to sensitize gallbladder cancer cells to gemcitabine [200].

Akt signaling pathway can be negatively regulated by phosphatase and tensin homolog (PTEN) [174, 198]. However, although PTEN is able to antagonize PI3K/Akt pathway due to its phospholipid 3-phosphatase activity, low expression or inactivation of this tumor suppressor can not adequately restrain overactivation of PI3K/Akt signaling and its downstream components. Indeed, downregulation of PTEN has been often detected in several tumors, including melanoma or breast cancer, due to mutations or deletions in the respective gene [76, 174, 198, 201]. As aberrant upregulation of Akt and its upstream molecules is a common feature in various human cancer types, development of inhibitors for targeting this pathway has received an immense attention in the past decade to overcome chemoresistance to different cytotoxic drugs, and thereby suppressing malignant progression [181, 185, 190, 197, 202-204]. Treatment of tumors combining standard chemotherapeutics with natural inhibitors of PI3K/Akt pathway components might be a promising strategy to chemosensitize cancer cells to cytotoxic drugs and improve clinical outcome.

4.6. ABERRANT REDOX HOMEOSTASIS. OVERACTIVATION OF NRF2

A critical point in determination of the fate of cancer cells is maintaining redox balance that is regulated by mitochondria which are the main production site of intracellular free radicals [95, 205]. Basal cellular levels of reactive oxygen species (ROS) serve as a physiological regulator of normal proliferation, while accumulation of ROS leads to oxidative stress in cells and is an endogenous source of DNA damage [95, 205-209]. Intracellular ROS levels are mainly controlled by glutathione (GSH) as one of the major endogenous antioxidants created by cells [116, 210]. Due to increased demand for energy production and important metabolic alterations, cancer cells are generally more active than normal cells in generation of ROS being therefore under constant oxidative stress [205, 211, 212]. Hence, cancer cells are more sensitive to further oxidative attack because exceeding their endurance, and treatment regimens which potentiate ROS levels can negatively impact the viability of malignant cells offering a therapeutic opportunity [207, 212-214]. Indeed, most of the chemotherapeutic drugs used in clinical settings, such as cisplatin, camptothecin, etoposide, doxorubicin, epirubicin, daunorubicin, mitoxantrone, 5-fluorouracil, gemcitabine, paclitaxel and bleomycin induce oxidative stress by generation of oxygen free radicals [96, 195, 208, 212, 215-

218]. Elevated ROS levels produced by drugs enhance cytotoxic activity of these antineoplastic agents via inducing mitochondrial apoptosis of tumor cells [96, 206, 208, 215]. Therefore, amplifying oxidative damage using natural compounds with prooxidative properties could be an attractive approach to improve susceptibility of cancer cells towards cytotoxicity of standard chemotherapeutics and overcome multidrug resistance phenomenon [206, 214, 216].

However, tumor cells have become highly adaptive to intrinsic oxidative stress by triggering complex cellular survival mechanisms to evade drug-induced cell killing, and progress [208, 212]. Nuclear factor (erythroid-derived 2)-like 2 (Nrf2) is an important transcription factor that plays a critical role in maintaining cellular redox homeostasis and protecting cells from oxidative and xenobiotic stresses by inducing the transcriptional activation of various cytoprotective and detoxification genes [8, 67, 176, 209, 212, 219-221]. Under normal unstressed conditions, Nrf2 molecules are mostly found in cytoplasm in all human tissues where they are anchored by Kelch-like ECH-associated protein 1 (Keap1) that is a major suppressor of Nrf2 and facilitates its degradation through the ubiquitin-proteasome pathway [11, 219, 221-223]. In response to oxidative stress, released Nrf2 translocates into the nucleus, binds to antioxidant responsive element (ARE) and regulates expression of its target genes, including heme-oxygenase-1 (HO-1) and NAD(P)H:quinone oxidoreductase (NQO1) [26, 219, 220, 223] (Figure 4.6). Because oxidative stress is implicated in the initiation of malignant transformation, activation of Nrf2 signaling pathway in normal healthy tissues leads to increase in cellular defense systems, such as antioxidant and phase II detoxification, and is considered as a useful chemopreventive mechanism [11, 176, 209, 220-222]. Conversely, upregulation of Nrf2 signaling pathway and its cytoprotective target products during the course of cancer treatment may be one of the causes of reducing the efficacy of different chemotherapeutic agents, acquisition of drug resistance and poor survival outcomes of patients [8, 176, 212, 214, 219, 220]. Indeed, significantly higher expression and oncogenic function of Nrf2 have been detected in many tumor types, including prostate, ovarian, breast, esophageal, pancreatic and lung cancers, neuroblastoma and hepatocellular carcinoma [8, 67, 209, 219-222]. In the case of head and neck cancer, resistance to cisplatin has been correlated with activation of Nrf2 pathway [209]; in breast cancer cells, activation of cytoprotective Nrf2 signaling has been associated with resistance to doxorubicin [223]. Moreover, based on recent reports, Nrf2 signaling pathway may regulate also the expression of MRP1 and MRP2 transporter genes, leading to drug efflux and lower effective concentrations of anticancer agents in tumor cells [26, 66, 212, 222]. Therefore, in clinical management of cancer, antioxidant and cytoprotective potential of Nrf2 signaling is considered as the dark side of Nrf2 pathway. Development of novel non-toxic inhibitors for Nrf2, preferably from natural sources, can be beneficial to augment cytotoxic responses of cancer cells to various chemotherapeutic drugs through generation of ROS and reverse drug resistance in different human tumor types [176, 212, 219, 220].

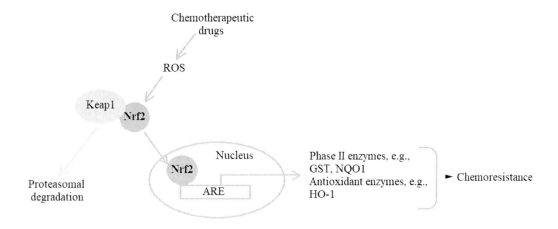

Figure 4.6. Cytoprotective action of nuclear factor (erythroid-derived 2)-like 2 (Nrf2) protecting cancer cells against cytotoxicity of chemotherapeutic drugs (ARE, antioxidant responsive element; GST, glutathione S-transferase; HO-1, heme oxygenase-1; Keap1, Kelch-like ECH-associated protein 1; NQO1, NAD(P)H:quinone oxidoreductase 1; ROS, reactive oxygen species).

4.7. OTHER MAJOR CELLULAR TARGETS INVOLVED IN CHEMORESISTANCE

4.7.1. Overexpression of Heat Shock Proteins

Heat shock proteins (Hsps) as survival factors are ubiquitously expressed in many types of cells and modulate a number of functions, including folding and unfolding of nascent proteins, protection against stress and other potentially harmful stimuli, and stimulation of immune response [102, 107, 154, 224, 225]. Hsps are classified according to their molecular mass into high molecular weight Hsps, including Hsp 70, and low molecular weight Hsps, such as Hsp27 [224, 225]. Malignant cells from a wide variety of tissue origin express abnormally high levels of one or more members of Hsps, where these proteins are implicated in increased DNA repair capacity, attenuated response to chemotherapy, development of drug resistance, tumor progression and unfavorable clinical prognosis [154, 156, 167, 224-228]. Indeed, elevated Hsp levels are believed to indicate poor clinical outcome in renal, gastric, prostate, breast, ovarian and endometrial tumors and it is possible that correlation between Hsp expression and therapeutic responses may be cancer type specific [226]. It has been also reported that cytotoxic anticancer agents can induce overexpression of specific Hsps in malignant cells, in order to survive the drug-induced stress, exhibiting an attempt to escape cell death mechanisms [224]. For instance, both Hsp27 and Hsp40 have been shown to be upregulated by exposure of hepatoma cells to carboplatin and 5-fluorouracil, whereas inhibition of expression of these proteins enhances cytotoxic activity of chemotherapeutic drugs [224]. Overexpression of Hsp27 has been correlated with poor prognosis and survival rate in patients with different cancers, including breast, ovarian, and head and neck tumors [224, 225]. Overexpression of Hsp70 has been related to drug resistance in breast, colon and pancreatic cancer cells, and associated with an adverse prognosis in patients suffering from non-small cell lung cancer [107, 154]. In fact, overexpression of Hsp70 confers resistance of pancreatic cancer to gemcitabine, probably via intervention of apoptosis induction [154]. Aberrant upregulation of a member of Hsp70 family, glucose-regulated protein 78 (GRP78), has been correlated with resistance of multiple cancer types to several chemotherapeutic agents, including etoposide, doxorubicin, paclitaxel and docetaxel, preventing malignant cells to undergo apoptotic death [229-232]. Accordingly, induction of downregulation of Hsps during chemotherapeutic treatment using novel safe and potent compounds might be an important strategy to suppress cancer cell survival, reverse resistance and sensitize tumors to standard cytotoxic drugs [154, 224].

4.7.2. Dysregulation of MicroRNAs

MicroRNAs (miRNAs) are small non-coding endogenous RNAs with lengths of 19-25 nucleotides that modulate gene expression via regulation of translation or degradation of target messenger RNAs (mRNAs) [160, 163, 233-235]. MiRNAs play an important role in regulation of a wide range of cellular processes. Their dysregulation contributes essentially to proliferation, angiogenesis, invasion, migration, apoptosis and autophagy of malignant cells, and affect also chemoresistance to several conventional anticancer drugs [160, 163, 233, 234, 236]. A single miRNA can simultaneously regulate multiple genes and cellular networks, making pharmacological targeting of dysregulated miRNAs especially attractive to reverse multidrug resistance phenomenon [160, 234]. Moreover, each type of malignant neoplasms might have a distinct miRNA profile allowing specific diagnostic and prognostic biomarkers [234, 235]. For instance, miR-25 has been described as an independent autophagy modulator with a certain role in development of drug resistance in breast tumors [160]. miR-34a has been detected to be substantially downregulated in paclitaxel resistant prostate cancer cells behaving as a tumor suppressor [236]. Also, miR-520b has been described as a tumor suppressor in various malignancies, such as breast, colon and liver tumors [163]. However, miR-21 has been shown to be overexpressed in docetaxel resistant metastatic prostate cancers [237] and similarly, miR-155 has been detected to be overexpressed in prostate cancer cells [235]. Accordingly, miRNAs have become important therapeutic targets for treatment of several human tumors and identification of non-toxic adjuvant compounds to modulate functioning of miRNAs during chemotherapy might be an important approach to circumvent drug resistance and restrain malignant progression [234].

4.7.3. Dysfunction of Mitogen-Activated Protein Kinases

There are three major subfamilies of mitogen-activated protein kinases (MAPKs), i.e., extracellular signal-regulated kinases (ERKs), c-Jun N-terminal kinases (JNKs) and p38 kinases; all involved in regulation of cellular survival responses, proliferation and death [13, 80, 102]. Dysregulation of MAPKs is a common feature for various malignancies and can also lead to resistance to standard chemotherapeutic drugs [13, 22, 62, 73, 189, 238]. Further research on molecular mechanisms of these enzymes in tumor cells are needed, as targeting their pathways might contribute to combating chemoresistance.

4.8. CANCER STEM CELLS

The clinical failure of chemotherapy, tumor relapse and metastasis are often attributed to the existence of a relatively small population of tumor initiating cells, called cancer stem cells (CSCs) or cells with stem-like properties (cancer stem-like cells, CSLCs), occurring in most human solid tumors and hematological malignancies [43, 159, 164, 236, 239-242]. These cells were first described in the context of leukemia and possess several unique features, such as self-renewal ability, pluripotency, unlimited proliferative capacity and refractoriness to conventional therapeutic regimens, including resistance to cytotoxic chemotherapeutic drugs [43, 159, 164, 225, 231, 236, 240-242]. The molecular mechanisms and complex signaling network controlling activities of CSCs and underlying multidrug resistance phenomenon have remained largely unknown. However, upregulation of membrane transporters P-gp and BCRP mediating the efflux of cytotoxic agents, acquisition of epithelial-mesenchymal transition (EMT) phenotype as well as overexpression of certain DNA repair proteins have been demonstrated to play important roles in chemoresistant behavior of CSCs, serving as stemness markers [1, 43, 225, 231, 241, 242]. As CSCs make a substantial contribution to drug resistance of human tumors, identification of novel non-toxic compounds and development of new combined strategies that target besides rapidly proliferating bulk tumor mass also CSCs may offer a great promise to increase therapeutic efficacy and expectedly cure cancer through eradicating the supposed roots of malignant neoplasms [1, 24, 159, 164, 225, 231, 241].

REFERENCES

[1] Zhang Y, Wang SX, Ma JW, Li HY, Ye JC, Xie SM, Du B, Zhong XY. EGCG inhibits properties of glioma stem-like cells and synergizes with temozolomide through downregulation of P-glycoprotein inhibition. *J Neurooncol* 2015; 121: 41-52.

[2] Chen P, Hu MD, Deng XF, Li B. Genistein reinforces the inhibitory effect of Cisplatin on liver cancer recurrence and metastasis after curative hepatectomy. *Asian Pac J Cancer Prev* 2013; 14: 759-64.

[3] Liu L, Ju Y, Wang J, Zhou R. Epigallocatechin-3-gallate promotes apoptosis and reversal of multidrug resistance in esophageal cancer cells. *Pathol Res Pract* 2017; 213: 1242-50.

[4] Farzaei MH, Bahramsoltani R, Rahimi R. Phytochemicals as adjunctive with conventional anticancer therapies. *Curr Pharm Des* 2016; 22: 4201-18.

[5] de Oliveira Junior RG, Christiane Adrielly AF, da Silva Almeida JRG, Grougnet R, Thiery V, Picot L. Sensitization of tumor cells to chemotherapy by natural products: A systematic review of preclinical data and molecular mechanisms. *Fitoterapia* 2018; 129: 383-400.

[6] Xu Z, Mei J, Tan Y. Baicalin attenuates DDP (cisplatin) resistance in lung cancer by downregulating MARK2 and p-Akt. *Int J Oncol* 2017; 50: 93-100.

[7] Mazumder ME, Beale P, Chan C, Yu JQ, Huq F. Epigallocatechin gallate acts synergistically in combination with cisplatin and designed trans-palladiums in ovarian cancer cells. *Anticancer Res* 2012; 32: 4851-60.

[8] Gao AM, Ke ZP, Shi F, Sun GC, Chen H. Chrysin enhances sensitivity of BEL-7402/ADM cells to doxorubicin by suppressing PI3K/Akt/Nrf2 and ERK/Nrf2 pathway. *Chem Biol Interact* 2013; 206: 100-8.

[9] Wen Y, Zhao RQ, Zhang YK, Gupta P, Fu LX, Tang AZ, Liu BM, Chen ZS, Yang DH, Liang G. Effect of Y6, an epigallocatechin gallate derivative, on reversing doxorubicin drug resistance in human hepatocellular carcinoma cells. *Oncotarget* 2017; 8: 29760-70.

[10] Daglioglu C. Enhancing tumor cell response to multidrug resistance with pH-sensitive quercetin and doxorubicin conjugated multifunctional nanoparticles. *Colloids Surf B Biointerfaces* 2017; 156: 175-85.

[11] Foygel K, Sekar TV, Paulmurugan R. Monitoring the antioxidant mediated chemosensitization and ARE-signaling in triple negative breast cancer therapy. *PLoS One* 2015; 10: e0141913.

[12] Mohan A, Narayanan S, Sethuraman S, Krishnan UM. Combinations of plant polyphenols & anti-cancer molecules: a novel treatment strategy for cancer chemotherapy. *Anticancer Agents Med Chem* 2013; 13: 281-95.

[13] Molavi O, Narimani F, Asiaee F, Sharifi S, Tarhriz V, Shayanfar A, Hejazi M, Lai R. Silibinin sensitizes chemo-resistant breast cancer cells to chemotherapy. *Pharm Biol* 2017; 55: 729-39.

[14] Wang H, Luo Y, Qiao T, Wu Z, Huang Z. Luteolin sensitizes the antitumor effect of cisplatin in drug-resistant ovarian cancer via induction of apoptosis and inhibition of cell migration and invasion. *J Ovarian Res* 2018; 11: 93.

[15] Catanzaro D, Gabbia D, Cocetta V, Biagi M, Ragazzi E, Montopoli M, Carrara M. Silybin counteracts doxorubicin resistance by inhibiting GLUT1 expression. *Fitoterapia* 2018; 124: 42-8.

[16] Kelly MG, Mor G, Husband A, O`Malley DM, Baker L, Azodi M, Schwartz PE, Rutherford TJ. Phase II evaluation of phenoxodiol in combination with cisplatin or paclitaxel in women with platinum/taxane-refractory/resistant epithelial ovarian, fallopian tube, or primary peritoneal cancers. *Int J Gynecol Cancer* 2011; 21: 633-9.

[17] Schumacher M, Hautzinger A, Rossmann A, Holzhauser S, Popovic D, Hertrampf A, Kuntz S, Boll M, Wenzel U. Chrysin blocks topotecan-induced apoptosis in Caco-2 cells in spite of inhibition of ABC-transporters. *Biochem Pharmacol* 2010; 80: 471-9.

[18] Xia YZ, Ni K, Guo C, Zhang C, Geng YD, Wang ZD, Yang L, Kong LY. Alopecurone B reverses doxorubicin-resistant human osteosarcoma cell line by inhibiting P-glycoprotein and NF-kappa B signaling. *Phytomedicine* 2015; 22: 344-51.

[19] Qian F, Wei D, Zhang Q, Yang S. Modulation of P-glycoprotein function and reversal of multidrug resistance by (-)-epigallocatechin gallate in human cancer cells. *Biomed Pharmacother* 2005; 59: 64-9.

[20] Wang Z, Yang L, Xia Y, Guo C, Kong L. Icariin enhances cytotoxicity of doxorubicin in human multidrug-resistant osteosarcoma cells by inhibition of ABCB1 and down-regulation of the PI3K/Akt pathway. *Biol Pharm Bull* 2015; 38: 277-84.

[21] Sun L, Chen W, Qu L, Wu J, Si J. Icaritin reverses multidrug resistance of HepG2/ADR human hepatoma cells via downregulation of MDR1 and P-glycoprotein expression. *Mol Med Rep* 2013; 8: 1883-7.

[22] Wang ZD, Wang RZ, Xia YZ, Kong LY, Yang L. Reversal of multidrug resistance by icaritin in doxorubicin-resistant human osteosarcoma cells. *Chin J Nat Med* 2018; 16: 20-8.

[23] Zhang FY, Du GJ, Zhang L, Zhang CL, Lu WL, Liang W. Naringenin enhances the anti-tumor effect of doxorubicin through selectively inhibiting the activity of multidrug resistance-associated proteins but not P-glycoprotein. *Pharm Res* 2009; 26: 914-25.

[24] Li S, Yuan S, Zhao Q, Wang B, Wang X, Li K. Quercetin enhances chemotherapeutic effect of doxorubicin against human breast cancer cells while reducing toxic side effects of it. *Biomed Pharmacother* 2018; 100: 441-7.

[25] An G, Morris ME. Effects of single and multiple flavonoids on BCRP-mediated accumulation, cytotoxicity and transport of mitoxantrone in vitro. *Pharm Res* 2010; 27: 1296-308.

[26] Wei X, Mo X, An F, Ji X, Lu Y. 2`,4`-Dihydroxy-6`-methoxy-3`,5`-dimethylchalcone, a potent Nrf2/ARE pathway inhibitor, reverses drug resistance by decreasing glutathione synthesis and drug efflux in BEL-7402/5-FU cells. *Food Chem Toxicol* 2018; 119: 252-9.

[27] Mohana S, Ganesan M, Agilan B, Karthikeyan R, Srithar G, Beaulah Mary R, Ananthakrishnan D, Velmurugan D, Rajendra Prasad N, Ambudkar SV. Screening dietary flavonoids for the reversal of P-glycoprotein-mediated multidrug resistance in cancer. *Mol Biosyst* 2016; 12: 2458-70.

[28] Hyun HB, Moon JY, Cho SK. Quercetin suppresses CYR61-mediated multidrug resistance in human gastric adenocarcinoma AGS cells. *Molecules* 2018; 23: E209.

[29] Iriti M, Kubina R, Cochis A, Sorrentino R, Varoni EM, Kabala-Dzik A, Azzimonti B, Dziedzic A, Rimondini L, Wojtyczka RD. Rutin, a quercetin glycoside, restores chemosensitivity in human breast cancer cells. *Phytother Res* 2017; 31: 1529-38.

[30] Brechbuhl HM, Kachadourian R, Min E, Chan D, Day BJ. Chrysin enhances doxorubicin-induced cytotoxicity in human lung epithelial cancer cell lines: the role of glutathione. *Toxicol Appl Pharmacol* 2012; 258: 1-9.

[31] Chen HJ, Chung YL, Li CY, Chang YT, Wang CCN, Lee HY, Lin HY, Hung CC. Taxifolin resensitizes multidrug resistance cancer cells via uncompetitive inhibition of P-glycoprotein function. *Molecules* 2018; 23: E3055.

[32] Zheng J, Asakawa T, Chen Y, Zheng Z, Chen B, Lin M, Liu T, Hu J. Synergistic effect of baicalin and adriamycin in resistant HL-60/ADM leukaemia cells. *Cell Physiol Biochem* 2017; 43: 419-30.

[33] Punia R, Raina K, Agarwal R, Singh RP. Acacetin enhances the therapeutic efficacy of doxorubicin in non-small-cell lung carcinoma cells. *PLoS One* 2017; 12: e0182870.

[34] Lv L, Liu C, Chen C, Yu X, Chen G, Shi Y, Qin F, Qu J, Qiu K, Li G. Quercetin and doxorubicin co-encapsulated biotin receptor-targeting nanoparticles for minimizing drug resistance in breast cancer. *Oncotarget* 2016; 7: 32184-99.

[35] Mohana S, Ganesan M, Rajendra Prasad N, Ananthakrishnan D, Velmurugan D. Flavonoids modulate multidrug resistance through wnt signaling in P-glycoprotein overexpressing cell lines. *BMC Cancer* 2018; 18: 1168.

[36] Li X, Wan L, Wang F, Pei H, Zheng L, Wu W, Ye H, Wang Y, Chen L. Barbigerone reverses multidrug resistance in breast MCF-7/ADR cells. *Phytother Res* 2018; 32: 733-40.

[37] Vittorio O, Le Grand M, Makharza SA, Curcio M, Tucci P, Iemma F, Nicoletta FP, Hampel S, Cirillo G. Doxorubicin synergism and resistance reversal in human neuroblastoma BE(2)C cell lines: An in vitro study with dextran-catechin nanohybrids. *Eur J Pharm Biopharm* 2018; 122: 176-85.

[38] Qian F, Ye CL, Wei DZ, Lu YH, Yang SL. In vitro and in vivo reversal of cancer cell multidrug resistance by 2`,4`-dihydroxy-6`-methoxy-3`,5`-dimethylchalcone. *J Chemother* 2005; 17: 309-14.

[39] Angelini A, Di Ilio C, Castellani ML, Conti P, Cuccurullo F. Modulation of multidrug resistance p-glycoprotein activity by flavonoids and honokiol in human doxorubicin- resistant sarcoma cells (MES-SA/DX-5): implications for natural sedatives as chemosensitizing agents in cancer therapy. *J Biol Regul Homeost Agents* 2010; 24: 197-205.

[40] Liang G, Tang A, Lin X, Li L, Zhang S, Huang Z, Tang H, Li QQ. Green tea catechins augment the antitumor activity of doxorubicin in an in vivo mouse model for chemoresistant liver cancer. *Int J Oncol* 2010; 37: 111-23.

[41] Borska S, Sopel M, Chmielewska M, Zabel M, Dziegiel P. Quercetin as a potential modulator of P-glycoprotein expression and function in cells of human pancreatic carcinoma line resistant to daunorubicin. *Molecules* 2010; 15: 857-70.

[42] Yang HY, Zhao L, Yang Z, Zhao Q, Qiang L, Ha J, Li ZY, You QD, Guo QL. Oroxylin A reverses multi-drug resistance of human hepatoma BEL7402/5-FU cells via downregulation of P-glycoprotein expression by inhibiting NF-κB signaling pathway. *Mol Carcinog* 2012; 51: 185-95.

[43] Li S, Zhao Q, Wang B, Yuan S, Wang X, Li K. Quercetin reversed MDR in breast cancer cells through down-regulating P-gp expression and eliminating cancer stem cells mediated by YB-1 nuclear translocation. *Phytother Res* 2018; 32: 1530-6.

[44] Gao H, Xie J, Peng J, Han Y, Jiang Q, Han M, Wang C. Hispidulin inhibits proliferation and enhances chemosensitivity of gallbladder cancer cells by targeting HIF-1α. *Exp Cell Res* 2015; 332: 236-46.

[45] Bansal T, Jaggi M, Khar RK, Talegaonkar S. Emerging significance of flavonoids as P-glycoprotein inhibitors in cancer chemotherapy. *J Pharm Pharm Sci* 2009; 12: 46-78.

[46] Khan M, Maryam A, Mehmood T, Zhang Y, Ma T. Enhancing activity of anticancer drugs in multidrug resistant tumors by modulating P-glycoprotein through dietary nutraceuticals. *Asian Pac J Cancer Prev* 2015; 16: 6831-9.

[47] Mei Y, Qian F, Wei D, Liu J. Reversal of cancer multidrug resistance by green tea polyphenols. *J Pharm Pharmacol* 2004; 56: 1307-14.

[48] Fatma S, Talegaonkar S, Igbal Z, Panda AK, Negi LM, Goswami DG, Tariq M. Novel flavonoid-based biodegradable nanoparticles for effective oral delivery of etoposide by P-glycoprotein modulation: an in vitro, ex vivo and in vivo investigations. *Drug Deliv* 2016; 23: 500-11.

[49] Zhang J, Luo Y, Zhao X, Li X, Li K, Chen D, Qiao M, Hu H, Zhao X. Co-delivery of doxorubicin and the traditional Chinese medicine quercetin using biotin-PEG2000-DSPE modified liposomes for the treatment of multidrug resistant breast cancer. *RSC Adv* 2016; 6: 113173.

[50] Scambia G, Ranelletti FO, Panici PB, De Vincenzo R, Bonanno G, Ferrandina G, Piantelli M, Bussa S, Rumi C, Cianfriglia M, Mancuso S. Quercetin potentiates the effect of adriamycin in a multidrug-resistant MCF-7 human breast-cancer cell line: P-glycoprotein as a possible target. *Cancer Chemother Pharmacol* 1994; 34: 459-64.

[51] Zhang S, Morris ME. Effects of the flavonoids biochanin A, morin, phloretin, and silymarin on P-glycoprotein-mediated transport. *J Pharmacol Exp Ther* 2003; 304: 1258-67.

[52] Borska S, Chmielewska M, Wysocka T, Drag-Zalesinska M, Zabel M, Dziegiel P. In vitro effect of quercetin on human gastric carcinoma: targeting cancer cells death and MDR. *Food Chem Toxicol* 2012; 50: 3375-83.

[53] Hussain SA, Marouf BH. Silibinin improves the cytotoxicity of methotrexate in chemo resistant human rhabdomyosarcoma cell lines. *Saudi Med J* 2013; 34: 1145-50.

[54] Sato A, Sekine M, Kobayashi M, Virgona N, Ota M, Yano T. Induction of the connexin 32 gene by epigallocatechin-3-gallate potentiates vinblastine-induced cytotoxicity in human renal carcinoma cells. *Chemotherapy* 2013; 59: 192-9.

[55] Yuan Z, Wang H, Hu Z, Huang Y, Yao F, Sun S, Wu B. Quercetin inhibits proliferation and drug resistance in KB/VCR oral cancer cells and enhances its sensitivity to vincristine. *Nutr Cancer* 2015; 67: 126-36.

[56] Choi CH, Sun KH, An CS, Yoo JC, Hahm KS, Lee IH, Sohng JK, Kim YC. Reversal of P-glycoprotein-mediated multidrug resistance by 5,6,7,3`,4`-pentamethoxyflavone (Sinensetin). *Biochem Biophys Res Commun* 2002; 295: 832-40.

[57] Narayanan S, Mony U, Vijaykumar DK, Koyakutty M, Paul-Prasanth B, Menon D. Sequential release of epigallocatechin gallate and paclitaxel from PLGA-casein core/shell nanoparticles sensitizes drug-resistant breast cancer cells. *Nanomedicine* 2015; 11: 1399-406.

[58] Zheng AW, Chen YQ, Zhao LQ, Feng JG. Myricetin induces apoptosis and enhances chemosensitivity in ovarian cancer cells. *Oncol Lett* 2017; 13: 4974-8.

[59] Zhou L, Liu P, Chen B, Wang Y, Wang X, Chiriva Internati M, Wachtel MS, Frezza EE. Silibinin restores paclitaxel sensitivity to paclitaxel-resistant human ovarian carcinoma cells. *Anticancer Res* 2008; 28: 1119-27.

[60] Mukhtar E, Adhami VM, Siddiqui IA, Verma AK, Mukhtar H. Fisetin enhances chemotherapeutic effect of cabazitaxel against human prostate cancer cells. *Mol Cancer Ther* 2016; 15: 2863-74.

[61] Lee E, Enomoto R, Suzuki C, Ohno M, Ohashi T, Miyauchi A, Tanimoto E, Maeda K, Hirano H, Yokoi T, Sugahara C. Wogonin, a plant flavone, potentiates etoposide-induced apoptosis in cancer cells. *Ann N Y Acad Sci* 2007; 1095: 521-6.

[62] Hemalswarya S, Doble M. Potential synergism of natural products in the treatment of cancer. *Phytother Res* 2006; 20: 239-49.

[63] Tran VH, Marks D, Duke RK, Bebawy M, Duke CC, Roufogalis BD. Modulation of P-glycoprotein-mediated anticancer drug accumulation, cytotoxicity, and ATPase activity by flavonoid interactions. *Nutr Cancer* 2011; 63: 435-43.

[64] Gyemant N, Tanaka M, Antus S, Hohmann J, Csuka O, Mandoky L, Molnar J. In vitro search for synergy between flavonoids and epirubicin on multidrug-resistant cancer cells. *In Vivo* 2005; 19: 367-74.

[65] Wu L, Yang W, Zhang SN, Lu JB. Alpinetin inhibits lung cancer progression and elevates sensitization drug-resistant lung cancer cells to cis-diammined dichloridoplatium. *Drug Des Devel Ther* 2015; 9: 6119-27.

[66] Wang Z, Sun X, Feng Y, Liu X, Zhou L, Sui H, Ji Q, E Q, Chen J, Wu L, Li Q. Dihydromyricetin reverses MRP2-mediated MDR and enhances anticancer activity induced by oxaliplatin in colorectal cancer cells. *Anticancer Drugs* 2017; 28: 281-8.

[67] Gao AM, Ke ZP, Wang JN, Yang JY, Chen SY, Chen H. Apigenin sensitizes doxorubicin-resistant hepatocellular carcinoma BEL-7402/ADM cells to doxorubicin via inhibiting PI3K/Akt/Nrf2 pathway. *Carcinogenesis* 2013; 34: 1806-14.

[68] Zhang S, Yang X, Morris ME. Flavonoids are inhibitors of breast cancer resistance protein (ABCG2)-mediated transport. *Mol Pharmacol* 2004; 65: 1208-16.

[69] Yoshikawa M, Ikegami Y, Sano K, Yoshida H, Mitomo H, Sawada S, Ishikawa T. Transport of SN-38 by the wild type of human ABC transporter ABCG2 and its inhibition by quercetin, a natural flavonoid. *J Exp Ther Oncol* 2004; 4: 25-35.

[70] Imai Y, Tsukahara S, Asada S, Sugimoto Y. Phytoestrogens/flavonoids reverse breast cancer resistance protein/ABCG2-mediated multidrug resistance. *Cancer Res* 2004; 64: 4346-52.

[71] Bueno Perez L, Pan L, Sass E, Gupta SV, Lehman A, Kinghorn AD, Lucas DM. Potentiating effect of the flavonolignan (-)-hydnocarpin in combination with vincristine in a sensitive and P-gp-expressing acute lymphoblastic leukemia cell line. *Phytother Res* 2013; 27: 1735-8.

[72] Chen Z, Huang C, Ma T, Jiang L, Tang L, Shi T, Zhang S, Zhang L, Zhu P, Li J, Shen A. Reversal effect of quercetin on multidrug resistance via FZD7/β-catenin pathway in hepatocellular carcinoma cells. *Phytomedicine* 2018; 43: 37-45.

[73] Ma W, Feng S, Yao X, Yuan Z, Liu L, Xie Y. Nobiletin enhances the efficacy of chemotherapeutic agents in ABCB1 overexpression cancer cells. *Sci Rep* 2015; 5: 18789.

[74] Jacobs H, Bast A, Peters GJ, van der Vijgh WJ, Haenen GR. The semisynthetic flavonoid monoHER sensitises human soft tissue sarcoma cells to doxorubicin-induced apoptosis via inhibition of nuclear factor-κB. *Br J Cancer* 2011; 104: 437-40.

[75] Cheng T, Liu J, Ren J, Huang F, Ou H, Ding Y, Zhang Y, Ma R, An Y, Liu J, Shi L. Green tea catechin-based complex micelles combined with doxorubicin to overcome cardiotoxicity and multidrug resistance. *Theranostics* 2016; 6: 1277-92.

[76] Li SZ, Qiao SF, Zhang JH, Li K. Quercetin increase the chemosensitivity of breast cancer cells to doxorubicin via PTEN/Akt pathway. *Anticancer Agents Med Chem* 2015; 15: 1185-9.

[77] Li J, Duan B, Guo Y, Zhou R, Sun J, Bie B, Yang S, Huang C, Yang J, Li Z. Baicalein sensitizes hepatocellular carcinoma cells to 5-FU and Epirubicin by activating apoptosis and ameliorating P-glycoprotein activity. *Biomed Pharmacother* 2018; 98: 806-12.

[78] Zhu X, Ji M, Han Y, Guo Y, Zhu W, Gao F, Yang X, Zhang C. PGRMC1-dependent autophagy by hyperoside induces apoptosis and sensitizes ovarian cancer cells to cisplatin treatment. *Int J Oncol* 2017; 50: 835-46.

[79] Chen FY, Cao LF, Wan HX, Zhang MY, Cai JY, Shen LJ, Zhong JH, Zhong H. Quercetin enhances adriamycin cytotoxicity through induction of apoptosis and regulation of mitogen-activated protein kinase/extracellular signal-regulated kinase/c-Jun N-terminal kinase signaling in multidrug-resistant leukemia K562 cells. *Mol Med Rep* 2015; 11: 341-8.

[80] Park CH, Han SE, Nam-Goong IS, Kim YI, Kim ES. Combined effects of baicalein and docetaxel on apoptosis in 8505c anaplastic thyroid cancer cells via downregulation of the ERK and Akt/mTOR pathways. *Endocrinol Metab (Seoul)* 2018; 33: 121-32.

[81] Guo XF, Liu JP, Ma SQ, Zhang P, Sun WD. Avicularin reversed multidrug-resistance in human gastric cancer through enhancing Bax and BOK expressions. *Biomed Pharmacother* 2018; 103: 67-74.

[82] Mor G, Fu HH, Alvero AB. Phenoxodiol, a novel approach for the treatment of ovarian cancer. *Curr Opin Investig Drugs* 2006; 7: 542-8.

[83] Yi JL, Shi S, Shen YL, Wang L, Chen HY, Zhu J, Ding Y. Myricetin and methyl eugenol combination enhances the anticancer activity, cell cycle arrest and apoptosis induction of cis-platin against HeLa cervical cancer cell lines. *Int J Clin Exp Pathol* 2015; 8: 1116-27.

[84] Mihaila M, Bostan M, Hotnog D, Ferdes M, Brasoveanu LL. Real-time analysis of quercetin, resveratrol and/or doxorubicin effects in MCF-7 cells. *Rom Biotechnol Lett* 2013; 18: 8106-14.

[85] Moon JY, Cho M, Ahn KS, Cho SK. Nobiletin induces apoptosis and potentiates the effects of the anticancer drug 5-fluorouracil in p53-mutated SNU-16 human gastric cancer cells. *Nutr Cancer* 2013; 65: 286-95.

[86] Motwani M, Jung C, Sirotnak FM, She Y, Shah MA, Gonen M, Schwartz GK. Augmentation of apoptosis and tumor regression by flavopiridol in the presence of CPT-11 in Hct116 colon cancer monolayers and xenografts. *Clin Cancer Res* 2001; 7: 4209-19.

[87] Yoshimizu N, Otani Y, Saikawa Y, Kubota T, Yoshida M, Furukawa T, Kumai K, Kameyama K, Fujii M, Yano M, Sato T, Ito A, Kitajima M. Anti-tumour effects of nobiletin, a citrus flavonoid, on gastric cancer include: antiproliferative effects, induction of apoptosis and cell cycle deregulation. *Aliment Pharmacol Ther* 2004; 20 Suppl1: 95-101.

[88] Marone M, D`Andrilli G, Das N, Ferlini C, Chatterjee S, Scambia G. Quercetin abrogates taxol-mediated signaling by inhibiting multiple kinases. *Exp Cell Res* 2001; 270: 1-12.

[89] Papazisis KT, Kalemi TG, Zambouli D, Geromichalos GD, Lambropoulos AF, Kotsis A, Boutis LL, Kortsaris AH. Synergistic effects of protein tyrosine kinase inhibitor genistein with camptothecins against three cell lines in vitro. *Cancer Lett* 2006; 233: 255-64.

[90] Demiroglu-Zergeroglu A, Ergene E, Ayvali N, Kuete V, Sivas H. Quercetin and Cisplatin combined treatment altered cell cycle and mitogen activated protein kinase expressions in malignant mesotelioma cells. *BMC Complement Altern Med* 2016; 16: 281.

[91] Li WG, Wang HQ. Inhibitory effects of Silibinin combined with doxorubicin in hepatocellular carcinoma; an in vivo study. *J BUON* 2016; 21: 917-24.

[92] Fornier MN, Rathkopf D, Shah M, Patil S, O`Reilly E, Tse AN, Hudis C, Lefkowitz R, Kelsen DP, Schwartz GK. Phase I dose-finding study of weekly docetaxel followed by flavopiridol for patients with advanced solid tumors. *Clin Cancer Res* 2007; 13: 5841-6.

[93] Abaza MS, Orabi KY, Al-Quattan E, Al-Attiyah RJ. Growth inhibitory and chemo-sensitization effects of naringenin, a natural flavanone purified from Thymus vulgaris, on human breast and colorectal cancer. *Cancer Cell Int* 2015; 15: 46.

[94] Kiartivich S, Wei Y, Liu J, Soiampornkul R, Li M, Zhang H, Dong J. Regulation of cytotoxicity and apoptosis-associated pathways contributes to the enhancement of efficacy of cisplatin by baicalein adjuvant in human A549 lung cancer cells. *Oncol Lett* 2017; 13: 2799-804.

[95] Namazi Sarvestani N, Sepehri H, Delphi L, Moridi Farimani M. Eupatorin and salvigenin potentiate doxorubicin-induced apoptosis and cell cycle arrest in HT-29 and SW948 human colon cancer cells. *Asian Pac J Cancer Prev* 2018; 19: 131-9.

[96] Lo YL, Wang W. Formononetin potentiates epirubicin-induced apoptosis via ROS production in HeLa cells in vitro. *Chem Biol Interact* 2013; 205: 188-97.

[97] Chuang-Xin L, Wen-Yu W, Yao C, Xiao-Yan L, Yun Z. Quercetin enhances the effects of 5-fluorouracil-mediated growth inhibition and apoptosis of esophageal cancer cells by inhibiting NF-κB. *Oncol Lett* 2012; 4: 775-8.

[98] Yang YI, Lee KT, Park HJ, Kim TJ, Choi YS, Shih IeM, Choi JH. Tectorigenin sensitizes paclitaxel-resistant human ovarian cancer cells through downregulation of the Akt and NFκB pathway. *Carcinogenesis* 2012; 33: 2488-98.

[99] Johnson JL, Gonzalez de Mejia E. Interactions between dietary flavonoids apigenin or luteolin and chemotherapeutic drugs to potentiate anti-proliferative effect on human pancreatic cancer cells, in vitro. *Food Chem Toxicol* 2013; 60: 83-91.

[100] Lin X, Tian L, Wang L, Li W, Xu Q, Xiao X. Antitumor effects and the underlying mechanism of licochalcone A combined with 5-fluorouracil in gastric cancer cells. *Oncol Lett* 2017; 13: 1695-701.

[101] Wang L, Feng J, Chen X, Guo W, Du Y, Wang Y, Zang W, Zhang S, Zhao G. Myricetin enhance chemosensitivity of 5-fluorouracil on esophageal carcinoma in vitro and in vivo. *Cancer Cell Int* 2014; 14: 71.

[102] Sharma H, Sen S, Singh N. Molecular pathways in the chemosensitization of cisplatin by quercetin in human head and neck cancer. *Cancer Biol Ther* 2005; 4: 949-55.

[103] Dhivya S, Khandelwal N, Abraham SK, Premkumar K. Impact of anthocyanidins on mitoxantrone-induced cytotoxicity and genotoxicity: An in vitro and in vivo analysis. *Integr Cancer Ther* 2016; 15: 525-34.

[104] Guo XF, Yang ZR, Wang J, Lei XF, Lv XG, Dong WG. Synergistic antitumor effect of puerarin combined with 5-fluorouracil on gastric carcinoma. *Mol Med Rep* 2015; 11: 2562-8.

[105] Jakubowicz-Gil J, Langner E, Badziul D, Wertel I, Rzeski W. Apoptosis induction in human glioblastoma multiforme T98G cells upon temozolomide and quercetin treatment. *Tumour Biol* 2013; 34: 2367-78.

[106] Yu S, Gong LS, Li NF, Pan YF, Zhang L. Galangin (GG) combined with cisplatin (DDP) to suppress human lung cancer by inhibition of STAT3-regulated NF-κB and Bcl-2/Bax signaling pathways. *Biomed Pharmacother* 2018; 97: 213-24.

[107] Lee SH, Lee EJ, Min KH, Hur GY, Lee SH, Lee SY, Kim JH, Shin C, Shim JJ, In KH, Kang KH, Lee SY. Quercetin enhances chemosensitivity to gemcitabine in lung cancer cells by inhibiting heat shock protein 70 expression. *Clin Lung Cancer* 2015; 16: e235-43.

[108] Zhang Y, Ge Y, Ping X, Yu M, Lou D, Shi W. Synergistic apoptotic effects of silibinin in enhancing paclitaxel toxicity in human gastric cancer cell lines. *Mol Med Rep* 2018; 18: 1835-41.

[109] Dai W, Gao Q, Qiu J, Yuan J, Wu G, Shen G. Quercetin induces apoptosis and enhances 5-FU therapeutic efficacy in hepatocellular carcinoma. *Tumour Biol* 2016; 37: 6307-13.

[110] Zhao Q, Wang J, Zou MJ, Hu R, Zhao L, Qiang L, Rong JJ, You QD, Guo QL. Wogonin potentiates the antitumor effects of low dose 5-fluorouracil against gastric cancer through induction of apoptosis by down-regulation of NF-kappaB and regulation of its metabolism. *Toxicol Lett* 2010; 197: 201-10.

[111] Yang MY, Wang CJ, Chen NF, Ho WH, Lu FJ, Tseng TH. Luteolin enhances paclitaxel-induced apoptosis in human breast cancer MDA-MB-231 cells by blocking STAT3. *Chem Biol Interact* 2014; 213: 60-8.

[112] Silasi DA, Alvero AB, Rutherford TJ, Brown D, Mor G. Phenoxodiol: pharmacology and clinical experience in cancer monotherapy and in combination with chemotherapeutic drugs. *Expert Opin Pharmacother* 2009; 10: 1059-67.

[113] Li X, Huang JM, Wang JN, Xiong XK, Yang XF, Zou F. Combination of chrysin and cisplatin promotes the apoptosis of Hep G2 cells by up-regulating p53. *Chem Biol Interact* 2015; 232: 12-20.

[114] Jiang L, Zhang Q, Ren H, Ma S, Lu C, Liu B, Liu J, Liang J, Li M, Zhu R. Dihydromyricetin enhances the chemo-sensitivity of nedaplatin via regulation of the p53/Bcl-2 pathway in hepatocellular carcinoma cells. *PLoS One* 2015; 10: e0124994.

[115] Tang Q, Ji F, Sun W, Wang J, Guo J, Guo L, Li Y, Bao Y. Combination of baicalein and 10-hydroxy camptothecin exerts remarkable synergetic anti-cancer effects. *Phytomedicine* 2016; 23: 1778-86.

[116] Singh M, Bhui K, Singh R, Shukla Y. Tea polyphenols enhance cisplatin chemosensitivity in cervical cancer cells via induction of apoptosis. *Life Sci* 2013; 93: 7-16.

[117] Xu GY, Tang XJ. Troxerutin (TXN) potentiated 5-Fluorouracil (5-Fu) treatment of human gastric cancer through suppressing STAT3/NF-κB and Bcl-2 signaling pathways. *Biomed Pharmacother* 2017; 92: 95-107.

[118] Wang G, Zhang J, Liu L, Sharma S, Dong Q. Quercetin potentiates doxorubicin mediated antitumor effects against liver cancer through p53/Bcl-xl. *PLoS One* 2012; 7: e51764.

[119] Ping SY, Hour TC, Lin SR, Yu DS. Taxol synergizes with antioxidants in inhibiting hormal refractory prostate cancer cell growth. *Urol Oncol* 2010; 28: 170-9.

[120] Jiang YY, Wang HJ, Wang J, Tashiro S, Onodera S, Ikejima T. The protective effect of silibinin against mitomycin C-induced intrinsic apoptosis in human melanoma A375-S2 cells. *J Pharmacol Sci* 2009; 111: 137-46.

[121] Singh M, Bhatnagar P, Mishra S, Kumar P, Shukla Y, Gupta KC. PLGA-encapsulated tea polyphenols enhance the chemotherapeutic efficacy of cisplatin

against human cancer cells and mice bearing Ehrlich ascites carcinoma. *Int J Nanomedicine* 2015; 10: 6789-809.

[122] Singh VK, Arora D, Satija NK, Khare P, Roy SK, Sharma PK. Intricatinol synergistically enhances the anticancerous activity of cisplatin in human A549 cells via p38 MAPK/p53 signalling. *Apoptosis* 2017; 22: 1273-86.

[123] Xu H, Yang T, Liu X, Tian Y, Chen X, Yuan R, Su S, Lin X, Du G. Luteolin synergizes the antitumor effects of 5-fluorouracil against human hepatocellular carcinoma cells through apoptosis induction and metabolism. *Life Sci* 2016; 144: 138-47.

[124] Mehnath S, Arjama M, Rajan M, Annamalai G, Jeyaraj M. Co-encapsulation of dual drug loaded in MLNPs: Implication on sustained drug release and effectively inducing apoptosis in oral carcinoma cells. *Biomed Pharmacother* 2018; 104: 661-71.

[125] Lo YL. A potential daidzein derivative enhances cytotoxicity of epirubicin on human colon adenocarcinoma Caco-2 cells. *Int J Mol Sci* 2012; 14: 158-76.

[126] Kluger HM, McCarthy MM, Alvero AB, Sznol M, Ariyan S, Camp RL, Rimm DL, Mor G. The X-linked inhibitor of apoptosis protein (XIAP) is up-regulated in metastatic melanoma, and XIAP cleavage by Phenoxodiol is associated with Carboplatin sensitization. *J Transl Med* 2007; 5: 6.

[127] Reiner T, de las Pozas A, Perez-Stable C. Sequential combinations of flavopiridol and docetaxel inhibit prostate tumors, induce apoptosis, and decrease angiogenesis in the Ggamma/T-15 transgenic mouse model of prostate cancer. *Prostate* 2006; 66: 1487-97.

[128] Sapi E, Alvero AB, Chen W, O`Malley D, Hao XY, Dwipoyono B, Garg M, Kamsteeg M, Rutherford T, Mor G. Resistance of ovarian carcinoma cells to docetaxel is XIAP dependent and reversible by phenoxodiol. *Oncol Res* 2004; 14: 567-78.

[129] Miyamoto M, Takano M, Aoyama T, Soyama H, Ishibashi H, Kato K, Iwahashi H, Takasaki K, Kuwahara M, Matuura H, Sakamoto T, Yoshikawa T, Furuya K. Phenoxodiol increases cisplatin sensitivity in ovarian clear cancer cells through XIAP down-regulation and autophagy inhibition. *Anticancer Res* 2018; 38: 301-6.

[130] Wall NR, O`Connor DS, Plescia J, Pommier Y, Altieri DC. Suppression of survivin phosphorylation on Thr35 by flavopiridol enhances tumor cell apoptosis. *Cancer Res* 2003; 63: 230-5.

[131] Zhuo W, Zhang L, Zhu Y, Zhu B, Chen Z. Fisetin, a dietary bioflavonoid, reverses acquired Cisplatin-resistance of lung adenocarcinoma cells through MAPK/Survivin/Caspase pathway. *Am J Transl Res* 2015; 7: 2045-52.

[132] Xu Y, Wang S, Chan HF, Lu H, Lin Z, He C, Chen M. Dihydromyricetin induces apoptosis and reverses drug resistance in ovarian cancer cells by p53-mediated downregulation of survivin. *Sci Rep* 2017; 7: 46060.

[133] Jiang YY, Yang R, Wang HJ, Huang H, Wu D, Tashiro S, Onodera S, Ikejima T. Mechanism of autophagy induction and role of autophagy in antagonizing mitomycin C-induced cell apoptosis in silibinin treated human melanoma A375-S2 cells. *Eur J Pharmacol* 2011; 659: 7-14.

[134] Tripathi R, Samadder T, Gupta S, Surolia A, Shaha C. Anticancer activity of a combination of cisplatin and fisetin in embryonal carcinoma cells and xenograft tumors. *Mol Cancer Ther* 2011; 10: 255-68.

[135] Cai X, Liu X. Inhibition of Thr-55 phosphorylation restores p53 nuclear localization and sensitizes cancer cells to DNA damage. *Proc Natl Acad Sci USA* 2008; 105: 16958-63.

[136] Shi R, Huang Q, Zhu X, Ong YB, Zhao B, Lu J, Ong CN, Shen HM. Luteolin sensitizes the anticancer effect of cisplatin via c-Jun NH2-terminal kinase-mediated p53 phosphorylation and stabilization. *Mol Cancer Ther* 2007; 6: 1338-47.

[137] Lee JJ, Koh KN, Park CJ, Jang S, Im HJ, Kim N. The combination of flavokawain B and daunorubicin induces apoptosis in human myeloid leukemic cells by modifying NF-κB. *Anticancer Res* 2018; 38: 2771-8.

[138] Xavier CP, Lima CF, Rohde M, Pereira-Wilson C. Quercetin enhances 5-fluorouracil-induced apoptosis in MSI colorectal cancer cells through p53 modulation. *Cancer Chemother Pharmacol* 2011; 68: 1449-57.

[139] Samuel T, Fadlalla K, Turner T, Yehualaeshet TE. The flavonoid quercetin transiently inhibits the activity of taxol and nocodazole through interference with the cell cycle. *Nutr Cancer* 2010; 62: 1025-35.

[140] Stearns ME, Wang M. Synergistic effects of the green tea extract epigallocatechin-3-gallate and taxane in eradication of malignant human prostate tumors. *Transl Oncol* 2011; 4: 147-56.

[141] Masuda M, Suzui M, Weinstein IB. Effects of epigallocatechin-3-gallate on growth, epidermal growth factor receptor signaling pathways, gene expression, and chemosensitivity in human head and neck squamous cell carcinoma cell lines. *Clin Cancer Res* 2001; 7: 4220-9.

[142] Budak-Alpdogan T, Chen B, Warrier A, Medina DJ, Moore D, Bertino JR. Retinoblastoma tumor suppressor gene expression determines the response to sequential flavopiridol and doxorubicin treatment in small-cell lung carcinoma. *Clin Cancer Res* 2009; 15: 1232-40.

[143] Varela-Castillo O, Cordero P, Gutierrez-Iglesias G, Palma I, Rubio-Gayosso I, Meaney E, Ramirez-Sanchez I, Villarreal F, Ceballos G, Najera N. Characterization of the cytotoxic effects of the combination of cisplatin and flavanol (-)-epicatechin on human lung cancer cell line A549. An isobolographic approach. *Exp Oncol* 2018; 40: 19-23.

[144] Chan JY, Tan BK, Lee SC. Scutellarin sensitizes drug-evoked colon cancer cell apoptosis through enhanced caspase-6 activation. *Anticancer Res* 2009; 29: 3043-7.

[145] Zhang S, Wang Y, Chen Z, Kim S, Iqbal S, Chi A, Ritenour C, Wang YA, Kucuk O, Wu D. Genistein enhances the efficacy of cabazitaxel chemotherapy in metastatic castration-resistant prostate cancer cells. *Prostate* 2013; 73: 1681-9.

[146] Ma L, Wang R, Nan Y, Li W, Wang Q, Jin F. Phloretin exhibits an anticancer effect and enhances the anticancer ability of cisplatin on non-small cell lung cancer cell lines by regulating expression of apoptotic pathways and matrix metalloproteinases. *Int J Oncol* 2016; 48: 843-53.

[147] Kuhar M, Sen S, Singh N. Role of mitochondria in quercetin-enhanced chemotherapeutic response in human non-small cell lung carcinoma H-520 cells. *Anticancer Res* 2006; 26: 1297-303.

[148] Isonishi S, Saitou M, Yasuda M, Ochiai K, Tanaka T. Enhancement of sensitivity to cisplatin by orobol is associated with increased mitochondrial cytochrome c release in human ovarian carcinoma cells. *Gynecol Oncol* 2003; 90: 413-20.

[149] Gaballah HH, Gaber RA, Mohamed DA. Apigenin potentiates the antitumor activity of 5-FU on solid Ehrlich carcinoma: Crosstalk between apoptotic and JNK-mediated autophagic cell death platforms. *Toxicol Appl Pharmacol* 2017; 316: 27-35.

[150] Pan XW, Li L, Huang Y, Huang H, Xu DF, Gao Y, Chen L, Ren JZ, Cao JW, Hong Y, Cui XG. Icaritin acts synergistically with epirubicin to suppress bladder cancer growth through inhibition of autophagy. *Oncol Rep* 2016; 35: 334-42.

[151] Suzuki R, Kang Y, Li X, Roife D, Zhang R, Fleming JB, Genistein potentiates the antitumor effect of 5-Fluorouracil by inducing apoptosis and autophagy in human pancreatic cancer cells. *Anticancer Res* 2014; 34: 4685-92.

[152] Chen L, Ye HL, Zhang G, Yao WM, Chen XZ, Zhang FC, Liang G. Autophagy inhibition contributes to the synergistic interaction between EGCG and doxorubicin to kill the hepatoma Hep3B cells. *PLoS One* 2014; 9: e85771.

[153] Zhang B, Yu X, Xia H. The flavonoid luteolin enhances doxorubicin-induced autophagy in human osteosarcoma U2OS cells. *Int J Clin Exp Med* 2015; 8: 15190-7.

[154] Hyun JJ, Lee HS, Keum B, Seo YS, Jeen YT, Chun HJ, Um SH, Kim CD. Expression of heat shock protein 70 modulates the chemoresponsiveness of pancreatic cancer. *Gut Liver* 2013; 7: 739-46.

[155] Xu XD, Zhao Y, Zhang M, He RZ, Shi XH, Guo XJ, Shi CJ, Peng F, Wang M, Shen M, Wang X, Li X, Qin RY. Inhibition of autophagy by deguelin sensitizes pancreatic cancer cells to doxorubicin. *Int J Mol Sci* 2017; 18: E370.

[156] Jakubowicz-Gil J, Langner E, Wertel I, Piersiak T, Rzeski W. Temozolomide, quercetin and cell death in the MOGGCCM astrocytoma cell line. *Chem Biol Interact* 2010; 188: 190-203.

[157] Klimaszewska-Wisniewska A, Halas-Wisniewska M, Tadrowski T, Gagat M, Grzanka D, Grzanka A. Paclitaxel and the dietary flavonoid fisetin: a synergistic

combination that induces mitotic catastrophe and autophagic cell death in A549 non-small cell lung cancer cells. *Cancer Cell Int* 2016; 16: 10.

[158] Ruela-de-Sousa RR, Fuhler GM, Blom N, Ferreira CV, Aoyama H, Peppelenbosch MP. Cytotoxicity of apigenin on leukemia cell lines: implications for prevention and therapy. *Cell Death Dis* 2010; 1: e19.

[159] Su YK, Huang WC, Lee WH, Bamodu OA, Zucha MA, Astuti I, Suwito H, Yeh CT, Lin CM. Methoxyphenyl chalcone sensitizes aggressive epithelial cancer to cisplatin through apoptosis induction and cancer stem cell eradication. *Tumour Biol* 2017; 39: 1010428317691689.

[160] Wang Z, Wang N, Liu P, Chen Q, Situ H, Xie T, Zhang J, Peng C, Lin Y, Chen J. MicroRNA-25 regulates chemoresistance-associated autophagy in breast cancer cells, a process modulated by the natural autophagy inducer isoliquiritigenin. *Oncotarget* 2014; 5: 7013-26.

[161] Hu F, Wei F, Wang Y, Wu B, Fang Y, Xiong B. EGCG synergizes the therapeutic effect of cisplatin and oxaliplatin through autophagic pathway in human colorectal cancer cells. *J Pharmacol Sci* 2015; 128: 27-34.

[162] Jakubowicz-Gil J, Langner E, Rzeski W. Kinetic studies of the effects of Temodal and quercetin on astrocytoma cells. *Pharmacol Rep* 2011; 63: 403-16.

[163] Gao AM, Zhang XY, Hu JN, Ke ZP. Apigenin sensitizes hepatocellular carcinoma cells to doxorubic through regulating miR-520b/ATG7 axis. *Chem Biol Interact* 2018; 280: 45-50.

[164] Erdogan S, Turkekul K, Serttas R, Erdogan Z. The natural flavonoid apigenin sensitizes human CD44+ prostate cancer stem cells to cisplatin therapy. *Biomed Pharmacother* 2017; 88: 210-7.

[165] Yang L, Wang Y, Guo H, Guo M. Synergistic anti-cancer effects of icariin and temozolomide in glioblastoma. *Cell Biochem Biophys* 2015; 71: 1379-85.

[166] Nazari M, Ghorbani A, Hekmat-Doost A, Jeddi-Tehrani M, Zand H. Inactivation of nuclear factor-κB by citrus flavanone hesperidin contributes to apoptosis and chemo-sensitizing effect in Ramos cells. *Eur J Pharmacol* 2011; 650: 526-33.

[167] Brito AF, Ribeiro M, Abrantes AM, Pires AS, Teixo RJ, Tralhao JG, Botelho MF. Quercetin in cancer treatment, alone or in combination with conventional therapeutics? *Curr Med Chem* 2015; 22: 3025-39.

[168] Shi DB, Li XX, Zheng HT, Li DW, Cai GX, Peng JJ, Gu WL, Guan ZQ, Xu Y, Cai SJ. Icariin-mediated inhibition of NF-κB activity enhances the in vitro and in vivo antitumour effect of 5-fluorouracil in colorectal cancer. *Cell Biochem Biophys* 2014; 69: 523-30.

[169] Zhang B, Shi ZL, Liu B, Yan XB, Feng J, Tao HM. Enhanced anticancer effect of gemcitabine by genistein in osteosarcoma: the role of Akt and nuclear factor-kappaB. *Anticancer Drugs* 2010; 21: 288-96.

[170] Singh RP, Mallikarjuna GU, Sharma G, Dhanalakshmi S, Tyagi AK, Chan DC, Agarwal C, Agarwal R. Oral silibinin inhibits lung tumor growth in athymic nude mice and forms a novel chemocombination with doxorubicin targeting nuclear factor kappaB-mediated inducible chemoresistance. *Clin Cancer Res* 2004; 10: 8641-7.

[171] Banerjee S, Zhang Y, Ali S, Bhuiyan M, Wang Z, Chiao PJ, Philip PA, Abbruzzese J, Sarkar FH. Molecular evidence for increased antitumor activity of gemcitabine by genistein in vitro and in vivo using an orthotopic model of pancreatic cancer. *Cancer Res* 2005; 65: 9064-72.

[172] Zhang DC, Liu JL, Ding YB, Xia JG, Chen GY. Icariin potentiates the antitumor activity of gemcitabine in gallbladder cancer by suppressing NF-κB. *Acta Pharmacol Sin* 2013; 34: 301-8.

[173] Wang Y, Miao H, Li W, Yao J, Sun Y, Li Z, Zhao L, Guo Q. CXCL12/CXCR4 axis confers adriamycin resistance to human chronic myelogenous leukemia and oroxylin A improves the sensitivity of K562/ADM cells. *Biochem Pharmacol* 2014; 90: 212-25.

[174] Zhao L, Sha YY, Zhao Q, Yao J, Zhu BB, Lu ZJ, You QD, Guo QL. Enhanced 5-fluorouracil cytotoxicity in high COX-2 expressing hepatocellular carcinoma cells by wogonin via the PI3K/Akt pathway. *Biochem Cell Biol* 2013; 91: 221-9.

[175] Bieg D, Sypniewski D, Nowak E, Bednarek I. Morin decreases galectin-3 expression and sensitizes ovarian cancer cells to cisplatin. *Arch Gynecol Obstet* 2018; 298: 1181-94.

[176] Xu X, Zhang X, Zhang Y, Yang L, Liu Y, Huang S, Lu L, Kong L, Li Z, Guo Q, Zhao L. Wogonin reversed resistant human myelogenous leukemia cells via inhibiting Nrf2 signaling by Stat3/NF-κB inactivation. *Sci Rep* 2017; 7: 39950.

[177] Manu KA, Shanmugam MK, Ramachandran L, Li F, Siveen KS, Chinnathambi A, Zayed ME, Alharbi SA, Arfuso F, Kumar AP, Ahn KS, Sethi G. Isorhamnetin augments the anti-tumor effect of capeciatbine through the negative regulation of NF-κB signaling cascade in gastric cancer. *Cancer Lett* 2015; 363: 28-36.

[178] Li Y, Ellis KL, Ali S, El-Rayes BF, Nedeljkovic-Kurepa A, Kucuk O, Philip PA, Sarkar FH. Apoptosis-inducing effect of chemotherapeutic agents is potentiated by soy isoflavone genistein, a natural inhibitor of NF-kappaB in BxPC-3 pancreatic cancer cell line. *Pancreas* 2004; 28: e90-5.

[179] Li Y, Ahmed F, Ali S, Philip PA, Kucuk O, Sarkar FH. Inactivation of nuclear factor kappaB by soy isoflavone genistein contributes to increased apoptosis induced by chemotherapeutic agents in human cancer cells. *Cancer Res* 2005; 65: 6934-42.

[180] Nessa MU, Beale P, Chan C, Yu JQ, Huq F. Synergism from combinations of cisplatin and oxaliplatin with quercetin and thymoquinone in human ovarian tumour models. *Anticancer Res* 2011; 31: 3789-97.

[181] Zhou L, Wu Y, Guo Y, Li Y, Li N, Yang Y, Qin X. Calycosin enhances some chemotherapeutic drugs inhibition of Akt signaling pathway in gastric cells. *Cancer Invest* 2017; 35: 289-300.

[182] Xu YY, Wu TT, Zhou SH, Bao YY, Wang QY, Fan J, Huang YP. Apigenin suppresses GLUT-1 and p-AKT expression to enhance the chemosensitivity to cisplatin of laryngeal carcinoma Hep-2 cells: an in vitro study. *Int J Clin Exp Pathol* 2014; 7: 3938-47.

[183] Liu D, Yan L, Wang L, Tai W, Wang W, Yang C. Genistein enhances the effect of cisplatin on the inhibition of non-small cell lung cancer A549 cell growth *in vitro* and *in vivo*. *Oncol Lett* 2014; 8: 2806-10.

[184] Strouch MJ, Milam BM, Melstrom LG, McGull JJ, Salabat MR, Ujiki MB, Ding XZ, Bentrem DJ. The flavonoid apigenin potentiates the growth inhibitory effects of gemcitabine and abrogates gemcitabine resistance in human pancreatic cancer cells. *Pancreas* 2009; 38: 409-15.

[185] Choi EJ, Kim GH. 5-Fluorouracil combined with apigenin enhances anticancer activity through induction of apoptosis in human breast cancer MDA-MB-453 cells. *Oncol Rep* 2009; 22: 1533-7.

[186] Satoh H, Nishikawa K, Suzuki K, Asano R, Virgona N, Ichikawa T, Hagiwara K, Yano T. Genistein, a soy isoflavone, enhances necrotic-like cell death in a breast cancer cell treated with a chemotherapeutic agent. *Res Commun Mol Pathol Pharmacol* 2003; 113-114: 149-58.

[187] Lei W, Mayotte JE, Levitt ML. Enhancement of chemosensitivity and programmed cell death by tyrosine kinase inhibitors correlates with EGFR expression in non-small cell lung cancer cells. *Anticancer Res* 1999; 19: 221-8.

[188] Zhang BY, Wang YM, Gong H, Zhao H, Lv XY, Yuan GH, Han SR. Isorhamnetin flavonoid synergistically enhances the anticancer activity and apoptosis induction by cis-platin and carboplatin in non-small cell lung carcinoma (NSCLC). *Int J Clin Exp Pathol* 2015; 8: 25-37.

[189] Zhang L, Yang X, Li X, Li C, Zhao L, Zhou Y, Hou H. Butein sensitizes HeLa cells to cisplatin through the AKT and ERK/p38 MAPK pathways by targeting FoxO3a. *Int J Mol Med* 2015; 36: 957-66.

[190] Yu M, Qi B, Xiaoxiang W, Xu J, Liu X. Baicalein increases cisplatin sensitivity of A549 lung adenocarcinoma cells via PI3K/Akt/NF-κB pathway. *Biomed Pharmacother* 2017; 90: 677-85.

[191] Liu M, Qi Z, Liu B, Ren Y, Li H, Yang G, Zhang Q. RY-2f, an isoflavone analog, overcomes cisplatin resistance to inhibit ovarian tumorigenesis via targeting the PI3K/AKT/mTOR signaling pathway. *Oncotarget* 2015; 6: 25281-94.

[192] Dia VP, Pangloli P. Epithelial-to-mesenchymal transition in paclitaxel-resistant ovarian cancer cells is downregulated by luteolin. *J Cell Physiol* 2017; 232: 391-401.

[193] Yang XW, Wang XL, Cao LQ, Jiang XF, Peng HP, Lin SM, Xue P, Chen D. Green tea polyphenol epigallocatehin-3-gallate enhances 5-fluorouracil-induced cell growth inhibition of hepatocellular carcinoma cells. *Hepatol Res* 2012; 42: 494-501.

[194] Hwang JT, Ha J, Park OJ. Combination of 5-fluorouracil and genistein induces apoptosis synergistically in chemo-resistant cancer cells through the modulation of AMPK and COX-2 signaling pathways. *Biochem Biophys Res Commun* 2005; 332: 433-40.

[195] Ha J, Zhao L, Zhao Q, Yao J, Zhu BB, Lu N, Ke X, Yang HY, Li Z, You QD, Guo QL. Oroxylin A improves the sensitivity of HT-29 human colon cancer cells to 5-FU through modulation of the COX-2 signaling pathway. *Biochem Cell Biol* 2012; 90: 521-31.

[196] Rebolleda N, Losada-Fernandez I, Perez-Chacon G, Castejon R, Rosado S, Morado M, Vallejo-Cremades MT, Martinez A, Vargas-Nunez JA, Perez-Aciego P. Synergistic activity of deguelin and fludarabine in cells from chronic lymphocytic leukemia patients and in the New Zealand Black murine model. *PLoS One* 2016; 11: e0154159.

[197] Li N, Zhang Z, Jiang G, Sun H, Yu D. Nobiletin sensitizes colorectal cancer cells to oxaliplatin by PI3K/Akt/MTOR pathway. *Front Biosci (Landmark Ed)* 2019; 24: 303-12.

[198] Chen F, Zhuang M, Zhong C, Peng J, Wang X, Li J, Chen Z, Huang Y. Baicalein reverses hypoxia-induced 5-FU resistance in gastric cancer AGS cells through suppression of glycolysis and the PTEN/Akt/HIF-1α signaling pathway. *Oncol Rep* 2015; 33: 457-63.

[199] Jung EU, Yoon JH, Lee YJ, Lee JH, Kim BH, Yu SJ, Myung SJ, Kim YJ, Lee HS. Hypoxia and retinoic acid-inducible NDRG1 expression is responsible for doxorubicin and retinoic acid resistance in hepatocellular carcinoma cells. *Cancer Lett* 2010; 298: 9-15.

[200] Li Y, Huang X, Huang Z, Feng J. Phenoxodiol enhances the antitumor activity of gemcitabine in gallbladder cancer through suppressing Akt/mTOR pathway. *Cell Biochem Biophys* 2014; 70: 1337-42.

[201] Shi H, Wu Y, Wang Y, Zhou M, Yan S, Chen Z, Gu D, Cai Y. Liquiritigenin potentiates the inhibitory effects of cisplatin on invasion and metastasis via downregulation of MMP-2/9 and PI3K/AKT signaling pathway in B16F10 melanoma cells and mice model. *Nutr Cancer* 2015; 67: 761-70.

[202] Bortul R, Tazzari PL, Billi AM, Tabellini G, Mantovani I, Cappellini A, Grafone T, Martinelli G, Conte R, Martelli AM. Deguelin, a PI3K/AKT inhibitor, enhances chemosensitivity of leukaemia cells with an active PI3K/AKT pathway. *Br J Haematol* 2005; 129: 677-86.

[203] Wang P, Henning SM, Heber D, Vadgama JV. Sensitization of docetaxel in prostate cancer cells by green tea and quercetin. *J Nutr Biochem* 2015; 26: 408-15.

[204] Arafa el-SA, Zhu Q, Barakat BM, Wani G, Zhao Q, El-Mahdy MA, Wani AA. Tangeretin sensitizes cisplatin-resistant human ovarian cancer cells through downregulation of phosphoinositide 3-kinase/Akt signaling pathway. *Cancer Res* 2009; 69: 8910-7.

[205] Kuhar M, Imran S, Singh N. Curcumin and quercetin combined with cisplatin to induce apoptosis in human laryngeal carcinoma Hep-2 cells through the mitochondrial pathway. *J Cancer Mol* 2007; 3: 121-8.

[206] Wang G, Zhang D, Yang S, Wang Y, Tang Z, Fu X. Co-administration of genistein with doxorubicin-loaded polypeptide nanoparticles weakens the metastasis of malignant prostate cancer by amplifying oxidative damage. *Biomater Sci* 2018; 6: 827-35.

[207] Hörmann V, Kumi-Diaka J, Durity M, Rathinavelu A. Anticancer activities of genistein-topotecan combination in prostate cancer cells. *J Cell Mol Med* 2012; 16: 2631-6.

[208] Hu XY, Liang JY, Guo XJ, Liu L, Guo YB. 5-Fluorouracil combined with apigenin enhances anticancer activity through mitochondrial membrane potential ($\Delta\Psi$m)-mediated apoptosis in hepatocellular carcinoma. *Clin Exp Pharmacol Physiol* 2015; 42: 146-53.

[209] Kim EH, Jang H, Shin D, Baek SH, Roh JL. Targeting Nrf2 with wogonin overcomes cisplatin resistance in head and neck cancer. *Apoptosis* 2016; 21: 1265-78.

[210] Kachadourian R, Leitner HM, Day BJ. Selected flavonoids potentiate the toxicity of cisplatin in human lung adenocarcinoma cells: a role for glutathione depletion. *Int J Oncol* 2007; 31: 161-8.

[211] Xu Y, Xin Y, Diao Y, Lu C, Fu J, Luo L, Yin Z. Synergistic effects of apigenin and paclitaxel on apoptosis of cancer cells. *PLoS One* 2011; 6: e29169.

[212] Qian C, Wang Y, Zhong Y, Tang J, Zhang J, Li Z, Wang Q, Hu R. Wogonin-enhanced reactive oxygen species-induced apoptosis and potentiated cytotoxic effects of chemotherapeutic agents by suppression Nrf2-mediated signaling in HepG2 cells. *Free Radic Res* 2014; 48: 607-21.

[213] Chan MM, Soprano KJ, Weinstein K, Fong D. Epigallocatechin-3-gallate delivers hydrogen peroxide to induce death of ovarian cancer cells and enhances their cisplatin susceptibility. *J Cell Physiol* 2006; 207: 389-96.

[214] Kim EH, Jang H, Roh JL. A novel polyphenol conjugate sensitizes cisplatin-resistant head and neck cancer cells to cisplatin via Nrf2 inhibition. *Mol Cancer Ther* 2016; 15: 2620-9.

[215] Akbas SH, Timur M, Ozben T. The effect of quercetin on topotecan cytotoxicity in MCF-7 and MDA-MB 231 human breast cancer cells. *J Surg Res* 2005; 125: 49-55.

[216] Meng L, Xia X, Yang Y, Ye J, Dong W, Ma P, Jin Y, Liu Y. Co-encapsulation of paclitaxel and baicalein in nanoemulsions to overcome multidrug resistance via oxidative stress augmentation and P-glycoprotein inhibition. *Int J Pharm* 2016; 513: 8-16.

[217] Chang YF, Chi CW, Wang JJ. Reactive oxygen species production is involved in quercetin-induced apoptosis in human hepatoma cells. *Nutr Cancer* 2006; 55: 201-9.

[218] Li N, Sun C, Zhou B, Xing H, Ma D, Chen G, Weng D. Low concentration of quercetin antagonizes the cytotoxic effects of anti-neoplastic drugs in ovarian cancer. *PLoS One* 2014; 9: e100314.

[219] Hou X, Bai X, Gou X, Zeng H, Xia C, Zhuang W, Chen X, Zhao Z, Huang M, Jin J. 3`,4`,5`,5,7-pentamethoxyflavone sensitizes Cisplatin-resistant A549 cells to Cisplatin by inhibition of Nrf2 pathway. *Mol Cells* 2015; 38: 396-401.

[220] Lim J, Lee SH, Cho S, Lee IS, Kang BY, Choi HJ. 4-methoxychalcone enhances cisplatin-induced oxidative stress and cytotoxicity by inhibiting the Nrf2/ARE-mediated defense mechanism in A549 lung cancer cells. *Mol Cells* 2013; 36: 340-6.

[221] Tang X, Wang H, Fan L, Wu X, Xin A, Ren H, Wang XJ. Luteolin inhibits Nrf2 leading to negative regulation of the Nrf2/ARE pathway and sensitization of human lung carcinoma A549 cells to therapeutic drugs. *Free Radic Biol Med* 2011; 50: 1599-609.

[222] Sabzichi M, Hamishehkar H, Ramezani F, Sharifi S, Tabasinezhad M, Pirouzpanah M, Ghanbari P, Samadi N. Luteolin-loaded phytosomes sensitize human breast carcinoma MDA-MB 231 cells to doxorubicin by suppressing Nrf2 mediated signalling. *Asian Pac J Cancer Prev* 2014; 15: 5311-6.

[223] Zhong Y, Zhang F, Sun Z, Zhou W, Li ZY, You QD, Guo QL, Hu R. Drug resistance associates with activation of Nrf2 in MCF-7/DOX cells, and wogonin reverses it by down-regulating Nrf2-mediated cellular defense response. *Mol Carcinog* 2013; 52: 824-34.

[224] Sharma A, Upadhyay AK, Bhat MK. Inhibition of Hsp27 and Hsp40 potentiates 5-fluorouracil and carboplatin mediated cell killing in hepatoma cells. *Cancer Biol Ther* 2009; 8: 2106-13.

[225] Chen SF, Nieh S, Jao SW, Liu CL, Wu CH, Chang YC, Yang CY, Lin YS. Quercetin suppresses drug-resistant spheres via the p38 MAPK-Hsp27 apoptotic pathway in oral cancer cells. *PLoS One* 2012; 7: e49275.

[226] Zanini C, Giribaldi G, Madili G, Carta F, Crescenzio N, Bisaro B, Doria A, Foglia L, di Montezemolo LC, Timeus F, Turrini F. Inhibition of heat shock proteins

(HSP) expression by quercetin and differential doxorubicin sensitization in neuroblastoma and Ewing`s sarcoma cell lines. *J Neurochem* 2007; 103: 1344-54.

[227] Jakubowicz-Gil J, Paduch R, Piersiak T, Glowniak K, Gawron A, Kandefer-Szerszen M. The effect of quercetin on pro-apoptotic activity of cisplatin in HeLa cells. *Biochem Pharmacol* 2005; 69: 1343-50.

[228] Sang DP, Li RJ, Lan Q. Quercetin sensitizes human glioblastoma cells to temozolomide in vitro via inhibition of Hsp27. *Acta Pharmacol Sin* 2014; 35: 832-8.

[229] Ermakova SP, Kang BS, Choi BY, Choi HS, Schuster TF, Ma WY, Bode AM, Dong Z. (-)-Epigallocatechin gallate overcomes resistance to etoposide-induced cell death by targeting the molecular chaperone glucose-regulated protein 78. *Cancer Res* 2006; 66: 9260-9.

[230] Luo T, Wang J, Yin Y, Hua H, Jing J, Sun X, Li M, Zhang Y, Jiang Y. (-)-Epigallocatechin gallate sensitizes breast cancer cells to paclitaxel in a murine model of breast carcinoma. *Breast Cancer Res* 2010; 12: R8.

[231] Wang N, Wang Z, Peng C, You J, Shen J, Han S, Chen J. Dietary compound isoliquiritigenin targets GRP78 to chemosensitize breast cancer stem cells via β-catenin/ABCG2 signaling. *Carcinogenesis* 2014; 35: 2544-54.

[232] Lim HA, Kim JH, Kim JH, Sung MK, Kim MK, Park JH, Kim JS. Genistein induces glucose-regulated protein 78 in mammary tumor cells. *J Med Food* 2006; 9: 28-32.

[233] Lu C, Wang H, Chen S, Yang R, Li H, Zhang G. Baicalein inhibits cell growth and increases cisplatin sensitivity of A549 and H460 cells via miR-424-3p and targeting PTEN/PI3K/Akt pathway. *J Cell Mol Med* 2018; 22: 2478-87.

[234] Zhou DH, Wang X, Feng Q. EGCG enhances the efficacy of cisplatin by downregulating hsa-miR-98-5p in NSCLC A549 cells. *Nutr Cancer* 2014; 66: 636-44.

[235] Li B, Jin X, Meng H, Hu B, Zhang T, Yu J, Chen S, Guo X, Wang W, Jiang W, Wang J. Morin promotes prostate cancer cells chemosensitivity to paclitaxel through miR-155/GATA3 axis. *Oncotarget* 2017; 8: 47849-60.

[236] Wen D, Peng Y, Lin F, Singh RK, Mahato RI. Micellar delivery of miR-34a modulator rubone and paclitaxel in resistant prostate cancer. *Cancer Res* 2017; 77: 3244-54.

[237] Ghasemi S, Lorigooini Z, Wibowo J, Amini-Khoei H. Tricin isolated from Allium atroviolaceum potentiated the effect of docetaxel on PC3 cell proliferation: role of miR-21. *Nat Prod Res* 2019; 33: 1828-31.

[238] Huang W, Wan C, Luo Q, Huang Z, Luo Q. Genistein-inhibited cancer stem cell-like properties and reduced chemoresistance of gastric cancer. *Int J Mol Sci* 2014; 15: 3432-43.

[239] Molavi O, Samadi N, Wu C, Lavasanifar A, Lai R. Silibinin suppresses NPM-ALK, potently induces apoptosis and enhances chemosensitivity in ALK-positive anaplastic large cell lymphoma. *Leuk Lymphoma* 2016; 57: 1154-62.

[240] Solomon LA, Ali S, Banerjee S, Munkarah AR, Morris RT, Sarkar FH. Sensitization of ovarian cancer cells to cisplatin by genistein: the role of NF-kappaB. *J Ovarian Res* 2008; 1: 9.

[241] Lee SH, Nam HJ, Kang HJ, Kwon HW, Lim YC. Epigallocatechin-3-gallate attenuates head and neck cancer stem cell traits through suppression of Notch pathway. *Eur J Cancer* 2013; 49: 3210-8.

[242] Hu FW, Yu CC, Hsieh PL, Liao YW, Lu MY, Chu PM. Targeting oral cancer stemness and chemoresistance by isoliquiritigenin-mediated GRP78 regulation. *Oncotarget* 2017; 8: 93912-23.

Chapter 5

PLANT FLAVONOIDS: THEIR NATURAL SOURCES, BIOAVAILABILITY AND ANTICANCER PROPERTIES

Due to several impediments of conventional chemotherapy, i.e., poor efficacy and adverse side effects, considerable attention has been focused on identification of naturally occurring bioactive molecules and their related synthetic analogues to prevent the development and progression of cancer without harming normal healthy tissues [1-15]. It has been indeed suggested that a large number of products from natural sources, dietary or non-dietary, hold the ability to induce death in diverse malignant cells from different human cancer types, whereas almost all stages of tumorigenesis can be affected by agents and extracts derived from various medicinal plants [1, 3, 6, 16-20].

The use of natural products as therapeutic agents has a very long history, especially in the traditional medicine in Asian countries [15, 21-26]. Isolation and characterization of novel bioactive substances from natural sources have been continued up to date within different drug discovery and drug development programs. As a result, more than 60% of all anticancer drugs approved for clinical use between 1982 and 2006 are either natural products or their semisynthetic derivatives [1, 18, 21, 25, 27-32]. For instance, camptothecin, paclitaxel, and vinca alkaloids vinblastine and vincristine are all originally obtained from plants, highlighting the crucial role of phytochemicals in development of anticancer drugs [3, 24, 26, 33, 34]. Nature has a great potential to provide scientists with a source of structures, on which basis most of the current cytotoxic anticancer drugs have been synthesized and probably will be produced also in the future [25]. Natural products are an inexhaustible resource not only for new structurally unique compounds but also agents with novel action mechanisms [35]. Moreover, phytochemicals may play important roles also in modulating the efficacy of existing therapies, in combination with standard drugs, to exhibit additive or synergistic therapeutic efficacies [3, 25, 36-38]. Therefore, investigation of natural compounds has gained several new insights and still represents a promising strategy for identification of novel potent therapeutic agents for clinical management of malignant disorders in the future, thereby limiting the global cancer burden. To be successful, these studies must be intensified [3, 13, 21, 39-42].

5.1. PLANT FLAVONOIDS AND THEIR STRUCTURAL DIVERSITY

Flavonoids are a large group of low molecular weight polyphenolic compounds synthesized by plants to provide bright colors to flowers and fruits, but also to protect plants against pathogen assaults and ultraviolet radiation [25, 43-46]. These plant secondary metabolites are regularly ingested by humans in significant quantities because of their abundant distribution in diverse plant-derived foods, such as fruits, vegetables, seeds, grains, spices, nuts, honey, natural beverages like tea, wine and juice, but also medicinal herbs and herbal supplements [1, 6, 7, 47-54]. Although flavonoids are considered as nonessential dietary factors, they are bioactive food components with various health benefits [55, 56]. Based on estimation of nutritionists, the average intake of flavonoids by humans in a normal diet is rather variable, being mostly about 1 gram per day [52, 56-60]. In addition, a number of flavonoids-containing dietary supplements and herbal products are nowadays available in the market and ingested in large quantities by both healthy individuals but also cancer patients in the form of complementary therapy [60-62].

The common structure of flavonoids, i.e., the flavan nucleus (C6-C3-C6), consists of two aromatic rings (A and B) linked through three carbon atoms heterocyclic ring C that is an oxygen containing pyran ring [15, 46, 61, 63-65] (Figure 5.1). Various substitutions on the basic skeleton are responsible for a great diversity of flavonoids in the nature; there are more than 8000 structurally different flavonoids described so far [61, 66-69]. At that, hydroxyl groups at the backbone generally increase the solubility of flavonoids, whereas methoxyl groups facilitate their permeability through cell membrane [70]. According to the structural peculiarities, especially variations in the hydroxylation pattern and different substitutions in the ring C, flavonoids are divided into six major subclasses: flavones, flavonols, flavanones, flavanols or catechins, isoflavones and anthocyanidins [2, 44, 46, 61, 65, 68, 71-74] (Figure 5.1). Chalcones as open-chain flavonoids are natural precursors for biosynthesis of flavonoids in plants [75-77].

Over the past decades, flavonoids have attracted significant scientific and therapeutic interest because of their diverse beneficial biological properties and promising health-promoting activities in humans. These compounds exert antioxidant, antibacterial, antiviral, antifungal, anti-inflammatory, anti-aging, anti-allergic, immunostimulatory, antidiabetic, antithrombotic, antiatherogenic, hypolipidemic, neuroprotective, hepatoprotective, nephroprotective, cardioprotective, analgesic and antipyretic effects, and have been also proposed as potential chemopreventive agents to suppress, prevent or reverse carcinogenesis [7, 37, 46-48, 57, 58, 71, 78-88]. Indeed, numerous epidemiological studies have confirmed the risk-lowering action of various flavonoids against different human cancer types in diverse populations [37, 89-93]. At that, biological effects and physiological activities of flavonoids largely depend on both their chemical structure as well as target cell types [46]. Therefore, flavonoids constitute a promising research direction for further treating the malignant neoplasms [94].

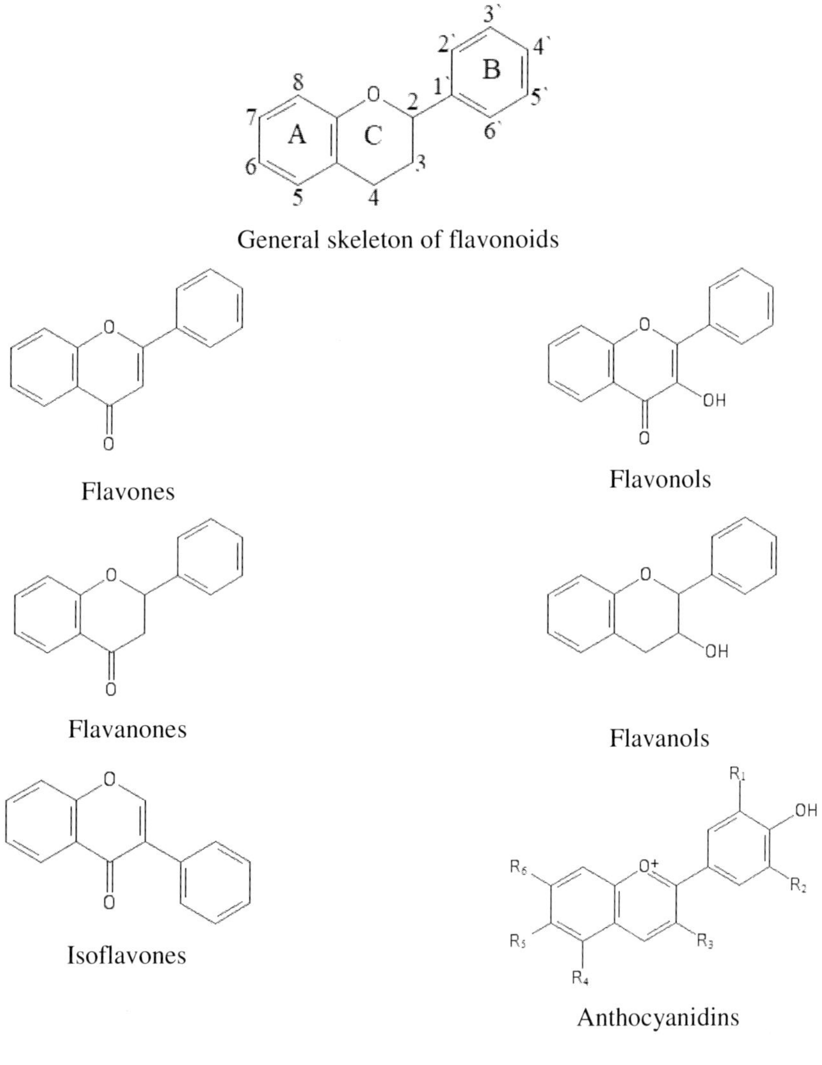

General skeleton of flavonoids

Flavones

Flavonols

Flavanones

Flavanols

Isoflavones

Anthocyanidins

Figure 5.1. Basic structure and classification of flavonoids.

5.2. NATURAL SOURCES OF THE MOST COMMON FLAVONOIDS

Flavonoids like apigenin, luteolin, quercetin, kaempferol, fisetin and myricetin are abundantly present in diverse fruits and vegetables being thus widely consumed by humans as an integral part of everyday diet. Flavonoids can be commonly found also in various medicinal herbs and different dietary supplements, such as green tea extracts, Ginkgo biloba, milk thistle, and soy isoflavones [52]. A concise overview about the major natural sources of most important flavonoids is presented in Table 5.1.

Quercetin is a ubiquitous flavonoid (flavonol) in normal human diet, found in a wide range of fruits and vegetables, with an estimated daily intake ranging from 4 to 68 mg (on the average of 25-30 mg) [6, 64, 65, 69, 95-103]. It is one of the most abundant dietary flavonoids, whereas its richest sources include onions (841 mg/kg in onion leaves, 50 mg/kg in white onion bulb) and apples (250 mg/kg in apple skin) [98, 104-106]. In fact, quercetin constitutes about 99% of total flavonoids found in apple peel [107, 108]. Currently, quercetin is available also in formulation of numerous dietary supplements purported to improve the general health and well-being [107, 109].

Catechins or flavanols are the main polyphenolic constituents of green tea leaves, including catechin, epicatechin (EC), epigallocatechin (EGC), epicatechin 3-gallate (ECG) and epigallocatechin 3-gallate (EGCG) [110-112]. The potential health benefits gained from consuming green tea and green tea extracts are often attributed to its most abundant and bioactive component, EGCG [40, 84, 113-115]. Actually, EGCG accounts for 10-15% of the total green tea, more than 40% of the total polyphenol mixture and about 80% of all catechins in green tea [42, 116, 117]. A cup of green tea prepared from 2.5 g of dried leaves may contain approximately 90 mg EGCG [106].

Genistein has attracted a wide interest because of its main natural origin, soybeans [28, 118-120]. This isoflavone is rich in traditional Asian diets containing plenty of soy products, such as miso or tofu [121]. The average daily intake of genistein in Asian countries is about 1.5-4.1 mg being significantly higher than the average consumption of soy isoflavones in Western Europe and the United States [120]. Genistein was first isolated from dyer's broom already in 1899 [122, 123] and is nowadays one of the most abundantly consumed flavonoids. In addition to food items, several preparations containing soy isoflavones are currently available in market as dietary supplements, such as Novasoy that is rich in genistein and another isoflavone, daidzein [124].

Silibinin, also known as silybin, is a flavonolignan derived from the seeds of milk thistle and is a major bioactive constituent of silymarin, a standardized milk thistle extract [21, 125-133]. Milk thistle has been used in traditional medicine already from ancient times and is today a popular dietary supplement widely consumed for treatment of liver diseases [12, 21, 132, 134-138]. Moreover, silymarin has been reported to be one of the most frequently used herbal preparations by cancer patients, on their own accord [130].

Many bioactive flavones have been derived also from the root of Baikal skullcap, including baicalein, baicalin, wogonin and oroxylin A [23, 139-142]. This herb has been widely used in traditional Chinese medicine for treatment of different conditions, including inflammatory and cancerous diseases [13, 79, 140, 143, 144]. Another valuable natural source containing a high spectrum of bioactive flavonoids is the plant genus

Table 5.1. Major natural sources of most important flavonoids

Flavonoid	Natural/dietary sources	Ref.
ANTHOCYANIDINS		
Pelargonidin	Berries	[44]
Malvidin	Berries and fruits, especially pomegranate	[44]
CHALCONES		
2`,4`-Dihydroxy-6`-methoxy-3`,5`-dimethylchalcone (DMC)	Buds of *Cleistocalyx operculatus* (Roxb.) Merr. et L.M.Perry	[216, 258, 302, 303]
Flavokawain B (FKB)	Kava root. *Alpinia pricei* Hayata	[30]
Isoliquiritigenin (ISL)	Shallot, bean sprouts. Root and stem of licorice species *Glycyrrhiza glabra* L., *Glycyrrhiza uralensis* Fisch. ex DC. and *Glycyrrhiza inflata* Bat.; *Spatholobus suberectus* Dunn	[18, 145, 146, 148, 210, 304]
Licochalcone A (LCA)	Root and rhizome of licorice species *Glycyrrhiza uralensis* Fisch. ex DC. and *Glycyrrhiza glabra* L.	[9, 145]
Phloretin	Apple, pear	[305]
FLAVANOLS		
Catechin	Green tea	[71]
Epicatechin (EC)	Cocoa, cacao beans, dark chocolate; green tea	[306, 307]
Epicatechin 3-gallate (ECG)	Green tea	[112, 307]
Epigallocatechin (EGC)	Green tea	[307]
Epigallocatechin 3-gallate (EGCG)	Green tea, green tea extracts	[40, 42, 84, 106, 112-117, 169, 212, 213, 253, 264, 307-313]
FLAVANONES		
Alpinetin	Zingiberaceous plants, such as *Alpinia katsumadae* Hayata	[220, 314]
Hesperetin	Citrus fruits	[165]
Hesperidin (vitamin P)	Citrus fruits, such as lemons and oranges	[48, 72]
Liquiritigenin	Licorice species *Glycyrrhiza uralensis* Fisch. ex DC.	[94, 147]
Naringenin	Citrus fruits, such as grapefruit	[152, 153]
Naringin	Citrus fruits, such as grapefruit	[154]
FLAVANONOLS		
Ampelopsin (dihydromyricetin, DHM)	Tender stem and leaves of vines *Ampelopsis cantoniensis* (Hook. & Arn.) K.Koch and *Ampelopsis grossedentata* (Hand.-Mazz.) W.T.Wang	[171, 315-317]

Table 5.1. (Continued)

Flavonoid	Natural/dietary sources	Ref.
	FLAVONES	
3',4',5',5,7-Pentamethoxyflavone (3',4',5',5,7-PMF)	Plants from citrus family, such as orange jessamine (*Murraya paniculata* (L.) Jack) and *Neoraputia magnifica* (Engler) M.Emmerich	[318]
Acacetin	Damiana (*Turnera diffusa* Willd. ex Schult.) and black locust (*Robinia pseudoacacia* L.)	[83]
Apigenin	Celery, parsley, tomatoes, beans, wheat sprouts, onions, oranges, grapefruit, red wine, tea, chamomile tea	[49, 162, 176, 265, 319]
Baicalein	Root of Baikal skullcap (*Scutellaria baicalensis* Georgi)	[13, 79, 139, 143, 255, 271, 291, 320-325]
Baicalin	Genus *Scutellaria*, such as Baikal skullcap (*Scutellaria baicalensis* Georgi) and blue skullcap (*Scutellaria lateriflora* L.)	[140, 144, 326]
Chrysin	Bee wax, honey, honeycomb, propolis; fruit skin. Blue passionflower (*Passiflora caerulea* L.)	[51, 87, 170, 249]
Eupatorin	*Salvia mirzayanii* Rech.f. & Esfand.	[7]
Hispidulin	Snow lotus (*Saussurea involucrata* Kar.) and roseleaf sage (*Salvia involucrata* Cav.)	[38, 327]
Luteolin	Celery, parsley, perilla leaf and seeds, rosemary, thyme, peppermint, broccoli, carrots, peppers (green pepper, sweet bell pepper), artichoke, cauliflower, cabbage, spinach, onion leaves, grapefruit, oranges, apple, honey, chamomile tea, pinophyte, pteridophyte, chrysanthemum flowers	[4, 36, 187, 218, 265, 328-331]
Nobiletin	Citrus fruits, such as orange and shiikuwasha (*Citrus depressa* Hayata); peel of mandarins (*Citrus reticulata* Blanco)	[150, 151, 332]
Oroxylin A	Root of Baikal skullcap (*Scutellaria baicalensis* Georgi)	[54, 142, 181, 333-335]
Salvigenin	*Salvia lachnocalyx* Hedge and *Salvia hydrangea* DC. ex Benth.	[7]
Scutellarin	*Erigeron breviscapus* (Vaniot) Hand.-Mazz.	[167]
Tangeretin	Citrus fruits	[149]
Vicenin-2 (VCN-2)	*Ocimum sanctum* Linn. (Tulsi)	[238]
Wogonin	Root of Baikal skullcap (*Scutellaria baicalensis* Georgi)	[141, 187, 203, 251, 269, 336-341]
	FLAVONOLS	
Fisetin	Strawberries, apple, persimmon, grape; onion, cucumber. Parrot tree (*Schotia brachypetala* Sond.), honey locust (*Gleditsia triacanthos* L.), smoke tree (*Cotinus coggygria* Scop.)	[2, 31, 266]
Galangin	Root of greater galangal (*Alpinia galanga* (L.) Willd.)	[222]
Hyperoside	Plants of the genera St. John's wort (*Hypericum*) and hawthorn (*Crataegus*)	[342]
Kaempferol	Vegetables, such as leek and broccoli	[62]
Morin	Figs, almond, sweet chestnut, old fustic. Originally isolated from white mulberry (*Morus alba* L.)	[211, 343]
Myricetin	Parsley, sweet potatoes, broad beans, grapes, oranges, berries, walnuts, red wine	[53, 344]
Quercetin	Celery, onion, kale, tomatoes, broccoli, leek, lettuce, apples (especially apple peel), grapes, lemons, blueberries, cranberries, honey, chamomile tea, red wine	[6, 65, 73, 96-100, 105-109, 156, 172]
Rutin (quercetin 3-rutinoside)	Onion, orange, lemon, apple, green tea	[345]
Troxerutin (TXN)	Japanese pagoda tree (*Sophora japonica* L.)	[346]

Flavonoid	Natural/dietary sources	Ref.
	FLAVONOLIGNANS	
Hydnocarpin	*Brucea javanica* (L.) Merr., *Hydnocarpus wightianus* Blume, *Verbascum sinaiticum* Benth.; species of *Berberis*	[347]
Silibinin (silybin)	Milk thistle seeds (*Silybum marianum* (L.) Gaertn.)	[12, 21, 27, 88, 125, 127-138, 166, 208, 234, 348, 349]
	FLAVONOSTILBENES	
Alopecurone B (ALOB)	*Sophora alopecuroides* L.	[17]
HOMOISOFLAVONOIDS		
Intricatinol (INT)	Root of *Caesalpinia digyna* Rottler	[3]
	ISOFLAVONES	
8-Hydroxydaidzein	Fermented products of soy germ	[350]
Calycosin	Herb Radix Astragali	[351]
Daidzein	Soybeans, soybean products	[153, 286]
Formononetin	Red clover, alfalfa, chick peas. Mongolian milkvetch (*Astragalus membranaceus* (Fisch.) Bunge), Chinese licorice (*Glycyrrhiza uralensis* Fisch. ex DC.)	[19, 352, 353]
Genistein	Soybeans, soybean products (tofu), red clover; fermentation broth of *Pseudomonas* sp. First isolated from dyer`s broom (*Genista tinctoria* L.) in 1899	[28, 118-124, 153, 160, 172, 223, 282-284, 286, 354-359]
Genistin	Soy	[120]
Orobol	*Streptomyces* spp.	[360, 361]
Puerarin	Root of kudzu (*Pueraria lobate* Ohwi)	[362, 363]
	PRENYLATED FLAVONOIDS	
Icariin	Genus *Epimedium*	[11, 41, 230, 364]
Icariside II	Genus *Epimedium*	[41, 268]
Icaritin (ICT)	Genus *Epimedium*	[8, 41, 85]
Isoxanthohumol (IXN)	Hops	[34]
	ROTENOIDS	
Deguelin	*Mundulea sericea* (Willd.) A.Chev., *Tephrosia vogelii* Hook.f., *Derris trifoliata* Lour.	[175, 179]

licorice. Chalcones isoliquiritigenin and licochalcone A as well as flavanone liquiritigenin have been isolated from the root of different licorice species [9, 94, 145-147]. The licorice plant has been used already for more than four millennia as a natural sweetener of foods and beverages, but also as medicinal herb against the different health problems, such as peptic ulcers, hepatitis and lung diseases [9, 145, 148].

In addition, structurally different bioactive flavonoids have been isolated from various citrus fruits. Flavanones hesperetin, hesperidin, naringenin and naringin, and polymethoxylated flavones tangeretin and nobiletin can be all abundantly found in different citrus fruits, including lemons, oranges and grapefruits [48, 72, 149-154].

As flavonoids have been an integral part of everyday diet and consumed as ingredients of medicinal plants already for millennia, the safety profiles of these plant compounds, including quercetin [64, 69, 73, 98, 101, 107, 155, 156], EGCG [84, 115, 157, 158], genistein [159, 160], apigenin [49, 161-164], hesperetin [165], hesperidin [72], naringenin [20], naringin [154], nobiletin [151] and silibinin [128, 132, 133, 135, 166], are empirically approved and confirmed, exerting no or low toxicity in human beings [47, 167]. The pharmacological safety of flavonoids has also been proven in numerous recent clinical trials and toxicological tests making these compounds ideal candidates for novel chemopreventive and anticancer agents [1, 12, 21, 37, 41, 168-171]. This is especially important considering a wide range of toxic side effects related to administration of traditional cytotoxic chemotherapeutic drugs. Moreover, flavonoids-containing natural products are generally also easily available and rather inexpensive [13, 42, 83, 115, 122, 154, 157, 172]. The last argument is crucial considering the fact that most cancer patients are under enormous economic pressure due to the very high cost of standard chemotherapeutic drugs [122]. Furthermore, according to the data of the World Health Organization (WHO), about 80% of people living in rural areas depend on medicinal plants as the primary health care system [26].

5.3. FLAVONOIDS AS POTENTIAL CHEMOTHERAPEUTIC AND CHEMOSENSITIZING AGENTS

5.3.1. Chemotherapeutic Potential of Flavonoids

Increasing evidence over the past few decades suggest that flavonoids exhibit various antitumor activities in cell culture studies and animal models of different human cancer types, including both solid tumors as well as hematological malignancies [4, 13, 135, 146, 173-176]. Flavonoids are able to induce cell cycle arrest, inhibit proliferation and exert proapoptotic action via intrinsic or extrinsic pathway in multiple neoplastic cells, behaving thus as cytotoxic agents [3, 6, 35, 37, 101, 122, 153, 162, 172, 177-185]. In addition, several flavonoids can suppress angiogenesis and metastasis, exert antiinvasive and antimigratory properties [35, 172, 173, 182, 183, 186-191]. Indeed, these phytochemicals have been shown to regulate the activity of matrix metalloproteinases (MMPs), reducing the expression of MMP-2 and/or MMP-9 [44, 168, 173]. Likewise, anti-inflammatory effects of some flavonoids can also contribute to their anticancer efficacy [23, 34, 44, 192]. There are still some controversies concerning the dual action of phytochemicals either as antioxidant or prooxidant agents, as this can essentially impact their functional role in cancer cells [15, 67, 173, 193, 194]. Apparently both flavonoid structure and concentration as well as molecular environment and cellular redox state determine the actual oxidative behavior of certain polyphenolic compounds [50, 75, 104, 193, 195-198]. For instance, EGCG has been shown to behave as antioxidant at low doses, i.e., at high nanomolar and low micromolar concentrations, and to induce generation of reactive oxygen species (ROS) and oxidative stress at higher levels [195, 199]. While antioxidant action of flavonoids has been related to their chemopreventive effects, their prooxidant action can probably induce the death of malignant cells being thus important in chemotherapy context [195, 198]. Overview of multifaceted anticancer properties of flavonoids is presented in Figure 5.2.

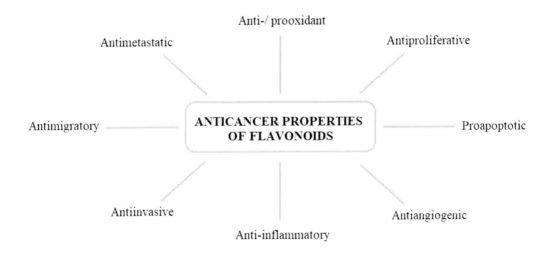

Figure 5.2. Multitargeting action of flavonoids in cancer cells.

The pleiotropic antitumor activities and underlying molecular mechanisms of flavonoids depend largely on differences in their chemical structure but also on types of malignant cells [76, 95, 182, 200]. Moreover, due to natural origin and safety of flavonoids, they usually selectively affect only cancer cells, with no obvious toxicity towards normal healthy tissues [3, 33, 44, 141, 186, 196, 201, 202]. Considering that development of effective anticancer therapy with negligible adverse effects is an important research direction in healthcare studies all over the world, flavonoids can be

98   Katrin Sak

regarded as ideal candidates for novel chemotherapeutic drugs for treatment of diverse human malignancies [5, 15, 200, 201, 203-206].

5.3.2. Flavonoids as Chemosensitizing Agents

Since chemoresistance is one of the most important hurdles in current cancer treatment resulting in tumor recurrence and poor clinical prognosis, extensive studies have focused on discovery of natural bioactive compounds with known action mechanisms to overcome multidrug resistance (MDR) phenotype [1, 67, 71, 205, 207-210]. Accordingly, a growing interest has been paid to flavonoids, which could sensitize malignant cells to standard chemotherapeutics and augment their cytotoxic activity in a broad spectrum of cancer types in order to achieve better clinical responses [43, 149, 187, 211-215]. At that, both their own anticancer properties as well as general safety profile and tolerability of flavonoids may contribute to increased cytotoxic activity and therapeutic benefits when co-administered with drugs approved for clinical use. Indeed, due to the presence in normal human diet and herbal medicines, flavonoids are generally safe and associated with low toxicity [172, 209, 216-218]. On the other hand, due to the extensive dietary intake of flavonoids by humans, it is crucial to know the potential effects of these phytochemicals on the efficacy of chemotherapeutic treatment [60, 219].

Several recent studies have revealed that a number of flavonoids may act in cooperation or in synergy with certain chemotherapeutic agents in different types of cancer cells, being active both in sensitive as well as resistant cells, enhancing the overall antitumor efficacy and sometimes even reversing cancer cell resistance to conventional drugs, with the ultimate goal to eradicate tumors [2, 21, 49, 53, 63, 65, 78, 96, 104, 119, 122, 141, 174, 207, 213, 219-228]. Moreover, such combinatorial therapy may allow to use reduced drug dosages to maintain therapeutic efficacy and thereby minimize systemic toxicity and decrease deleterious and undesirable side effects associated with application of chemotherapeutic agents, implying improved quality of life of patients [3, 11, 28, 44, 63, 78, 87, 107, 119, 120, 176, 198, 207, 229, 230]. Therefore, plant-derived flavonoids have been proposed as potentially valuable adjuvants for cancer chemotherapy. However, differently from chemopreventive and also chemotherapeutic action of flavonoids, their use as MDR modulators and chemosensitizers is still a recent, innovative and fast-growing discipline currently under intensive exploration [15, 35, 63, 223, 231, 232].

As described in the Chapter 4, cancer chemoresistance is a complex phenomenon, comprising multiple cellular mechanisms all contributing to lowered clinical response to different conventional drugs. Combinatorial studies with flavonoids have revealed modulation of various intracellular targets and regulation of different signaling pathways by these phytochemicals, thereby sensitizing tumor cells to cytotoxic agents currently used in clinical practice [35, 46, 64, 73, 98, 156, 232-235]. In fact, flavonoids can increase the chemosensitivity of drugs by suppressing proliferation and potentiating tumor cell killing through inducing apoptosis and/or activating alternative signaling pathways related to cell death [7, 12, 31, 35, 143, 169, 172, 198, 236, 237], modulating metabolism and biodistribution of chemotherapeutics [34, 209, 232, 238], affecting the expression of drug targets in cancer cells, or regulating different cellular cascades involved in cancer cell survival and drug resistance mechanisms [35, 195, 232]. Indeed, several flavonoids have been reported to be able to inhibit phosphoinositide 3-kinase (PI3K)/protein kinase B (Akt) pathway and suppress nuclear factor-κB (NF-κB) activity resulting in downregulation of respective gene products and thereby improving efficacy of chemotherapeutic drugs [15, 46, 72, 159, 195, 230, 239-242]. In addition, some flavonoids have been reported as potent nuclear factor (erythroid-derived 2)-like 2 (Nrf2) inhibitors, also reversing resistance of cancer cells to antineoplastic drugs [100, 170, 187, 217, 218, 243]. Certain plant flavonoids have been shown to behave as suppressors of epidermal growth factor receptor (EGFR) activation [121, 244, 245], downregulators of different heat shock proteins (Hsps) [246-248] or inhibitors of proteasome [46], thus contributing to their chemosensitizing activity. Also, repressive effect of flavonoids on cancer stem cells (CSCs) has been described [43, 210].

Last but not least, flavonoids can modulate ABC transporters, i.e., inhibit P-glycoprotein (P-gp), multidrug resistance-associated proteins (MRPs) 1 and 2, and breast cancer resistance protein (BCRP), by a number of different ways to reduce the efflux and increase intracellular accumulation of different chemotherapeutic drugs in cancer cells, thereby serving as promising MDR reversing agents [17, 61, 152, 249-258]. Indeed, due to their low toxicity and well tolerability in human beings, natural products have been proposed as potential candidates for fourth generation P-gp inhibitors [256, 259], whereas the effects produced by some of these compounds have been shown to be even comparable to those of the first generation P-gp inhibitors like verapamil and cyclosporin A [74]. Flavonoids are able to regulate the cell surface expression, posttranslational modification and transport function of ABC transporters [17, 74, 106, 109, 151, 249, 250, 259-261]. The latter event can be achieved through an inhibitory effect of these phytochemicals on ATPase activity by interaction with nucleotide binding domains of efflux pumps [73, 74, 249, 250]. In addition, certain flavonoids can directly interact with substrate binding site and competitively inhibit ABC transporters functioning [73, 249]. All these mechanisms make an essential contribution to chemosensitization of tumor cells towards conventional chemotherapeutic agents by different plant flavonoids, exhibiting a potential clinical importance and representing as possible lead compounds for novel MDR modulators. At that, structurally diverse flavonoids interact rather differently with ABC transporters and certain structural requirements are necessary for effective suppression of P-gp action by flavonoids. As chalcones, flavonols and flavones have been reported to be the most active P-gp inhibitors, isoflavones and flavanones usually reveal significantly lower binding affinity to P-gp efflux pump [54, 74, 259]. Furthermore, the inhibitory effects of methoxylated flavones on P-gp function have been suggested to be related to the number of methoxyl groups on their skeleton [262].

Altogether, considering the ability of plant flavonoids to simultaneously affect multiple signaling pathways and exhibit pleiotropic molecular effects, they are suitable candidates to serve as partners for traditional chemotherapeutic agents to overcome drug resistance in many human tumor types, providing a novel promising strategy for improving clinical outcome of cancer treatment [7, 35, 49, 98, 107, 174, 263]. However, few recent studies have revealed that besides various beneficial effects exerted by flavonoids when co-administered with conventional chemotherapeutic drugs, these plant metabolites might also exert unfavorable detrimental activities in certain combinations and specific malignant cell types, resulting in attenuated therapeutic efficacy and promoting tumor progression [15, 66, 195, 198, 264]. Such undesirable activities may proceed from strong antioxidant properties of flavonoids as most chemotherapeutic drugs mediate their cytotoxic effects through prooxidant action [66, 103, 265] or activation instead of inhibiting P-gp mediated drug transport, thereby increasing drug resistance in certain biological systems [261]. One of the important factors determining such negative effects can probably include concentrations of interacting compounds. Hence, flavonoids might impact the efficacy of clinically used antineoplastic agents synergistically, additively or antagonistically [66, 110, 172, 238], whereas adverse interactions between flavonoids and drugs are of particular concern for patients consuming high levels of flavonoids containing food products, affecting the course of chemotherapeutic treatment and clinical outcome. Therefore, the Chapter 6 of this book is devoted to specific interactions between structurally diverse flavonoids and different chemotherapeutic cytotoxic drugs in a wide range of studied cancer cell types, with the aim to present desired favorable combinations but also to highlight undesired antagonistic co-effects which should be avoided by patients to not militate against their clinical treatment and achieve the best therapeutic outcome. Although increasing evidence suggest that flavonoids could be used also for protection of normal cells from therapy-associated toxicities and drug-induced damage [65, 110, 209, 266], this issue is out of focus in the current book.

Therefore, finding of appropriate flavonoid combinations is an important goal for complementary treatment of specific cancer types, whereas this approach could supposedly lead to a breakthrough in clinical management of malignant disorders in the future [15, 117, 172, 174, 215, 267-269].

5.4. METABOLIC CONVERSION OF FLAVONOIDS IN THE HUMAN BODY

Despite promising results on multifaceted anticancer action of flavonoids described *in vitro* cell culture and *in vivo* animal models, none of these agents have reached the actual clinical application to treat patients so far, being lost in translation [15, 127]. Reasons behind this situation include poor aqueous solubility, low stability in body fluids, low oral bioavailability, and fast and extensive metabolic conversion of flavonoids before entering systemic circulation [15, 47, 51, 61, 70, 109, 128, 160, 190, 218, 226, 270-274]. In addition, poor permeability across the cells also restricts the use of these plant polyphenols in current therapeutic protocols [100, 168, 218]. In plant-based food items, flavonoids are prevalently present in the form of different glycosides which pass through the small intestine and are hydrolyzed by intestinal enzymes and enterobacteria to the respective aglycones before their absorption into epithelial cells of the intestinal tract [46, 55, 64, 65, 69, 74, 120, 154]. Thereafter, flavonoids undergo a rapid and extensive metabolic conversion in the small intestine and the liver to various methylated, sulfated and glucuronidated conjugates, which reach the bloodstream [1, 46, 65, 78]. As a result, only minimal amounts of parent flavonoids and considerably higher levels of their metabolites can be detected in the plasma, whereas the possible bioactivity of metabolic conjugates is still only scarcely known [64, 78, 169, 238, 275]. It is believed that free hydroxyl moieties on polyphenolic backbone are one of the major reasons of low bioavailability, being subject to extensive phase II conjugation. Indeed, methylated flavonoids with blocked hydroxyl groups are generally considered to have improved pharmacokinetic properties compared to parental compounds [61, 276]. Flavonoids have been found in a wide range of human tissues, including lungs, testes, prostate, breast, kidneys, heart and liver, suggesting that these phytochemicals can affect various physiological and pathophysiological processes [57]. Moreover, as small molecules, they are able to cross even the blood-brain barrier [277]. Flavonoids are mainly excreted from the body through the biliary system and to a less extent, also via urinary elimination. In the colon, flavonoids are degraded by microbes to phenolic acids which further undergo fecal excretion [64, 65, 128]. The simplified scheme depicting metabolic conversion of flavonoids in the human body is presented in Figure 5.3.

Due to an extensive metabolism, the plasma concentrations of different flavonoids upon ingestion of plant-based foods commonly remain rather low, in the nanomolar or lower micromolar range, revealing also some interindividual variations in dosages, absorption and conversion. For instance, baseline levels of quercetin usually vary between 50 and 80 nM [78]. According to a recent study with healthy volunteers supplemented with 50, 100 or 150 mg/day of quercetin administered per oral route for 2 weeks, plasma levels of this flavonol were measured to be 145 nM, 217 nM and 380 nM, respectively [103]. After supplementation with over 1 g/day of quercetin for 4 weeks, the baseline concentration increased to 1.5 µM [78]. From a daily dose of 1.5 g, serum concentrations of 10 µM have been attained [98]. Moreover, following an intravenous infusion of 100 mg quercetin, plasma doses up to 12 µM have been reported without any obvious side effects [278-281]. Likewise, the highest achievable blood levels of genistein after intake of diets rich in soy and soy products remain below 10 µM, reaching maximally 4-5 µM [121, 282-284]. Based on a series of human trials, steady state plasma concentrations of isoflavones (genistein and daidzein) between 3 and 6 µM have been reported following feeding of 4 months old infants with soy-based milk formulas [285, 286]. Somewhat higher levels can be attained with dietary supplements. While the mean blood concentrations of genistein in human volunteers ingesting 240 mg of this isoflavone for 2 weeks were about 0.66 µM, the plasma levels of 9.2-10 µM have been measured in prostate cancer patients after taking genistein supplements at a dose of 600 mg daily [223]. Plasma concentrations of EGCG observed after drinking several cups of tea or receiving an oral dose of green tea extracts remain in the range of about 0.2-2 µM [111, 287-289]. In fact, maximal serum concentrations of EGCG were reported to be 1.7 µM after an oral intake of one polyphenon E tablet (a green tea extract containing 400 mg of EGCG) by healthy human volunteers [110]. Similarly, the mean peak plasma levels of hesperetin were detected around 2.7 µM after administering a single oral dose of 135 mg hesperetin to healthy adults [165] and plasma levels of apigenin as low as about 0.12 µM were measured following intake of 2 g blanched parsley per kilogram of body weight of healthy subjects [290].

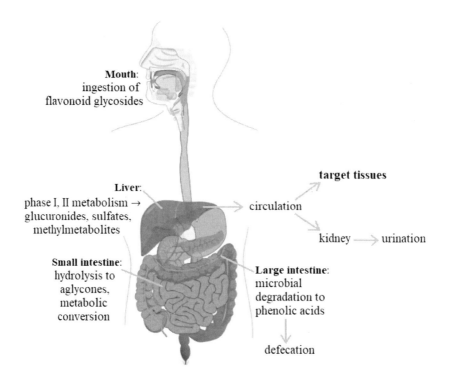

Figure 5.3. Metabolic conversion of flavonoids in the human body.

Overall, the doses of flavonoids at which their pleiotropic anticancer activities have been described in numerous *in vitro* and *in vivo* experiments commonly remain in the range over 10-20 µM, being much higher than the levels achievable via the normal human diet [39, 54, 71, 98, 103, 107, 121, 205, 227, 240, 290, 291]. Thus, ingestion of flavonoids may not provide the concentrations required for their anticancer efficacy at the site of action and thereby may not justify the use of dietary flavonoids as sole chemotherapeutic agents for treatment of different types of human cancers [158, 205, 275, 285, 286, 292]. Nevertheless, these low concentrations may still be sufficient to achieve significant synergistic cytotoxic effects on certain malignant cells when combined with conventional chemotherapeutic drugs [285, 286]. Therefore, it is reasonable to think that the main role of flavonoids can be to augment the therapeutic efficacy of standard antineoplastic agents used in clinical settings. Last but not least, the current knowledge about the actual doses of flavonoids in specific tissues is still limited as conjugated metabolites might be converted back to the bioactive aglycone forms in the target cancerous cells [153, 223].

The successful application of flavonoids in the clinical settings still awaits strategies to circumvent low bioavailability issue and develop efficient drug delivery systems. Therefore, further studies are highly needed to attain and maintain the effective therapeutic concentrations of flavonoids in tumor cells [51, 190]. One way to achieve this goal is to increase the stability and bioavailability of natural flavonoids via synthetic modifications. In this regard, a prodrug of EGCG has been developed by protecting its reactive hydroxyl groups by peracetate moieties [293]. Another attractive possibility comprises implementation of nanotechnological strategy.

5.5. NANOTECHNOLOGICAL APPROACH TO OVERCOME THE CURRENT LIMITATIONS FOR THERAPEUTIC USE OF FLAVONOIDS

Recent studies have shown that bioavailability and effectiveness of different flavonoids might be enhanced by encapsulating them in nanoparticles, thus improving the potential clinical application [3, 57, 144, 264, 294]. Such innovative nanotechnological approach exhibits several unique advantages, such as high drug loading for poorly soluble agents, improvement of pharmacokinetic parameters by controlled drug release and increased stability, better pharmacodynamic effects, and low preparation costs [144, 214, 218, 271, 274]. Due to their small size, rapid mobility and enhanced penetration, nanoparticles can be made available for selective targeting to tumors, thereby accumulating in malignant tissue and delivering higher levels of anticancer agents to tumor cells [109, 128, 144, 190, 266, 270]. In this way, concentrations of flavonoids in the range used in numerous experimental cancer cell models can be achieved in *in vivo* conditions to exert enhanced antitumor efficacy [266].

Various types of non-toxic biodegradable nano-sized carriers have been used to encapsulate dietary flavonoids, including lipid-based vehicles (liposomes, solid lipid nanoparticles, nanoemulsions) and polymer-based vehicles (nanospheres, nanocapsules, micelles, inclusion complexes) [70, 190, 250, 271, 295]. Coating with polyethylene glycol (PEG) has been introduced to extend the circulation time of nanocarriers in the bloodstream and prevent leakage of encapsulated bioactive agent [272, 295-297]. Besides their passive targeting via the enhanced permeability and retention (EPR) effect, nanocarriers can undergo also functionalized active targeting by conjugating them with certain ligands (for instance biotin, folic acid, hyaluronic acid, antibodies) which bind to overexpressed receptors or antigens on the surface of malignant cells, thus facilitating the selective accumulation and allowing increased therapeutic efficacy of anticancer agents in tumor cells without any obvious adverse reactions [109, 272, 298-300]. Furthermore, nanoparticles can concurrently deliver multiple types of agents with different anticancer mechanisms, such as a traditional chemotherapeutic drug with a natural chemosensitizer like efflux pump inhibitor, proapoptotic agent or antiangiogenic compound, to exhibit synergistic antitumor action [87, 109, 191, 214, 270]. As conventional anticancer drugs and natural MDR modulators usually possess different pharmacokinetic properties, they may not reach the same cancer cell at the same time at the ideal molar ratio after systemic administration *in vivo*, leading to probable loss of encouraging results observed in *in vitro* combinational experiments [109, 250, 255]. Co-administration of chemotherapeutic drugs and natural flavonoids using nanoparticle-mediated delivery systems can result in their co-localization in tumor cell, providing thus a smart solution for *in vivo* emerging obstacles and circumventing translational loss of therapeutic application of flavonoids. Combined nanoparticle-mediated delivery of flavonoids and conventional antineoplastic drugs could serve as an innovative paradigm for enhancing the cytotoxic potency while concomitantly limiting the unwanted toxicity of chemotherapeutics [190, 296, 301]. Therefore, multifunctional combinational nanoformulations might provide plentiful novel options to reverse drug resistance and improve therapeutic efficacy, by opening a new avenue for more potent and selective anticancer treatment modalities in the future.

REFERENCES

[1]   Jia WZ, Zhao JC, Sun XL, Yao ZG, Wu HL, Xi ZQ. Additive anticancer effects of chrysin and low dose cisplatin in human malignant glioma cell (U87) proliferation and evaluation of the mechanistic pathway. *J BUON* 2015; 20: 1327-36.

[2]   Zhuo W, Zhang L, Zhu Y, Zhu B, Chen Z. Fisetin, a dietary bioflavonoid, reverses acquired Cisplatin-resistance of lung adenocarcinoma cells through MAPK/Survivin/Caspase pathway. *Am J Transl Res* 2015; 7: 2045-52.

[3] Singh VK, Arora D, Satija NK, Khare P, Roy SK, Sharma PK. Intricatinol synergistically enhances the anticancerous activity of cisplatin in human A549 cells via p38 MAPK/p53 signalling. *Apoptosis* 2017; 22: 1273-86.

[4] Ryu S, Park S, Lim W, Song G. Effects of luteolin on canine osteosarcoma: Suppression of cell proliferation and synergy with cisplatin. *J Cell Physiol* 2019; 234: 9504-14.

[5] Liu M, Qi Z, Liu B, Ren Y, Li H, Yang G, Zhang Q. RY-2f, an isoflavone analog, overcomes cisplatin resistance to inhibit ovarian tumorigenesis via targeting the PI3K/AKT/mTOR signaling pathway. *Oncotarget* 2015; 6: 25281-94.

[6] Mihaila M, Bostan M, Hotnog D, Ferdes M, Brasoveanu LL. Real-time analysis of quercetin, resveratrol and/or doxorubicin effects in MCF-7 cells. *Rom Biotechnol Lett* 2013; 18: 8106-14.

[7] Namazi Sarvestani N, Sepehri H, Delphi L, Moridi Farimani M. Eupatorin and salvigenin potentiate doxorubicin-induced apoptosis and cell cycle arrest in HT-29 and SW948 human colon cancer cells. *Asian Pac J Cancer Prev* 2018; 19: 131-9.

[8] Pan XW, Li L, Huang Y, Huang H, Xu DF, Gao Y, Chen L, Ren JZ, Cao JW, Hong Y, Cui XG. Icaritin acts synergistically with epirubicin to suppress bladder cancer growth through inhibition of autophagy. *Oncol Rep* 2016; 35: 334-42.

[9] Lin X, Tian L, Wang L, Li W, Xu Q, Xiao X. Antitumor effects and the underlying mechanism of licochalcone A combined with 5-fluorouracil in gastric cancer cells. *Oncol Lett* 2017; 13: 1695-701.

[10] Wang L, Feng J, Chen X, Guo W, Du Y, Wang Y, Zang W, Zhang S, Zhao G. Myricetin enhance chemosensitivity of 5-fluorouracil on esophageal carcinoma in vitro and in vivo. *Cancer Cell Int* 2014; 14: 71.

[11] Zhang DC, Liu JL, Ding YB, Xia JG, Chen GY. Icariin potentiates the antitumor activity of gemcitabine in gallbladder cancer by suppressing NF-κB. *Acta Pharmacol Sin* 2013; 34: 301-8.

[12] Hussain SA, Marouf BH. Silibinin improves the cytotoxicity of methotrexate in chemo resistant human rhabdomyosarcoma cell lines. *Saudi Med J* 2013; 34: 1145-50.

[13] Park CH, Han SE, Nam-Goong IS, Kim YI, Kim ES. Combined effects of baicalein and docetaxel on apoptosis in 8505c anaplastic thyroid cancer cells via downregulation of the ERK and Akt/mTOR pathways. *Endocrinol Metab (Seoul)* 2018; 33: 121-32.

[14] Chavoshi H, Vahedian V, Saghaei S, Pirouzpanah MB, Raeisi M, Samadi N. Adjuvant therapy with silibinin improves the efficacy of paclitaxel and cisplatin in MCF-7 breast cancer cells. *Asian Pac J Cancer Prev* 2017; 18: 2243-7.

[15] Mohan A, Narayanan S, Sethuraman S, Krishnan UM. Combinations of plant polyphenols & anti-cancer molecules: a novel treatment strategy for cancer chemotherapy. *Anticancer Agents Med Chem* 2013; 13: 281-95.

[16] Cai X, Liu X. Inhibition of Thr-55 phosphorylation restores p53 nuclear localization and sensitizes cancer cells to DNA damage. *Proc Natl Acad Sci USA* 2008; 105: 16958-63.

[17] Xia YZ, Ni K, Guo C, Zhang C, Geng YD, Wang ZD, Yang L, Kong LY. Alopecurone B reverses doxorubicin-resistant human osteosarcoma cell line by inhibiting P-glycoprotein and NF-kappa B signaling. *Phytomedicine* 2015; 22: 344-51.

[18] Chen X, Wu Y, Jiang Y, Zhou Y, Wang Y, Yao Y, Yi C, Gou L, Yang J. Isoliquiritigenin inhibits the growth of multiple myeloma via blocking IL-6 signaling. *J Mol Med (Berl)* 2012; 90: 1311-9.

[19] Liu Q, Sun Y, Zheng JM, Yan XL, Chen HM, Chen JK, Huang HQ. Formononetin sensitizes glioma cells to doxorubicin through preventing EMT via inhibition of histone deacetylase 5. *Int J Clin Exp Pathol* 2015; 8: 6434-41.

[20] Abaza MS, Orabi KY, Al-Quattan E, Al-Attiyah RJ. Growth inhibitory and chemo-sensitization effects of naringenin, a natural flavanone purified from Thymus vulgaris, on human breast and colorectal cancer. *Cancer Cell Int* 2015; 15: 46.

[21] Catanzaro D, Gabbia D, Cocetta V, Biagi M, Ragazzi E, Montopoli M, Carrara M. Silybin counteracts doxorubicin resistance by inhibiting GLUT1 expression. *Fitoterapia* 2018; 124: 42-8.

[22] Chen FY, Cao LF, Wan HX, Zhang MY, Cai JY, Shen LJ, Zhong JH, Zhong H. Quercetin enhances adriamycin cytotoxicity through induction of apoptosis and regulation of mitogen-activated protein kinase/extracellular signal-regulated kinase/c-Jun N-terminal kinase signaling in multidrug-resistant leukemia K562 cells. *Mol Med Rep* 2015; 11: 341-8.

[23] Wang HW, Lin CP, Chiu JH, Chow KC, Kuo KT, Lin CS, Wang LS. Reversal of inflammation-associated dihydrodiol dehydrogenases (AKR1C1 and AKR1C2) overexpression and drug resistance in nonsmall cell lung cancer cells by wogonin and chrysin. *Int J Cancer* 2007; 120: 2019-27.

[24] Desai UN, Shah KP, Mirza SH, Panchal DK, Parikh SK, Rawal RM. Enhancement of the cytotoxic effects of cytarabine in synergism with hesperidine and silibinin in acute myeloid leukemia: An in-vitro approach. *J Cancer Res Ther* 2015; 11: 352-7.

[25] Hemalswarya S, Doble M. Potential synergism of natural products in the treatment of cancer. *Phytother Res* 2006; 20: 239-49.

[26] Simoben CV, Ibezim A, Ntie-Kang F, Nwodo JN, Lifongo LL. Exploring cancer therapeutics with natural products from African medicinal plants, Part I: Xanthones, quinones, steroids, coumarins, phenolics and other classes of compounds. *Anticancer Agents Med Chem* 2015; 15: 1092-111.

[27] Ho BY, Lin CH, Apaya MK, Chao WW, Shyur LF. Silibinin and paclitaxel cotreatment significantly suppress the activity and lung metastasis of triple

negative 4T1 mammary tumor cell in mice. *J Tradit Complement Med* 2011; 2: 301-11.

[28] Chen P, Hu MD, Deng XF, Li B. Genistein reinforces the inhibitory effect of Cisplatin on liver cancer recurrence and metastasis after curative hepatectomy. *Asian Pac J Cancer Prev* 2013; 14: 759-64.

[29] Yunos NM, Beale P, Yu JQ, Huq F. Synergism from the combination of oxaliplatin with selected phytochemicals in human ovarian cancer cell lines. *Anticancer Res* 2011; 31: 4283-9.

[30] Lee JJ, Koh KN, Park CJ, Jang S, Im HJ, Kim N. The combination of flavokawain B and daunorubicin induces apoptosis in human myeloid leukemic cells by modifying NF-κB. *Anticancer Res* 2018; 38: 2771-8.

[31] Sung B, Pandey MK, Aggarwal BB. Fisetin, an inhibitor of cyclin-dependent kinase 6, down-regulates nuclear factor-kappaB-regulated cell proliferation, antiapoptotic and metastatic gene products through the suppression of TAK-1 and receptor-interacting protein-regulated IkappaBalpha kinase activation. *Mol Pharmacol* 2007; 71: 1703-14.

[32] Farzaei MH, Bahramsoltani R, Rahimi R. Phytochemicals as adjunctive with conventional anticancer therapies. *Curr Pharm Des* 2016; 22: 4201-18.

[33] Jiang L, Zhang Q, Ren H, Ma S, Lu C, Liu B, Liu J, Liang J, Li M, Zhu R. Dihydromyricetin enhances the chemo-sensitivity of nedaplatin via regulation of the p53/Bcl-2 pathway in hepatocellular carcinoma cells. *PLoS One* 2015; 10: e0124994.

[34] Krajnovic T, Kaluderovic GN, Wessjohann LA, Mijatovic S, Maksimovic-Ivanic D. Versatile antitumor potential of isoxanthohumol: Enhancement of paclitaxel activity in vivo. *Pharmacol Res* 2016; 105: 62-73.

[35] de Oliveira Junior RG, Christiane Adrielly AF, da Silva Almeida JRG, Grougnet R, Thiery V, Picot L. Sensitization of tumor cells to chemotherapy by natural products: A systematic review of preclinical data and molecular mechanisms. *Fitoterapia* 2018; 129: 383-400.

[36] Wang H, Luo Y, Qiao T, Wu Z, Huang Z. Luteolin sensitizes the antitumor effect of cisplatin in drug-resistant ovarian cancer via induction of apoptosis and inhibition of cell migration and invasion. *J Ovarian Res* 2018; 11: 93.

[37] Kuhar M, Imran S, Singh N. Curcumin and quercetin combined with cisplatin to induce apoptosis in human laryngeal carcinoma Hep-2 cells through the mitochondrial pathway. *J Cancer Mol* 2007; 3: 121-8.

[38] Wang Y, Liu W, He X, Fei Z. Hispidulin enhances the anti-tumor effects of temozolomide in glioblastoma by activating AMPK. *Cell Biochem Biophys* 2015; 71: 701-6.

[39] Flores-Perez A, Marchat LA, Sanchez LL, Romero-Zamora D, Arechaga-Ocampo E, Ramirez-Torres N, Chavez JD, Carlos-Reyes A, Astudillo-de la Vega H, Ruiz-

Garcia E, Gonzales-Perez A, Lopez-Camarillo C. Differential proteomic analysis reveals that EGCG inhibits HDGF and activates apoptosis to increase the sensitivity of non-small cells lung cancer to chemotherapy. *Proteomics Clin Appl* 2016; 10: 172-82.

[40] Wen Y, Zhao RQ, Zhang YK, Gupta P, Fu LX, Tang AZ, Liu BM, Chen ZS, Yang DH, Liang G. Effect of Y6, an epigallocatechin gallate derivative, on reversing doxorubicin drug resistance in human hepatocellular carcinoma cells. *Oncotarget* 2017; 8: 29760-70.

[41] Wang ZD, Wang RZ, Xia YZ, Kong LY, Yang L. Reversal of multidrug resistance by icaritin in doxorubicin-resistant human osteosarcoma cells. *Chin J Nat Med* 2018; 16: 20-8.

[42] Tang SN, Fu J, Shankar S, Srivastava RK. EGCG enhances the therapeutic potential of gemcitabine and CP690550 by inhibiting STAT3 signaling pathway in human pancreatic cancer. *PLoS One* 2012; 7: e31067.

[43] Erdogan S, Turkekul K, Serttas R, Erdogan Z. The natural flavonoid apigenin sensitizes human CD44+ prostate cancer stem cells to cisplatin therapy. *Biomed Pharmacother* 2017; 88: 210-7.

[44] Dhivya S, Khandelwal N, Abraham SK, Premkumar K. Impact of anthocyanidins on mitoxantrone-induced cytotoxicity and genotoxicity: An in vitro and in vivo analysis. *Integr Cancer Ther* 2016; 15: 525-34.

[45] Yang SF, Yang WE, Chang HR, Chu SC, Hsieh YS. Luteolin induces apoptosis in oral squamous cancer cells. *J Dent Res* 2008; 87: 401-6.

[46] Shen M, Chan TH, Dou QP. Targeting tumor ubiquitin-proteasome pathway with polyphenols for chemosensitization. *Anticancer Agents Med Chem* 2012; 12: 891-901.

[47] Seguin J, Brulle L, Boyer R, Lu YM, Ramos Romano M, Touil YS, Scherman D, Bessodes M, Mignet N, Chabot GG. Liposomal encapsulation of the natural flavonoid fisetin improves bioavailability and antitumor efficacy. *Int J Pharm* 2013; 444: 146-54.

[48] Hosseinimehr SJ, Jalayer Z, Naghshvar F, Mahmoudzadeh A, Hesperidin inhibits cyclophosphamide-induced tumor growth delay in mice. *Integr Cancer Ther* 2012; 11: 251-6.

[49] Liu R, Ji P, Liu B, Qiao H, Wang X, Zhou L, Deng T, Ba Y. Apigenin enhances the cisplatin cytotoxic effect through p53-modulated apoptosis. *Oncol Lett* 2017; 13: 1024-30.

[50] He F, Wang Q, Zheng XL, Yan JQ, Yang L, Sun H, Hu LN, Lin Y, Wang X. Wogonin potentiates cisplatin-induced cancer cell apoptosis through accumulation of intracellular reactive oxygen species. *Oncol Rep* 2012; 28: 601-5.

[51] Brechbuhl HM, Kachadourian R, Min E, Chan D, Day BJ. Chrysin enhances doxorubicin-induced cytotoxicity in human lung epithelial cancer cell lines: the role of glutathione. *Toxicol Appl Pharmacol* 2012; 258: 1-9.

[52] Zhang S, Morris ME. Effects of the flavonoids biochanin A, morin, phloretin, and silymarin on P-glycoprotein-mediated transport. *J Pharmacol Exp Ther* 2003; 304: 1258-67.

[53] Zheng AW, Chen YQ, Zhao LQ, Feng JG. Myricetin induces apoptosis and enhances chemosensitivity in ovarian cancer cells. *Oncol Lett* 2017; 13: 4974-8.

[54] Go WJ, Ryu JH, Qiang F, Han HK. Evaluation of the flavonoid oroxylin A as an inhibitor of P-glycoprotein-mediated cellular efflux. *J Nat Prod* 2009; 72: 1616-9.

[55] Guo XF, Liu JP, Ma SQ, Zhang P, Sun WD. Avicularin reversed multidrug-resistance in human gastric cancer through enhancing Bax and BOK expressions. *Biomed Pharmacother* 2018; 103: 67-74.

[56] Ramachandran L, Manu KA, Shanmugam MK, Li F, Siveen KS, Vali S, Kapoor S, Abbasi T, Surana R, Smoot DT, Ashktorab H, Tan P, Ahn KS, Yap CW, Kumar AP, Sethi G. Isorhamnetin inhibits proliferation and invasion and induces apoptosis through the modulation of peroxisome proliferator-activated receptor γ activation pathway in gastric cancer. *J Biol Chem* 2012; 287: 38028-40.

[57] Hagen RM, Chedea VS, Mintoff CP, Bowler E, Morse HR, Ladomery MR. Epigallocatechin-3-gallate promotes apoptosis and expression of the caspase 9a splice variant in PC3 prostate cancer cells. *Int J Oncol* 2013; 43: 194-200.

[58] Sharma H, Sen S, Singh N. Molecular pathways in the chemosensitization of cisplatin by quercetin in human head and neck cancer. *Cancer Biol Ther* 2005; 4: 949-55.

[59] Critchfield JW, Welsh CJ, Phang JM, Yeh GC. Modulation of adriamycin accumulation and efflux by flavonoids in HCT-15 colon cells. Activation of P-glycoprotein as a putative mechanism. *Biochem Pharmacol* 1994; 48: 1437-45.

[60] Zhang S, Yang X, Morris ME. Flavonoids are inhibitors of breast cancer resistance protein (ABCG2)-mediated transport. *Mol Pharmacol* 2004; 65: 1208-16.

[61] An G, Morris ME. Effects of single and multiple flavonoids on BCRP-mediated accumulation, cytotoxicity and transport of mitoxantrone in vitro. *Pharm Res* 2010; 27: 1296-308.

[62] Nakatsuma A, Fukami T, Suzuki T, Furuishi T, Tomono K, Hidaka S. Effects of kaempferol on the mechanisms of drug resistance in the human glioblastoma cell line T98G. *Pharmazie* 2010; 65: 379-83.

[63] Iriti M, Kubina R, Cochis A, Sorrentino R, Varoni EM, Kabala-Dzik A, Azzimonti B, Dziedzic A, Rimondini L, Wojtyczka RD. Rutin, a quercetin glycoside, restores chemosensitivity in human breast cancer cells. *Phytother Res* 2017; 31: 1529-38.

[64] Chen C, Zhou J, Ji C. Quercetin: a potential drug to reverse multidrug resistance. *Life Sci* 2010; 87: 333-8.

[65] Brito AF, Ribeiro M, Abrantes AM, Pires AS, Teixo RJ, Tralhao JG, Botelho MF. Quercetin in cancer treatment, alone or in combination with conventional therapeutics? *Curr Med Chem* 2015; 22: 3025-39.

[66] Nadova S, Miadokova E, Cipak L. Flavonoids potentiate the efficacy of cytarabine through modulation of drug-induced apoptosis. *Neoplasma* 2007; 54: 202-6.

[67] Li J, Wang Y, Lei JC, Hao Y, Yang Y, Yang CX, Yu JQ. Sensitisation of ovarian cancer cells to cisplatin by flavonoids from Scutellaria barbata. *Nat Prod Res* 2014; 28: 683-9.

[68] Limtrakul P, Khantamat O, Pintha K. Inhibition of P-glycoprotein function and expression by kaempferol and quercetin. *J Chemother* 2005; 17: 86-95.

[69] Czepas J, Gwozdzinski K. The flavonoid quercetin: possible solution for anthracycline-induced cardiotoxicity and multidrug resistance. *Biomed Pharmacother* 2014; 68: 1149-59.

[70] Hyun HB, Moon JY, Cho SK. Quercetin suppresses CYR61-mediated multidrug resistance in human gastric adenocarcinoma AGS cells. *Molecules* 2018; 23: E209.

[71] Kuo CY, Zupko I, Chang FR, Hunyadi A, Wu CC, Weng TS, Wang HC. Dietary flavonoid derivatives enhance chemotherapeutic effect by inhibiting the DNA damage response pathway. *Toxicol Appl Pharmacol* 2016; 311: 99-105.

[72] Nazari M, Ghorbani A, Hekmat-Doost A, Jeddi-Tehrani M, Zand H. Inactivation of nuclear factor-κB by citrus flavanone hesperidin contributes to apoptosis and chemo-sensitizing effect in Ramos cells. *Eur J Pharmacol* 2011; 650: 526-33.

[73] Borska S, Chmielewska M, Wysocka T, Drag-Zalesinska M, Zabel M, Dziegiel P. In vitro effect of quercetin on human gastric carcinoma: targeting cancer cells death and MDR. *Food Chem Toxicol* 2012; 50: 3375-83.

[74] Bansal T, Jaggi M, Khar RK, Talegaonkar S. Emerging significance of flavonoids as P-glycoprotein inhibitors in cancer chemotherapy. *J Pharm Pharm Sci* 2009; 12: 46-78.

[75] Kachadourian R, Leitner HM, Day BJ. Selected flavonoids potentiate the toxicity of cisplatin in human lung adenocarcinoma cells: a role for glutathione depletion. *Int J Oncol* 2007; 31: 161-8.

[76] Lim J, Lee SH, Cho S, Lee IS, Kang BY, Choi HJ. 4-methoxychalcone enhances cisplatin-induced oxidative stress and cytotoxicity by inhibiting the Nrf2/ARE-mediated defense mechanism in A549 lung cancer cells. *Mol Cells* 2013; 36: 340-6.

[77] Fonseca J, Marques S, Silva PM, Brandao P, Cidade H, Pinto MM, Bousbaa H. Prenylated chalcone 2 acts as an antimitotic agent and enhances the chemosensitivity of tumor cells to paclitaxel. *Molecules* 2016; 21: E982.

[78] Jakubowicz-Gil J, Langner E, Rzeski W. Kinetic studies of the effects of Temodal and quercetin on astrocytoma cells. *Pharmacol Rep* 2011; 63: 403-16.

[79] Lee SW, Song GS, Kwon CH, Kim YK. Beneficial effect of flavonoid baicalein in cisplatin-induced cell death of human glioma cells. *Neurosci Lett* 2005; 382: 71-5.

[80] Yang Z, Liu Y, Liao J, Gong C, Sun C, Zhou X, Wei X, Zhang T, Gao Q, Ma D, Chen G. Quercetin induces endoplasmic reticulum stress to enhance cDDP cytotoxicity in ovarian cancer: involvement of STAT3 signaling. *FEBS J* 2015; 282: 1111-25.

[81] Cipak L, Berczeliova E, Paulikova H. Effects of flavonoids on glutathione and glutathione-related enzymes in cisplatin-treated L1210 leukemia cells. *Neoplasma* 2003; 50: 443-6.

[82] Ferreira de Oliveira JMP, Pacheco AR, Coutinho L, Oliveira H, Pinho S, Almeida L, Fernandes E, Santos C. Combination of etoposide and fisetin results in anti-cancer efficiency against osteosarcoma cell models. *Arch Toxicol* 2018; 92: 1205-14.

[83] Punia R, Raina K, Agarwal R, Singh RP. Acacetin enhances the therapeutic efficacy of doxorubicin in non-small-cell lung carcinoma cells. *PLoS One* 2017; 12: e0182870.

[84] Liu L, Ju Y, Wang J, Zhou R. Epigallocatechin-3-gallate promotes apoptosis and reversal of multidrug resistance in esophageal cancer cells. *Pathol Res Pract* 2017; 213: 1242-50.

[85] Sun L, Chen W, Qu L, Wu J, Si J. Icaritin reverses multidrug resistance of HepG2/ADR human hepatoma cells via downregulation of MDR1 and P-glycoprotein expression. *Mol Med Rep* 2013; 8: 1883-7.

[86] Coutinho L, Oliveira H, Pacheco AR, Almeida L, Pimentel F, Santos C, Ferreira de Oliveira JM. Hesperetin-etoposide combinations induce cytotoxicity in U2OS cells: Implications on therapeutic developments for osteosarcoma. *DNA Repair (Amst)* 2017; 50: 36-42.

[87] Mehnath S, Arjama M, Rajan M, Annamalai G, Jeyaraj M. Co-encapsulation of dual drug loaded in MLNPs: Implication on sustained drug release and effectively inducing apoptosis in oral carcinoma cells. *Biomed Pharmacother* 2018; 104: 661-71.

[88] Elhag R, Mazzio EA, Soliman KF. The effect of silibinin in enhancing toxicity of temozolomide and etoposide in p53 and PTEN-mutated resistant glioma cell lines. *Anticancer Res* 2015; 35: 1263-9.

[89] Sak K. Intake of individual flavonoids and risk of carcinogenesis: Overview of epidemiological evidence. *Nutr Cancer* 2017; 69: 1119-50.

[90] Sak K. Epidemiological evidences on dietary flavonoids and breast cancer risk: A narrative review. *Asian Pac J Cancer Prev* 2017; 18: 2309-28.

[91] Sak K. Dietary flavonoids and colorectal cancer: Evidence from epidemiological studies. *Int Arch Clin Pharmacol* 2017; 3: 012.

[92] Sak K. Current epidemiological knowledge about the role of flavonoids in prostate carcinogenesis. *Exp Oncol* 2017; 39: 98-105.

[93] Sak K. Role of flavonoids in prevention of gynecological cancers: Epidemiological clues. *Curr Women`s Health Rev* 2017; 13: 103-13.

[94] Shi H, Wu Y, Wang Y, Zhou M, Yan S, Chen Z, Gu D, Cai Y. Liquiritigenin potentiates the inhibitory effects of cisplatin on invasion and metastasis via downregulation of MMP-2/9 and PI3K/AKT signaling pathway in B16F10 melanoma cells and mice model. *Nutr Cancer* 2015; 67: 761-70.

[95] Zhang X, Guo Q, Chen J, Chen Z. Quercetin enhances cisplatin sensitivity of human osteosarcoma cells by modulating microRNA-217-KRAS axis. *Mol Cells* 2015; 38: 638-42.

[96] Jakubowicz-Gil J, Langner E, Wertel I, Piersiak T, Rzeski W. Temozolomide, quercetin and cell death in the MOGGCCM astrocytoma cell line. *Chem Biol Interact* 2010; 188: 190-203.

[97] Jakubowicz-Gil J, Paduch R, Piersiak T, Glowniak K, Gawron A, Kandefer-Szerszen M. The effect of quercetin on pro-apoptotic activity of cisplatin in HeLa cells. *Biochem Pharmacol* 2005; 69: 1343-50.

[98] Daker M, Ahmad M, Khoo AS. Quercetin-induced inhibition and synergistic activity with cisplatin – a chemotherapeutic strategy for nasopharyngeal carcinoma cells. *Cancer Cell Int* 2012; 12: 34.

[99] Chen SF, Nieh S, Jao SW, Liu CL, Wu CH, Chang YC, Yang CY, Lin YS. Quercetin suppresses drug-resistant spheres via the p38 MAPK-Hsp27 apoptotic pathway in oral cancer cells. *PLoS One* 2012; 7: e49275.

[100] Minaei A, Sabzichi M, Ramezani F, Hamishehkar H, Samadi N. Co-delivery with nano-quercetin enhances doxorubicin-mediated cytotoxicity against MCF-7 cells. *Mol Biol Rep* 2016; 43: 99-105.

[101] Du G, Lin H, Yang Y, Zhang S, Wu X, Wang M, Ji L, Lu L, Yu L, Han G. Dietary quercetin combining intratumoral doxorubicin injection synergistically induces rejection of established breast cancer in mice. *Int Immunopharmacol* 2010; 10: 819-26.

[102] Zhu B, Yu L, Yue Q. Co-delivery of vincristine and quercetin by nanocarriers for lymphoma combination chemotherapy. *Biomed Pharmacother* 2017; 91: 287-94.

[103] Li N, Sun C, Zhou B, Xing H, Ma D, Chen G, Weng D. Low concentration of quercetin antagonizes the cytotoxic effects of anti-neoplastic drugs in ovarian cancer. *PLoS One* 2014; 9: e100314.

[104] Heeba GH, Mahmoud ME. Dual effects of quercetin in doxorubicin-induced nephrotoxicity in rats and its modulation of the cytotoxic activity of doxorubicin on human carcinoma cells. *Environ Toxicol* 2016; 31: 624-36.

[105] Wang P, Henning SM, Heber D, Vadgama JV. Sensitization of docetaxel in prostate cancer cells by green tea and quercetin. *J Nutr Biochem* 2015; 26: 408-15.

[106] Khan M, Maryam A, Mehmood T, Zhang Y, Ma T. Enhancing activity of anticancer drugs in multidrug resistant tumors by modulating P-glycoprotein through dietary nutraceuticals. *Asian Pac J Cancer Prev* 2015; 16: 6831-9.

[107] Samuel T, Fadlalla K, Mosley L, Katkoori V, Turner T, Manne U. Dual-mode interaction between quercetin and DNA-damaging drugs in cancer cells. *Anticancer Res* 2012; 32: 61-71.

[108] Samuel T, Fadlalla K, Turner T, Yehualaeshet TE. The flavonoid quercetin transiently inhibits the activity of taxol and nocodazole through interference with the cell cycle. *Nutr Cancer* 2010; 62: 1025-35.

[109] Lv L, Liu C, Chen C, Yu X, Chen G, Shi Y, Qin F, Qu J, Qiu K, Li G. Quercetin and doxorubicin co-encapsulated biotin receptor-targeting nanoparticles for minimizing drug resistance in breast cancer. *Oncotarget* 2016; 7: 32184-99.

[110] Rudolfova P, Hanusova V, Skalova L, Bartikova H, Matouskova P, Bousova I. Effect of selected catechins on doxorubicin antiproliferative efficacy and hepatotoxicity in vitro. *Acta Pharm* 2014; 64: 199-209.

[111] Qiao J, Gu C, Shang W, Du J, Yin W, Zhu M, Wang W, Han M, Lu W. Effect of green tea on pharmacokinetics of 5-fluorouracil in rats and pharmacodynamics in human cell lines in vitro. *Food Chem Toxicol* 2011; 49: 1410-5.

[112] Liang G, Tang A, Lin X, Li L, Zhang S, Huang Z, Tang H, Li QQ. Green tea catechins augment the antitumor activity of doxorubicin in an in vivo mouse model for chemoresistant liver cancer. *Int J Oncol* 2010; 37: 111-23.

[113] Mayr C, Wagner A, Neureiter D, Pichler M, Jakab M, Illig R, Berr F, Kiesslich T. The green tea catechin epigallocatechin gallate induces cell cycle arrest and shows potential synergism with cisplatin in biliary tract cancer cells. *BMC Complement Altern Med* 2015; 15: 194.

[114] Ermakova SP, Kang BS, Choi BY, Choi HS, Schuster TF, Ma WY, Bode AM, Dong Z. (-)-Epigallocatechin gallate overcomes resistance to etoposide-induced cell death by targeting the molecular chaperone glucose-regulated protein 78. *Cancer Res* 2006; 66: 9260-9.

[115] Chen L, Ye HL, Zhang G, Yao WM, Chen XZ, Zhang FC, Liang G. Autophagy inhibition contributes to the synergistic interaction between EGCG and doxorubicin to kill the hepatoma Hep3B cells. *PLoS One* 2014; 9: e85771.

[116] Yang XW, Wang XL, Cao LQ, Jiang XF, Peng HP, Lin SM, Xue P, Chen D. Green tea polyphenol epigallocatehin-3-gallate enhances 5-fluorouracil-induced cell growth inhibition of hepatocellular carcinoma cells. *Hepatol Res* 2012; 42: 494-501.

[117] Xu F, Zhen YS. (-)-Epigallocatechin-3-gallate enhances anti-tumor effect of cytosine arabinoside on HL-60 cells. *Acta Pharmacol Sin* 2003; 24: 163-8.

[118] Wietrzyk J, Mazurkiewicz M, Madej J, Dzimira S, Grynkiewicz G, Radzikowski C, Opolski A. Genistein alone or combined with cyclophosphamide may stimulate

16/C transplantable mouse mammary cancer growth. *Med Sci Monit* 2004; 10: BR414-9.

[119] Liu D, Yan L, Wang L, Tai W, Wang W, Yang C. Genistein enhances the effect of cisplatin on the inhibition of non-small cell lung cancer A549 cell growth *in vitro* and *in vivo*. *Oncol Lett* 2014; 8: 2806-10.

[120] Hörmann V, Kumi-Diaka J, Durity M, Rathinavelu A. Anticancer activities of genistein-topotecan combination in prostate cancer cells. *J Cell Mol Med* 2012; 16: 2631-6.

[121] Satoh H, Nishikawa K, Suzuki K, Asano R, Virgona N, Ichikawa T, Hagiwara K, Yano T. Genistein, a soy isoflavone, enhances necrotic-like cell death in a breast cancer cell treated with a chemotherapeutic agent. *Res Commun Mol Pathol Pharmacol* 2003; 113-114: 149-58.

[122] Xue JP, Wang G, Zhao ZB, Wang Q, Shi Y. Synergistic cytotoxic effect of genistein and doxorubicin on drug-resistant human breast cancer MCF-7/Adr cells. *Oncol Rep* 2014; 32: 1647-53.

[123] Wietrzyk J, Boratynski J, Grynkiewicz G, Ryczynski A, Radzikowski C, Opolski A. Antiangiogenic and antitumour effects in vivo of genistein applied alone or combined with cyclophosphamide. *Anticancer Res* 2001; 21: 3893-6.

[124] El-Rayes BF, Philip PA, Sarkar FH, Shields AF, Ferris AM, Hess K, Kaseb AO, Javle MM, Varadhachary GR, Wolff RA, Abbruzzese JL. A phase II study of isoflavones, erlotinib, and gemcitabine in advanced pancreatic cancer. *Invest New Drugs* 2011; 29: 694-9.

[125] Jiang YY, Yang R, Wang HJ, Huang H, Wu D, Tashiro S, Onodera S, Ikejima T. Mechanism of autophagy induction and role of autophagy in antagonizing mitomycin C-induced cell apoptosis in silibinin treated human melanoma A375-S2 cells. *Eur J Pharmacol* 2011; 659: 7-14.

[126] Jiang YY, Wang HJ, Wang J, Tashiro S, Onodera S, Ikejima T. The protective effect of silibinin against mitomycin C-induced intrinsic apoptosis in human melanoma A375-S2 cells. *J Pharmacol Sci* 2009; 111: 137-46.

[127] Giacomelli S, Gallo D, Apollonio P, Ferlini C, Distefano M, Morazzoni P, Riva A, Bombardelli E, Mancuso S, Scambia G. Silybin and its bioavailable phospholipid complex (IdB 1016) potentiate in vitro and in vivo the activity of cisplatin. *Life Sci* 2002; 70: 1447-59.

[128] Molavi O, Samadi N, Wu C, Lavasanifar A, Lai R. Silibinin suppresses NPM-ALK, potently induces apoptosis and enhances chemosensitivity in ALK-positive anaplastic large cell lymphoma. *Leuk Lymphoma* 2016; 57: 1154-62.

[129] Yurtcu E, Darcansov Iseri O, Iffet Sahin F. Effects of silymarin and silymarin-doxorubicin applications on telomerase activity of human hepatocellular carcinoma cell line HepG2. *J BUON* 2015; 20: 555-61.

[130] Yurtcu E, Iseri Ö, Sahin F. Genotoxic and cytotoxic effects of doxorubicin and silymarin on human hepatocellular carcinoma cells. *Hum Exp Toxicol* 2014; 33: 1269-76.

[131] Zhang Y, Ge Y, Ping X, Yu M, Lou D, Shi W. Synergistic apoptotic effects of silibinin in enhancing paclitaxel toxicity in human gastric cancer cell lines. *Mol Med Rep* 2018; 18: 1835-41.

[132] Li J, Li B, Xu WW, Chan KW, Guan XY, Qin YR, Lee NP, Chan KT, Law S, Tsao SW, Cheung AL. Role of AMPK signaling in mediating the anticancer effects of silibinin in esophageal squamous cell carcinoma. *Expert Opin Ther Targets* 2016; 20: 7-18.

[133] Colombo V, Lupi M, Falcetta F, Forestieri D, D`Incalci M, Ubezio P. Chemotherapeutic activity of silymarin combined with doxorubicin or paclitaxel in sensitive and multidrug-resistant colon cancer cells. *Cancer Chemother Pharmacol* 2011; 67: 369-79.

[134] Tyagi AK, Singh RP, Agarwal C, Chan DC, Agarwal R. Silibinin strongly synergizes human prostate carcinoma DU145 cells to doxorubicin-induced growth inhibition, G2-M arrest, and apoptosis. *Clin Cancer Res* 2002; 8: 3512-9.

[135] Pashaei-Asl F, Pashaei-Asl R, Khodadadi K, Akbarzadeh A, Ebrahimie E, Pashaiasl M. Enhancement of anticancer activity by silibinin and paclitaxel combination on the ovarian cancer. *Artif Cells Nanomed Biotechnol* 2018; 46: 1483-7.

[136] Zhou L, Liu P, Chen B, Wang Y, Wang X, Chiriva Internati M, Wachtel MS, Frezza EE. Silibinin restores paclitaxel sensitivity to paclitaxel-resistant human ovarian carcinoma cells. *Anticancer Res* 2008; 28: 1119-27.

[137] Flaig TW, Su LJ, Harrison G, Agarwal R, Glode LM. Silibinin synergizes with mitoxantrone to inhibit cell growth and induce apoptosis in human prostate cancer cells. *Int J Cancer* 2007; 120: 2028-33.

[138] Sadava D, Kane SE. Silibinin reverses drug resistance in human small-cell lung carcinoma cells. *Cancer Lett* 2013; 339: 102-6.

[139] Tang Q, Ji F, Sun W, Wang J, Guo J, Guo L, Li Y, Bao Y. Combination of baicalein and 10-hydroxy camptothecin exerts remarkable synergetic anti-cancer effects. *Phytomedicine* 2016; 23: 1778-86.

[140] Zheng J, Asakawa T, Chen Y, Zheng Z, Chen B, Lin M, Liu T, Hu J. Synergistic effect of baicalin and adriamycin in resistant HL-60/ADM leukaemia cells. *Cell Physiol Biochem* 2017; 43: 419-30.

[141] Kim EH, Jang H, Shin D, Baek SH, Roh JL. Targeting Nrf2 with wogonin overcomes cisplatin resistance in head and neck cancer. *Apoptosis* 2016; 21: 1265-78.

[142] Wang Y, Miao H, Li W, Yao J, Sun Y, Li Z, Zhao L, Guo Q. CXCL12/CXCR4 axis confers adriamycin resistance to human chronic myelogenous leukemia and

oroxylin A improves the sensitivity of K562/ADM cells. *Biochem Pharmacol* 2014; 90: 212-25.

[143] Kiartivich S, Wei Y, Liu J, Soiampornkul R, Li M, Zhang H, Dong J. Regulation of cytotoxicity and apoptosis-associated pathways contributes to the enhancement of efficacy of cisplatin by baicalein adjuvant in human A549 lung cancer cells. *Oncol Lett* 2017; 13: 2799-804.

[144] Li S, Wang L, Li N, Liu Y, Su H. Combination lung cancer chemotherapy: Design of a pH-sensitive transferrin-PEG-Hz-lipid conjugate for the co-delivery of docetaxel and baicalin. *Biomed Pharmacother* 2017; 95: 548-55.

[145] Zhao H, Yuan X, Li D, Chen H, Jiang J, Wang Z, Sun X, Zheng Q. Isoliquiritigen enhances the antitumour activity and decreases the genotoxic effect of cyclophosphamide. *Molecules* 2013; 18: 8786-98.

[146] Patricia Moreno-Londono A, Bello-Alvarez C, Pedraza-Chaverri J. Isoliquiritigenin pretreatment attenuates cisplatin induced proximal tubular cells (LLC-PK1) death and enhances the toxicity induced by this drug in bladder cancer T24 cell line. *Food Chem Toxicol* 2017; 109: 143-54.

[147] Wu W, Xia Q, Luo RJ, Lin ZQ, Xue P. In vitro study of the antagonistic effect of low-dose liquiritigenin on gemcitabine-induced capillary leak syndrome in pancreatic adenocarcinoma via inhibiting ROS-mediated signalling pathways. *Asian Pac J Cancer Prev* 2015; 16: 4369-76.

[148] Wang Z, Wang N, Liu P, Chen Q, Situ H, Xie T, Zhang J, Peng C, Lin Y, Chen J. MicroRNA-25 regulates chemoresistance-associated autophagy in breast cancer cells, a process modulated by the natural autophagy inducer isoliquiritigenin. *Oncotarget* 2014; 5: 7013-26.

[149] Arafa el-SA, Zhu Q, Barakat BM, Wani G, Zhao Q, El-Mahdy MA, Wani AA. Tangeretin sensitizes cisplatin-resistant human ovarian cancer cells through downregulation of phosphoinositide 3-kinase/Akt signaling pathway. *Cancer Res* 2009; 69: 8910-7.

[150] Li N, Zhang Z, Jiang G, Sun H, Yu D. Nobiletin sensitizes colorectal cancer cells to oxaliplatin by PI3K/Akt/MTOR pathway. *Front Biosci (Landmark Ed)* 2019; 24: 303-12.

[151] Ma W, Feng S, Yao X, Yuan Z, Liu L, Xie Y. Nobiletin enhances the efficacy of chemotherapeutic agents in ABCB1 overexpression cancer cells. *Sci Rep* 2015; 5: 18789.

[152] Zhang FY, Du GJ, Zhang L, Zhang CL, Lu WL, Liang W. Naringenin enhances the anti-tumor effect of doxorubicin through selectively inhibiting the activity of multidrug resistance-associated proteins but not P-glycoprotein. *Pharm Res* 2009; 26: 914-25.

[153] Imai Y, Tsukahara S, Asada S, Sugimoto Y. Phytoestrogens/flavonoids reverse breast cancer resistance protein/ABCG2-mediated multidrug resistance. *Cancer Res* 2004; 64: 4346-52.

[154] Kanno S, Shouji A, Hirata R, Asou K, Ishikawa M. Effects of naringin on cytosine arabinoside (Ara-C)-induced cytotoxicity and apoptosis in P388 cells. *Life Sci* 2004; 75: 353-65.

[155] Du G, Lin H, Wang M, Zhang S, Wu X, Lu L, Ji L, Yu L. Quercetin greatly improved therapeutic index of doxorubicin against 4T1 breast cancer by its opposing effects on HIF-1α in tumor and normal cells. *Cancer Chemother Pharmacol* 2010; 65: 277-87.

[156] Maciejczyk A, Surowiak P. Quercetin inhibits proliferation and increases sensitivity of ovarian cancer cells to cisplatin and paclitaxel. *Ginekol Pol* 2013; 84: 590-5.

[157] Mei Y, Wei D, Liu J. Reversal of multidrug resistance in KB cells with tea polyphenol antioxidant capacity. *Cancer Biol Ther* 2005; 4: 468-73.

[158] Stearns ME, Amatangelo MD, Varma D, Sell C, Goodyear SM. Combination therapy with epigallocatechin-3-gallate and doxorubicin in human prostate tumor modeling studies: inhibition of metastatic tumor growth in severe combined immunodeficiency mice. *Am J Pathol* 2010; 177: 3169-79.

[159] Banerjee S, Zhang Y, Ali S, Bhuiyan M, Wang Z, Chiao PJ, Philip PA, Abbruzzese J, Sarkar FH. Molecular evidence for increased antitumor activity of gemcitabine by genistein in vitro and in vivo using an orthotopic model of pancreatic cancer. *Cancer Res* 2005; 65: 9064-72.

[160] Löhr JM, Karimi M, Omazic B, Kartalis N, Verbeke CS, Berkenstam A, Frödin JE. A phase I dose escalation trial of AXP107-11, a novel multi-component crystalline form of genistein, in combination with gemcitabine in chemotherapy-naive patients with unresectable pancreatic cancer. *Pancreatology* 2016; 16: 640-5.

[161] Gaballah HH, Gaber RA, Mohamed DA. Apigenin potentiates the antitumor activity of 5-FU on solid Ehrlich carcinoma: Crosstalk between apoptotic and JNK-mediated autophagic cell death platforms. *Toxicol Appl Pharmacol* 2017; 316: 27-35.

[162] Lee SH, Ryu JK, Lee KY, Woo SM, Park JK, Yoo JW, Kim YT, Yoon YB. Enhanced anti-tumor effect of combination therapy with gemcitabine and apigenin in pancreatic cancer. *Cancer Lett* 2008; 259: 39-49.

[163] Chan LP, Chou TH, Ding HY, Chen PR, Chiang FY, Kuo PL, Liang CH. Apigenin induces apoptosis via tumor necrosis factor receptor- and Bcl-2-mediated pathway and enhances susceptibility of head and neck squamous cell carcinoma to 5-fluorouracil and cisplatin. *Biochim Biophys Acta* 2012; 1820: 1081-91.

[164] Choi EJ, Kim GH. 5-Fluorouracil combined with apigenin enhances anticancer activity through induction of apoptosis in human breast cancer MDA-MB-453 cells. *Oncol Rep* 2009; 22: 1533-7.

[165] Yu Y, Kong R, Cao H, Yin Z, Liu J, Nan X, Phan AT, Ding T, Zhao H, Wong STC. Two birds, one stone: hesperetin alleviates chemotherapy-induced diarrhea and potentiates tumor inhibition. *Oncotarget* 2018; 9: 27958-73.

[166] Molavi O, Narimani F, Asiaee F, Sharifi S, Tarhriz V, Shayanfar A, Hejazi M, Lai R. Silibinin sensitizes chemo-resistant breast cancer cells to chemotherapy. *Pharm Biol* 2017; 55: 729-39.

[167] Chan JY, Tan BK, Lee SC. Scutellarin sensitizes drug-evoked colon cancer cell apoptosis through enhanced caspase-6 activation. *Anticancer Res* 2009; 29: 3043-7.

[168] Ramadass SK, Anantharaman NV, Subramanian S, Sivasubramanian S, Madhan B. Paclitaxel/epigallocatechin gallate coloaded liposome: a synergistic delivery to control the invasiveness of MDA-MB-231 breast cancer cells. *Colloids Surf B Biointerfaces* 2015; 125: 65-72.

[169] Lang M, Henson R, Braconi C, Patel T. Epigallocatechin-gallate modulates chemotherapy-induced apoptosis in human cholangiocarcinoma cells. *Liver Int* 2009; 29: 670-7.

[170] Gao AM, Ke ZP, Shi F, Sun GC, Chen H. Chrysin enhances sensitivity of BEL-7402/ADM cells to doxorubicin by suppressing PI3K/Akt/Nrf2 and ERK/Nrf2 pathway. *Chem Biol Interact* 2013; 206: 100-8.

[171] Zhu H, Luo P, Fu Y, Wang J, Dai J, Shao J, Yang X, Chang L, Weng Q, Yang B, He Q. Dihydromyricetin prevents cardiotoxicity and enhances anticancer activity induced by adriamycin. *Oncotarget* 2015; 6: 3254-67.

[172] Lewandowska U, Gorlach S, Owczarek K, Hrabec E, Szewczyk K. Synergistic interactions between anticancer chemotherapeutics and phenolic compounds and anticancer synergy between polyphenols. *Postepy Hig Med Dosw (Online)* 2014; 68: 528-40.

[173] Ma L, Wang R, Nan Y, Li W, Wang Q, Jin F. Phloretin exhibits an anticancer effect and enhances the anticancer ability of cisplatin on non-small cell lung cancer cell lines by regulating expression of apoptotic pathways and matrix metalloproteinases. *Int J Oncol* 2016; 48: 843-53.

[174] Tripathi R, Samadder T, Gupta S, Surolia A, Shaha C. Anticancer activity of a combination of cisplatin and fisetin in embryonal carcinoma cells and xenograft tumors. *Mol Cancer Ther* 2011; 10: 255-68.

[175] Wang A, Wang W, Chen Y, Ma F, Wei X, Bi Y. Deguelin induces PUMA-mediated apoptosis and promotes sensitivity of lung cancer cells (LCCs) to doxorubicin (Dox). *Mol Cell Biochem* 2018; 442: 177-86.

[176] Strouch MJ, Milam BM, Melstrom LG, McGull JJ, Salabat MR, Ujiki MB, Ding XZ, Bentrem DJ. The flavonoid apigenin potentiates the growth inhibitory effects

of gemcitabine and abrogates gemcitabine resistance in human pancreatic cancer cells. *Pancreas* 2009; 38: 409-15.

[177] Borska S, Gebarowska E, Wysocka T, Drag-Zalesinska M, Zabel M. The effects of quercetin vs cisplatin on proliferation and the apoptotic process in A549 and SW1271 cell lines in in vitro conditions. *Folia Morphol (Warsz)* 2004; 63: 103-5.

[178] Li QC, Liang Y, Hu GR, Tian Y. Enhanced therapeutic efficacy and amelioration of cisplatin-induced nephrotoxicity by quercetin in 1,2-dimethyl hydrazine-induced colon cancer in rats. *Indian J Pharmacol* 2016; 48: 168-71.

[179] Xu XD, Zhao Y, Zhang M, He RZ, Shi XH, Guo XJ, Shi CJ, Peng F, Wang M, Shen M, Wang X, Li X, Qin RY. Inhibition of autophagy by deguelin sensitizes pancreatic cancer cells to doxorubicin. *Int J Mol Sci* 2017; 18: E370.

[180] Kuhar M, Sen S, Singh N. Role of mitochondria in quercetin-enhanced chemotherapeutic response in human non-small cell lung carcinoma H-520 cells. *Anticancer Res* 2006; 26: 1297-303.

[181] Zhong Y, Zhang F, Sun Z, Zhou W, Li ZY, You QD, Guo QL, Hu R. Drug resistance associates with activation of Nrf2 in MCF-7/DOX cells, and wogonin reverses it by down-regulating Nrf2-mediated cellular defense response. *Mol Carcinog* 2013; 52: 824-34.

[182] Lee SH, Lee EJ, Min KH, Hur GY, Lee SH, Lee SY, Kim JH, Shin C, Shim JJ, In KH, Kang KH, Lee SY. Quercetin enhances chemosensitivity to gemcitabine in lung cancer cells by inhibiting heat shock protein 70 expression. *Clin Lung Cancer* 2015; 16: e235-43.

[183] Shen J, Tai YC, Zhou J, Stephen Wong CH, Cheang PT, Fred Wong WS, Xie Z, Khan M, Han JH, Chen CS. Synergistic antileukemia effect of genistein and chemotherapy in mouse xenograft model and potential mechanism through MAPK signaling. *Exp Hematol* 2007; 35: 75-83.

[184] Li S, Zhao Q, Wang B, Yuan S, Wang X, Li K. Quercetin reversed MDR in breast cancer cells through down-regulating P-gp expression and eliminating cancer stem cells mediated by YB-1 nuclear translocation. *Phytother Res* 2018; 32: 1530-6.

[185] Zhang BY, Wang YM, Gong H, Zhao H, Lv XY, Yuan GH, Han SR. Isorhamnetin flavonoid synergistically enhances the anticancer activity and apoptosis induction by cis-platin and carboplatin in non-small cell lung carcinoma (NSCLC). *Int J Clin Exp Pathol* 2015; 8: 25-37.

[186] Wang Y, Wang H, Zhang W, Shao C, Xu P, Shi CH, Shi JG, Li YM, Fu Q, Xue W, Lei YH, Gao JY, Wang JY, Gao XP, Li JQ, Yuan JL, Zhang YT. Genistein sensitizes bladder cancer cells to HCPT treatment in vitro and in vivo via ATM/NF-κB/IKK pathway-induced apoptosis. *PLoS One* 2013; 8: e50175.

[187] Xu X, Zhang X, Zhang Y, Yang L, Liu Y, Huang S, Lu L, Kong L, Li Z, Guo Q, Zhao L. Wogonin reversed resistant human myelogenous leukemia cells via inhibiting Nrf2 signaling by Stat3/NF-κB inactivation. *Sci Rep* 2017; 7: 39950.

[188] Wu H, Xin Y, Xu C, Xiao Y. Capecitabine combined with (-)-epigallocatechin-3-gallate inhibits angiogenesis and tumor growth in nude mice with gastric cancer xenografts. *Exp Ther Med* 2012; 3: 650-4.

[189] Ruela-de-Sousa RR, Fuhler GM, Blom N, Ferreira CV, Aoyama H, Peppelenbosch MP. Cytotoxicity of apigenin on leukemia cell lines: implications for prevention and therapy. *Cell Death Dis* 2010; 1: e19.

[190] Singh M, Bhatnagar P, Mishra S, Kumar P, Shukla Y, Gupta KC. PLGA-encapsulated tea polyphenols enhance the chemotherapeutic efficacy of cisplatin against human cancer cells and mice bearing Ehrlich ascites carcinoma. *Int J Nanomedicine* 2015; 10: 6789-809.

[191] Mendes LP, Gaeti MP, de Avila PH, de Sousa Vieira M, Dos Santos Rodrigues B, de Avila Marcelino RI, Dos Santos LC, Valadares MC, Lima EM. Multicompartimental nanoparticles for co-encapsulation and multimodal drug delivery to tumor cells and neovasculature. *Pharm Res* 2014; 31: 1106-19.

[192] Fujiki H, Suganuma M. Green tea: an effective synergist with anticancer drugs for tertiary cancer prevention. *Cancer Lett* 2012; 324: 119-25.

[193] Xu Y, Xin Y, Diao Y, Lu C, Fu J, Luo L, Yin Z. Synergistic effects of apigenin and paclitaxel on apoptosis of cancer cells. *PLoS One* 2011; 6: e29169.

[194] Hu XY, Liang JY, Guo XJ, Liu L, Guo YB. 5-Fluorouracil combined with apigenin enhances anticancer activity through mitochondrial membrane potential ($\Delta\Psi$m)-mediated apoptosis in hepatocellular carcinoma. *Clin Exp Pharmacol Physiol* 2015; 42: 146-53.

[195] Lecumberri E, Dupertuis YM, Miralbell R, Pichard C. Green tea polyphenol epigallocatechin-3-gallate (EGCG) as adjuvant in cancer therapy. *Clin Nutr* 2013; 32: 894-903.

[196] Papiez MA, Bukowska-Strakova K, Krzysciak W, Baran J. (-)-Epicatechin enhances etoposide-induced antileukaemic effect in rats with acute myeloid leukaemia. *Anticancer Res* 2012; 32: 2905-13.

[197] Akbas SH, Timur M, Ozben T. The effect of quercetin on topotecan cytotoxicity in MCF-7 and MDA-MB 231 human breast cancer cells. *J Surg Res* 2005; 125: 49-55.

[198] Mahbub AA, Le Maitre CL, Haywood-Small SL, Cross NA, Jordan-Mahy N. Polyphenols act synergistically with doxorubicin and etoposide in leukaemia cell lines. *Cell Death Discov* 2015; 1: 15043.

[199] Yunos NM, Beale P, Yu JQ, Huq F. Synergism from sequenced combinations of curcumin and epigallocatechin-3-gallate with cisplatin in the killing of human ovarian cancer cells. *Anticancer Res* 2011; 31: 1131-40.

[200] Ghasemi S, Lorigooini Z, Wibowo J, Amini-Khoei H. Tricin isolated from Allium atroviolaceum potentiated the effect of docetaxel on PC3 cell proliferation: role of miR-21. *Nat Prod Res* 2019; 33: 1828-31.

[201] Donia TIK, Gerges MN, Mohamed TM. Amelioration effect of Egyptian sweet orange hesperidin on Ehrlich ascites carcinoma (EAC) bearing mice. *Chem Biol Interact* 2018; 285: 76-84.

[202] Liu P, Feng J, Sun M, Yuan W, Xiao R, Xiong J, Huang X, Xiong M, Chen W, Yu X, Sun Q, Zhao X, Zhang Q, Shao L. Synergistic effects of baicalein with gemcitabine or docetaxel on the proliferation, migration and apoptosis of pancreatic cancer cells. *Int J Oncol* 2017; 51: 1878-86.

[203] Enomoto R, Koshiba C, Suzuki C, Lee E. Wogonin potentiates the antitumor action of etoposide and ameliorates its adverse effects. *Cancer Chemother Pharmacol* 2011; 67: 1063-72.

[204] Li X, Huang JM, Wang JN, Xiong XK, Yang XF, Zou F. Combination of chrysin and cisplatin promotes the apoptosis of Hep G2 cells by up-regulating p53. *Chem Biol Interact* 2015; 232: 12-20.

[205] Tyagi T, Treas JN, Mahalingaiah PK, Singh KP. Potentiation of growth inhibition and epigenetic modulation by combination of green tea polyphenol and 5-aza-2`-deoxycytidine in human breast cancer cells. *Breast Cancer Res Treat* 2015; 149: 655-68.

[206] Chang HR, Chen PN, Yang SF, Sun YS, Wu SW, Hung TW, Lian JD, Chu SC, Hsieh YS. Silibinin inhibits the invasion and migration of renal carcinoma 786-O cells in vitro, inhibits the growth of xenografts in vivo and enhances chemosensitivity to 5-fluorouracil and paclitaxel. *Mol Carcinog* 2011; 50: 811-23.

[207] Yu M, Qi B, Xiaoxiang W, Xu J, Liu X. Baicalein increases cisplatin sensitivity of A549 lung adenocarcinoma cells via PI3K/Akt/NF-κB pathway. *Biomed Pharmacother* 2017; 90: 677-85.

[208] Li WG, Wang HQ. Inhibitory effects of Silibinin combined with doxorubicin in hepatocellular carcinoma; an in vivo study. *J BUON* 2016; 21: 917-24.

[209] Klimaszewska-Wisniewska A, Halas-Wisniewska M, Tadrowski T, Gagat M, Grzanka D, Grzanka A. Paclitaxel and the dietary flavonoid fisetin: a synergistic combination that induces mitotic catastrophe and autophagic cell death in A549 non-small cell lung cancer cells. *Cancer Cell Int* 2016; 16: 10.

[210] Wang N, Wang Z, Peng C, You J, Shen J, Han S, Chen J. Dietary compound isoliquiritigenin targets GRP78 to chemosensitize breast cancer stem cells via β-catenin/ABCG2 signaling. *Carcinogenesis* 2014; 35: 2544-54.

[211] Bieg D, Sypniewski D, Nowak E, Bednarek I. Morin decreases galectin-3 expression and sensitizes ovarian cancer cells to cisplatin. *Arch Gynecol Obstet* 2018; 298: 1181-94.

[212] Mazumder ME, Beale P, Chan C, Yu JQ, Huq F. Epigallocatechin gallate acts synergistically in combination with cisplatin and designed trans-palladiums in ovarian cancer cells. *Anticancer Res* 2012; 32: 4851-60.

[213] Zhou DH, Wang X, Feng Q. EGCG enhances the efficacy of cisplatin by downregulating hsa-miR-98-5p in NSCLC A549 cells. *Nutr Cancer* 2014; 66: 636-44.

[214] Dash TK, Konkimalla VB. Formulation and optimization of doxorubicin and biochanin A combinational liposomes for reversal of chemoresistance. *AAPS PharmSciTech* 2017; 18: 1116-24.

[215] Yang YI, Lee KT, Park HJ, Kim TJ, Choi YS, Shih IeM, Choi JH. Tectorigenin sensitizes paclitaxel-resistant human ovarian cancer cells through downregulation of the Akt and NFκB pathway. *Carcinogenesis* 2012; 33: 2488-98.

[216] Wei X, Mo X, An F, Ji X, Lu Y. 2`,4`-Dihydroxy-6`-methoxy-3`,5`-dimethylchalcone, a potent Nrf2/ARE pathway inhibitor, reverses drug resistance by decreasing glutathione synthesis and drug efflux in BEL-7402/5-FU cells. *Food Chem Toxicol* 2018; 119: 252-9.

[217] Gao AM, Ke ZP, Wang JN, Yang JY, Chen SY, Chen H. Apigenin sensitizes doxorubicin-resistant hepatocellular carcinoma BEL-7402/ADM cells to doxorubicin via inhibiting PI3K/Akt/Nrf2 pathway. *Carcinogenesis* 2013; 34: 1806-14.

[218] Sabzichi M, Hamishehkar H, Ramezani F, Sharifi S, Tabasinezhad M, Pirouzpanah M, Ghanbari P, Samadi N. Luteolin-loaded phytosomes sensitize human breast carcinoma MDA-MB 231 cells to doxorubicin by suppressing Nrf2 mediated signalling. *Asian Pac J Cancer Prev* 2014; 15: 5311-6.

[219] Cipak L, Rauko P, Miadokova E, Cipakova I, Novotny L. Effects of flavonoids on cisplatin-induced apoptosis of HL-60 and L1210 leukemia cells. *Leuk Res* 2003; 27: 65-72.

[220] Wu L, Yang W, Zhang SN, Lu JB. Alpinetin inhibits lung cancer progression and elevates sensitization drug-resistant lung cancer cells to cis-diammined dichloridoplatium. *Drug Des Devel Ther* 2015; 9: 6119-27.

[221] Wang X, Jiang P, Wang P, Yang CS, Wang X, Feng Q. EGCG enhances cisplatin sensitivity by regulating expression of the copper and cisplatin influx transporter CTR1 in ovary cancer. *PLoS One* 2015; 10: e0125402.

[222] Yu S, Gong LS, Li NF, Pan YF, Zhang L. Galangin (GG) combined with cisplatin (DDP) to suppress human lung cancer by inhibition of STAT3-regulated NF-κB and Bcl-2/Bax signaling pathways. *Biomed Pharmacother* 2018; 97: 213-24.

[223] Hu XJ, Xie MY, Kluxen FM, Diel P. Genistein modulates the anti-tumor activity of cisplatin in MCF-7 breast and HT-29 colon cancer cells. *Arch Toxicol* 2014; 88: 625-35.

[224] Zhao JL, Zhao J, Jiao HJ. Synergistic growth-suppressive effects of quercetin and cisplatin on HepG2 human hepatocellular carcinoma cells. *Appl Biochem Biotechnol* 2014; 172: 784-91.

[225] Gao AM, Zhang XY, Hu JN, Ke ZP. Apigenin sensitizes hepatocellular carcinoma cells to doxorubic through regulating miR-520b/ATG7 axis. *Chem Biol Interact* 2018; 280: 45-50.

[226] Vittorio O, Le Grand M, Makharza SA, Curcio M, Tucci P, Iemma F, Nicoletta FP, Hampel S, Cirillo G. Doxorubicin synergism and resistance reversal in human neuroblastoma BE(2)C cell lines: An in vitro study with dextran-catechin nanohybrids. *Eur J Pharm Biopharm* 2018; 122: 176-85.

[227] Staedler D, Idrizi E, Kenzaoui BH, Juillerat-Jeanneret L. Drug combinations with quercetin: doxorubicin plus quercetin in human breast cancer cells. *Cancer Chemother Pharmacol* 2011; 68: 1161-72.

[228] Kasala ER, Bodduluru LN, Barua CC, Gogoi R. Chrysin and its emerging role in cancer drug resistance. *Chem Biol Interact* 2015; 236: 7-8.

[229] Shervington A, Pawar V, Menon S, Thakkar D, Patel R. The sensitization of glioma cells to cisplatin and tamoxifen by the use of catechin. *Mol Biol Rep* 2009; 36: 1181-6.

[230] Shi DB, Li XX, Zheng HT, Li DW, Cai GX, Peng JJ, Gu WL, Guan ZQ, Xu Y, Cai SJ. Icariin-mediated inhibition of NF-κB activity enhances the in vitro and in vivo antitumour effect of 5-fluorouracil in colorectal cancer. *Cell Biochem Biophys* 2014; 69: 523-30.

[231] Rastegar H, Ahmadi Ashtiani H, Anjarani S, Bokaee S, Khaki A, Javadi L. The role of milk thistle extract in breast carcinoma cell line (MCF-7) apoptosis with doxorubicin. *Acta Med Iran* 2013; 51; 591-8.

[232] Garg AK, Buchholz TA, Aggarwal BB. Chemosensitization and radiosensitization of tumors by plant polyphenols. *Antioxid Redox Signal* 2005; 7: 1630-47.

[233] Mukhtar E, Adhami VM, Siddiqui IA, Verma AK, Mukhtar H. Fisetin enhances chemotherapeutic effect of cabazitaxel against human prostate cancer cells. *Mol Cancer Ther* 2016; 15: 2863-74.

[234] Raina K, Agarwal R. Combinatorial strategies for cancer eradication by silibinin and cytotoxic agents: efficacy and mechanisms. *Acta Pharmacol Sin* 2007; 28: 1466-75.

[235] Singh M, Bhui K, Singh R, Shukla Y. Tea polyphenols enhance cisplatin chemosensitivity in cervical cancer cells via induction of apoptosis. *Life Sci* 2013; 93: 7-16.

[236] Xavier CP, Lima CF, Rohde M, Pereira-Wilson C. Quercetin enhances 5-fluorouracil-induced apoptosis in MSI colorectal cancer cells through p53 modulation. *Cancer Chemother Pharmacol* 2011; 68: 1449-57.

[237] Yang MY, Wang CJ, Chen NF, Ho WH, Lu FJ, Tseng TH. Luteolin enhances paclitaxel-induced apoptosis in human breast cancer MDA-MB-231 cells by blocking STAT3. *Chem Biol Interact* 2014; 213: 60-8.

[238] Nagaprashantha LD. Vatsyayan R, Singhal J, Fast S, Roby R, Awasthi S, Singhal SS. Anti-cancer effects of novel flavonoid vicenin-2 as a single agent and in synergistic combination with docetaxel in prostate cancer. *Biochem Pharmacol* 2011; 82: 1100-9.

[239] Nessa MU, Beale P, Chan C, Yu JQ, Huq F. Synergism from combinations of cisplatin and oxaliplatin with quercetin and thymoquinone in human ovarian tumour models. *Anticancer Res* 2011; 31: 3789-97.

[240] Johnson JL, Dia VP, Wallig M, Gonzalez de Mejia E. Luteolin and gemcitabine protect against pancreatic cancer in an orthotopic mouse model. *Pancreas* 2015; 44: 144-51.

[241] Li Y, Ahmed F, Ali S, Philip PA, Kucuk O, Sarkar FH. Inactivation of nuclear factor kappaB by soy isoflavone genistein contributes to increased apoptosis induced by chemotherapeutic agents in human cancer cells. *Cancer Res* 2005; 65: 6934-42.

[242] Sarkar FH, Li Y. Using chemopreventive agents to enhance the efficacy of cancer therapy. *Cancer Res* 2006; 66: 3347-50.

[243] Chian S, Li YY, Wang XJ, Tang XW. Luteolin sensitizes two oxaliplatin-resistant colorectal cancer cell lines to chemotherapeutic drugs via inhibition of the Nrf2 pathway. *Asian Pac J Cancer Prev* 2014; 15: 2911-6.

[244] Lei W, Mayotte JE, Levitt ML. Enhancement of chemosensitivity and programmed cell death by tyrosine kinase inhibitors correlates with EGFR expression in non-small cell lung cancer cells. *Anticancer Res* 1999; 19: 221-8.

[245] Lee R, Kim YJ, Lee YJ, Chung HW. The selective effect of genistein on the toxicity of bleomycin in normal lymphocytes and HL-60 cells. *Toxicology* 2004; 195: 87-95.

[246] Zanini C, Giribaldi G, Madili G, Carta F, Crescenzio N, Bisaro B, Doria A, Foglia L, di Montezemolo LC, Timeus F, Turrini F. Inhibition of heat shock proteins (HSP) expression by quercetin and differential doxorubicin sensitization in neuroblastoma and Ewing`s sarcoma cell lines. *J Neurochem* 2007; 103: 1344-54.

[247] Hyun JJ, Lee HS, Keum B, Seo YS, Jeen YT, Chun HJ, Um SH, Kim CD. Expression of heat shock protein 70 modulates the chemoresponsiveness of pancreatic cancer. *Gut Liver* 2013; 7: 739-46.

[248] Sharma A, Upadhyay AK, Bhat MK. Inhibition of Hsp27 and Hsp40 potentiates 5-fluorouracil and carboplatin mediated cell killing in hepatoma cells. *Cancer Biol Ther* 2009; 8: 2106-13.

[249] Schumacher M, Hautzinger A, Rossmann A, Holzhauser S, Popovic D, Hertrampf A, Kuntz S, Boll M, Wenzel U. Chrysin blocks topotecan-induced apoptosis in Caco-2 cells in spite of inhibition of ABC-transporters. *Biochem Pharmacol* 2010; 80: 471-9.

[250] Fatma S, Talegaonkar S, Igbal Z, Panda AK, Negi LM, Goswami DG, Tariq M. Novel flavonoid-based biodegradable nanoparticles for effective oral delivery of etoposide by P-glycoprotein modulation: an in vitro, ex vivo and in vivo investigations. *Drug Deliv* 2016; 23: 500-11.

[251] Lee E, Enomoto R, Koshiba C, Hirano H. Inhibition of P-glycoprotein by wogonin is involved with the potentiation of etoposide-induced apoptosis in cancer cells. *Ann N Y Acad Sci* 2009; 1171: 132-6.

[252] Li X, Wan L, Wang F, Pei H, Zheng L, Wu W, Ye H, Wang Y, Chen L. Barbigerone reverses multidrug resistance in breast MCF-7/ADR cells. *Phytother Res* 2018; 32: 733-40.

[253] Qian F, Wei D, Zhang Q, Yang S. Modulation of P-glycoprotein function and reversal of multidrug resistance by (-)-epigallocatechin gallate in human cancer cells. *Biomed Pharmacother* 2005; 59: 64-9.

[254] Mohana S, Ganesan M, Rajendra Prasad N, Ananthakrishnan D, Velmurugan D. Flavonoids modulate multidrug resistance through wnt signaling in P-glycoprotein overexpressing cell lines. *BMC Cancer* 2018; 18: 1168.

[255] Meng L, Xia X, Yang Y, Ye J, Dong W, Ma P, Jin Y, Liu Y. Co-encapsulation of paclitaxel and baicalein in nanoemulsions to overcome multidrug resistance via oxidative stress augmentation and P-glycoprotein inhibition. *Int J Pharm* 2016; 513: 8-16.

[256] Chen HJ, Chung YL, Li CY, Chang YT, Wang CCN, Lee HY, Lin HY, Hung CC. Taxifolin resensitizes multidrug resistance cancer cells via uncompetitive inhibition of P-glycoprotein function. *Molecules* 2018; 23: E3055.

[257] Delmas D, Xiao J. Natural polyphenols properties: chemopreventive and chemosensitizing activities. *Anticancer Agents Med Chem* 2012; 12: 835.

[258] Huang HY, Niu JL, Lu YH. Multidrug resistance reversal effect of DMC derived from buds of Cleistocalyx operculatus in human hepatocellular tumor xenograft model. *J Sci Food Agric* 2012; 92: 135-40.

[259] Mohana S, Ganesan M, Agilan B, Karthikeyan R, Srithar G, Beaulah Mary R, Ananthakrishnan D, Velmurugan D, Rajendra Prasad N, Ambudkar SV. Screening dietary flavonoids for the reversal of P-glycoprotein-mediated multidrug resistance in cancer. *Mol Biosyst* 2016; 12: 2458-70.

[260] Yuan Z, Wang H, Hu Z, Huang Y, Yao F, Sun S, Wu B. Quercetin inhibits proliferation and drug resistance in KB/VCR oral cancer cells and enhances its sensitivity to vincristine. *Nutr Cancer* 2015; 67: 126-36.

[261] Tran VH, Marks D, Duke RK, Bebawy M, Duke CC, Roufogalis BD. Modulation of P-glycoprotein-mediated anticancer drug accumulation, cytotoxicity, and ATPase activity by flavonoid interactions. *Nutr Cancer* 2011; 63: 435-43.

[262] Ohtani H, Ikegawa T, Honda Y, Kohyama N, Morimoto S, Shoyama Y, Juichi M, Naito M, Tsuruo T, Sawada Y. Effects of various methoxyflavones on vincristine

uptake and multidrug resistance to vincristine in P-gp-overexpressing K562/ADM cells. *Pharm Res* 2007; 24: 1936-43.

[263] Klimaszewska-Wisniewska A, Halas-Wisniewska M, Grzanka A, Grzanka D. Evaluation of anti-metastatic potential of the combination of fisetin with paclitaxel on A549 non-small cell lung cancer cells. *Int J Mol Sci* 2018; 19: E661.

[264] Luo T, Wang J, Yin Y, Hua H, Jing J, Sun X, Li M, Zhang Y, Jiang Y. (-)-Epigallocatechin gallate sensitizes breast cancer cells to paclitaxel in a murine model of breast carcinoma. *Breast Cancer Res* 2010; 12: R8.

[265] Johnson JL, Gonzalez de Mejia E. Interactions between dietary flavonoids apigenin or luteolin and chemotherapeutic drugs to potentiate anti-proliferative effect on human pancreatic cancer cells, in vitro. *Food Chem Toxicol* 2013; 60: 83-91.

[266] Smith ML, Murphy K, Doucette CD, Greenshields AL, Hoskin DW. The dietary flavonoid fisetin causes cell cycle arrest, caspase-dependent apoptosis, and enhanced cytotoxicity of chemotherapeutic drugs in triple-negative breast cancer cells. *J Cell Biochem* 2016; 117: 1913-25.

[267] Xu H, Yang T, Liu X, Tian Y, Chen X, Yuan R, Su S, Lin X, Du G. Luteolin synergizes the antitumor effects of 5-fluorouracil against human hepatocellular carcinoma cells through apoptosis induction and metabolism. *Life Sci* 2016; 144: 138-47.

[268] Wu J, Guan M, Wong PF, Yu H, Dong J, Xu J. Icariside II potentiates paclitaxel-induced apoptosis in human melanoma A375 cells by inhibiting TLR4 signaling pathway. *Food Chem Toxicol* 2012; 50: 3019-24.

[269] Wang T, Gao J, Yu J, Shen L. Synergistic inhibitory effect of wogonin and low-dose paclitaxel on gastric cancer cells and tumor xenografts. *Chin J Cancer Res* 2013; 25: 505-13.

[270] Daglioglu C. Enhancing tumor cell response to multidrug resistance with pH-sensitive quercetin and doxorubicin conjugated multifunctional nanoparticles. *Colloids Surf B Biointerfaces* 2017; 156: 175-85.

[271] Liu Q, Li J, Pu G, Zhang F, Liu H, Zhang Y. Co-delivery of baicalein and doxorubicin by hyaluronic acid decorated nanostructured lipid carriers for breast cancer therapy. *Drug Deliv* 2016; 23: 1364-8.

[272] Zhang J, Luo Y, Zhao X, Li X, Li K, Chen D, Qiao M, Hu H, Zhao X. Co-delivery of doxorubicin and the traditional Chinese medicine quercetin using biotin-PEG2000-DSPE modified liposomes for the treatment of multidrug resistant breast cancer. *RSC Adv* 2016; 6: 113173.

[273] Cote B, Carlson LJ, Rao DA, Alani AWG. Combinatorial resveratrol and quercetin polymeric micelles mitigate doxorubicin induced cardiotoxicity in vitro and in vivo. *J Control Release* 2015; 213: 128-33.

[274] Liao B, Ying H, Yu C, Fan Z, Zhang W, Shi J, Ying H, Ravichandran N, Xu Y, Yin J, Jiang Y, Du Q. (-)-Epigallocatechin gallate (EGCG)-nanoethosomes as a

transdermal delivery system for docetaxel to treat implanted human melanoma cell tumors in mice. *Int J Pharm* 2016; 512: 22-31.

[275] Wong MY, Chiu GN. Simultaneous liposomal delivery of quercetin and vincristine for enhanced estrogen-receptor-negative breast cancer treatment. *Anticancer Drugs* 2010; 21: 401-10.

[276] Goto H, Yanagimachi M, Goto S, Takeuchi M, Kato H, Yokosuka T, Kajiwara R, Yokota S. Methylated chrysin reduced cell proliferation, but antagonized cytotoxicity of other anticancer drugs in acute lymphoblastic leukemia. *Anticancer Drugs* 2012; 23: 417-25.

[277] Pyrko P, Schönthal AH, Hofman FM, Chen TC, Lee AS. The unfolded protein response regulator GRP78/BiP as a novel target for increasing chemosensitivity in malignant gliomas. *Cancer Res* 2007; 67: 9809-16.

[278] Hoffman R, Graham L, Newlands ES. Enhanced anti-proliferative action of busulphan by quercetin on the human leukaemia cell line K562. *Br J Cancer* 1989; 59: 347-8.

[279] Teofili L, Pierelli L, Iovino MS, Leone G, Scambia G, De Vincenzo R, Benedetti-Panici P, Menichella G, Macri E, Piantelli M, Ranelletti FO, Larocca LM. The combination of quercetin and cytosine arabinoside synergistically inhibits leukemic cell growth. *Leuk Res* 1992; 16: 497-503.

[280] Scambia G, Ranelletti FO, Panici PB, De Vincenzo R, Bonanno G, Ferrandina G, Piantelli M, Bussa S, Rumi C, Cianfriglia M, Mancuso S. Quercetin potentiates the effect of adriamycin in a multidrug-resistant MCF-7 human breast-cancer cell line: P-glycoprotein as a possible target. *Cancer Chemother Pharmacol* 1994; 34: 459-64.

[281] Scambia G, Ranelletti FO, Benedetti Panici P, Paintelli M, Bonanno G, De Vincenzo R, Ferrandina G, Maggiano N, Capelli A, Mancuso S. Inhibitory effect of quercetin on primary ovarian and endometrial cancers and synergistic activity with cis-diamminedichloroplatinum (II). *Gynecol Oncol* 1992; 45: 13-9.

[282] Tamura S, Bito T, Ichihashi M, Ueda M. Genistein enhances the cisplatin-induced inhibition of cell growth and apoptosis in human malignant melanoma cells. *Pigment Cell Res* 2003; 16: 470-6.

[283] Lim HA, Kim JH, Kim JH, Sung MK, Kim MK, Park JH, Kim JS. Genistein induces glucose-regulated protein 78 in mammary tumor cells. *J Med Food* 2006; 9: 28-32.

[284] Marverti G, Andrews PA. Stimulation of cis-diamminedichloroplatinum(II) accumulation by modulation of passive permeability with genistein: an altered response in accumulation-defective resistant cells. *Clin Cancer Res* 1996; 2: 991-9.

[285] Khoshyomn S, Nathan D, Manske GC, Osler TM, Penar PL. Synergistic effect of genistein and BCNU on growth inhibition and cytotoxicity of glioblastoma cells. *J Neurooncol* 2002; 57: 193-200.

[286] Khoshyomn S, Manske GC, Lew SM, Wald SL, Penar PL. Synergistic action of genistein and cisplatin on growth inhibition and cytotoxicity of human medulloblastoma cells. *Pediatr Neurosurg* 2000; 33: 123-31.

[287] Masuda M, Suzui M, Weinstein IB. Effects of epigallocatechin-3-gallate on growth, epidermal growth factor receptor signaling pathways, gene expression, and chemosensitivity in human head and neck squamous cell carcinoma cell lines. *Clin Cancer Res* 2001; 7: 4220-9.

[288] Masuda M, Suzui M, Lim JT, Weinstein IB. Epigallocatechin-3-gallate inhibits activation of HER-2/neu and downstream signaling pathways in human head and neck and breast carcinoma cells. *Clin Cancer Res* 2003; 9: 3486-91.

[289] Zhang Q, Wei D, Liu J. In vivo reversal of doxorubicin resistance by (-)-epigallocatechin gallate in a solid human carcinoma xenograft. *Cancer Lett* 2004; 208: 179-86.

[290] Angelini A, Di Ilio C, Castellani ML, Conti P, Cuccurullo F. Modulation of multidrug resistance p-glycoprotein activity by flavonoids and honokiol in human doxorubicin- resistant sarcoma cells (MES-SA/DX-5): implications for natural sedatives as chemosensitizing agents in cancer therapy. *J Biol Regul Homeost Agents* 2010; 24: 197-205.

[291] Chen YJ, Wu CS, Shieh JJ, Wu JH, Chen HY, Chung TW, Chen YK, Lin CC. Baicalein triggers mitochondria-mediated apoptosis and enhances the antileukemic effect of vincristine in childhood acute lymphoblastic leukemia CCRF-CEM cells. *Evid Based Complement Alternat Med* 2013: 2013: 124747.

[292] Lim HK, Kim KM, Jeong SY, Choi EK, Jung J. Chrysin increases the therapeutic efficacy of docetaxel and mitigates docetaxel-induced edema. *Integr Cancer Ther* 2017; 16: 496-504.

[293] Davenport A, Frezza M, Shen M, Ge Y, Huo C, Chan TH, Dou QP. Celastrol and an EGCG pro-drug exhibit potent chemosensitizing activity in human leukemia cells. *Int J Mol Med* 2010; 25: 465-70.

[294] Singh M, Bhatnagar P, Srivastava AK, Kumar P, Shukla Y, Gupta KC. Enhancement of cancer chemosensitization potential of cisplatin by tea polyphenols poly(lactide-co-glycolide) nanoparticles. *J Biomed Nanotechnol* 2011; 7: 202.

[295] Sak K, Everaus H. Nanotechnological approach to improve the bioavailability of dietary flavonoids with chemopreventive and anticancer properties. *In*: Grumezescu AM, ed. Nutraceuticals. Nanotechnology in the Agri-Food Industry, Vol.4. Elsevier 2016, pp. 427-79.

[296] Hu J, Wang J, Wang G, Yao Z, Dang X. Pharmacokinetics and antitumor efficacy of DSPE-PEG2000 polymeric liposomes loaded with quercetin and temozolomide: Analysis of their effectiveness in enhancing the chemosensitization of drug-resistant glioma cells. *Int J Mol Med* 2016; 37: 690-702.

[297] Wen D, Peng Y, Lin F, Singh RK, Mahato RI. Micellar delivery of miR-34a modulator rubone and paclitaxel in resistant prostate cancer. *Cancer Res* 2017; 77: 3244-54.

[298] Tsai LC, Hsieh HY, Lu KY, Wang SY, Mi FL. EGCG/gelatin-doxorubicin gold nanoparticles enhance therapeutic efficacy of doxorubicin for prostate cancer treatment. *Nanomedicine (Lond)* 2016; 11: 9-30.

[299] Vittorio O, Brandl M, Cirillo G, Spizzirri UG, Picci N, Kavallaris M, Iemma F, Hampel S. Novel functional cisplatin carrier based on carbon nanotubes-quercetin nanohybrid induces synergistic anticancer activity against neuroblastoma in vitro. *RSC Adv* 2014; 4: 31378.

[300] Li J, Zhang J, Wang Y, Liang X, Wusiman Z, Yin Y, Shen Q. Synergistic inhibition of migration and invasion of breast cancer cells by dual docetaxel/quercetin-loaded nanoparticles via Akt/MMP-9 pathway. *Int J Pharm* 2017; 523: 300-9.

[301] Narayanan S, Mony U, Vijaykumar DK, Koyakutty M, Paul-Prasanth B, Menon D. Sequential release of epigallocatechin gallate and paclitaxel from PLGA-casein core/shell nanoparticles sensitizes drug-resistant breast cancer cells. *Nanomedicine* 2015; 11: 1399-406.

[302] Qian F, Ye CL, Wei DZ, Lu YH, Yang SL. In vitro and in vivo reversal of cancer cell multidrug resistance by 2`,4`-dihydroxy-6`-methoxy-3`,5`-dimethylchalcone. *J Chemother* 2005; 17: 309-14.

[303] Huang HY, Niu JL, Zhao LM, Lu YH. Reversal effect of 2`,4`-dihydroxy-6`-methoxy-3`,5`-dimethylchalcone on multi-drug resistance in resistant human hepatocellular carcinoma cell line BEL-7402/5-FU. *Phytomedicine* 2011; 18: 1086-92.

[304] Hu FW, Yu CC, Hsieh PL, Liao YW, Lu MY, Chu PM. Targeting oral cancer stemness and chemoresistance by isoliquiritigenin-mediated GRP78 regulation. *Oncotarget* 2017; 8: 93912-23.

[305] Yang KC, Tsai CY, Wang YJ, Wei PL, Lee CH, Chen JH, Wu CH, Ho YS. Apple polyphenol phloretin potentiates the anticancer actions of paclitaxel through induction of apoptosis in human hep G2 cells. *Mol Carcinog* 2009; 48: 420-31.

[306] Varela-Castillo O, Cordero P, Gutierrez-Iglesias G, Palma I, Rubio-Gayosso I, Meaney E, Ramirez-Sanchez I, Villarreal F, Ceballos G, Najera N. Characterization of the cytotoxic effects of the combination of cisplatin and flavanol (-)-epicatechin on human lung cancer cell line A549. An isobolographic approach. *Exp Oncol* 2018; 40: 19-23.

[307] Suganuma M, Saha A, Fujiki H. New cancer treatment strategy using combination of green tea catechins and anticancer drugs. *Cancer Sci* 2011; 102: 317-23.

[308] Chan MM, Soprano KJ, Weinstein K, Fong D. Epigallocatechin-3-gallate delivers hydrogen peroxide to induce death of ovarian cancer cells and enhances their cisplatin susceptibility. *J Cell Physiol* 2006; 207: 389-96.

[309] Huang W, Ding L, Huang Q, Hu H, Liu S, Yang X, Hu X, Dang Y, Shen S, Li J, Ji X, Jiang S, Liu JO, Yu L. Carbonyl reductase 1 as a novel target of (-)-epigallocatechin gallate against hepatocellular carcinoma. *Hepatology* 2010; 52: 703-14.

[310] Saiko P, Steinmann MT, Schuster H, Graser G, Bressler S, Giessrigl B, Lackner A, Grusch M, Krupitza G, Bago-Horvath Z, Jaeger W, Fritzer-Szekeres M, Szekeres T. Epigallocatechin gallate, ellagic acid, and rosmarinic acid perturb dNTP pools and inhibit de novo DNA synthesis and proliferation of human HL-60 promyelocytic leukemia cells: Synergism with arabinofuranosylcytosine. *Phytomedicine* 2015; 22: 213-22.

[311] Garcia-Vilas JA, Quesada AR, Medina MA. Screening of synergistic interactions of epigallocatechin-3-gallate with antiangiogenic and antitumor compounds. *Synergy* 2016; 3: 5-13.

[312] Hu F, Wei F, Wang Y, Wu B, Fang Y, Xiong B. EGCG synergizes the therapeutic effect of cisplatin and oxaliplatin through autophagic pathway in human colorectal cancer cells. *J Pharmacol Sci* 2015; 128: 27-34.

[313] Hwang JT, Ha J, Park IJ, Lee SK, Baik HW, Kim YM, Park OJ. Apoptotic effect of EGCG in HT-29 colon cancer cells via AMPK signal pathway. *Cancer Lett* 2007; 247: 115-21.

[314] Tang B, Du J, Wang J, Tan G, Gao Z, Wang Z, Wang L. Alpinetin suppresses proliferation of human hepatoma cells by the activation of MKK7 and elevates sensitization to cis-diammined dichloridoplatium. *Oncol Rep* 2012; 27: 1090-6.

[315] Lu L, Yang LN, Wang XX, Song CL, Qin H, Wu YJ. Synergistic cytotoxicity of ampelopsin sodium and carboplatin in human non-small cell lung cancer cell line SPC-A1 by G1 cell cycle arrested. *Chin J Integr Med* 2017; 23: 125-31.

[316] Wang Z, Sun X, Feng Y, Liu X, Zhou L, Sui H, Ji Q, E Q, Chen J, Wu L, Li Q. Dihydromyricetin reverses MRP2-mediated MDR and enhances anticancer activity induced by oxaliplatin in colorectal cancer cells. *Anticancer Drugs* 2017; 28: 281-8.

[317] Xu Y, Wang S, Chan HF, Lu H, Lin Z, He C, Chen M. Dihydromyricetin induces apoptosis and reverses drug resistance in ovarian cancer cells by p53-mediated downregulation of survivin. *Sci Rep* 2017; 7: 46060.

[318] Hou X, Bai X, Gou X, Zeng H, Xia C, Zhuang W, Chen X, Zhao Z, Huang M, Jin J. 3`,4`,5`,5,7-pentamethoxyflavone sensitizes Cisplatin-resistant A549 cells to Cisplatin by inhibition of Nrf2 pathway. *Mol Cells* 2015; 38: 396-401.

[319] Xu YY, Wu TT, Zhou SH, Bao YY, Wang QY, Fan J, Huang YP. Apigenin suppresses GLUT-1 and p-AKT expression to enhance the chemosensitivity to

cisplatin of laryngeal carcinoma Hep-2 cells: an in vitro study. *Int J Clin Exp Pathol* 2014; 7: 3938-47.

[320] Lu C, Wang H, Chen S, Yang R, Li H, Zhang G. Baicalein inhibits cell growth and increases cisplatin sensitivity of A549 and H460 cells via miR-424-3p and targeting PTEN/PI3K/Akt pathway. *J Cell Mol Med* 2018; 22: 2478-87.

[321] Chen F, Zhuang M, Zhong C, Peng J, Wang X, Li J, Chen Z, Huang Y. Baicalein reverses hypoxia-induced 5-FU resistance in gastric cancer AGS cells through suppression of glycolysis and the PTEN/Akt/HIF-1α signaling pathway. *Oncol Rep* 2015; 33: 457-63.

[322] Pan Q, Xue M, Xiao SS, Wan YJ, Xu DB. A combination therapy with baicalein and taxol promotes mitochondria-mediated cell apoptosis: Involving in Akt/β-catenin signaling pathway. *DNA Cell Biol* 2016; 35: 646-56.

[323] Akmal Y, Senthil M, Yan J, Xing Q, Wang Y, Somlo G, Yim J. Combination of a natural compound (baicalein) and paclitaxel results in synergistic apoptosis in mouse breast cancer cells. *J Surg Res* 2011; 165: 218-9.

[324] Wang W, Xi M, Duan X, Wang Y, Kong F. Delivery of baicalein and paclitaxel using self-assembled nanoparticles: synergistic antitumor effect in vitro and in vivo. *Int J Nanomedicine* 2015; 10: 3737-50.

[325] Li J, Duan B, Guo Y, Zhou R, Sun J, Bie B, Yang S, Huang C, Yang J, Li Z. Baicalein sensitizes hepatocellular carcinoma cells to 5-FU and Epirubicin by activating apoptosis and ameliorating P-glycoprotein activity. *Biomed Pharmacother* 2018; 98: 806-12.

[326] Xu Z, Mei J, Tan Y. Baicalin attenuates DDP (cisplatin) resistance in lung cancer by downregulating MARK2 and p-Akt. *Int J Oncol* 2017; 50: 93-100.

[327] Gao H, Xie J, Peng J, Han Y, Jiang Q, Han M, Wang C. Hispidulin inhibits proliferation and enhances chemosensitivity of gallbladder cancer cells by targeting HIF-1α. *Exp Cell Res* 2015; 332: 236-46.

[328] Qu Q, Qu J, Guo Y, Zhou BT, Zhou HH. Luteolin potentiates the sensitivity of colorectal cancer cell lines to oxaliplatin through the PPARγ/OCTN2 pathway. *Anticancer Drugs* 2014; 25: 1016-27.

[329] Sato Y, Sasaki N, Saito M, Endo N, Kugawa F, Ueno A. Luteolin attenuates doxorubicin-induced cytotoxicity to MCF-7 human breast cancer cells. *Biol Pharm Bull* 2015; 38: 703-9.

[330] Dia VP, Pangloli P. Epithelial-to-mesenchymal transition in paclitaxel-resistant ovarian cancer cells is downregulated by luteolin. *J Cell Physiol* 2017; 232: 391-401.

[331] Tang X, Wang H, Fan L, Wu X, Xin A, Ren H, Wang XJ. Luteolin inhibits Nrf2 leading to negative regulation of the Nrf2/ARE pathway and sensitization of human lung carcinoma A549 cells to therapeutic drugs. *Free Radic Biol Med* 2011; 50: 1599-609.

[332] Moon JY, Cho M, Ahn KS, Cho SK. Nobiletin induces apoptosis and potentiates the effects of the anticancer drug 5-fluorouracil in p53-mutated SNU-16 human gastric cancer cells. *Nutr Cancer* 2013; 65: 286-95.

[333] Yang HY, Zhao L, Yang Z, Zhao Q, Qiang L, Ha J, Li ZY, You QD, Guo QL. Oroxylin A reverses multi-drug resistance of human hepatoma BEL7402/5-FU cells via downregulation of P-glycoprotein expression by inhibiting NF-κB signaling pathway. *Mol Carcinog* 2012; 51: 185-95.

[334] Ha J, Zhao L, Zhao Q, Yao J, Zhu BB, Lu N, Ke X, Yang HY, Li Z, You QD, Guo QL. Oroxylin A improves the sensitivity of HT-29 human colon cancer cells to 5-FU through modulation of the COX-2 signaling pathway. *Biochem Cell Biol* 2012; 90: 521-31.

[335] Zhao L, Chen Z, Wang J, Yang L, Zhao Q, Wang J, Qi Q, Mu R, You QD, Guo QL. Synergistic effect of 5-fluorouracil and the flavanoid oroxylin A on HepG2 human hepatocellular carcinoma and on H22 transplanted mice. *Cancer Chemother Pharmacol* 2010; 65: 481-9.

[336] Hong ZP, Wang LG, Wang HJ, Ye WF, Wang XZ. Wogonin exacerbates the cytotoxic effect of oxaliplatin by inducing nitrosative stress and autophagy in human gastric cancer cells. *Phytomedicine* 2018; 39: 168-75.

[337] Fu P, Du F, Liu Y, Hong Y, Yao M, Zheng S. Wogonin increases doxorubicin sensitivity by down-regulation of IGF-1R/AKT signaling pathway in human breast cancer. *Cell Mol Biol (Noisy-le-grand)* 2015; 61: 123-7.

[338] Zhao Q, Wang J, Zou MJ, Hu R, Zhao L, Qiang L, Rong JJ, You QD, Guo QL. Wogonin potentiates the antitumor effects of low dose 5-fluorouracil against gastric cancer through induction of apoptosis by down-regulation of NF-kappaB and regulation of its metabolism. *Toxicol Lett* 2010; 197: 201-10.

[339] Zhao L, Sha YY, Zhao Q, Yao J, Zhu BB, Lu ZJ, You QD, Guo QL. Enhanced 5-fluorouracil cytotoxicity in high COX-2 expressing hepatocellular carcinoma cells by wogonin via the PI3K/Akt pathway. *Biochem Cell Biol* 2013; 91: 221-9.

[340] Lee E, Enomoto R, Suzuki C, Ohno M, Ohashi T, Miyauchi A, Tanimoto E, Maeda K, Hirano H, Yokoi T, Sugahara C. Wogonin, a plant flavone, potentiates etoposide-induced apoptosis in cancer cells. *Ann N Y Acad Sci* 2007; 1095: 521-6.

[341] Qian C, Wang Y, Zhong Y, Tang J, Zhang J, Li Z, Wang Q, Hu R. Wogonin-enhanced reactive oxygen species-induced apoptosis and potentiated cytotoxic effects of chemotherapeutic agents by suppression Nrf2-mediated signaling in HepG2 cells. *Free Radic Res* 2014; 48: 607-21.

[342] Zhu X, Ji M, Han Y, Guo Y, Zhu W, Gao F, Yang X, Zhang C. PGRMC1-dependent autophagy by hyperoside induces apoptosis and sensitizes ovarian cancer cells to cisplatin treatment. *Int J Oncol* 2017; 50: 835-46.

[343] Li B, Jin X, Meng H, Hu B, Zhang T, Yu J, Chen S, Guo X, Wang W, Jiang W, Wang J. Morin promotes prostate cancer cells chemosensitivity to paclitaxel through miR-155/GATA3 axis. *Oncotarget* 2017; 8: 47849-60.

[344] Yi JL, Shi S, Shen YL, Wang L, Chen HY, Zhu J, Ding Y. Myricetin and methyl eugenol combination enhances the anticancer activity, cell cycle arrest and apoptosis induction of cis-platin against HeLa cervical cancer cell lines. *Int J Clin Exp Pathol* 2015; 8: 1116-27.

[345] Zhang P, Sun S, Li N, Ho ASW, Kiang KMY, Zhang X, Cheng YS, Poon MW, Lee D, Pu JKS, Leung GKK. Rutin increases the cytotoxicity of temozolomide in glioblastoma via autophagy inhibition. *J Neurooncol* 2017; 132: 393-400.

[346] Xu GY, Tang XJ. Troxerutin (TXN) potentiated 5-Fluorouracil (5-Fu) treatment of human gastric cancer through suppressing STAT3/NF-κB and Bcl-2 signaling pathways. *Biomed Pharmacother* 2017; 92: 95-107.

[347] Bueno Perez L, Pan L, Sass E, Gupta SV, Lehman A, Kinghorn AD, Lucas DM. Potentiating effect of the flavonolignan (-)-hydnocarpin in combination with vincristine in a sensitive and P-gp-expressing acute lymphoblastic leukemia cell line. *Phytother Res* 2013; 27: 1735-8.

[348] Scambia G, De Vincenzo R, Ranelletti FO, Panici PB, Ferrandina G, D`Agostino G, Fattorossi A, Bombardelli E, Mancuso S. Antiproliferative effect of silybin on gynaecological malignancies: synergism with cisplatin and doxorubicin. *Eur J Cancer* 1996; 32A: 877-82.

[349] Tyagi AK, Agarwal C, Chan DC, Agarwal R. Synergistic anti-cancer effects of silibinin with conventional cytotoxic agents doxorubicin, cisplatin and carboplatin against human breast carcinoma MCF-7 and MDA-MB468 cells. *Oncol Rep* 2004; 11: 493-9.

[350] Lo YL. A potential daidzein derivative enhances cytotoxicity of epirubicin on human colon adenocarcinoma Caco-2 cells. *Int J Mol Sci* 2012; 14: 158-76.

[351] Zhou L, Wu Y, Guo Y, Li Y, Li N, Yang Y, Qin X. Calycosin enhances some chemotherapeutic drugs inhibition of Akt signaling pathway in gastric cells. *Cancer Invest* 2017; 35: 289-300.

[352] Lee H, Lee D, Kang KS, Song JH, Choi YK. Inhibition of intracellular ROS accumulation by formononetin attenuates cisplatin-mediated apoptosis in LLC-PK1 cells. *Int J Mol Sci* 2018; 19: E813.

[353] Lo YL, Wang W. Formononetin potentiates epirubicin-induced apoptosis via ROS production in HeLa cells in vitro. *Chem Biol Interact* 2013; 205: 188-97.

[354] Wietrzyk J, Opolski A, Madej J, Radzikowski C. Antitumour and antimetastatic effect of genistein alone or combined with cyclophosphamide in mice transplanted with various tumours depends on the route of tumour transplantation. *In Vivo* 2000; 14: 357-62.

[355] Monti E, Sinha BK. Antiproliferative effect of genistein and adriamycin against estrogen-dependent and -independent human breast carcinoma cell lines. *Anticancer Res* 1994; 14: 1221-6.

[356] Hwang JT, Ha J, Park OJ. Combination of 5-fluorouracil and genistein induces apoptosis synergistically in chemo-resistant cancer cells through the modulation of AMPK and COX-2 signaling pathways. *Biochem Biophys Res Commun* 2005; 332: 433-40.

[357] Zhang B, Shi ZL, Liu B, Yan XB, Feng J, Tao HM. Enhanced anticancer effect of gemcitabine by genistein in osteosarcoma: the role of Akt and nuclear factor-kappaB. *Anticancer Drugs* 2010; 21: 288-96.

[358] Zhang S, Wang Y, Chen Z, Kim S, Iqbal S, Chi A, Ritenour C, Wang YA, Kucuk O, Wu D. Genistein enhances the efficacy of cabazitaxel chemotherapy in metastatic castration-resistant prostate cancer cells. *Prostate* 2013; 73: 1681-9.

[359] Pons DG, Nadal-Serrano M, Torrens-Mas M, Oliver J, Roca P. The phytoestrogen genistein affects breast cancer cells treatment depending on the ERα/ERβ ratio. *J Cell Biochem* 2016; 117: 218-29.

[360] Isonishi S, Saitou M, Yasuda M, Ochiai K, Tanaka T. Enhancement of sensitivity to cisplatin by orobol is associated with increased mitochondrial cytochrome c release in human ovarian carcinoma cells. *Gynecol Oncol* 2003; 90: 413-20.

[361] Shiotsuka S, Isonishi S. Differential sensitization by orobol in proliferating and quiescent human ovarian carcinoma cells. *Int J Oncol* 2001; 18: 337-42.

[362] Wang J, Yang ZR, Guo XF, Song J, Zhang JX, Wang J, Dong WG. Synergistic effects of puerarin combined with 5-fluorouracil on esophageal cancer. *Mol Med Rep* 2014; 10: 2535-41.

[363] Guo XF, Yang ZR, Wang J, Lei XF, Lv XG, Dong WG. Synergistic antitumor effect of puerarin combined with 5-fluorouracil on gastric carcinoma. *Mol Med Rep* 2015; 11: 2562-8.

[364] Wang Z, Yang L, Xia Y, Guo C, Kong L. Icariin enhances cytotoxicity of doxorubicin in human multidrug-resistant osteosarcoma cells by inhibition of ABCB1 and down-regulation of the PI3K/Akt pathway. *Biol Pharm Bull* 2015; 38: 277-84.

Chapter 6

EFFECTS OF PLANT FLAVONOIDS ON CHEMOTHERAPEUTIC EFFICACY OF CANCER DRUGS

Increasing evidence suggest that plant-derived bioactive polyphenolic components, especially structurally different flavonoids, can affect the therapeutic efficacy of conventional anticancer agents. There are hundreds of studies published in this field in the scientific literature, whereas interactions between flavonoids and chemotherapeutic drugs might be additive to synergistic, but also antagonistic. As flavonoids-containing plant-based food products constitute an important part of the everyday diet of human beings, but considering also the fact that diet is a potentially modifiable factor in the behavioral choices of cancer patients, knowledge about the modulation of antitumor efficiency of chemotherapeutic drugs by addition of different flavonoids is of vital importance to contribute to the best therapeutic outcome, while simultaneously not contravening the drug action, just due to lack of information. Therefore, in the following subchapters currently available evidence-based data about the interactions of flavonoids and chemotherapeutics in different cancer models are compiled. At present, these data are predominantly preclinical with only a very few clinical trials performed to date. However, these preclinical findings, obtained both *in vitro* with cancer cell lines as well as *in vivo* animal models, clearly highlight the combinations which are worth of further therapeutic development due to strong synergistic anticancer effects, but also bring forth the antagonistic combinations which should be avoided by patients suffering from certain tumors during the active treatment phase with specific antineoplastic drugs.

In this book, the term "chemotherapeutic drug" comprises traditional cytotoxic anticancer agents, i.e., drugs which act on the DNA (alkylating drugs, platinum compounds and topoisomerase inhibitors), antimetabolites and drugs which target microtubules. Agents used in hormonal anticancer therapy, targeted biological therapy, differentiating agents and modern immunomodulating drugs are not covered in this book. The following sections are built up according to the general classification of cytotoxic drugs, whereas the practical use of assembled material is facilitated by presentation of the Subject Index both by specific drugs as well as certain flavonoids in the end of the book.

Some restrictions were set when gathering the data presented in this book. First, only the cytotoxic chemotherapeutic drugs that are officially approved are involved, excluding the anticancer agents still studied in the clinical trials. At that, interactions of flavonoids with three commonly used cytotoxic drugs, i.e., cisplatin, doxorubicin and paclitaxel, have been most often studied in different preclinical cancer models and therefore, these results deserve also longer discussions. Second, interactions with only pure flavonoid entities are considered, leaving out the plant extracts and mixtures of polyphenolic compounds, such as green tea extract or flavonoid mixture silymarin, as in those cases it is not clear which natural compound exactly affects the chemotherapeutic efficacy. In addition, findings on monomeric flavonoids, and not their oligomeric or polymeric counterparts like proanthocyanidins, are compiled in the analysis. Also, only natural flavonoids, and not their semisynthetic derivatives, are involved. Regarding to the cancer systems, interactions of flavonoids and cytotoxic drugs explored in both solid tumor cell lines as well as leukemia cell lines, and in animal models carrying diverse types of malignancies are under consideration. Besides malignant cells derived from human neoplasms, also cell lines isolated from tumors evolved in mice or dogs are regarded as experimental model systems. Last but not least, only the data describing the role of flavonoids on anticancer efficacy or clinical responsiveness of cytotoxic agents are involved in this book, leaving out the works analyzing merely the influences of flavonoids on pharmacokinetic profile, bioavailability properties or toxic side effects caused by the drugs.

The following subchapters clearly show that natural dietary flavonoids affect chemosensitivity of traditional cytotoxic drugs not only in resistant cancer cells, but also in drug sensitive parental malignant cells, through modulating various molecular targets and regulating different cellular signaling pathways. These mechanisms are shortly described in the text, but are more thoroughly summarized in the respective Tables and Figures added to this chapter. For those readers, who are not familiar with the cellular biology and physiology or are not interested in the molecular mechanisms underlying the coeffects, the most important information about the interactions between dietary flavonoids and antineoplastic agents is presented in the end of each subsection as a paragraph distinguished by italics. Most importantly, antagonistic combinations are specifically highlighted in the boxes ibidem, with the warnings to cancer patients suffering from certain tumor types. Intake of the plant-based food products or dietary supplements rich in these contraindicated flavonoids during the active treatment phase with specific anticancer drugs might decrease or even abolish the therapeutic efficacy, impair clinical outcome, worsen the overall prognosis and survival time. Knowledge of these combinations enables patients to make well-informed and conscious choices concerning their diet during the treatment period.

Finally, it is important to re-emphasize that following sections are written based on the findings obtained in preclinical settings, i.e., cancer cell lines and xenograft tumor models in experimental animals. With no doubt, further investigations and especially, clinical trials, are urgently needed with the aim to enhance the anticancer efficacy applying synergistic combinations of cytotoxic drugs and plant-derived non-toxic flavonoids, allowing to achieve therapeutic responses in significantly lower drug doses with substantially milder adverse side effects. Altogether, it would mean improved quality of life and prolonged survival time to patients fighting against different cancer types.

6.1. Drugs Which Act on the DNA

6.1.1. Alkylating Drugs

Alkylating agents are the oldest antineoplastic drugs used in cancer treatment, applied against both solid tumors as well as hematological malignancies [1]. The fundamental common point for these agents is the alkylation reaction, whereas the therapeutic potential comes from ability to induce cell death via intervention of DNA integrity in fast proliferating malignant tissues [1, 2].

6.1.1.1. Cyclophosphamide (CY)

Cyclophosphamide (CY) is extensively used in current chemotherapeutic protocols. It is a cytotoxic alkylating drug that is effectively applied as the first-line agent against a variety of cancers, including breast cancer, cervical cancer, small cell lung cancer, leukemia and non-Hodgkin`s lymphoma [3, 4]. CY itself is a prodrug that must be first converted to its active metabolite in the liver. CY is activated by hepatic cytochrome P450 (CYP) enzymes to form 4-hydroxycyclophosphamide (4HO-CY) which enters systemic circulation, is transported to malignant cells by erythrocytes and leads to DNA cross-linking [4]. Despite its effectiveness, CY exerts a wide range of severe and life-threatening adverse side effects, mainly bone marrow toxicity and serious infections, limiting its clinical use [3, 4]. In addition, it has been shown that CY may cause temporary or occasionally even permanent sterility [3]. Moreover, a few secondary cancer cases have also been associated with the administration of CY; whereas in rats, CY was shown to be able to induce the formation of urinary bladder tumors [3]. Therefore, it is necessary to identify adjuvant compounds that could reduce the harmful side effects of CY without any decrease in its antitumor efficacy [3, 4].

Abundantly occurring plant flavonol *fisetin* could increase the cytotoxicity of the active CY metabolite 4HO-CY in human triple negative breast cancer (TNBC) cell lines MDA-MB-231 and MDA-MB-468, allowing thus to attain increased sensitivity to tumor cell killing by reduced drug doses. Such chemosensitization may comprise blockade of several signaling pathways that are crucial for survival and constitutively active in malignant cells [5] (Table 6.1). Combined treatment with CY and fisetin also resulted in a marked improvement in antitumor activity *in vivo* conditions using Lewis lung carcinoma (LLC)-bearing mice [6, 7] (Table 6.2). Fisetin augmented both the inhibitory effect of CY on tumor growth as well as the decrease in microvessel density (MVD), i.e., antiangiogenic action, while revealing only low or no systemic toxicity [6]. Moreover, co-treatment of LLC-bearing mice with CY and liposomal fisetin formulation resulted in a significant improvement in tumor growth delay compared to CY monotherapy, whereas using of liposomal fisetin instead of its free form allowed about six-fold reduction of fisetin dose (from 223 mg/kg for the free form to 35 mg/kg for liposomal conjugation) related to the marked increase in its bioavailability [7] (Table 6.2). Another flavonol, *rutin* (quercetin 3-O-rutinoside), reversed the multidrug resistance (MDR) phenotype and chemosensitized human TNBC cells MDA-MB-231 towards the cytotoxic action of CY via suppression of the activity of P-glycoprotein (P-gp) and breast cancer resistance protein (BCRP) efflux pumps. As a result, significantly lower dosages of CY induced the therapeutically significant effects, thereby strongly reducing the dose-dependent toxicity level of this drug. However, in estrogen receptor and progesterone receptor positive human breast cancer cell line MCF-7, rutin did not further increase the anticancer efficacy of CY. Compared to the overexpression of efflux pumps on the surface of MDA-MB-231 cells, they are only poorly expressed in MCF-7 cell membrane [8] (Table 6.1). The potential adjuvant role of daily oral dosage of *quercetin* aglycone in the third-line CY oral treatment protocol was studied in a patient with metastatic urothelial carcinoma of the bladder, resulting in a complete radiologic response with prolonged progression-free survival, minimal toxicity and marked antifatigue effect [9]. Therefore, the combinations of CY with non-toxic dietary flavonols could be beneficial in the treatment of different solid tumors, and certainly deserve further studies for optimization of schedule, dosages and pharmaceutical formulations to improve the treatment regimens currently used in clinical settings.

Flavanone *naringenin* enhanced the sensitivity of both human breast cancer cell line HTB26 and human colorectal cancer cell line SW1116 to CY [10] (Table 6.1). However, co-administration of CY with the glycoside form of citrus flavanone hesperetin, i.e., *hesperidin* or hesperetin 7-rutinoside, led to quite opposite results. In murine colon carcinoma cells CT-26 bearing mice, hesperidin interacted with CY to inhibit its anticancer efficacy and significantly attenuated CY-induced tumor growth suppression, leading to increase in tumor volume as compared to CY monotreated mice. This unfavorable action can be caused by inhibition of cytochrome P450 enzymes by hesperidin, thereby modulating the pharmacokinetics of CY and reducing activation of CY in the liver to its active metabolite 4HO-CY. Also, anticancer effects of CY can be impaired by blocking of the reactive oxygen species (ROS) formation by antioxidant action of hesperidin. It is well known that the active metabolite of CY, 4HO-CY, generates ROS to cause oxidative DNA damage and death of tumor cells. Accordingly, intake of fruits rich in hesperidin, such as citrus fruits, might have undesired effects on the efficacy of CY in the treatment of patients suffering from colon cancer and therefore, any hesperidin-containing fruits should be excluded from their diet during the active phase chemotherapy with CY [4] (Table 6.2). Similarly, a methylated flavone, *5,7-dimethoxyflavone (5,7-DMF)*, was shown to antagonize the CY cytotoxic activity in several human acute lymphoblastic leukemia (ALL) cell lines, YCUB-2, YCUB-5 and YCUB-6. Thus, combined use of CY with 5,7-DMF is also not recommended [11] (Table 6.1).

In vivo results of combined treatment with CY and soy isoflavone *genistein* revealed some dependence on the route of tumor transplantation to mice, i.e., the site of tumor growth, besides the certain tumor type (Table 6.2). In murine mammary gland tumor cells 16/C bearing mice, genistein did not significantly affect the tumor growth inhibition by CY, regardless of the localization of primary tumor (subcutaneous or direct inoculation of tumor cells into the mammary gland of mice) [12]. In Lewis lung cancer cells LL_2 bearing mice, genistein and CY exhibited additive antiangiogenic activity [13] and enhanced antimetastatic effects by reducing the number of lung colonies and tumor recurrence rate in subcutaneous but not intravenous injection model [14, 15]. Although in murine melanoma cells B16 bearing mice no effect of genistein on antiangiogenic action of CY was described [13], synergistic effects of both agents in combined treatment on life span prolongation of animals were still observed, regardless of the route of tumor inoculation, i.e., either intraperitoneal, intravenous or intradermal injection [15]. However, in another study, the tumor recurrence rate and mean weight of recurrent tumors were both increased by combined treatment of B16 melanoma cells bearing mice with CY and genistein as compared to CY monotherapy [14], suggesting that concerning the therapeutic efficacy it may be better for melanoma patients to avoid the exposure to soy products during treatment with CY (Table 6.2).

The only chalcone studied so far in combination with CY treatment, *isoliquiritigenin*, exerted enhanced antitumor effects both in *in vitro* and *in vivo* models of murine cervical cancer cells U14, by significantly inhibiting the tumor growth [3] (Table 6.1, Table 6.2).

According to the current experimental findings it is recommended for cancer patients *not to consume* dietary products or dietary supplements rich in following plant flavonoids during the active chemotherapeutic treatment phase with **cyclophosphamide**:

- **5,7-dimethoxyflavone** in acute lymphoblastic leukemia
- **hesperidin** in colon cancer
- **genistein** in melanoma

Table 6.1. Effects of flavonoids on anticancer action of cyclophosphamide (CY) and 4-hydroxyperoxycyclophosphamide (4HO-CY) *in vitro* conditions

Drug	Flavonoid	Biological system	Direction of combination	Effects	Ref.
CY, 1 mg/ml	Isoliquiritigenin, 20 and 25 μg/ml	U14 murine **cervical** cancer cell line	↑	Increase in CY-induced cell proliferation inhibition, increase in colony formation inhibition	[3]
CY, 0.01 nM-10 μM	Naringenin, 1 mM	HTB26 human **breast** cancer cell line	↑	Increase in CY-induced cytotoxicity	[10]
CY, 0.01 nM-10 μM	Naringenin, 1 mM	SW1116 human **colorectal** cancer cell line	↑	Increase in CY-induced cytotoxicity	[10]
CY, 20 μM	Rutin, 20 μM	MDA-MB-231 human TN **breast** cancer cell line	↑	Increase in CY-induced cytotoxicity, inhibition of P-gp and BCRP pumps	[8]
CY, 20 μM	Rutin, 20 μM	MCF-7 human ER- and PR-positive, HER2-negative **breast** cancer cell line	~	No effect on CY anticancer efficacy	[8]
4HO-CY	5,7-DMF	YCUB-2 human acute lymphoblastic **leukemia** (ALL) cell line	↓	Antagonism at ratios of 20:1 and 40:1 (5,7-DMF:4HO-CY), additivity at ratios of 10:1, 80:1 and 160:1	[11]
4HO-CY	5,7-DMF	YCUB-5 human acute lymphoblastic **leukemia** (ALL) cell line	↓	Antagonism with 4HO-CY	[11]
4HO-CY	5,7-DMF	YCUB-6 human acute lymphoblastic **leukemia** (ALL) cell line	↓	Antagonism at ratios of 10:1 and 20:1 (5,7-DMF:4HO-CY), additivity at ratios of 40:1, 80:1 and 160:1	[11]
4HO-CY, 0.25-4 μg/ml	Fisetin, 25 μM	MDA-MB-231 human TN **breast** cancer cell line, p53-deficient	↑	Increase in 4HO-CY-induced cytotoxicity	[5]
4HO-CY, 0.25-4 μg/ml	Fisetin, 25 μM	MDA-MB-468 human TN **breast** cancer cell line, p53-deficient	↑	Increase in 4HO-CY-induced cytotoxicity	[5]

BCRP, breast cancer resistance protein; ER, estrogen receptor; HER2, human epidermal growth factor receptor 2; P-gp, P-glycoprotein; PR, progesterone receptor; TN, triple negative.

Table 6.2. Effects of flavonoids on anticancer action of cyclophosphamide (CY) *in vivo* conditions

Drug	Flavonoid	Biological system	Direction of combination	Effects	Ref.
CY, 30 mg/kg, s.c., on days 4, 5, 7, 8	Fisetin, 223 mg/kg, i.p., on days 4-8, 11, 12 and 14	LLC murine Lewis **lung** carcinoma tumor fragments injected s.c. bilaterally into flanks of C57BL/5J female mice	↑	Increase in CY-induced tumor growth inhibition, decline in tumor volumes, decrease in MVD	[6]
CY, 30 mg/kg, s.c., 12 consecutive days	Fisetin, liposomal, 35 mg/kg, i.p., 12 consecutive days	LLC murine Lewis **lung** carcinoma tumor fragments implanted s.c. bilaterally into flanks of female 8w old C57BL/6J mice	↑	Improvement of tumor growth delay, decrease in tumor volumes	[7]
CY, 100 mg/kg, i.p., on day 4 or 12	Genistein, 100 mg/kg, i.p., 3 days after CY for 10 days	16/C murine **mammary gland** cancer cells inoculated s.c. into the right flank region of 12-16w old female C3H/IiW mice	~	No significant effect on CY-induced tumor growth inhibition	[12]
CY, 100 mg/kg, i.p., on day 4 or 12	Genistein, 100 mg/kg, i.p., 3 days after CY for 10 days	16/C murine **mammary gland** cancer cells inoculated orthotopically into mammary fat pad of 12-16w old female C3H/IiW mice	~	No significant effect on CY-induced tumor growth inhibition; increase in ER and PR expression	[12]
CY, 100 mg/kg, on day after inoculation	Genistein, 100 mg/kg, on day 4 after CY for 12 days	LL₂ Lewis **lung** cancer cells inoculated s.c. into 12-16w old (C57BL/6 x DBA/2)F1 male mice	~ ↑	No effect on CY-induced cytostatic activity; additive antiangiogenic effect	[13]
CY, 100 mg/kg, i.p., on day after inoculation	Genistein, 100 mg/kg, i.p., on day after CY for 10 days	LL₂ Lewis **lung** cancer cells inoculated s.c. into 12-16w old male (C57BL/6 x DBA/2)F1 mice	↑	Potentiation of CY-induced decrease in lung colonies number, decrease in mean weight of recurrent tumors	[14]
CY, 100 mg/kg, i.p., on day 4 after inoculation	Genistein, 100 mg/kg, i.p., on day 4 after CY for 10 days	LL₂ Lewis **lung** cancer cells inoculated s.c. into the right flank region of 12-16w old male (C57BL/6 x DBA/2)F1 mice	↑	Increase in CY-induced tumor growth inhibition, decrease in lung colonies number	[15]
CY, 100 mg/kg, i.p., on day 4 after inoculation	Genistein, 100 mg/kg, i.p., on day 4 after CY for 10 days	LL₂ Lewis **lung** cancer cells inoculated i.v. into the lateral tail vein of 12-16w old male (C57BL/6 x DBA/2)F1 mice	~	No increase in CY-induced antitumor effect	[15]
CY, 100 mg/kg, on day after inoculation	Genistein, 100 mg/kg, on day 4 after CY for 12 days	B16 **melanoma** cells inoculated s.c. into 12-16w old male (C57BL/6 x DBA/2)F1 mice	~	No effect on CY-induced cytostatic or antiangiogenic activity	[13]
CY, 100 mg/kg, i.p., on day after inoculation	Genistein, 100 mg/kg, i.p., on day after CY for 10 days	B16F-10 **melanoma** cells inoculated s.c. into the right flank region of 12-16w old male (C57BL/6 x DBA/2)F1 mice	↓	Increase in primary tumor recurrence % and mean weight of recurrent tumors	[14]
CY, 100 mg/kg, i.p., on day 4 after inoculation	Genistein, 100 mg/kg, i.p., on day 4 after CY for 10 days	B16F-10 **melanoma** cells inoculated i.p. into 12-16w old male (C57BL/6 x DBA/2)F1 mice	↑	Increase in CY-induced antitumor effect, increase in life span of mice	[15]
CY, 100 mg/kg, i.p., on day 4 after inoculation	Genistein, 100 mg/kg, i.p., on day 4 after CY for 10 days	B16F-10 **melanoma** cells inoculated i.v. into 12-16w old male (C57BL/6 x DBA/2)F1 mice	↑	Increase in CY-induced antitumor effect, decrease in metastatic colonies number	[15]
CY, 100 mg/kg, i.p., on day 4 after inoculation	Genistein, 100 mg/kg, i.p., on day 4 after CY for 10 days	B16F-10 **melanoma** cells inoculated i.d. into the right flank region of 12-16w old male (C57BL/6 x DBA/2)F1 mice	↑	Increase in CY-induced antitumor effect, increase in primary tumor growth inhibition	[15]
CY, 25 mg/kg, i.p.	Hesperidin, 200 mg/kg, oral gavage	CT-26 murine **colon** carcinoma cells injected i.d. into the right flank of BALB/c mice	↓	Reduction of CY-induced antitumor effects, increase in tumor volume	[4]
CY, 40 mg/kg, i.p., on day 1 after inoculation	Isoliquiritigenin, 5, 10 or 20 mg/kg, orally, for 10 days	U14 murine **cervical** cancer cells implanted s.c. into 5-7w old female SPF KM mice	↑	Increase in CY-induced antitumor activity, increase in tumor growth inhibition	[3]

ER, estrogen receptor; MVD, microvessel density; PR, progesterone receptor.

6.1.1.2. Temozolomide (TMZ)

Temozolomide (TMZ) is an orally delivered alkylating drug that in combination with surgery and radiation is the current standard of care for patients with glioblastoma multiforme (GBM) [16-18]. TMZ, a dacarbazine (DTIC) derivative, is a second-generation alkylating agent that is indicated for the treatment of adult patients with newly diagnosed malignant gliomas, but is approved also for the treatment of brain metastases from various malignancies and has proven clinical activity against melanoma [16, 19, 20]. TMZ is able to effectively cross the blood-brain barrier and enter the cerebrospinal fluid, requiring no hepatic metabolism for activation [20-23]. Its action is associated with the ability to damage DNA through formation of O^6-methylguanine in genomic DNA and subsequent substitution of cytosine by thymine during DNA replication. This alerts the mismatch repair (MMR) mechanism, which recognizes the mispaired thymine [19]. Consequently, glioma cells respond to TMZ by undergoing G2/M phase arrest and ultimately induce the cell death through apoptosis or autophagy [17, 18, 21, 22, 24]. Off-target toxicities of TMZ include reproductive and neurotoxicity [25]. However, high expression of different resistance proteins often reduces the therapeutic efficacy of TMZ and leads to poor clinical response [17, 26, 27]. Resistance to TMZ in GBM patients has been linked predominantly to increased expression of O^6-methylguanine DNA methyltransferase (MGMT) or acquisition of MMR deficiency [17, 19, 27]. Mutagenic properties of TMZ have also been observed to promote the emergence of potentially resistant tumor cell clones [27]. Moreover, there are probably many more factors that regulate chemosensitivity to TMZ. Accordingly, despite its well tolerability, TMZ has limited clinical efficacy and provides only a small and unsatisfactory extension of median survival time [16, 19, 22, 23]. Moreover, the higher response (35%) in WHO grade III anaplastic astrocytomas in comparison with the low response rate in grade IV brain tumors (6-8%) suggests a possible trend of enhancing efficacy in lower grade tumors [22]. Therefore, more efficient therapeutic regimens and novel strategies to attenuate resistance and potentiate antitumor action of TMZ are urgently needed to prolong survival and improve clinical outcome of GBM patients.

The major polyphenolic green tea constituent, flavanol *epigallocatechin 3-gallate (EGCG)*, was shown to behave as an important chemosensitizer for glioblastoma cells towards cytotoxic action of TMZ via different molecular mechanisms. Experimental evidence suggests that EGCG is able to pass through the blood-brain barrier and is active across this border. It is well described that glioblastoma cells, but not normal brain tissue, express elevated levels of glucose-regulated protein 78 (GRP78) that contributes to chemoresistance phenotype. GRP78 as an endoplasmic reticulum chaperone protein is a key prosurvival component of the endoplasmic reticulum stress (ERS) response system, whereas increased GRP78 activity can lead to suppression of caspase-mediated cell death pathways. Indeed, expression levels of GRP78 have been inversely correlated with tumor aggressiveness and median survival time of GBM patients representing not only a potential prognostic marker but also a novel chemosensitizing target [16, 19]. Although EGCG alone did not substantially affect the survival of glioblastoma cells up to high 100 μM concentration, ten-fold lower doses of this flavanol synergistically enhanced the therapeutic efficacy of TMZ in several human glioma cell lines, such as LN229, U87 and U251 resulting in apoptotic cell death. At that, EGCG blocked the TMZ-induced increase in GRP78 levels and eliminated key prosurvival protective feature of the ERS response [16, 19] (Table 6.3). These results were confirmed also in orthotopic mouse models of malignant gliomas, i.e., by injecting U87 or U251 cells directly into the rodent brain. Combined treatment with EGCG and TMZ led to a significantly improved therapeutic response as compared to TMZ monotherapy, including life extension of rodents. The level of prosurvival GRP78 was decreased when TMZ was combined with EGCG making at least a partial contribution to chemosensitizing ability of this green tea flavanol [16] (Table 6.4). Moreover, GRP78 is definitely not the sole molecular target for EGCG in glioma cells, as this flavanol was able to significantly downregulate P-glycoprotein (P-gp) expression in glioma stem-like cells derived from human glioblastoma cell line U87, thereby reversing resistance to TMZ [26] (Table 6.3). Thus, inclusion of EGCG in the treatment regimen of TMZ can increase the therapeutic efficacy of this DNA damaging drug to eliminate residual malignant cells after surgical resection and increase the effectiveness of glioma chemotherapy.

Abundantly occurring plant flavonol *quercetin* was also reported to potentiate the therapeutic efficacy of TMZ in various human glioma cells. In human astrocytoma cell line MOGGCCM, quercetin augmented TMZ-induced cell death in a concentration dependent manner. At low doses (5 μM), quercetin potentiated proautophagic effects of TMZ, while higher flavonoid concentrations (30 μM) switched autophagy to mitochondrial apoptosis with activation of caspase-3, release of cytochrome c and reduced mitochondrial membrane potential. This was accompanied by suppression of heat shock proteins (Hsps) 27 and 72 expression. In addition, combined treatment with TMZ and quercetin efficiently inhibited migratory phenotype that is one of the important features responsible for glioma invasiveness [21, 22]. In human glioblastoma cell lines U87 and U251, 30 μM quercetin was also able to enhance the TMZ-induced cell growth inhibition and apoptosis, besides suppression of Hsp27 expression, thereby increasing the chemosensitivity towards TMZ. The TMZ-caused upregulation of Hsp27 may confer chemoresistant phenotype of glioblastoma cells that was reversed by quercetin treatment [17]. Significantly increased mitochondrial apoptosis after combined treatment with TMZ and quercetin was observed also in human glioblastoma cell line T98G as compared to TMZ monotreatment [24]. Moreover, the cytotoxic effects of TMZ and quercetin co-loaded into nanoliposomes were superior to those detected with either agents alone in both U87 and TMZ-resistant U87 cells. Considering the short half-life of TMZ after its oral administration (less than 2 hours) the achievement of effective therapeutic concentrations at the tumor site may be impeded and development of nanoformulations is especially relevant [25] (Table 6.3). Therefore, TMZ co-administered with quercetin seems to be a potent and promising therapeutic combination which might be useful for clinical management of high-grade malignant gliomas. Moreover, quercetin can be a convenient adjuvant to therapeutic regimens of TMZ also for melanoma treatment. Indeed, quercetin abrogated chemoresistance to TMZ and caused more than additive induction of apoptosis in human melanoma cells DB-1. As this effect involved modulation of p53 family proteins, no significant enhancement of apoptosis was observed in p53 mutant human melanoma cell line SK Mel 28 [20] (Table 6.3). Glycoside form of quercetin, *rutin* or quercetin 3-O-rutinoside, enhanced the cytotoxic efficacy of TMZ in different human glioblastoma cell lines, such as U87, U251 and D54, and in U87 cells bearing mice models (subcutaneous or intracranial), leading to decrease in both tumor volumes and tumor weights as compared to TMZ monotherapy. This flavonoid could cross blood-brain barrier, suppress TMZ-induced and c-Jun N-terminal kinase (JNK)-mediated cytoprotective autophagy, and augment apoptotic cell death and therapeutic efficacy of TMZ. Therefore, rutin might serve as a chemosensitizer of TMZ for the treatment of GBM patients [18] (Table 6.3 and Table 6.4).

A natural methylated flavone *hispidulin* potentiated the antitumor activity of TMZ in human glioblastoma cell line SHG44 by inhibiting cell proliferation, increasing cell cycle arrest and inducing apoptosis. Such synergistic cytotoxic action was mediated via activation of AMP-activated protein kinase (AMPK) and inhibition of downstream mammalian target of rapamycin (mTOR) survival pathway, leading to downregulation of antiapoptotic protein B-cell lymphoma 2 (Bcl-2) and representing hispidulin as a potential chemosensitizing agent of TMZ in GBM treatment [27] (Table 6.3).

Inclusion of a prenylated flavonoid glycoside, *icariin*, in combinational treatment with TMZ also led to a synergistic enhancement of antitumor activity in human glioblastoma U87 cells. This action was, at least in part, mediated by suppression of nuclear factor-κB (NF-κB) activity resulting in enhanced apoptosis as compared to TMZ monotherapy. Combined treatment also potentiated the TMZ-induced inhibition of cell migration and invasion capacities [23] (Table 6.3). Flavonolignan *silibinin* was effective in potentiating the cytotoxic efficacy of TMZ in diverse human glioma cell lines LN229, TR-LN229 and U87 [28] (Table 6.3). Thus, natural compounds like icariin or silibinin which could pass through blood-brain barrier may be ideal chemosensitizers of TMZ in GBM therapy.

Table 6.3. Effects of flavonoids on anticancer action of temozolomide (TMZ) *in vitro* conditions

Drug	Flavonoid	Biological system	Direction of combination	Effects	Ref.
TMZ, 20, 40 μM	EGCG, 10, 20 μM	LN229 human **glioblastoma** cell line	↑	Increase in TMZ-induced cytotoxicity and apoptosis, inhibition of GRP78, increase in CHOP	[16]
TMZ, 20, 40 μM	EGCG, 10, 20 μM	U87 human **glioblastoma** cell line, wild-type p53	↑	Increase in TMZ-induced cytotoxicity and apoptosis, inhibition of GRP78, increase in CHOP	[16]
TMZ, 20, 40 μM	EGCG, 10, 20 μM	U251 human **glioblastoma** cell line, mutant p53	↑	Slight synergism in TMZ-induced cytotoxicity (CI 0.85-0.89) and apoptosis, inhibition of GRP78, increase in CHOP	[16]
TMZ, 20, 40 μM	EGCG, 10, 20 μM	U251 human **glioma** cell line	↑	Increase in chemosensitivity to TMZ, suppression of GRP78	[19]
TMZ, 100 μM	EGCG, 100 μM	Glioma stem-like cells derived from U87 human **glioblastoma** cell line, MDR, TMZ-resistant	↑	Increase in TMZ-induced cell viability reduction, downregulation of P-gp	[26]
TMZ, 100 μM	Hispidulin, 40 μM	SHG44 human **glioblastoma** cell line	↑	Synergism in TMZ-induced cell growth inhibition (CI 0.584), increase in apoptosis and G2 phase cell cycle arrest. Activation of AMPK, decrease in mTOR activity, downregulation of Bcl-2	[27]
TMZ, 200 μM	Icariin, 10 μM	U87MG human **glioblastoma** cell line	↑	Synergism in antitumor effect (CI 0.694). Increase in apoptosis (caspase-3 activation, PARP cleavage), inhibition of cell migration and invasion. Suppression of NF-κB activity	[23]
TMZ, 100 μM	Quercetin, 5, 30 μM	MOGGCCM human **brain astrocytoma** cell line, WHO grade III	↑	Potentiation of TMZ pro-autophagic effect at 5 μM quercetin (increase in LC3II). Switch of autophagy to synergistic apoptosis at 30 μM (caspase-3 activation, cyt c release, decrease in ΔΨm); downregulation of Hsp27 and Hsp72. Inhibition of migratory phenotype	[22]
TMZ, 100 μM	Quercetin, 5, 15, 30 μM	MOGGCCM human **brain astrocytoma** cell line	↑	Induction of autophagy at 5μM quercetin (increase in LC3II). Increase in apoptosis at 15 and 30 μM (caspase-3 activation, cyt c release)	[21]
TMZ, 50 μM	Quercetin, 50 μM	T98G human **glioblastoma** multiforme cell line	↑	Increase in apoptosis (decrease in ΔΨm, cyt c release, caspases-3/-9 activation)	[24]
TMZ, 100, 200, 400 μM	Quercetin, 30 μM	U251 human **glioblastoma** cell line	↑	Increase in TMZ-induced cell growth inhibition and apoptosis (caspase-3 activation), inhibition of Hsp27	[17]

Table 6.3. (Continued)

Drug	Flavonoid	Biological system	Direction of combination	Effects	Ref.
TMZ, 100, 200, 400 μM	Quercetin, 30 μM	U87 human **glioblastoma** cell line	↑	Increase in TMZ-induced cell growth inhibition and apoptosis (caspase-3 activation), inhibition of Hsp27	[17]
TMZ, 25, 50, 100 μM, co-loaded into PEGylated NLs	Quercetin, 25, 50, 100 μM, co-loaded into PEGylated NLs	U87 human **glioma** cell line	↑	Decrease in cell viability, induction of apoptosis	[25]
TMZ, 6.25-200 μM, co-loaded into PEGylated NLs	Quercetin, 6.25-200 μM, co-loaded into PEGylated NLs	U87/TR human **glioma** cell line, TMZ-resistant	↑	Decrease in cell viability	[25]
TMZ, 400 μM	Quercetin, 75 μM	DB-1 human **melanoma** cell line, wild-type p53	↑	Increase in apoptosis (increase in Bax, PARP cleavage), induction of ΔNp73 translocation out of nucleus associated with increased p53 transcriptional activity	[20]
TMZ, 400 μM	Quercetin, 75 μM	SK Mel 28 human **melanoma** cell line, mutant p53	~	No increase in apoptosis	[20]
TMZ, 63-1000 μM	Rutin, 50, 100, 200 μM	D54-MG human **glioblastoma** cell line	↑	Increase in TMZ-induced cytotoxicity. Blocking of TMZ-induced JNK activity resulting in decreased autophagy and increased apoptosis (upregulation of caspase-3)	[18]
TMZ, 63-1000 μM	Rutin, 50, 100, 200 μM	U251-MG human **glioblastoma** cell line	↑	Increase in TMZ-induced cytotoxicity	[18]
TMZ, 63-1000 μM	Rutin, 50, 100, 200 μM	U87-MG human **glioblastoma** cell line	↑	Increase in TMZ-induced cytotoxicity. Blocking of TMZ-induced JNK activity resulting in decreased autophagy and increased apoptosis (upregulation of caspase-3)	[18]
TMZ, 0-50 μM	Silibinin, 50 μM	LN229 human **glioma** cell line, mutant p53	↑	Potentiation of TMZ-induced cytotoxicity	[28]
TMZ, 0-50 μM	Silibinin, 50 μM	TR-LN229 human **glioma** cell line, mutant p53, TMZ-resistant	↑	Potentiation of TMZ-induced cytotoxicity	[28]
TMZ, 0-50 μM	Silibinin, 50 μM	U87 human **glioma** cell line, mutant PTEN	↑	Additive effect on TMZ-induced cytotoxicity	[28]

AMPK, AMP-activated protein kinase; Bax, Bcl-2-associated X protein; Bcl-2, B-cell lymphoma 2; CHOP, CCAAT/enhancer binding protein homologues protein; CI, combination index; cyt c, cytochrome c; GRP78, glucose-regulated protein 78; Hsp, heat shock protein; JNK, c-Jun N-terminal kinase; mTOR, mammalian target of rapamycin; NF-κB, nuclear factor-κB; NL, nanoliposome; P-gp, P-glycoprotein; PARP, poly(ADP-ribose)polymerase; PTEN, phosphatase and tensin homolog; ΔΨm, mitochondrial membrane potential.

Table 6.4. Effects of flavonoids on anticancer action of temozolomide (TMZ) *in vivo* conditions

Drug	Flavonoid	Biological system	Direction of combination	Effects	Ref.
TMZ, 5 mg/kg, by gavage, 14 days cycles (7 days with/7 days without)	EGCG, 50 mg/kg, by gavage, 14 days cycles (7 days with/7 days without)	U87 human **glioblastoma** cells injected intracranially into the right frontal lobe of brain of athymic mice	↑	Increase in TMZ-induced antitumor effect, prolongation of mice survival. Blocking of TMZ-induced increase in GRP78, enhancement of CHOP level	[16]
TMZ, 5 mg/kg, by gavage, 14 days cycles (7 days with/7 days without)	EGCG, 50 mg/kg, by gavage, 14 days cycles (7 days with/7 days without)	U251 human **glioblastoma** cells injected intracranially into the right frontal lobe of brain of athymic mice	↑	Increase in TMZ-induced antitumor effect, prolongation of mice survival. Blocking of TMZ-induced increase in GRP78, enhancement of CHOP level	[16]
TMZ, 55 mg/kg, orally, thrice a week for 2 weeks	Rutin, 20 mg/kg, i.p., for 18 days	U87-MG human **glioblastoma** cells injected s.c. into the flank of 6w old male nude BALB/c athymic mice	↑	Increase in TMZ-induced reduction of tumor volume and weight. Blocking of TMZ-induced JNK activity resulting in decreased autophagy and increased apoptosis (upregulation of caspase-3)	[18]
TMZ, 55 mg/kg, orally, thrice a week for 2 weeks	Rutin, 20 mg/kg, i.p., for 18 days	U87-MG human **glioblastoma** cells with luciferase injected intracranially into the right frontal lobe of 6w old male nude BALB/c athymic mice	↑	Increase in TMZ-induced reduction of tumor sizes	[18]

CHOP, CCAAT/enhancer binding protein homologues protein; GRP78, glucose-regulated protein 78; JNK, c-Jun N-terminal kinase.

Based on the knowledge that malignant gliomas are among the most chemoresistant tumors and TMZ chemotherapy is one of the least impressive therapeutic regimens for cancer patients in general, demonstrations that flavonoids like EGCG, quercetin, rutin, hispidulin, icariin and silibinin can achieve chemosensitization towards TMZ is of particular clinical importance. As depicted in Figure 6.1, flavonoids act on multiple targets and modulate different cellular signaling pathways associated with chemoresistance to TMZ. It is also essential to mention that up to now, no antagonistic interactions between dietary flavonoids and TMZ on drug chemotherapeutic efficacy have been reported.

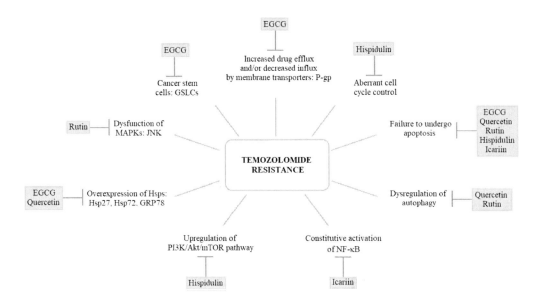

Figure 6.1. Cellular mechanisms contributing to temozolomide resistance and their blocking by plant flavonoids (Akt, protein kinase B; GRP78, glucose-regulated protein 78; GSLCs, glioma stem-like cells; Hsp, heat shock protein; JNK, c-Jun N-terminal kinase; MAPK, mitogen-activated protein kinase; mTOR, mammalian target of rapamycin; NF-κB, nuclear factor-κB; P-gp, P-glycoprotein; PI3K, phosphoinositide 3-kinase).

6.1.1.3. Dacarbazine (DTIC)

Dacarbazine (DTIC) is a DNA binding alkylating agent that has been used for treatment of melanoma already for decades [29, 30]. Its antitumor activities result from methylation of nucleic acids or direct DNA damage resulting in arrest of cell growth and subsequent cell death. Production of O^6-methylguanine by DTIC would generate DNA replication forks and further lead to the formation of O^6-methylguanine thymine mispair, eventually inducing apoptosis in cells subjected to DTIC treatment [29, 30]. However, monotherapy with DTIC has resulted only in moderate response rates ranging from 11 to 25%; patients usually survive only a short time and are often faced with DTIC-caused liver and lung toxicities [29, 30]. Therefore, it is crucial to identify novel bioactive adjuvant agents to DTIC and develop more efficient combination strategies to gain higher response rates and improve survival of melanoma patients.

Dietary flavonoid *quercetin* was demonstrated to sensitize human melanoma cells to DTIC and stimulated apoptotic cell death. This potentiating effect was further increased by overexpression of the catalytic enzyme tyrosinase in melanoma cells that promotes an ataxia telangiectasia mutated (ATM)-dependent p53 upregulation and subsequent DNA damage response by quercetin, complementing thus DTIC cytotoxicity. Therefore, the chemosensitization effect was most potent in wild-type p53 cells. Tyrosinase is usually overexpressed in melanoma tumors and is also used as a tumor marker. Moreover, prooxidant properties of quercetin could also contribute to its cytotoxic action in combination with DTIC [29] (Table 6.5). Enhanced response to DTIC has also been observed in combination with the green tea flavanol *EGCG* in highly metastatic murine melanoma B16 cells (B16-F3m clone) bearing mice. Combinational treatment of rodents with DTIC and EGCG led to an augmented antimetastatic efficacy, resulting in increased suppression of the number of pulmonary metastases as compared to DTIC monotherapy [30].

As clinical management of patients with metastatic melanoma has still remained unsatisfactory, experimental findings showing the chemosensitizing capacity of certain flavonoids can be of potential importance. Both quercetin and EGCG might be used as adjuvant agents in combination with DTIC to improve the DTIC response rates and therapeutic efficacy for combating melanoma progression and metastasis.

6.1.1.4. Chlorambucil (CMB)

Chlorambucil (CMB) is a cytotoxic alkylating agent that is mainly used for the treatment of lymphoproliferative disorders, such as chronic lymphocytic leukemia and Hodgkin and non-Hodgkin lymphomas [1]. CMB acts as a DNA cross-linker, interfering with DNA replication and causing DNA damage [31]. DNA lesions further induce the cell cycle arrest and apoptosis.

Several plant-derived flavonoids, such as *quercetin, morin, butein* and *2`-hydroxychalcone* augmented the cytotoxic activity of CMB in human colon adenocarcinoma COLO 320HSR cells [31]. This potentiation effect was partly explained by the suppression of efflux of monochloromonoglutathionyl CMB (MG-CMB), the major glutathione conjugate of CMB, out of the colon cancer cells. In addition, these four natural polyphenols were also able to inhibit the activity of glutathione S-transferase (GST) in tumor cells [31]. GSTs constitute of family of drug-metabolizing enzymes that participate in the detoxification process of many chemotherapeutic drugs, including CMB, by enhancing the glutathione conjugation. Overexpression of these enzymes has been detected in numerous drug-resistant cells contributing to resistance against certain anticancer agents like CMB [31, 32] (Table 6.5).

Table 6.5. Effects of flavonoids on anticancer action of other alkylating drugs *in vitro* conditions

Drug	Flavonoid	Biological system	Direction of combination	Effects	Ref.
DTIC, 200-800 µg/ml	Quercetin, 25, 75 µM	DB-1 human **melanoma** cell line, DTIC-resistant	↑	Increase in DTIC-induced apoptosis. Further sensitization of cells by tyrosinase overexpression promoting ATM-dependent p53 phosphorylation	[29]
DTIC, 200-800 µg/ml	Quercetin, 25, 75 µM	SK Mel 5 human **melanoma** cell line, wild-type p53	↑	Increase in DTIC-induced apoptosis. Further sensitization of cells by tyrosinase overexpression promoting ATM-dependent p53 phosphorylation	[29]
DTIC, 200-800 µg/ml	Quercetin, 25, 75 µM	SK Mel 28 human **melanoma** cell line, mutant p53	↑	Increase in DTIC-induced apoptosis	[29]
CMB, 5-20 µM	2`-Hydroxychalcone, 10 µM	COLO 320HSR human **colon** adenocarcinoma cell line	↑	Potentiation of CMB cytotoxicity. Inhibition of GST activity and efflux of CMB GSH conjugate (MG-CMB)	[31]
CMB, 5-20 µM	Butein, 10 µM	COLO 320HSR human **colon** adenocarcinoma cell line	↑	Potentiation of CMB cytotoxicity. Inhibition of GST activity and efflux of CMB GSH conjugate (MG-CMB)	[31]
CMB, 5-20 µM	Morin, 10 µM	COLO 320HSR human **colon** adenocarcinoma cell line	↑	Potentiation of CMB cytotoxicity. Inhibition of GST activity and efflux of CMB GSH conjugate (MG-CMB)	[31]
CMB, 5-20 µM	Quercetin, 10 µM	COLO 320HSR human **colon** adenocarcinoma cell line	↑	Potentiation of CMB cytotoxicity. Inhibition of GST activity and efflux of CMB GSH conjugate (MG-CMB)	[31]
BCNU, 5-50 µM	Genistein, 4 µM	C6 rat **glioma** cell line	↑	Increase in BCNU-induced growth inhibition and decrease in clonogenic survival	[33]
BCNU, 1-10 µM	Genistein, 4 µM	U87 human **glioblastoma** multiforme cell line	↑	Increase in BCNU-induced growth inhibition and decrease in clonogenic survival	[33]
Busulfan, 0-200 µM	Quercetin, 0-100 µM	K562 human chronic myeloid **leukemia** cell line	↑	Synergism in antiproliferative action	[34]
MMC, 50 µM	EGC, 1 µM	Mz-ChA-1 human malignant cholangiocytes derived from metastatic **gallbladder** cancer	~	No effect on MMC-induced cytotoxicity	[37]
MMC, 50 µM	EGCG, 1 µM	Mz-ChA-1 human malignant cholangiocytes derived from metastatic **gallbladder** cancer	↑	Increase in MMC-induced apoptosis	[37]
MMC, 0.2-125 µg/ml	Quercetin, 40, 80, 160 µM	BEL/5-FU human **hepatocellular** carcinoma cell line, MDR BEL-7402 cells	↑	Increase in MMC-induced cytotoxicity; downregulation of ABCB1, ABCC1, ABCC2, decrease in FZD7 and β-catenin expression	[38]
MMC, 20 µg/ml	Silibinin, 50-200 µM	A375-S2 human **melanoma** cell line	↓	Promotion of survival. Antagonism in MMC-induced intrinsic apoptosis through increasing the expression of SIRT1 and inhibiting p53 (attenuation of MMC-induced decrease in Bcl-2, blocking of Bax and cyt c translocation, amelioration of $\Delta\Psi$m loss, reduction of MMC-induced activation of caspases-9/-3)	[35]
MMC, 40 µg/ml	Silibinin, 150 µM	A375-S2 human **melanoma** cell line	↓	Suppression of MMC-induced cell growth inhibition. Induction of autophagy (by suppressing p53 and triggering NF-κB activation) to facilitate cell survival	[39]

ABC, ATP-binding cassette; ATM, ataxia telangiectasia mutated; Bax, Bcl-2-associated X protein; Bcl-2, B-cell lymphoma 2; cyt c, cytochrome c; FZD7, Frizzled homolog protein 7; GSH, glutathione; GST, glutathione S-transferase; MDR, multidrug resistance; MG-CMB, monochloromonoglutathionyl CMB; NF-κB, nuclear factor-κB; SIRT1, sirtuin 1; $\Delta\Psi$m, mitochondrial membrane potential.

Thus, certain plant flavonoids, including quercetin and morin, may provide adjunctive effects to chemotherapeutic efficacy of CMB, by retaining the drug in tumor cells and increasing its cytotoxicity.

6.1.1.5. Carmustine (BCNU)

Carmustine (BCNU) is an important agent for the treatment of primary and secondary brain tumors, but is also approved for multiple myelomas, lymphomas and melanoma [1]. However, its use is limited by severe and life-threatening toxicities, including myelosuppression, pulmonary and hepatic toxicity [33].

Soy isoflavone *genistein* was observed to significantly increase the BCNU-induced growth suppression and cytotoxicity in human glioblastoma cell line U87 and rat glioma cell line C6, whereas apoptotic cell death was probably not involved in the mechanisms underlying this potentiation. The possible implication of such combined treatment may be a decrease in the recommended dosage of BCNU accompanied with a reduction of devastating side effects of this chemotherapeutic drug [33] (Table 6.5).

Genistein could be administered as an adjuvant therapy for treatment of malignant gliomas with BCNU enhancing the antiproliferative and cytotoxic action.

6.1.1.6. Busulfan

Busulfan is an alkylating antineoplastic agent that was initially approved for treatment of chronic myeloid leukemia (CML). Nowadays the use of this drug is limited due to resistance; patients receiving busulfan for CML ultimately relapsed since the malignant clone remained unremoved [34].

Quercetin was found to synergistically enhance the antiproliferative activity of busulfan in human CML cell line K562, allowing to achieve similar therapeutic effects at significantly lower drug doses. For instance, 6 μM busulfan combined with 18 μM quercetin was as effective as 13 μM busulfan alone in inducing inhibition of cell proliferation [34] (Table 6.5).

6.1.1.7. Mitomycin C (MMC)

Mitomycin C (MMC) is a DNA damaging chemotherapeutic drug that is actually an antitumor antibiotic [1, 35]. This drug requires reductive transformation of its quinone groups to produce active metabolites which are able to generate alkylating DNA adducts and reactive oxygen species [36]. MMC is indicated for the clinical treatment of gastric, colorectal, pancreatic and breast tumors.

Green tea catechin *EGCG*, but not its structurally related flavanol *epigallocatechin (EGC)*, was able to sensitize human cholangiocarcinoma cells Mz-ChA-1 to MMC-induced apoptosis [37]. Also, the sensitivity of multidrug resistant (MDR) BEL-7402 human hepatocellular carcinoma cells, BEL/5-FU, towards MMC was increased by 1.36-2.51-fold when the drug was combined with *quercetin*. At that, quercetin suppressed the expression and function of P-gp (ABCB1), MRP1 (ABCC1) and MRP2 (ABCC2) efflux pumps via blocking of frizzled homolog protein 7 (FZD7)/β-catenin signaling pathway. Thus, inclusion of quercetin in the MMC-based treatment regimen of hepatocellular carcinoma might contribute to reversal of MDR phenotype [38] (Table 6.5).

On the contrary, flavonolignan *silibinin* exhibited a protective effect against MMC-induced cell death in human melanoma cell line A375-S2. Silibinin substantially suppressed MMC-initiated mitochondrial apoptosis and promoted survival of malignant cells. Such cytoprotective action was p53-dependent as the increase in p53 expression caused by MMC treatment was alleviated by silibinin. Moreover, the level of sirtuin 1 (SIRT1) that deacetylates p53 to reduce its stability was increased [35]. Furthermore, suppression of p53 by silibinin triggered NF-κB activation and thereby induced autophagy. Such silibinin-induced autophagy attenuated MMC-triggered apoptosis and facilitated survival of human melanoma cells [39] (Table 6.5). As silibinin antagonized the MMC-induced cytotoxic response in human melanoma cells, dietary supplements containing this flavonolignan should be avoided by melanoma patients receiving MMC treatment (Figure 6.2).

According to the current experimental findings it is recommended for cancer patients *not to consume* dietary products or dietary supplements rich in following plant flavonoids during the active chemotherapeutic treatment phase with **mitomycin C**:
- **silibinin** in melanoma

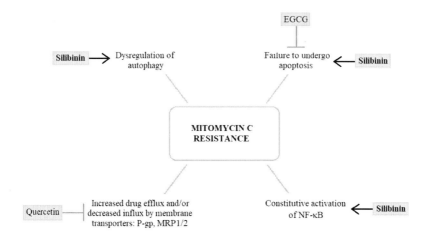

Figure 6.2. Modulation of mitomycin C resistance by plant flavonoids (MRP, multidrug resistance-associated protein; NF-κB, nuclear factor-κB; P-gp, P-glycoprotein).

Altogether, dietary flavonoids modulate the therapeutic efficacy of alkylating anticancer agents in a drug dependent and tumor type and stage dependent manner, whereas this effect can include both desired chemosensitization but also undesired increase in chemoresistance. Therefore, caution is always needed when cancer patients decide to consume dietary supplements containing flavonoids on their own accord.

6.1.2. Platinum Drugs

Platinum compounds bind covalently to DNA and form both intrastrand and interstrand crosslinks between guanine bases. These platinum-DNA adducts further suppress DNA replication and transcription resulting in cell cycle arrest and apoptotic cell death [2, 40, 41]. The first hint to antiproliferative potential of platinum complexes originates from 1965 when it was demonstrated that a current between platinum electrodes caused inhibition of *Escherichia coli* replication due to formation of platinum-containing agents in the presence of ammonium and chloride ions. This discovery brought about synthesis and testing of numerous platinum compounds against different experimental malignant models, leading to preparation of cisplatin (CDDP), carboplatin (CBP), nedaplatin (NDP) and oxaliplatin (OXA) with a great clinical efficacy [2]. The platinum drugs have generally a broad antineoplastic activity against epithelial tumors and have been used over the past 30 years for treatment of various cancers, including head and neck, lung, esophagus, colon, bladder, ovarian and testicular tumors [2, 42-44]. However, besides severe side effects, acquired resistance of cancer cells to cytotoxicity of platinum drugs still impedes the antitumor efficacy of these widely used chemotherapeutic agents limiting their clinical success, whereas different defense mechanisms contribute to this process [2, 44, 45]. Therefore, novel safe compounds, preferentially from natural origin, are highly needed to augment the therapeutic efficacy and overcome resistance associated with clinical use of platinum drugs.

6.1.2.1. Cisplatin (CDDP)

Cisplatin (cis-diamminedichloroplatinum (II), CDDP) was the first platinum-containing molecule introduced in clinical chemotherapy and due to its widespread use, it is known as the "penicillin of cancer" [46, 47]. CDDP is a very old antineoplastic compound that was first described already in 1844 and was approved by the Food and Drug Administration (FDA) in 1978 [48-51]. This commonly used DNA-damaging anticancer agent has demonstrated therapeutic properties against various types of human malignancies, including head and neck, breast, ovarian, cervical, endometrial, testicular, prostate, bladder, lung, pancreatic, esophageal, gastric and colorectal cancers, hepatocellular carcinoma, melanoma and also relapsed lymphoma [40, 48, 52-65]. CDDP is used alone, or in combination with radiotherapy or other chemotherapeutic drugs [50, 51, 61, 66-68]. CDDP forms intrastrand adducts or crosslinks between purine bases within DNA, inducing oxidative stress, unrepairable DNA damage, cell cycle arrest and ultimately leading to apoptosis and necrosis in cancer cells [46, 48, 50, 51, 53, 54, 57, 64,

66, 68-71]. The CDDP-triggered DNA damage signals involve activation of several cellular pathways, such as p53, p73 and mitogen-activated protein kinases (MAPKs) [41, 72]. Although many tumors initially demonstrate a good therapeutic responsiveness to CDDP, drug resistance eventually develops, contributes to disease relapse and metastasis, resulting in the failure of clinical application of CDDP [50, 53, 55, 56, 68, 73, 74]. Moreover, many patients are also intrinsically resistant to CDDP-based therapies [59, 75-77]. Complex multifactorial mechanisms underlie tumor resistance to CDDP, including reduced drug transport, decreased cellular drug accumulation, elevated cellular detoxification, changes in DNA repair efficacy and alterations in apoptotic cell death pathways [70, 72, 78-81]. To date, there are still no efficient pharmacological agents available to overcome complex resistance to CDDP in clinical settings [73]. Furthermore, the clinical use of CDDP is limited also by its moderate to severe adverse side effects in normal healthy tissues, including nephrotoxicity, gastrointestinal toxicity, hepatotoxicity, allergic reactions, myelosuppression, peripheral neuropathy and ototoxicity [2, 54, 60, 63, 64, 66, 69, 71]. CDDP-induced renal toxicity is related to increased production of reactive oxygen species (ROS) and decreased antioxidant defense system in kidney, posing the major limitation on drug dosage and administration frequency. In fact, kidney is the main organ responsible for elimination of CDDP from the body and due to its accumulation in the renal tubular cells, concentration of CDDP in kidney is about five times higher than in the blood plasma conferring renal dysfunction [51, 60, 64, 78, 82]. Thus, hardly controlled comorbidities accompany the clinical application of CDDP, whereas no agents contributing to protection against these undesirable side effects have been developed [69]. Therefore, novel safe compounds, preferably from natural sources, that selectively augment cytotoxicity of CDDP in malignant cells allowing to reduce its dosage could be clinically attractive in adjuvant chemotherapy to overcome drug resistance and decrease toxicity [50, 64, 67, 68, 75, 77, 83]. Combined treatment with such chemosensitizing agents might lead to improved clinical outcome, prolonged survival and better quality of life of patients.

Dietary abundant flavonol *quercetin* was shown to modulate the cytotoxic efficacy of CDDP in several different ways in various malignant cells (Table 6.6 and Table 6.7). In murine leukemia L1210 cells, quercetin synergistically enhanced cytotoxicity of CDDP and induced apoptosis, associated at least partly with the changes in cellular redox state [84-86]. In human promyelocytic leukemia HL-60 cells, quercetin potentiated CDDP-induced apoptosis only in the case of pretreatment of cells with this flavonol, but not in simultaneous or posttreatment with quercetin [86]. Based on so far published preclinical data, increasing intake of quercetin is beneficial to triple negative breast cancer (TNBC) patients who are receiving CDDP chemotherapy. In human TNBC cells MDA-MB-231, quercetin suppressed the activation of DNA damage response pathway when

Table 6.6. Effects of flavonoids on anticancer action of cisplatin (CDDP) *in vitro* conditions

Drug	Flavonoid	Biological system	Direction of combination	Effects	Ref.
CDDP, 1 μM	(-)-Catechin, 10, 20 μM	MDA-MB-231 human TN **breast** cancer cell line	↑	Enhancement of clonogenic cell growth decrease, inhibition of CDDP-induced Chk1 phosphorylation	[87[
CDDP, 4 μM	(s)-Equol, 10 nM	D283 Med human **medulloblastoma** cell line	↓	Decrease in CDDP-induced cytotoxicity, decrease in caspase-3 activity	[134]
CDDP, 20 μM	2`,5`-DHC, 20 μM	A549 human **lung** adenocarcinoma cell line	↑	Potentiation of CDDP-induced cytotoxicity. Induction of GSH depletion, exacerbation of CDDP-induced mitochondrial dysfunction	[147]
CDDP, 5-400 μM	3`,4`,5`,5,7-PMF, 10, 25, 50 μM	A549/CDDP human **lung** cancer cell line, CDDP-resistant	↑	Potentiation of CDDP-induced apoptosis (cleavage of PARP1 and caspase-3), downregulation of Nrf2	[156]
CDDP, 100 μM	4-MC, 5 μg/ml	A549 human **lung** cancer cell line	↑	Increase in CDDP-induced cytotoxicity, accelerated generation of ROS, increase in apoptosis through inhibition of Nrf2/ARE signaling	[83]
CDDP, 120 μM	5,7,4`-trihydroxy-6-methoxyflavanone, 10 μM	OVCAR-3 human **ovarian** cancer cell line, CDDP-resistant	~	No effect on CDDP-induced decrease in cell viability	[112]
CDDP, 120 μM	5,7,4`-trihydroxy-8-methoxyflavanone, 120 μM	OVCAR-3 human **ovarian** cancer cell line, CDDP-resistant	↑	Increase in CDDP-induced cell viability reduction	[112]
CDDP	Alopecurone B, 10 μM	MG-63-DOX human **osteosarcoma** cell line, DOX-resistant	↑	Increase in sensitivity to CDDP, 4.54-fold decrease in IC_{50} of CDDP	[235]
CDDP, 20 μg/ml	Alpinetin, 60 μg/ml	HepG2 human **hepatic** cancer cell line	↑	Increase in CDDP-induced cell growth inhibition	[52]
CDDP	Alpinetin, 200 μM	A549/CDDP human **lung** cancer cell line, CDDP-resistant	↑	Reversal of CDDP resistance; decrease in MRP1, MRP5 and P-gp proteins	[160]
CDDP, 1, 2 μM	Apigenin, 5, 10 μM	L1210 murine **leukemia** cell line	↓	Decrease in CDDP-induced cytotoxicity	[84]
CDDP, 2.5, 5, 10 μM	Apigenin, 30 μM	MCF-7 human **breast** cancer cell line, wild-type p53	↑	Increase in CDDP-induced cytotoxicity (in p53-dependent manner)	[53]
CDDP, 2.5, 5, 10 μM	Apigenin, 30 μM	HCT 116 human **colorectal** cancer cell line, wild-type p53	↑	Increase in CDDP-induced cytotoxicity (in p53-dependent manner)	[53]
CDDP, 5 μg/ml	Apigenin, 10, 40, 160 μM	Hep-2 human **laryngeal** carcinoma cell line	↑	Increase in CDDP-induced cell growth suppression. Inhibition of GLUT-1 and p-Akt expression	[55]
CDDP, 10-100 μM	Apigenin, 5 μM	SCC25 human **head and neck** squamous cell carcinoma cell line	↑	Synergism in cell proliferation inhibition (CI<1)	[141]
CDDP, 2.5, 5, 10 μM	Apigenin, 30 μM	A549 human **lung** cancer cell line, wild-type p53	↑	Increase in CDDP-induced cytotoxicity. Promotion of Erk/MAPK activation and p53 accumulation, increase in apoptosis (cleavage of caspases-3/-9 and PARP, increase in Bax)	[53]

Table 6.6. (Continued)

Drug	Flavonoid	Biological system	Direction of combination	Effects	Ref.
CDDP, 2.5, 5, 10 µM	Apigenin, 30 µM	H1299 human **lung** cancer cell line, p53-null	~	No effect on CDDP-induced cytotoxicity	[53]
CDDP, 120 µM	Apigenin, 60 µM	OVCAR-3 human **ovarian** cancer cell line, CDDP-resistant	~	No effect on CDDP-induced cell viability reduction	[112]
CDDP, 10 µM	Apigenin, 15 µM	BxPC-3 human **pancreatic** cancer cell line	↑	Increase in CDDP-induced inhibitory potential	[140]
CDDP, 1.56-100 µM	Apigenin, 15 µM	CD44⁻ CSCs derived from PC3 human **prostate** cancer cell line	↑	Increase in CDDP cytotoxicity, 3.4-fold decrease in CDDP IC_{50}. Potentiation of apoptosis (increase in caspase-8, Apaf-1, p53; decrease in Bcl-2, sharpin, survivin); suppression of p-PI3K, p-AKT and NF-κB. Prevention of cell migration (decrease in Snail)	[54]
CDDP, 2.5, 5, 10 µM	Apigenin, 30 µM	HeLa human **cervical** cancer cell line, wild-type p53	↑	Increase in CDDP-induced cytotoxicity (in p53-dependent manner)	[53]
CDDP, 1.25-160 µM	Avicularin, 10 µM	SGC-7901/DDP human **gastric** cancer cell line, CDDP-resistant	↑	Increase in CDDP-induced cytotoxicity, decrease in colony formation ability. Increase in apoptosis (cleavage of caspases-3/-9 and PARP, increase in Bax and BOK, decrease in Bcl-2)	[56]
CDDP, 300 µM	Baicalein, 2, 5, 10 µM	A172 human **glioma** cell line	↓	Protection against CDDP cytotoxicity. Prevention of CDDP-induced apoptosis (inhibition of ΔΨm decrease, Bax and caspase increase, and cyt c release)	[151]
CDDP, 2-32 µM	Baicalein, 40 µM	A549 human non-small cell **lung** cancer cell line	↑	Increase in CDDP-induced cell viability reduction. Downregulation of miR-424-3p, upregulation of PTEN	[149]
CDDP, 7 µg/ml	Baicalein, 25, 50 µM	A549 human **lung** adenocarcinoma cell line	↑	Increase in CDDP-induced apoptosis (decrease in Bcl-2, increase in Bax and caspase-3). Inhibition of TNF-α and IL-6 secretion	[48]
CDDP, 20-320 µM	Baicalein, 100 µM	A549/CDDP human **lung** adenocarcinoma cell line, CDDP-resistant	↑	Reversal of resistance to CDDP. Suppression of PI3K/Akt/NF-κB pathway leading to conversion of EMT to MET and inhibition of NF-κB-mediated antiapoptotic proteins, induction of apoptosis	[150]
CDDP, 2-32 µM	Baicalein, 40 µM	H460 human non-small cell **lung** cancer cell line	↑	Increase in CDDP-induced cell viability reduction. Downregulation of miR-424-3p, upregulation of PTEN	[149]
CDDP, 0.5 µM	Baicalein, 0.1 µM	Cx26-HeLa human **cervical** cancer cell line, Cx26-transfected	↑	Increase in CDDP-induced cytotoxicity in high-density cultures with functional GJs, enhancement of GJIC	[49]

Drug	Flavonoid	Biological system	Direction of combination	Effects	Ref.
CDDP, 1-8 μg/ml	Baicalin, 8 μg/ml	A549 human lung cancer cell line	↑↓	Dosage- and time-dependent effect: antagonism in proliferation inhibition at 24h. Additive to synergistic increase in CDDP (4 and 8 μg/ml)-induced antiproliferation at 48h; suppression of invasion	[40]
CDDP, 1-8 μg/ml	Baicalin, 8 μg/ml	A549/DDP human **lung** cancer cell line, CDDP-resistant	↑↓	Dosage- and time-dependent effect: antagonism in proliferation inhibition at 24h. Additive to synergistic increase in CDDP (4 and 8 μg/ml)-induced antiproliferative effect at 48h; suppression of invasion; downregulation of MARK2 and p-Akt	[40]
CDDP, 20 μM	Butein, 20 μM	HeLa human **cervical** carcinoma cell line	↑	Increase in CDDP-induced cell growth inhibition and apoptosis, induction of G1 phase cell cycle arrest. Inhibition of activation of AKT and ERK/p38 MAPK pathways by targeting FoxO3a (increase in p27 and Bax, decrease in cyclin D1 and Bcl-2)	[168]
CDDP, 20 μg/ml	Calycosin, 10 μg/ml	SGC7901 human **gastric** cancer cell line	↑	Potentiation of CDDP-induced proliferation inhibition. Increase in G1 phase cell cycle arrest (decrease in cyclin D1, CDK4/6) and apoptosis (decrease in Bcl-2, increase in caspase-3 and Bax). Suppression of invasion and migration (decrease in MMP-2/-9), inhibition of p-Akt	[139]
CDDP, 20 μg/ml	Calycosin, 10 μg/ml	BGC823 human **gastric** cancer cell line	↑	Potentiation of CDDP-induced proliferation inhibition. Decrease in cyclin D1, CDK4/6 and Bcl-2, increase in caspase-3 and Bax. Suppression of invasion and migration (decrease in MMP-2/-9), inhibition of p-Akt	[139]
CDDP, 20 μg/ml	Calycosin, 10 μg/ml	NCI-N87 human **gastric** cancer cell line	↑	Potentiation of CDDP-induced proliferation inhibition. Decrease in cyclin D1, CDK4/6 and Bcl-2, increase in caspase-3 and Bax. Suppression of invasion and migration (decrease in MMP-2/-9), inhibition of p-Akt	[139]
CDDP, 2 μM	Chrysin, 40 μM	U87 human **glioma** cell line	↑	Increase in growth inhibition and apoptosis, loss of $\Delta\Psi m$	[146]
CDDP, 5 μg/ml	Chrysin, 20, 40 μM	HepG2 human **liver** cancer cell line, wild-type p53	↑	Promotion of apoptosis (increase in Bax and DR5, decrease in Bcl-2, activation of caspases-3/-8/-9, PARP cleavage, cyt c release). Increase in phosphorylation and accumulation of p53 through activating ERK1/2	[57]

Table 6.6. (Continued)

Drug	Flavonoid	Biological system	Direction of combination	Effects	Ref.
CDDP, 20 μM	Chrysin, 20 μM	A549 human **lung** adenocarcinoma cell line	↑	Potentiation of CDDP-induced cytotoxicity; induction of GSH depletion, exacerbation of mitochondrial dysfunction (cyt c release)	[147]
CDDP, 250 μM	Chrysin, 2.5, 10, 20 μM	HL-60 human promyelocytic **leukemia** cell line	~	No effect on CDDP-induced cytotoxicity	[86]
CDDP, 1, 2 μM	Chrysin, 5, 10 μM	L1210 murine **leukemia** cell line	↓	Decrease in CDDP-induced cytotoxicity	[84]
CDDP, 0.25-75 μg/ml, in dual multilayer NPs	Chrysin, 0.25-75 μg/ml, in dual multilayer NPs	KB human **oral** cancer cell line	↑	Potentiation of cytotoxicity. Increase in ROS and apoptosis (decrease in ΔΨm, cyt c release, upregulation of Bax and caspase-3, downregulation of Bcl-2)	[148]
CDDP, 4 μM	Daidzein, 10 nM	D283 Med human **medulloblastoma** cell line	↓	Inhibition of CDDP-induced cytotoxicity, decrease in caspase-3 activity	[134]
CDDP, 7 μM	EGCG, 4.5, 9, 18 μM, encapsulated into PLGA NPs	THP1 human acute monocytic **leukemia** cell line	↑	Increase in CDDP-induced antiproliferative activity and apoptosis	[116]
CDDP	EGCG, encapsulated in PLGA NPs	THP-1 human acute monocytic **leukemia** cell line	↑	Increase in CDDP anticancer potential	[117]
CDDP, 10-50 μM	EGCG, 100 μM	1321N1 human **glioma** cell line, grade II astrocytoma	↑	Increase in CDDP-induced cell viability reduction. Inhibition of telomerase expression	[124]
CDDP, 10-50 μM	EGCG, 100 μM	U87-MG human high-grade **glioma** cell line	↑	Increase in CDDP-induced cell viability reduction. Inhibition of telomerase expression	[124]
CDDP, 5-20 μM	EGCG, 50 μM	MDA-MB231 human TN **breast** cancer cell line	↑	Increase in CDDP-induced apoptosis, activation of Nrf2 signaling	[120]
CDDP, 2.5-20 μM	EGCG, 25, 50, 100 μM	DLD-1 human **colorectal** adenocarcinoma cell line	↑	Synergism in cytotoxicity (CI<1). Induction of autophagy (accumulation of LC3-II, increase om AVOs, formation of autophagosome)	[121]
CDDP, 2.5-20 μM	EGCG, 25, 50, 100 μM	HT-29 human **colorectal** adenocarcinoma cell line	↑	Synergism in cytotoxicity (CI<1). Induction of autophagy (accumulation of LC3-II, increase om AVOs, formation of autophagosome)	[121]
CDDP, 40 μM	EGCG, 20, 50 μM	BDC human **bile duct** carcinoma cell line	↑	Synergism in cytotoxicity (CI 0.66 at 20 μM, 0.49 at 50 μM EGCG)	[122]
CDDP, 40 μM	EGCG, 20, 50 μM	CCSW-1 human **bile duct** carcinoma cell line	↓	Antagonism in cytotoxicity (CI 1.21 at 20 μM, 1.26 at 50 μM EGCG)	[122]
CDDP, 40 μM	EGCG, 20, 50 μM	EGI-1 human **bile duct** carcinoma cell line	↓	Antagonism in cytotoxicity (CI 3.43 at 20 μM, 1.56 at 50 μM EGCG)	[122]

Drug	Flavonoid	Biological system	Direction of combination	Effects	Ref.
CDDP, 40 μM	EGCG, 20, 50 μM	GBC human **gallbladder** cancer cell line	↑	Synergism in cytotoxicity (CI 0.62 at 20 μM, 0.42 at 50 μM EGCG)	[122]
CDDP, 40 μM	EGCG, 20, 50 μM	MzChA-1 human **gallbladder** cancer cell line	↑	Moderate synergism in cytotoxicity (CI 0.85 at 20 μM, 0.83 at 50 μM EGCG)	[122]
CDDP, 40 μM	EGCG, 20, 50 μM	MzChA-2 human **gallbladder** cancer cell line	↑	Synergism in cytotoxicity (CI 0.49 at 20 μM, 0.68 at 50 μM EGCG)	[122]
CDDP, 40 μM	EGCG, 20, 50 μM	TFK-1 human **bile duct** carcinoma cell line	↑	Synergism in cytotoxicity (CI 0.59 at 20 μM, 0.49 at 50 μM EGCG)	[122]
CDDP, 5, 10, 20 μM	EGCG, 5 μM	HNSC CSCs human **head and neck** squamous carcinoma CSCs isolated from a patient	↑	Sensitization to CDDP. Increase in cleaved caspase-3, downregulation of ABCC2 and ABCG2; inhibition of Notch1 signaling	[123]
CDDP, 32.5 μM	EGCG, 174, 348, 522 μM	A549 human **lung** carcinoma cell line	↑	Increase in CDDP-induced cytotoxicity. Decrease in HDGF, increase in apoptosis (disruption of $\Delta\Psi$m, activation of caspases-3/-9)	[113]
CDDP, 5-30 μM	EGCG, 20 μM	A549 human non-small cell **lung** cancer cell line	↑	Synergism in cell growth inhibition (CI 0.72) and colony formation suppression. Increase in apoptosis, elevation of CTR1, promotion of Pt accumulation and enhancement of DNA-Pt adduct concentration in cells	[79]
CDDP, 10-40 μM	EGCG, 10 μM	A549 human non-small cell **lung** cancer cell line	↑	Increase in CDDP efficacy, downregulation of hsa-miR-98-5p followed by increase in p53	[75]
CDDP, 5 μM	EGCG, 3, 6, 12 μM, encapsulated into PLGA NPs	A549 human **lung** adenocarcinoma cell line	↑	Increase in CDDP-induced antiproliferative activity and apoptosis (decrease in $\Delta\Psi$m; increase in Bax/Bcl-2 ratio, PARP cleavage, cyt c release, caspases-9/-3). Increase in ROS, suppression of CDDP-induced NF-κB activation and downregulation of its corresponding genes (cyclin D1, VEGF, MMP-9)	[116]
CDDP	EGCG, encapsulated in PLGA NPs	A549 human **lung** carcinoma cell line	↑	Increase in inhibition of NF-κB activation, cyclin D1, MMP-9 and VEGF; potentiation of apoptosis (cleavage of caspases-3/-9, induction of Bax/Bcl-2 ratio)	[117]
CDDP, 10-50 μM	EGCG, 20 μM	A549/cDDP human non-small cell **lung** cancer cell line, CDDP-resistant	↑	Increase in CDDP-induced growth inhibition. Promotion of Pt and DNA-Pt adduct absorption, elevation of CTR1 expression; CTR1 regulated by NEAT1/hsa-miR-98-5p axis	[79]
CDDP, 2 μg/ml	EGCG, 50 μM	A549/DDP human **lung** adenocarcinoma cell line, CDDP-resistant	↑	Reversal of CDDP resistance, increase in apoptosis and G1 phase cell cycle arrest. Inhibition of DNMT and HDAC, reversal of hypermethylated status and downregulated expression of GAS1, TIMP4, ICAM1, WISP2 genes	[114]

Table 6.6. (Continued)

Drug	Flavonoid	Biological system	Direction of combination	Effects	Ref.
CDDP, 5-30 μM	EGCG, 20 μM	H1299 human non-small cell **lung** cancer cell line	↑	Synergism in cell growth inhibition (CI 0.65). Increase in CTR1 levels	[79]
CDDP, 5-30 μM	EGCG, 20 μM	H460 human non-small cell **lung** cancer cell line	↑	Synergism in cell growth inhibition (CI 0.78). Increase in CTR1 levels	[79]
CDDP, 10-40 μM	EGCG, 10 μM	LTEP-α-2 human non-small cell **lung** cancer cell line	↑	Increase in CDDP efficacy	[75]
CDDP, 10-40 μM	EGCG, 10, 20 μM	NCI-H460 human non-small cell **lung** cancer cell line	↓	Attenuation of CDDP efficacy. Upregulation of hsa-miR-98-5p	[75]
CDDP, 0.08-1.25 μM	EGCG, 1.97-21.98 μM	A2780 human **ovarian** cancer cell line	↑↓	Synergism in efficacy when CDDP added 4h before EGCG; increase in CDDP cellular accumulation and binding to DNA. Antagonism when EGCG added 4h before CDDP	[118]
CDDP	EGCG	A2780 human **ovarian** cancer cell line	↑↓	Schedule-dependent effect: Strongest synergism when CDDP added 4h before EGCG; increase in CDDP cellular accumulation and binding to DNA. Least synergism (often antagonism) when EGCG added 4h or 24h before CDDP	[58]
CDDP	EGCG	A2780cisR human **ovarian** cancer cell line, CDDP-resistant	↑↓	Schedule-dependent effect: Strongest synergism when CDDP added 4h before EGCG; increase in CDDP cellular accumulation and binding to DNA. Least synergism (often antagonism) when EGCG added 4h or 24h before CDDP	[58]
CDDP	EGCG	A2780ZD0473R human **ovarian** cancer cell line, CDDP-resistant	↑↓	Schedule-dependent effect: Strongest synergism when CDDP added 4h before EGCG; increase in CDDP cellular accumulation and binding to DNA. Least synergism (often antagonism) when EGCG added before CDDP	[58]
CDDP, 0.99-15.87 μM	EGCG, 1.33-21.34 μM	A2780cisR human **ovarian** cancer cell line, CDDP-resistant	↑	Strongest synergism when CDDP added before EGCG; increase in CDDP cellular accumulation and binding to DNA. Synergism also at co-treatment and adding EGCG before CDDP	[118]
CDDP, 50-350 μg/ml	EGCG, 20 μM	C200 human **ovarian** cancer cell line, CDDP-resistant	↑	Increase in CDDP potency. Increase in oxidative stress	[78[
CDDP, 0.5-4 μg/ml	EGCG, 10 μM	CAOV3 human **ovarian** cancer cell line	↑	Increase in CDDP potency. Increase in oxidative stress	[78]

Drug	Flavonoid	Biological system	Direction of combination	Effects	Ref.
CDDP, 5-40 μM	EGCG, 10 μM	OVCAR3 human **ovarian** cancer cell line	↑	2.7-fold decrease in CDDP IC_{50}, inhibition of colony growth. Potentiation of apoptosis, increase in CDDP and DNA-Pt adducts accumulation, promotion of CTR1 level, inhibition of CDDP-induced CTR1 degradation	[70]
CDDP, 1-4 μg/ml	EGCG, 10 μM	SKOV3 human **ovarian** cancer cell line	↑	Increase in CDDP potency. Increase in oxidative stress	[78]
CDDP, 5-40 μM	EGCG, 10 μM	SKOV3 human **ovarian** cancer cell line	↑	1.6-fold decrease in CDDP IC_{50}, inhibition of colony growth. Potentiation of apoptosis, promotion of CTR1 level, inhibition of CDDP-induced CTR1 degradation	[70]
CDDP, 2.5, 5 μM	EGCG, 1, 25 μM	PC3 human androgen-independent **prostate** cancer cell line	↑	Increase in apoptosis (promotion of expression of caspase-9 proapoptotic splice isoform)	[46]
CDDP, 8.6 μM	EGCG, 30 μM	LMS **leiomyosarcoma** cell line, from Wistar rats	↑~	Increase in cytotoxicity and apoptosis when EGCG added 24h before CDDP. No effect at simultaneous treatment or adding CDDP 24h before EGCG	[66]
CDDP, 10 μg/ml	EGCG, 10 μg/ml	HeLa human **cervical** cancer cell line, HPV18-positive	↑	About 3-fold decrease in CDDP IC_{50}, increase in apoptosis (decrease in ΔΨm, cyt c release, downregulation of Bcl-2, upregulation of p53 and Bax, activation of caspases-9/-3, PARP cleavage). Increase in ROS, decrease in cellular GSH content. Inhibition of CDDP-induced NF-κB activation and pAkt level, decrease in cyclin D1	[119]
CDDP, 4 μM	EGCG, 2.75, 5.5, 11 μM, encapsulated into PLGA NPs	HeLa human **cervical** cancer cell line	↑	Increase in CDDP-induced antiproliferative activity and apoptosis	[116]
CDDP	EGCG, encapsulated in PLGA NPs	HeLa human **cervical** carcinoma cell line	↑	Increase in CDDP anticancer potential	[117]
CDDP, 10 μg/ml	EGCG, 15 μg/ml	SiHa human **cervical** cancer cell line, HPV16-positive	↑	About 3-fold decrease in CDDP IC_{50}, increase in caspase-dependent apoptosis (decrease in ΔΨm). Increase in ROS, decrease in cellular GSH content	[119]
CDDP, 0.72, 1.45 μM	Epicatechin, 1.9, 3.75 μM	A549 human **lung** adenocarcinoma cell line	↑	Synergism in cell growth inhibition (CI<1), promotion of apoptosis	[69]
CDDP, 1 μM	Fisetin, 10, 20 μM	MDA-MB-231 human TN **breast** cancer cell line	↑	Increase in sensitivity to CDDP, decrease in clonogenic cell growth. Inhibition of CDDP-induced Cdk1 phosphorylation	[87[
CDDP, 0.25-8 μg/ml	Fisetin, 25 μM	MDA-MB-231 human TN **breast** cancer cell line, p53-deficient	↑	Increase in CDDP-induced cytotoxicity	[5]
CDDP, 0.25-8 μg/ml	Fisetin, 25 μM	MDA-MB-468 human TN **breast** cancer cell line, p53-deficient	↑	Increase in CDDP-induced cytotoxicity	[5]

Table 6.6. (Continued)

Drug	Flavonoid	Biological system	Direction of combination	Effects	Ref.
CDDP, 10 μM	Fisetin, 40 μM	A549-CR human **lung** adenocarcinoma cell line, CDDP-resistant	↑	Reversal of CDDP resistance, induction of apoptosis (increase in caspases-3/-8, cyt c release). Inhibition of MAPK pathway and survivin expression	[59]
CDDP, 10 μg/ml	Fisetin, 25 μM	H1299 human **lung** adenocarcinoma cell line	↑	Increase in CDDP-induced cytotoxicity	[105]
CDDP, 5 μg/ml	Fisetin, 20 μM	NT2/D1 human pluripotent cell line derived from **teratocarcinoma**, active p53	↑	Synergism in cytotoxicity (CI 0.65). Potentiation of apoptosis (increase in FasL, activation of caspases-3/-7/-8/-9, increase in Bak, truncation of Bid, loss of $\Delta\Psi$m, cyt c release, PARP cleavage); increase in p53 and p21, decrease in cyclin B1 and survivin	[106]
CDDP, 25 μM	Formononetin, 12.5-100 μM	CaSKi human **cervical** cancer cell line	~	No effect on CDDP efficacy	[60]
CDDP, 25 μM	Formononetin, 12.5-100 μM	HeLa human **cervical** cancer cell line	~	No effect on CDDP efficacy	[60]
CDDP, 25 μM	Formononetin, 12.5-100 μM	SiHa human **cervical** cancer cell line	~	No effect on CDDP efficacy	[60]
CDDP, 250 μM	Galangin, 2.5, 10, 20 μM	HL-60 human promyelocytic **leukemia** cell line	↓~	Decrease in CDDP-induced apoptosis when pretreated with galangin 40min before CDDP. No effect when posttreated with galangin	[86]
CDDP, 1, 2 μM	Galangin, 5, 10 μM	L1210 murine **leukemia** cell line	↓	Decrease in CDDP-induced cytotoxicity	[84]
CDDP, 4 μM	Galangin, 10 μM	L1210 murine **leukemia** cell line	~	No effect on total GSH level	[85]
CDDP, 1-2 μM	Galangin, 5-10 μM	L1210 murine **leukemia** cell line	↓	Antagonism in cytotoxicity (CI>1)	[86]
CDDP, 20 μM	Galangin, 0.5-40 μM	A549 human **lung** cancer cell line	↑	Potentiation of CDDP-suppressed proliferation. Inhibition of migration and colony formation, induction of apoptosis; inhibition of NF-κB (p65) activation	[61]
CDDP, 20 μM	Galangin, 0.5-40 μM	A549/DDP human **lung** cancer cell line, CDDP-resistant	↑	Potentiation of CDDP-suppressed proliferation. Inhibition of migration and colony formation, induction of intrinsic and extrinsic apoptosis through bcl-2 suppression and inactivation of NF-κB/STAT3 pathway (cyt c release, upregulation of caspases-3/-8/-9, PARP cleavage, decrease in Bcl-2, increase in Bax and tBid)	[61]
CDDP, 20 μM	Galangin, 0.5-40 μM	SPC-A1 human **lung** cancer cell line	↑	Potentiation of CDDP-suppressed proliferation. Inhibition of NF-κB (p65) activation	[61]
CDDP, 20 μM	Galangin, 0.5-40 μM	SPC-A1/DDP human **lung** cancer cell line, CDDP-resistant	↑	Potentiation of CDDP-suppressed proliferation. Induction of apoptosis (increase in caspase-3, PARP cleavage), inactivation of NF-κB/STAT3 pathway	[61]

Drug	Flavonoid	Biological system	Direction of combination	Effects	Ref.
CDDP, 0.5 µM	Genistein, 6 µM	CRL-8805 human **medulloblastoma** cell line	↑	Increase in inhibition of growth and clonogenic survival	[135]
CDDP, 4 µM	Genistein, 10 nM	D283 Med human **medulloblastoma** cell line	↓	Inhibition of CDDP cytotoxic action, decrease in caspase-3 activity	[134]
CDDP, 0.05 µM	Genistein, 6 µM	HTB-186 human **medulloblastoma** cell line	↑	Increase in inhibition of growth and clonogenic survival	[135]
CDDP, 0.5 µM	Genistein, 6 µM	MED-1 human **medulloblastoma** cell line	↑	Increase in inhibition of growth and clonogenic survival	[135]
CDDP, 10 µM	Genistein, 1 µM	MCF-7 human **breast** cancer cell line, high ERα/ERβ ratio	↓	Inhibition of sensitivity to CDDP. Decrease in ROS, increase in MnSOD, decrease in apoptosis, increase in G2/M phase cell proportion	[130]
CDDP, 5 µM	Genistein, 1, 10, 100 µM	MCF-7 human **breast** cancer cell line, ERα-positive, ERβ-negative	↓↑	Antagonism in CDDP-induced growth inhibition at 1 and 10 µM genistein; suppression of apoptosis (increase in Bcl-2). Additive effect at 100 µM genistein	[129]
CDDP, 10 µM	Genistein, 1 µM	T47D human **breast** cancer cell line, low ERα/ERβ ratio	~	No effect on CDDP-induced cytotoxicity	[130]
CDDP, 5 µM	Genistein, 10, 100 µM	HT-29 human **colon** cancer cell line, faint ERα, ERβ-negative	↓↑	Antagonism in CDDP-induced growth inhibition at 10 µM genistein; suppression of apoptosis (increase in Bcl-2). Additive effect at 100 µM genistein	[129]
CDDP, 2.5-40 µM	Genistein, 10-160 µM	HCCLM3 human highly metastatic **hepatocellular** carcinoma cell line	↑	Potentiation of proliferation inhibition; abolishment of CDDP-induced MMP-2 upregulation	[133]
CDDP	Genistein	A549 human non-small cell **lung** cancer cell line	↑	Potentiation of CDDP-induced growth inhibition and apoptosis (increase in caspases-3/-8/-10); suppression of PI3K/AKT pathway	[125]
CDDP, 500 nM	Genistein, 15 µM	H460 human **lung** cancer cell line	↑	Synergism in cell growth inhibition (CI 0.709), increase in apoptosis	[62]
CDDP, 1 µg/ml	Genistein, 25 µg/ml	NCI-H358 human non-small cell **lung** cancer cell line, weak EGFR	~	No effect on CDDP activity	[126]
CDDP, 1 µg/ml	Genistein, 40 µg/ml	NCI-H596 human non-small cell **lung** cancer cell line, strong EGFR	↑	Increase in CDDP-induced antiproliferative effects. Inhibition of EGFR phosphorylation, induction of apoptosis (PARP cleavage)	[126]
CDDP, 1 µg/ml	Genistein, 20 µM	A101D human **melanoma** cell line	↑	Augmentation of CDDP-induced cell growth inhibition. Increase in apoptosis (decrease in bcl-2, bcl-xl; increase in Apaf-1 protein), induction of p21 and p27 expression	[136]

Table 6.6. (Continued)

Drug	Flavonoid	Biological system	Direction of combination	Effects	Ref.
CDDP, 1 μg/ml	Genistein, 20 μM	HM3KO human **melanoma** cell line	↑	Augmentation of CDDP-induced cell growth inhibition. Increase in apoptosis (decrease in bcl-2, bcl-xl; increase in Apaf-1 protein)	[136]
CDDP, 1 μg/ml	Genistein, 20 μM	MeWo human **melanoma** cell line	↑	Augmentation of CDDP-induced cell growth inhibition. Increase in apoptosis (decrease in bcl-2, bcl-xl; increase in Apaf-1 protein)	[136]
CDDP, 1 μg/ml	Genistein, 20 μM	p22 human **melanoma** cell line	↑	Augmentation of CDDP-induced cell growth inhibition. Increase in apoptosis (decrease in bcl-2, bcl-xl; increase in Apaf-1 protein)	[136]
CDDP, 1 μg/ml	Genistein, 20 μM	p39 human **melanoma** cell line	↑	Augmentation of CDDP-induced cell growth inhibition. Increase in apoptosis (decrease in bcl-2, bcl-xl; increase in Apaf-1 protein)	[136]
CDDP, 0-5 μM	Genistein, 40 μM	2008 human **ovarian** carcinoma cell line	↑	8.2-fold decrease in CDDP IC_{50}, intracellular accumulation of CDDP	[127]
CDDP, 0-50 μM	Genistein, 5-50 μM	2008 C13 human **ovarian** carcinoma cell line, CDDP-resistant, wild-type p53	↑	Reversal of CDDP resistance, increase in CDDP cellular uptake	[73]
CDDP, 250 nM	Genistein, 10 μM	A2780 human **ovarian** cancer cell line	↑	Potentiation of cell viability inhibition. Increase in apoptosis (PARP cleavage, downregulation of Bcl-2, Bcl-xl, survivin, cIAP1), decrease in NF-κB DNA binding activity	[128]
CDDP, 0-100 μM	Genistein, 40 μM	C13* human **ovarian** carcinoma cell line, CDDP-resistant 2008 cells	↑	4.7-fold decrease in CDDP IC_{50}, intracellular accumulation of CDDP	[127]
CDDP, 250 nM	Genistein, 25 μM	C200 human **ovarian** cancer cell line, CDDP-resistant A2780 cells	↑	Potentiation of cell viability inhibition. Increase in apoptosis (PARP cleavage, downregulation of Bcl-2, Bcl-xl, survivin, cIAP1), decrease in NF-κB DNA binding activity	[128]
CDDP, 0-50 μM	Genistein, 5-50 μM	CP70 human **ovarian** cancer cell line, CDDP-resistant, mutant p53	↑	Reversal of resistance	[73]
CDDP, 0-50 μM	Genistein, 5-50 μM	OVCAR 8 human **ovarian** cancer cell line, CDDP-resistant, mutant p53	~	No effect on CDDP resistance	[73]
CDDP, 100 nM	Genistein, 30 μM	BxPC-3 human **pancreatic** cancer cell line	↑	Synergism in growth inhibition (CI 0.731). Increase in apoptosis, abrogation of drug-induced NF-κB DNA-binding activity	[62]

Drug	Flavonoid	Biological system	Direction of combination	Effects	Ref.
CDDP, 100 nM	Genistein, 30 μM	BxPC-3 human **pancreatic** cancer cell line	↑	Increase in CDDP-induced growth inhibition and apoptosis, abrogation of CDDP-induced NF-κB activation	[132]
CDDP, 100 nM	Genistein, 30 μM	PC-3 human **prostate** cancer cell line	↑	Synergism in growth inhibition (CI 0.861). Increase in apoptosis (upregulation of p21WAF1 expression, downregulation of survivin, Bcl-2, Bcl-xL), abrogation of drug-induced NF-κB DNA binding activity	[62]
CDDP, 0.25-1 μg/ml	Genistein, 15 μM	MGC-803 human **gastric** cancer cell line	↑	Decrease in resistance to CDDP, inhibition of ABCG2 and ERK1/2	[131]
CDDP, 0.01-0.5 μg/ml	Hesperidin	Primary **endometrial** cancer cells	~	No effect on CDDP antiproliferative activity	[90]
CDDP, 1 μg/ml	Hesperidin, 1 μM	OVCA 433 human **ovarian** cancer cell line	~	No effect on CDDP antiproliferative activity	[91]
CDDP, 0.01-0.5 μg/ml	Hesperidin	Primary **ovarian** cancer cells	~	No effect on CDDP antiproliferative activity	[90]
CDDP, 20 μM	Hyperoside, 100 μM	SKOV3 human **ovarian** cancer cell line, overexpressing PGRMC1	↑	Increase in chemosensitivity. Promotion of autophagy by co-localization of CDDP-induced PGRMC1 with LC-3B, induction of apoptosis	[111]
CDDP, 10, 20 μM	Intricatinol, 25, 50 μM	A549 human non-small cell **lung** carcinoma cell line	↑	Additivity to synergism in cytotoxicity, decrease in clonogenicity, augmentation of intrinsic apoptosis (increase in Bax/Bcl-2 ratio, loss of ΔΨm, cyt c release, cleavage of caspases-3/-9 and PARP1); increase in p53, p38 MAPK. Suppression of migration	[42]
CDDP, 5-100 μM	Isoliquiritigenin, 25, 50 μM	OECM1-CSC human **oral** squamous cancer cell line, CSCs	↑	Potentiation of CDDP action, downregulation of ABCG2, increase in suppression of colony formation and invasion. Decrease in GRP78	[169]
CDDP, 5-100 μM	Isoliquiritigenin, 25, 50 μM	SAS-CSC human **oral** squamous cancer cell line, CSCs	↑	Inhibition of CSCs number, downregulation of ABCG2, increase in suppression of colony formation and invasion. Decrease in GRP78	[169]
CDDP, 100 μM	Isoliquiritigenin, 5, 15, 25 μM	T24 human **bladder** cancer cell line	↑↓	Synergism in cell death at 15 μM (CI 0.58) and 25 μM isoliquiritigenin (CI 0.65). Antagonism with 5 μM isoliquiritigenin (CI 1.71)	[51]
CDDP, 0.5 μM	Isorhamnetin, 25 μM	A549 human non-small cell **lung** cancer cell line	↑	Potentiation of growth inhibition, increase in apoptosis (loss of ΔΨm, activation of caspases-3/-9, PARP cleavage), aberrant microtubule disruption, increase in G2/M phase cell cycle arrest, suppression of migration	[107]
CDDP, 0.94-15 μM	Isoxanthohumol, 5.75-23 μM	A375 human **melanoma** cell line	↓	Antagonism in CDDP anticancer efficacy	[171]
CDDP, 0.94-15 μM	Isoxanthohumol, 5.75-23 μM	B16 murine **melanoma** cell line	↓	Antagonism in CDDP anticancer efficacy	[171]

Table 6.6. (Continued)

Drug	Flavonoid	Biological system	Direction of combination	Effects	Ref.
CDDP	Kaempferol, 20 μM	T98G human **glioblastoma** cell line, no P-gp	↓	Decrease in cytotoxicity, 3-fold increase in CDDP IC_{50}. Increase in MRP1 and GST-π, decrease in MPR2 protein, increase in GST activity	[109]
CDDP, 40, 80 μM	Kaempferol, 20 μM	OVCAR-3 human **ovarian** cancer cell line, CDDP-resistant	↑	Increase in cell viability suppression. Inhibition of ABCC6 and cMyc transcription, upregulation of CDKN1A mRNA; promotion of apoptosis	[110]
CDDP, 2 μM	Liquiritigenin, 25-200 μM	B16F10 murine **melanoma** cell line	↑	Increase CDDP-induced cell viability reduction and inhibition of migration and invasion. Downregulation of MMP-2/-9, PI3K and p-AKT, upregulation of PTEN	[159]
CDDP, 1, 2 μM	Luteolin, 5, 10 μM	L1210 murine **leukemia** cell line	↑	Potentiation of CDDP cytotoxicity, increase in apoptosis	[84]
CDDP, 10 μM	Luteolin, 20 μM	D17 canine **osteosarcoma** cell line	↑	Increase CDDP-induced antiproliferative effect	[145]
CDDP, 10 μM	Luteolin, 20 μM	DSN canine **osteosarcoma** cell line	↑	Increase CDDP-induced antiproliferative effect	[145]
CDDP, 2, 5, 10 μg/ml	Luteolin, 40 μM	HCT116 human **colorectal** cancer cell line, wild-type p53	↑	Expedition and increase in CDDP-induced apoptosis (cleavage of caspase-3 and PARP, Bax mitochondrial translocation, cyt c release), stabilization of p53 protein via JNK activation and p53 phosphorylation	[142]
CDDP, 3-30 μg/ml	Luteolin, 5 μM	HCT116-OX human **colorectal** cancer cell line, OXA-resistant	↑	Synergism in anticancer activity (CI<1), 3.7-fold decrease in CDDP IC_{50}. Inhibition of Nrf2 pathway	[143]
CDDP, 10 μg/ml	Luteolin, 40 μM	HT29 human **colorectal** cancer cell line, mutant p53	~	No effect on CDDP-induced apoptosis	[142]
CDDP, 3-30 μg/ml	Luteolin, 5 μM	SW620-OX human **colorectal** cancer cell line, OXA-resistant	↑	Synergism in anticancer activity (CI<1), 1.9-fold decrease in CDDP IC_{50}. Inhibition of Nrf2 pathway	[143]
CDDP, 10 μg/ml	Luteolin, 20 μM	Hep3B human **liver** cancer cell line, mutant p53	~	No effect on CDDP-induced apoptosis	[142]
CDDP, 2, 5, 10 μg/ml	Luteolin, 20 μM	HepG2 human **liver** cancer cell line, wild-type p53	↑	Expedition and increase in CDDP-induced apoptosis	[142]
CDDP, 2, 5, 10 μg/ml	Luteolin, 40 μM	CNE1 human **nasopharyngeal** cancer cell line	↑	Expedition and increase in CDDP-induced apoptosis	[142]
CDDP, 2 μg/ml	Luteolin, 10, 50, 100 μM	CAOV3/DDP human **ovarian** cancer cell line, CDDP-resistant	↑	Additive to synergistic increase in CDDP-induced antiproliferative effect and apoptosis (decrease in Bcl-2); inhibition of migration and invasion	[80]
CDDP, 120 μM	Luteolin, 20 μM	OVCAR-3 human **ovarian** cancer cell line, CDDP-resistant	~	No effect on cell viability	[112]

Drug	Flavonoid	Biological system	Direction of combination	Effects	Ref.
CDDP, 10 μM	Luteolin, 15 μM	BxPC-3 human **pancreatic** cancer cell line	↑	Increase in CDDP inhibitory potential	[140]
CDDP	Luteolin	AGS human **gastric** cancer cell line	↑	Synergism in cell growth inhibition (CI<1)	[144]
CDDP, 3.125-50 μM	Morin, 100-250 μM	SK-OV-3 human **ovarian** cancer cell line, CDDP-resistant	↑↓	Dose- and schedule-dependent effect: synergism at low CDDP and low morin doses, additivity at high CDDP and low morin doses, antagonism at high CDDP and high morin doses (simultaneous treatment); additivity at low CDDP and antagonism at high CDDP when pretreated with morin before coincubation	[71]
CDDP, 3.125-50 μM	Morin, 100-250 μM	TOV-21G human **ovarian** cancer cell line, grade 3	↑↓	Dose- and schedule-dependent effect: synergism at low, additivity at medium, antagonism at high CDDP doses (simultaneous treatment); antagonism when pretreated with morin before coincubation	[71]
CDDP, 1 μM	Myricetin, 60 μM	HeLa human **cervical** cancer cell line	↑	Potentiation of cell growth inhibition and apoptosis ($\Delta\Psi$m loss, increase in caspase-3 activity), increase in G0/G1 phase cell cycle arrest	[67]
CDDP, 25-100 μM	Myricetin, 100 μM	SiHa human **cervical** cancer cell line, HPV-positive	↑	Reactivation of E6-compromised apoptotic pathway (increase in p53 and caspases-3/-7 activity)	[108]
CDDP, 0.1 nM-1 mM	Naringenin, 1 mM	HTB26 human **breast** cancer cell line	↑	Increase in CDDP-induced cytotoxicity	[10]
CDDP, 0.1 nM-1 mM	Naringenin, 1 mM	SW1116 human **colorectal** cancer cell line	↑	Increase in CDDP-induced cytotoxicity	[10]
CDDP	Nobiletin, 20, 60, 200 μM	MKN-45 human **stomach** cancer cell line	↑↓	Schedule-dependent effect: synergism when CDDP added after nobiletin, additivity when CDDP added before nobiletin, antagonism with simultaneous treatment	[157]
CDDP	Nobiletin, 20, 60, 200 μM	TMK-1 human **gastric** cancer cell line	↑↓	Schedule-dependent effect: synergism when CDDP added after nobiletin, additivity when CDDP added before nobiletin, antagonism with simultaneous treatment	[157]
CDDP	Orobol, 0.1 mM	2008 human **ovarian** cancer cell line	↑	2.3-fold increase in sensitivity to CDDP, potentiation of apoptosis (decrease in Bcl-2, release of cyt c)	[137]
CDDP, 0.5-2.5 μM	Orobol, 0.1 mM	2008 human **ovarian** cancer cell line	↑	2.2-fold increase in sensitivity of proliferating cells to CDDP (decrease in $\Delta\Psi$m)	[138]
CDDP, 0.5-25 μM	Orobol, 0.1 mM	2008/C13*5.25 human **ovarian** cancer cell line, CDDP-resistant	↑	2.4-fold decrease in CDDP IC_{50}	[138]
CDDP	Orobol, 0.1 mM	2008/C13*5.25 (C13) human **ovarian** cancer cell line, CDDP-resistant	↑	3.1-fold increase in sensitivity to CDDP, potentiation of apoptosis (decrease in Bcl-2, release of cyt c)	[137]
CDDP, 5 μg/ml	Phloretin, 50 μg/ml	A549 human **lung** cancer cell line	↑	Increase in antiproliferation effect and apoptosis	[170]
CDDP, 5 μg/ml	Phloretin, 50 μg/ml	Calu-1 human **lung** cancer cell line	↑	Increase in antiproliferation effect and apoptosis	[170]
CDDP, 5 μg/ml	Phloretin, 50 μg/ml	H520 human **lung** cancer cell line	↑	Decrease in Bcl-2, increase in cleaved caspases-3/-9; decrease in MMP-2/-9 proteins	[170]

Table 6.6. (Continued)

Drug	Flavonoid	Biological system	Direction of combination	Effects	Ref.
CDDP, 5 µg/ml	Phloretin, 50 µg/ml	H838 human **lung** cancer cell line	↑	Decrease in Bcl-2, increase in cleaved caspases-3/-9; decrease in MMP-2/-9 proteins	[170]
CDDP, 1-4 µM	Protoapigenone, 0.1, 0.5 µM	MDA-MB-231 human **breast** adenocarcinoma cell line	↑	Decrease in clonogenic survival; inhibition of CDDP-induced activation of ATR targets Chk1 and FANCD2, inducing replication stress via inhibition of ATR signaling	[158]
CDDP, 1-4 µM	Protoapigenone, 0.05, 0.1 µM	A549 human **lung** adenocarcinoma cell line	↑	Decrease in clonogenic survival; inhibition of CDDP-induced activation of ATR targets Chk1 and FANCD2, inducing replication stress via inhibition of ATR signaling	[158]
CDDP, 250 µM	Quercetin, 2.5, 10, 20 µM	HL-60 human promyelocytic **leukemia** cell line	↑~	Increase in CDDP-induced apoptosis when pretreated with quercetin 40min before CDDP. No effect with simultaneous treatment or posttreatment with quercetin	[86]
CDDP, 1, 2 µM	Quercetin, 5, 10 µM	L1210 murine **leukemia** cell line	↑	Increase in CDDP-induced cytotoxicity and apoptosis	[84]
CDDP, 4 µM	Quercetin, 10 µM	L1210 murine **leukemia** cell line	↑	Increase in total GSH level	[85]
CDDP, 1-2 µM	Quercetin, 5-10 µM	L1210 murine **leukemia** cell line	↑	Synergism in cell death (CI<1), increase in apoptosis	[86]
CDDP, 2-12 µM	Quercetin, 5 µM	143B human **osteosarcoma** cell line	↑	1.5-fold decrease in CDDP IC_{50}. Increase in apoptosis, upregulation of miR-217, downregulation of its target KRAS level	[102]
CDDP, 1 µM	Quercetin, 5, 10, 20 µM	MDA-MB-231 human TN **breast** cancer cell line	↑	Decrease in clonogenic cell growth; inhibition of CDDP-induced Chk1 phosphorylation	[87]
CDDP, 0.03-30 µM	Quercetin, 6.6 µM	MDA-MB-468 human TN **breast** cancer cell line; no ER, PR and HER2 expression	↑	Restoring CDDP cytotoxicity in CYP1B1-transfected cells, inhibition of CYP1B1 enzyme	[88]
CDDP, 0.01-10 µM	Quercetin, 5-100 µM	Walker rat **breast** carcinoma cells	↑	Synergism in antiproliferation (CI<1)	[89]
CDDP, 0.01-0.5 µg/ml	Quercetin, 0.1, 1 µM	Primary **endometrial** cancer cells	↑	Synergism in antiproliferation (CI<1), inhibition of colony formation	[90]
CDDP, 2.5 µg/ml	Quercetin, 40 µM	HeP2 human **laryngeal** carcinoma cell line	↑	Increase in apoptosis via acting by separate pathways (decrease in Bcl-2, Bcl-xL, survivin; increase in Bax, caspases-3/-8/-9 activities, cyt c release), decrease in pAkt, HSP70, telomerase activity and Ki-67	[97]
CDDP, 2.5 µg/ml	Quercetin, 40 µM	Hep-2 human **laryngeal** carcinoma cell line	↑	Increase in CDDP-induced apoptosis (decrease in Bcl-2, Bcl-Xl; increase in Bax, caspase-3 activity, cyt c release)	[98]

Drug	Flavonoid	Biological system	Direction of combination	Effects	Ref.
CDDP, 10 μM	Quercetin, 50 μM	HepG2 human **hepatocellular** carcinoma cell line	↑	Potentiation of cell growth suppression and apoptosis (cleavage of caspase-3 and PARP), increase in p21 and p53	[76]
CDDP, 500 ng/ml	Quercetin, 5, 10 μM	A549 human **pulmonary** adenocarcinoma cell line	↑	Augmentation of CDDP-induced antiproliferation and apoptosis	[99]
CDDP, 5 μg/ml	Quercetin, 40 μM	NCI-H-520 human non-small cell **lung** carcinoma cell line	↑	Increase in CDDP-induced apoptosis (decrease in Bcl-Xl, Bcl-2; increase in Bax, nuclear AIF, caspase-3 activity, cyt c release)	[100]
CDDP, 500 ng/ml	Quercetin, 5, 10 μM	SW1271 human small cell **lung** cancer cell line	↑	Augmentation of CDDP-induced antiproliferation and apoptosis	[99]
CDDP, 5, 10 μg/ml	Quercetin, 50 μM	SPC111 human malignant **mesothelioma** cell line	~	No significant effect on CDDP efficacy	[101]
CDDP, 5, 10 μg/ml	Quercetin, 50 μM	SPC212 human malignant **mesothelioma** cell line	↑	Increase in CDDP-induced antiproliferation, S phase cell cycle arrest and caspases-3/-9 activities	[101]
CDDP, 10 μM	Quercetin, 100 μM	DRSPs from SCC25 human **tongue** cancer cell line	↑	Increase in CDDP-induced growth reduction and apoptosis (cleavage of caspase-3 and PARP), downregulation of p-Hsp27, inhibition of migration and invasion, reversal of EMT-related markers (increase in E-cadherin, decrease in vimentin, Twist-1, fascin-1)	[74]
CDDP, 4-16 μg/ml	Quercetin, 85-340 μM	C666-1 human **nasopharyngeal** cancer cell line, EBV-positive	↑	Synergism in cytotoxicity (CI<1)	[82]
CDDP, 0.75-6 μg/ml	Quercetin, 41.25-320 μM	HK1 human **nasopharyngeal** cancer cell line, EBV-negative	↑	Synergism in cytotoxicity (CI<1)	[82]
CDDP, 0.1-1 μM	Quercetin, 2-16 μM, in PMAA_CNT nanocomposite	IMR-32 human **neuroblastoma** cell line	↑	Additivity or synergism in cell growth inhibition	[47]
CDDP, 0.26-4.09 μM	Quercetin, 9.08-145.22 μM	A2780 human **ovarian** cancer cell line	↑	Synergism in anticancer efficacy (CI 0.72-0.94)	[43]
CDDP, 1.66-26.52 μM	Quercetin, 10.38-166.1 μM	A2780cisR human **ovarian** cancer cell line, CDDP-resistant	↑	Synergism in anticancer efficacy (CI 0.27-0.46)	[43]
CDDP, 166.6 μM	Quercetin, 1, 5 μM	A2780P human **ovarian** cancer cell line	↑	Increase in sensitivity to CDDP	[94]
CDDP, 80 μM	Quercetin, 5-30 μM	C13* human **ovarian** cancer cell line, CDDP-resistant 2008 cells	↓	Decrease in CDDP cytotoxicity and apoptosis. Reduction of CDDP-induced oxidative injury and DNA damage, decrease in ROS, increase in expression of antioxidant enzymes. Additive effect at 100 μM quercetin	[95]

Table 6.6. (Continued)

Drug	Flavonoid	Biological system	Direction of combination	Effects	Ref.
CDDP, 20-80 μM	Quercetin, 20 μM	C13* human **ovarian** cancer cell line, CDDP-resistant 2008 cells	↑	Increase in CDDP-induced cytotoxicity. Eliciting ERS-mediated inhibition of STAT3 pathway accompanied by downregulation of BCL-2 and mitochondrial apoptosis (activation of caspases-9/-3, PARP cleavage)	[44]
CDDP, 2 μg/ml	Quercetin, 5-20 μM	CAOV3 human **ovarian** cancer cell line	↑	Increase in sensitivity to CDDP	[92]
CDDP, 166.6 μM	Quercetin, 1, 5 μM	EFO27 human **ovarian** cancer cell line	~	No effect on sensitivity to CDDP	[94]
CDDP, 0.01-2.5 μg/ml	Quercetin, 0.01-2.5 μM	OVCA 433 human **ovarian** cancer cell line	↑	Increase in CDDP-induced cell growth inhibition	[91]
CDDP, 166.6 μM	Quercetin, 1, 5 μM	OVCAR-3 human **ovarian** cancer cell line	↑	Increase in sensitivity to CDDP	[94]
CDDP, 120 μM	Quercetin, 30 μM	OVCAR-3 human **ovarian** cancer cell line, CDDP-resistant	~	No effect on cell viability	[112]
CDDP, 15, 60 μg/ml	Quercetin, 10 μg/ml	OVCAR-8 human **ovarian** cancer cell line, mutant p53	↑	Increase in CDDP-induced cytotoxicity	[93]
CDDP, 0.01-0.5 μg/ml	Quercetin, 0.1, 1 μM	Primary **ovarian** cancer cells	↑	Synergism in antiproliferation (CI<1), inhibition of colony formation	[90]
CDDP, 20-80 μM	Quercetin, 20 μM	P-ris primary **ovarian** cancer cells	↑	Increase in CDDP-induced cytotoxicity. Eliciting ERS-mediated inhibition of STAT3 pathway accompanied by downregulation of BCL-2 and mitochondrial apoptosis (activation of caspases-9/-3, PARP cleavage)	[44]
CDDP, 80 μM	Quercetin, 5-30 μM	SKOV3 human **ovarian** cancer cell line	↓	Decrease in CDDP-induced cytotoxicity. Increase in cytotoxicity at 100 μM quercetin	[95]
CDDP, 2 μg/ml	Quercetin, 5-20 μM	SKOV3 human **ovarian** cancer cell line	↑	Increase in sensitivity to CDDP	[92]
CDDP, 166.6 μM	Quercetin, 1, 5 μM	SKOV-3 human **ovarian** cancer cell line	~	No effect on sensitivity to CDDP	[94]
CDDP, 15, 60 μg/ml	Quercetin, 10 μg/ml	SKOV-3 human **ovarian** cancer cell line, mutant p53	↑	Increase in CDDP-induced cytotoxicity	[93]
CDDP, 10 μg/ml	Quercetin, 15 μg/ml	HeLa human **cervix** adenocarcinoma cell line	↑	Sequence-dependent effect: Strongest apoptosis when quercetin added before CDDP (activation of caspase-3); decrease in Hsp72 and MRP	[96]
CDDP, 0.01-0.5 μg/ml	Rutin	Primary **endometrial** cancer cells	~	No effect on CDDP-induced antiproliferation	[90]
CDDP, 1 μg/ml	Rutin, 1 μM	OVCA 433 human **ovarian** cancer cell line	~	No effect on CDDP-induced cell growth inhibition	[90]
CDDP, 0.01-0.5 μg/ml	Rutin	Primary **ovarian** cancer cells	~	No effect on CDDP-induced antiproliferation	[90]
CDDP, 120 μM	Scutellarein, 60 μM	OVCAR-3 human **ovarian** cancer cell line, CDDP-resistant	↑	Increase in cell viability inhibition	[112]

Drug	Flavonoid	Biological system	Direction of combination	Effects	Ref.
CDDP, 120 μM	Scutellarin, 60 μM	OVCAR-3 human **ovarian** cancer cell line, CDDP-resistant	↑	Increase in cell viability inhibition	[112]
CDDP, 3-12 μM	Scutellarin, 50-200 μM	PC3 human **prostate** cancer cell line	↑	Increase in CDDP-induced cytotoxicity and colony inhibition. Induction of DNA breaks, increase in frequency of DNA damage	[77]
CDDP, 1-5 μM	Silibinin, 150 μM	MCF-7 human **breast** cancer cell line	↑	Synergism in antiproliferation (CI<1), increase in apoptosis (decrease in Bcl-2; increase in Bax, p53, BRCA1 and ATM)	[161]
CDDP, 0.2-2 μg/ml	Silibinin, 25-100 μM	MCF-7 human estrogen-dependent **breast** cancer cell line	↑	Synergism in cell growth inhibition (CI<1)	[162]
CDDP, 1 μg/ml	Silibinin, 200 μM	MDA-MB-435/DOX human **breast** cancer cell line, DOX-resistant	↑	Synergism in cytotoxicity (CI 0.54)	[163]
CDDP, 0.2-2 μg/ml	Silibinin, 25-100 μM	MDA-MB468 human estrogen-independent **breast** cancer cell line	↑	Synergism in cell growth inhibition (CI<1)	[162]
CDDP, 10 μM	Silibinin, 15 μM	KYSE270 human **esophageal** squamous cell carcinoma cell line	↑	Synergism in cell proliferation inhibition (CI 0.480)	[65]
CDDP	Silibinin, 12.5-200 μM	H69 human small-cell **lung** carcinoma cell line	~	No effect on CDDP-induced cytotoxicity	[167]
CDDP	Silibinin, 12.5-200 μM	VPA17 human small-cell **lung** carcinoma cell line, VP-16-resistant, overexpressing P-gp	~	No effect on CDDP-induced cytotoxicity	[167]
CDDP, 0.001-100 μM	Silibinin, 1, 10 μM	A2780 human **ovarian** cancer cell line	↑	1.43- and 1.90-fold decrease in CDDP IC_{50} at 1 and 10 μM silibinin	[165]
CDDP, 0.1-1 μg/ml	Silibinin, 0.1, 1 μM	A2780 human **ovarian** cancer cell line, ER-negative, type II EBS positive	↑	Synergism in growth inhibition (CI<1)	[164]
CDDP, 0.1-1 μg/ml	Silibinin, 0.1, 1 μM	A2780/CDDP human **ovarian** cancer cell line, CDDP-resistant	↑	Synergism in cell growth inhibition (CI<1)	[164]
CDDP, 0.001-100 μM	Silibinin, 1, 10 μM	A2780/CDDP human **ovarian** cancer cell line, CDDP-resistant	~	No effect on CDDP antitumor activity	[165]
CDDP, 2 μg/ml	Silibinin, 50, 75, 100 μM	DU145 human advanced **prostate** cancer cell line	↑	Increase in growth inhibition, G2/M phase cell cycle arrest (decrease in cdc2, cyclin B1, cdc25C; increase in Chk1, wee1), apoptosis (cleavage of caspases-3/-9/-7 and PARP, cyt c release)	[166]
CDDP, 120 μM	Spiraeoside, 60 μM	OVCAR-3 human **ovarian** cancer cell line, CDDP-resistant	↑	Increase in CDDP-induced cell viability reduction	[112]

Table 6.6. (Continued)

Drug	Flavonoid	Biological system	Direction of combination	Effects	Ref.
CDDP, 1.5-6 µM	Tangeretin, 25-150 µM	2008/C13 human **ovarian** cancer cell line, CDDP-resistant	↑	Increase in CDDP-induced cytotoxicity and apoptosis (PARP cleavage, activation of caspases-7/-3). Downregulation of p-Akt and its substrates (NF-κB, p-GSK-3β, p-BAD). Synergism when pretreated with tangeretin for 24h (CI 0.5-0.7), additivity when posttreated with tangeretin (CI 1-1.1)	[81]
CDDP, 1.5-6 µM	Tangeretin, 25-150 µM	A2780/CP70 human **ovarian** cancer cell line, CDDP-resistant	↑	Increase in CDDP-induced cytotoxicity and apoptosis (PARP cleavage, activation of caspases-7/-3), arrest of cells in G2/M phase (decrease in Cdc25C, cyclin B1; increase in p53). Inhibition of PI3K/Akt pathway, downregulation of downstream NF-κB, p-GSK-3β, p-BAD. Synergism when pretreated with tangeretin for 24h (CI 0.5-0.7), additivity when posttreated with tangeretin (CI 1-1.1)	[81]
CDDP, 30 µM	Wogonin, 10 µM	HL-60 human **leukemia** cell line	?	No effect on CDDP-induced apoptosis	[154]
CDDP, 30 µM	Wogonin, 10 µM	Jurkat human **leukemia** cell line	?	No effect on CDDP-induced apoptosis	[154]
CDDP, 5, 7.5, 10 µM	Wogonin, 30 µM	AMC-HN4-cisR human **head and neck** cancer cell line, CDDP-resistant	↑	Increase in CDDP-induced cytotoxicity. Targeting Nrf2-mediated oxidative stress response, increase in apoptosis via Bax, PUMA and PARP cleavage (activation of caspase, decrease in ΔΨm)	[68]
CDDP, 5, 10, 15 µM	Wogonin, 30 µM	AMC-HN9-cisR human **head and neck** cancer cell line, CDDP-resistant	↑	Increase in CDDP-induced cytotoxicity	[68]
CDDP, 25, 50, 100 µg/ml	Wogonin, 20, 40, 60 µM	HepG2 human **hepatocellular** carcinoma cell line, wild-type p53	↑	Potentiation of CDDP-induced cytotoxicity. suppression of Nrf2	[152]
CDDP, 5, 7.5, 10 µM	Wogonin, 5, 10, 20 µM	A549 human non-small cell **lung** cancer cell line	↑	Increase in CDDP-induced cytotoxicity and apoptosis (activation of caspase-3, PARP cleavage), potentiation of H_2O_2 accumulation	[72]
CDDP	Wogonin	A549 human **lung** cancer cell line	?	No effect on CDDP-induced cytotoxicity	[153]
CDDP, 120 µM	Wogonin, 30 µM	OVCAR-3 human **ovarian** cancer cell line, CDDP-resistant	?	No effect on cell viability	[112]
CDDP	Wogonin	BGC-823 human **gastric** cancer cell line	↑	Synergism in cell growth inhibition (CI<1), increase in apoptosis	[155]
CDDP	Wogonin	HGC-27 human **gastric** cancer cell line	↑	Synergism in cell growth inhibition, increase in apoptosis	[155]
CDDP	Wogonin	MGC-803 human **gastric** cancer cell line	↑	Synergism in cell growth inhibition (CI<1), increase in apoptosis	[155]

Drug	Flavonoid	Biological system	Direction of combination	Effects	Ref.
CDDP	Wogonin	MKN-45 human **gastric** cancer cell line	↑	Synergism in cell growth inhibition, increase in apoptosis	[155]
CDDP, 5, 7.5, 10 μM	Wogonin, 5, 10, 20 μM	HeLa human **cervical** cancer cell line	↑	Increase in CDDP-induced cytotoxicity and apoptosis (activation of caspase-3, PARP cleavage), potentiation of H_2O_2 accumulation	[72]

ABC, ATP-binding cassette; AIF, apoptosis-inducing factor; Akt, protein kinase B; Apaf-1, apoptotic protease activating factor 1; ARE, antioxidant responsive element; ATM, ataxia telangiectasia mutated; ATR, ATM and Rad3-related; AVO, acidic vesicular organelle; Bad, Bcl-2-associated death promoter; Bak, Bcl-2 homologous antagonist/killer; Bax, Bcl-2-associated X protein; Bcl-2, B-cell lymphoma 2; Bcl-xl, B-cell lymphoma-extra large; Bid, BH3 interacting-domain death agonist; BOK, Bcl-2 related ovarian killer; BRCA, breast cancer gene; Cdk, cyclin-dependent kinase; CDKN1A, cyclin dependent kinase inhibitor 1A; Chk, checkpoint kinase; CI, combination index; CNT, CNT carbon nanotubes; CSC, cancer stem cell; CTR1, copper transporter 1; Cx, connexin; CYP, cytochrome P450; cyt c, cytochrome c; DHC, dihydroxychalcone; DNMT, DNA methyltransferase; DR, death receptor; DRSP, drug-resistant sphere; EBS, estrogen binding sites; EBV, Epstein-Barr Virus; EGFR, epidermal growth factor receptor; EMT, epithelial-mesenchymal transition; ER, estrogen receptor; ERK, extracellular signal-regulated kinase; ERS, endoplasmic reticulum stress; FANCD2, Fanconi anemia group D2; FasL, Fas ligand; Fox, Forkhead box; GJ, gap junction; GJIC, GJ intercellular communication; GLUT, glucose transporter; GRP, glucose-regulated protein; GSH, glutathione; GSK, glycogen synthase kinase; GST, glutathione S-transferase; HDAC, histone deacetylase; HDGF, hepatoma-derived growth factor; HER2 (erbB2), human epidermal growth factor receptor 2; HPV, human papillomavirus; Hsp, heat shock protein; IL, interleukin; JNK, c-Jun N-terminal kinase; MAPK, mitogen-activated protein kinase; MARK2, microtubule affinity-regulating kinase 2; MC, methoxychalcone; MET, mesenchymal-epithelial transition; miR, microRNA; MMP, matrix metalloproteinase; MnSOD, manganese superoxide dismutase; MRP, multidrug resistance-associated protein; NEAT, nuclear enriched abundant transcript; NF-κB, nuclear factor-κB; NP, nanoparticle; Nrf2, nuclear factor (erythroid-derived 2)-like 2; PARP, poly (ADP-ribose) polymerase; P-gp, P-glycoprotein; PGMRC1, progesterone receptor membrane component 1; PI3K, phosphoinositide 3-kinase; PLGA, poly(lactic-co-glycolic acid); PMAA, PMAA polymethacrylic acid; PMF, pentamethoxyflavone; PR, progesterone receptor; Pt, platinum; PTEN, phosphatase and tensin homolog; PUMA, p53 upregulated modulator of apoptosis; ROS, reactive oxygen species; STAT3, signal transducer and activator of transcription 3; tBid, truncated Bid; TN, triple negative; TNF-α, tumor necrosis factor-α; ΔΨm, ΔΨm mitochondrial membrane potential.

Table 6.7. Effects of flavonoids on anticancer action of cisplatin (CDDP) *in vivo* conditions

Drug	Flavonoid	Biological system	Direction of combination	Effects	Ref.
CDDP, 2 mg/kg, weekly for 4 weeks	Alpinetin, 50 mg/kg, weekly for 4 weeks	A549/CDDP human **lung** cancer cells injected s.c. into the right groin area of 5-6w old male nude mice	↑	Sensitization to CDDP treatment, decrease in tumor sizes and weight	[160]
CDDP, 2 mg/kg, i.v., 3 doses at 3-days intervals from 3 days after inoculation	Apigenin, 25 mg/kg, i.p., daily	B16-BL6 murine **melanoma** cells injected i.m. into the gastrocnemius muscle of 6-8w old female C57BL/6N mice	↑	Increase in CDDP-induced inhibition on tumor growth	[104]
CDDP, 5 mg/kg, i.p., every 3 days for 4 weeks	Avicularin, 5 mg/kg, i.p., daily for 4 weeks	SGC-7901/DDP human **gastric** cancer cells injected s.c. into the right flank of 6-8w old male nude mice	↑	Sensitization to CDDP treatment, decrease in tumor volume and weight. Induction of apoptosis (increase in Bax, BOK, cleaved caspase-3 and PARP), decrease in Ki-67	[56]
CDDP, 3 mg/kg, twice weekly	Baicalein, 3 mg/kg, i.p., daily	A549 human **lung** cancer cells (stably expressing firefly, A549-luc) implanted into the left armpit of 4-6w old female nude BALB/c mice	↑	Decrease in average radiance, decrease in tumor weight	[149]
CDDP, 5 mg/kg, i.p., every other day for 3 weeks	Baicalein, 5 mg/kg, i.p., daily	A549/CDDP human **lung** cancer cells injected s.c. into the right armpit of 4-6w old male BALB/c-nu mice	↑	Sensitization to CDDP treatment, reduction of tumor growth, decrease in tumor volume	[150]
CDDP, 2 mg/kg, i.p., every 2 days for 3 weeks	Butein, 2 mg/kg, i.p., every 2 days for 3 weeks	HeLa human **cervical** cancer cells injected s.c. into the flanks of 6-7w old female nude mice	↑	Suppression of tumor growth, decrease in tumor volume. Increase in FoxO3a expression	[168]
CDDP, 100 mg/kg, in dual multilayer NPs, thrice a week	Chrysin, 100 mg/kg, in dual multilayer NPs, thrice a week	DMBA-induced **oral** tumors in 8-10w old male golden Syrian hamsters	↑	Decrease in tumor incidence and burden, regression of tumor volume	[148]
CDDP, 10 µg/mouse, i.p., on days 1, 7, 14	EGCG, 20 µg/mouse, for 15 days, encapsulated in PLGA-NPs	EAC murine **mammary** adenocarcinoma cells injected i.p. into Swiss albino mice	↑	Increase in CDDP antitumor potential, decrease in tumor volume. Prolongation of %ILS, increase in mean survival time	[116]
CDDP, 5 mg/kg, on days 0, 5 and 11	EGCG, 100 mg/kg, on days 0, 5 and 11	MDA-MB231 human **breast** cancer cells implanted in the left and right flanks of mice	↑	Increase in CDDP-induced tumor growth reduction	[120]
CDDP, 10 µM, pretreatment before inoculation	EGCG, 5 µM, pretreatment before inoculation	Pretreated CSCs from **head and neck** cancer injected s.c. into the flank of 8w old female BALB/c nude mice	↑	Inhibition of tumor formation, increase in apoptotic cells	[123]
CDDP, i.p., as single dose	EGCG, i.p., daily	A549 human **lung** cancer cells injected s.c. into the right hind limb of 5-7w old female BALB/c nude mice	↑	Increase in CDDP-induced growth inhibition, decrease in tumor volume. Rebalancing of Ang-1/Ang-2 levels, affecting angiogenesis, IFP and oxygenation	[115]

Drug	Flavonoid	Biological system	Direction of combination	Effects	Ref.
CDDP, 5 mg/kg, i.p., every three days	EGCG, 20 mg/kg, i.p., every three days	A549 human **lung** cancer cells injected s.c. in the front dorsum of 4-5w old female BALB/c nude mice	↑	Sensitization to CDDP treatment. Repression of Ki-67, stimulation of CTR1 expression via NEAT1/hsa-mir-98-5p axis; promotion of CDDP absorption in tumor tissues	[79]
CDDP, 5 mg/kg, i.p., twice a week for 2 weeks	EGCG, 20 mg/kg, i.p., twice a week for 2 weeks, day before CDDP	A549 human **lung** cancer cells injected into the dorsal of 4w old female BALB/c nude mice	↑	Increase in CDDP-induced growth inhibition, decrease in tumor size. Decrease in hsa-miR-98-5p in tumors	[75]
CDDP, 2.5 mg/kg, i.p., twice a week	EGCG, 10 mg/kg, i.p., on days 1-3	A549/DDP human **lung** cancer cells inoculated s.c. into the right flank of BALB/c nu/nu mice	↑	Reversal of resistance to CDDP, inhibition of tumor growth. Demethylation of GAS1, TIMP4, ICAM1 and WISP2 genes, restoration of their expression	[114]
CDDP, 2 mg/kg, i.v., 3 doses at 3-days intervals from 3 days after inoculation	EGCG, i.p., daily	B16-FL6 murine **melanoma** cells injected i.m. into the gastrocnemius muscle of 6-8w old female C57BL/6N mice	↑	Increase in CDDP-induced inhibition of tumor growth	[104]
CDDP, 5 mg/kg, i.p., once a week	EGCG, 20 mg/kg, i.p., twice a week	OVCAR3 human **ovarian** cancer cells injected s.c. into the dorsum of 3-5w old female BALB/c nude mice	↑	Increase in CDDP-induced tumor growth repression. Increase in CTR1 expression, inhibition of CDDP-induced CTR1 degradation	[70]
CDDP, 1.5 mg/kg, i.p., for 10 days	Fisetin, 1 mg/kg, i.p., for 10 days	NT2/D1 human **teratocarcinoma** cells implanted into 6w old athymic nude mice	↑	Increase in CDDP-induced tumor regression and apoptosis (TUNEL positive cells), decrease in tumor size	[106]
CDDP, 5 mg/kg, i.p., 2-days intervals for 4 weeks	Galangin, 10 mg/kg, i.p., 2-days intervals for 4 weeks	A549/DDP human **lung** cancer cells injected s.c. into the right oxter of 5w old male athymic nude mice	↑	Suppression of tumor growth. Reduction of p-STAT3-, p-NF-κB- and bcl-2-positive cells in tumor sections, cleavage of caspase-3 and PARP	[61]
CDDP, 2 mg/kg, i.p., daily for 7 days from 3 days after hepatectomy	Genistein, 2 mg/kg, i.p., daily for 4 weeks from 3 days after hepatectomy	HCCLM3 human **hepatocellular** carcinoma cells injected s.c. in axilla area of 4-6w old BALB/c nu/nu mice, implantation of tumor pieces into single lobe of other mice, curative hepatectomy after 10 days	↑	Reinforcing of CDDP-induced inhibition on tumor recurrence and pulmonary metastasis after curative hepatectomy, decrease in volume of recurrent foci. Abolishment of CDDP-upregulated MMP-2 expression	[133]
CDDP, 5 mg/kg, on day one	Genistein, 500 µg/kg, on days 1-5	A549 human **lung** cancer cells injected i.p. into the 4-5w old female BALB/c nude mice	↑	Inhibition of tumor growth, decrease in tumor weight and volume	[125]
CDDP, 5 mg/kg, i.p., daily for 15 days	Licochalcone A, 1 mg/kg, oral gavage, daily for 15 days	CT-26 murine colon cancer cells injected s.c. into the right flanks of 5w old Balb/c male mice	~	No effect on CDDP-induced therapeutic efficacy	[63]

Table 6.7. (Continued)

Drug	Flavonoid	Biological system	Direction of combination	Effects	Ref.
CDDP, 1.5 mg/kg, i.p., once every 3 days	Liquiritigenin, 5, 10 or 20 mg/kg, i.g., daily	B16F10 murine **melanoma** cells injected into the tail vein of 6-8w old female C57BL/6 black mice	↑	Increase in CDDP-induced antitumor action, suppression of lung metastasis. Downregulation of MMP-2/-9, PI3K, p-Akt; upregulation of PTEN	[159]
CDDP, 1.25 mg/kg, i.p., thrice weekly	Luteolin, 40 mg/kg, i.p., thrice weekly	HCT116 human **colorectal** cancer cells inoculated s.c. in the two sides of flanks of 5-6w old female BALB/c nude mice	↑	Increase in CDDP therapeutic activity, decrease in tumor weight. Upregulation of p53 protein	[142]
CDDP, 3 mg/kg, i.p., daily	Luteolin, 10, 20 or 40 mg/kg, by gavage, daily for 5 days	CAOV3/DDP human **ovarian** cancer cells inoculated s.c. into 5-6w old female BALB/c nude mice	↑	Increase in CDDP-induced growth reduction, decrease in tumor volume and weight. Increase in apoptosis	[80]
CDDP, 2 mg/kg, i.p., every 4 days	Protoapigenone, 0.2 mg/kg, i.p., every 4 days	MDA-MB-231 human **breast** cancer cells injected s.c. into the right flank of female nude BALB/cAnN-Foxn1nu/Crl Narl mice	~	No effect on sensitivity to CDDP	[158]
CDDP, 7.5 mg/kg, i.p., 3 doses at 12th, 16th, 20th week	Quercetin, 50 mg/kg, i.p., daily, before a week of DMH exposure	**Colon** cancer induced by s.c. injection of DMH to male Sprague-Dawley rats	↑	Improvement of CDDP anticancer activity, decrease in the number of ACF	[64]
CDDP, 3 mg/kg, i.p., on days 1, 4, 7	Quercetin, 20 mg/kg, i.p., on days 1, 4, 7	LXFL 529 human large-cell **lung** carcinoma cells implanted s.c. into both flanks of athymic nude NMRI mice	↑	Increase in CDDP-induced tumor growth reduction	[103]
CDDP, 2 mg/kg, i.v., 3 doses at 3-days intervals from 3 days after inoculation	Quercetin, i.p., daily	B16-BL6 murine **melanoma** cells injected i.m. into the gastrocnemius muscle of 6-8w old female C57BL/6N mice	↑	Increase in CDDP-induced inhibition on tumor growth	[104]
CDDP	Quercetin	DRSPs from SCC25 human **oral** cancer cells injected s.c. into 6w old male BALB/c nude mice	↑	Attenuation of DRSPs tumorigenicity, increase in CDDP-induced tumor growth inhibition. Downregulation of p-Hsp27, reversal of EMT phenomenon (decrease in vimentin, Twist-1, fascin-1; increase in E-cadherin)	[74]
CDDP, 4 mg/kg, i.p., every 4 days	Quercetin, 20 mg/kg, i.p., daily	C13* human **ovarian** cancer cells injected s.c. into the flanks of 4-6w old athymic BALB/c-nu nude mice	↓	Reduction of CDDP therapeutic efficacy, promotion of cancer growth, increase in tumor sizes and weight. Enhancement of SOD1 expression, prevention of ROS-induced damage	[95]

Drug	Flavonoid	Biological system	Direction of combination	Effects	Ref.
CDDP, 3 mg/kg, i.p., weekly, one day after quercetin	Quercetin, 40 mg/kg, i.p., weekly	C13* human **ovarian** cancer cells injected s.c. into the right supra scapula region of 4-6w old female nude athymic BALB/c-nu mice	↑	Increase in CDDP-induced antitumor effect, decrease in tumor growth. Increase in ERS marker proteins (GRP78, CHOP), repression of STAT3 phosphorylation, lowering of BCL-2 and elevation of apoptosis	[44]
CDDP, 2 mg/kg, i.p., twice weekly	Silibinin, 25 mg/kg, oral, daily	KYSE270 human **esophageal** cancer cells injected s.c. into the left flank of 6-8w old nude mice	↑	Synergism in tumor size decrease (CI 0.273)	[65]
CDDP, 4 mg/kg, i.p., for 3 doses or 1.5 mg/kg for 4 doses	Silipide, 450 mg/kg, p.o., for 3 or 4 doses	A2780 human **ovarian** cancer cells injected s.c. in the right flank of female athymic nude HSD mice	↑	Potentiation of CDDP-induced antitumor activity	[165]
CDDP, 5 mg/kg, i.p., weekly	Wogonin, 50 mg/kg, i.p., daily	AMC-HN4-cisR human **head and neck** cancer cells injected s.c. into the flank of 6w old athymic BALB/c male nude mice	↑	Increase in CDDP-induced growth suppression, decrease in tumor volume and weight. Promotion of apoptosis (increase in cPARP, PUMA, pp53), decrease in Nrf2 expression	[68]
CDDP, 5 mg/kg, i.p., weekly	Wogonin, 50 mg/kg, i.p., daily	AMC-HN9-cisR human **head and neck** cancer cells injected s.c. into the flank of 6w old athymic BALB/c male nude mice	↑	Increase in CDDP-induced growth suppression, decrease in tumor volume and weight; increase in apoptosis	[68]

ACF, aberrant crypt foci; Akt, protein kinase B; Ang, angiopoietin; Bax, Bcl-2-associated X protein; Bcl-2, B-cell lymphoma 2; BOK, Bcl-2 related ovarian killer; CHOP, CCAAT/enhancer binding protein homologues protein; CI, combination index; CTR1, copper transporter 1; DMBA, 7,12-dimethylbenz[a] anthracene; DMH, 1,2-dimethyl hydrazine; DRSP, drug-resistant sphere; EAC, Ehrlich ascites carcinoma; EMT, epithelial-mesenchymal transition; ERS, endoplasmic reticulum stress; Fox, Forkhead box; GRP, glucose-regulated protein; Hsp, heat shock protein; IFP, interstitial fluid pressure; ILS, increase in the life span; miR, microRNA; MMP, matrix metalloproteinase; NEAT, nuclear enriched abundant transcript; NF-κB, nuclear factor-κB; Nrf2, nuclear factor (erythroid-derived 2)-like 2; PARP, poly (ADP-ribose) polymerase; PI3K, phosphoinositide 3-kinase; PTEN, phosphatase and tensin homolog; PUMA, p53 upregulated modulator of apoptosis; SOD, superoxide dismutase; STAT3, signal transducer and activator of transcription 3; TUNEL, terminal deoxynucleotidyl transferase dUTP nick end labeling.

administered with DNA-damaging chemotherapeutic drug and enhanced the sensitivity of cells to CDDP [87]. In another TNBC cell line, MDA-MB-468, quercetin reversed CDDP resistance by suppressing overexpression of cytochrome P450 1B1 (CYP1B1) enzyme [88]. Moreover, cotreatment of Walker rat breast carcinoma cells with quercetin and CDDP led to a synergistic antiproliferative effect [89]. Simultaneous treatment with quercetin and CDDP resulted in a synergistic suppression of proliferation also in human primary endometrial and ovarian tumor cells, with a CDDP potentiation ranging from 1.5- to 30-fold [90]. Significant increase in anticancer efficacy of CDDP by addition of quercetin was detected also in several human ovarian cancer cell lines. In A2780 and its CDDP-resistant subline A2780cisR, the greatest synergism was observed when flavonol was added 2 hours before chemotherapeutic drug; the intracellular drug accumulation and drug-DNA binding level were also highest with this sequence regimen [43]. Quercetin sensitized also OVCA 433 cells to CDDP and augmented the inhibitory effect on cell growth [91]. In CAOV3, OVCAR-8 and SKOV-3 lines, pretreatment with quercetin significantly suppressed the viability of CDDP-treated cells and enhanced cytotoxic response [92, 93]. In CDDP-resistant 2008 cells (C13*) and primary ovarian cancer cells P-ris, 12 hours pretreatment with quercetin significantly enhanced CDDP cytotoxicity by promoting endoplasmic reticulum stress (ERS) and lowering the threshold of mitochondrial apoptosis pathway. In addition, pre-administration of quercetin followed by drug intervention potentiated the antitumor effect of CDDP also in nude mice bearing C13* ovarian cancer xenografts leading to higher apoptosis levels and decrease in tumor growth [44]. Although simultaneous treatment with quercetin increased the sensitivity of A2780P and OVCAR-3 ovarian cancer cells to CDDP, with this regimen, this phytochemical did not affect the efficacy of CDDP in EFO27 and SKOV3 human ovarian cancer cells [94]. Moreover, cotreatment of C13* and SKOV3 cells with CDDP and low concentrations of quercetin (5-30 μM) was even shown to attenuate the cytotoxicity and proapoptotic activity of CDDP via reduced production of intracellular ROS level, upregulation of endogenous antioxidant enzymes and inhibition of ROS-induced injury, resulting in increased resistance to CDDP. Such antagonistic effect was confirmed also in xenogeneic model of C13* bearing mice, where combined treatment with quercetin and CDDP prevented ROS-induced oxidative damage, reduced therapeutic efficacy of CDDP and promoted ovarian cancer progression [95]. Although there are some controversies about the role of quercetin on CDDP efficacy in preclinical models of ovarian cancer, the current data point to the possibility that pretreatment of ovarian cancer cells with quercetin might be beneficial in potentiating the therapeutic efficacy of CDDP against ovarian tumors. Because acquired resistance to CDDP is one of the major causes of mortality of ovarian cancer patients [93], these observations can be particularly interesting from the clinical point of view. However, simultaneous addition of quercetin and CDDP may lead to antagonistic effect suggesting that supplementation of this phytochemical in ovarian cancer patients during CDDP chemotherapy certainly needs caution [95]. In another type of gynecological tumors, human cervical carcinoma cell line HeLa, the extent of apoptotic response depended on the succession of quercetin and cisplatin, as preincubation of cells with quercetin followed by chemotherapeutic drug exerted the most efficient cell death correlated with inhibition of Hsp72 and MRPs expression [96]. In drug-resistant spheres (DRSPs) from human tongue cancer cell line SCC25, quercetin combined with CDDP suppressed the overexpression of phosphorylated Hsp27, altered epithelial-mesenchymal transition (EMT) signature and promoted apoptosis, resulting in sensitization of cells to CDDP treatment. Quercetin attenuated tumorigenicity of DRSPs also in xenogeneic mouse model leading to potentiation of CDDP-induced tumor growth inhibition and decrease in drug resistance [74]. In human laryngeal HeP2 cells, quercetin and CDDP were shown to act by separate pathways which interact synergistically leading to enhanced apoptotic cell death [97, 98]. Synergistic enhancement of CDDP-induced cytotoxicity in combination with quercetin was detected also in human nasopharyngeal carcinoma cell lines C666-1 and HK1, irrespective of the expression of Epstein-Barr virus (EBV) in these tumor tissues [82]. In human lung cancer cell lines A549 and H-520 (non-small cell lung cancer) and SW1271 (small cell lung cancer), combined use of quercetin and CDDP led to an augmentation of chemotherapeutic efficacy promoting antiproliferative activity and apoptotic dell death [99, 100]. Quercetin also enhanced the sensitivity of human hepatocellular carcinoma HepG2 cells, neuroblastoma IMR-32 cells, malignant mesothelioma SPC212 cells and human osteosarcoma 143B cells to CDDP as compared to single agent treatments [47, 76, 101, 102]. In 143B cells, quercetin upregulated a tumor suppressor miR-217 expression and promoted apoptotic cell death, suggesting that co-administration of CDDP and quercetin might improve the treatment of osteosarcoma [102] (Table 6.6). Several animal studies also confirmed the chemosensitizing properties of quercetin towards CDDP treatment. In 1,2-dimethyl hydrazine (DMH) hydrochloride-induced colon cancer in rats, quercetin enhanced antitumor activity of CDDP by reducing the multiplicity of colon carcinoma precursors (aberrant crypt foci) compared to treatment with both agents alone, besides amelioration of nephrotoxicity [64]. In addition, quercetin enhanced the activity of CDDP also against lung tumor in established human lung carcinoma LXFL 529 cells bearing mice resulting in reduced tumor growth [103]. In murine melanoma B16-BL6 cells implanted into mice, quercetin significantly increased the inhibitory action of CDDP on melanoma growth [104] (Table 6.7).

Thus, quercetin can act as a good chemoadjuvant along with CDDP, depending on the tumor type, treatment regimen and dosages. The above-described results indicate complexity of modulation of CDDP efficacy by quercetin, due to involvement of multiple signaling pathways and mechanisms associated with drug resistance. Pleiotropic action of quercetin might be of therapeutic benefit and its inclusion may improve the prognosis of patients treated with CDDP. However, simultaneous administration of quercetin and CDDP may still be contraindicated leading to increase in the survival of ovarian cancer

180   *Katrin Sak*

cells and aggravation of drug resistance, needing a special attention by ovarian tumor patients who decide to consume plant-based dietary supplements on a voluntary basis.

Although the effects of other natural flavonols on chemotherapeutic activity of CDDP have been studied considerably less than interactions with quercetin, the data show that chemomodulation of malignant cells to CDDP can probably involve targeting of multiple signaling pathways that are critical for cancer cell survival. *Fisetin* increased CDDP-induced cytotoxicity and decreased cell growth of TN breast cancer lines MDA-MB-231 and MDA-MB-468, suggesting that consumption of food items rich in fisetin might be beneficial to breast cancer patients who receive CDDP treatment [5, 87]. Combined treatment of CDDP-resistant human lung cancer A549-CR cells with fisetin and CDDP led to enhanced apoptotic response and reversal of acquired drug resistance that was possibly, at least partly, mediated by suppression of aberrant activation of MAPK signaling pathways and downregulation of survivin protein [59]. Fisetin potentiated CDDP-induced cytotoxicity also in another human lung adenocarcinoma cell line H1299 [105]. In human embryonal carcinoma NT2/D1 cells, presence of fisetin in CDDP chemotherapy increased cytotoxic response inducing both intrinsic and extrinsic apoptosis, enhanced tumor suppressor protein p53 and its downstream target p21, and decreased survivin and cyclin B1 expression. Similarly, in NT2/D1 mouse xenograft model, combined treatment resulted in potentiation of tumor regression. Such combination therapy can obviously reduce effective treatment doses of CDDP as compared to monotherapy and thereby limit toxic side effects of this most widely used chemotherapeutic agent [106] (Table 6.6 and Table 6.7). Combination of flavonol *isorhamnetin* and CDDP led to a greater effect in cell cycle arrest at G2/M phase, suppression of cancer cell growth and invasion, and inducing of mitochondrial apoptosis compared to single drug treatment in human lung cancer A549 cells [107] (Table 6.6). Flavonol *myricetin* and CDDP augmented each other in inducing growth inhibition and apoptosis in human cervical cancer HeLa cells. Combined treatment also enhanced the number of cancer cells in G0/G1 phase [67]. Myricetin sensitized also another human papillomavirus (HPV)-positive cervical cancer cell line SiHa to CDDP-induced cytotoxic activity, while this dietary phytochemical did not affect CDDP efficacy in HPV-negative cervical cancer cells. Myricetin restored the missing signaling components in both intrinsic (p53) and extrinsic apoptotic cascades (caspase-8 and Fas-associated death domain) by destabilizing and/or disturbing the functions of respective virus protein [108]. As current therapies to treat HPV-associated malignancies are rather limited and cervical cancer tends to be relatively resistant to conventional anticancer drugs, myricetin combination with CDDP may provide a potential clinical chemotherapeutic approach for management of cervical cancer in the future (Table 6.6). The presence of another flavonol *galangin* promoted the ability of CDDP to induce growth inhibition and apoptosis in human lung cancer cell lines A549 and SPC-A1 as well as their CDDP-resistant sublines A549/DDP and SPC-A1/DDP. Cotreatment with galangin and CDDP inactivated NF-κB pathway which was associated with STAT3 phosphorylation. Similarly, in mice xenograft model of A549/DDP cells, the combined treatment augmented tumor growth inhibition compared to CDDP monotherapy, showing that galangin in combination with CDDP is of therapeutic value to treat human lung tumors resistant to CDDP [61]. However, preincubation of human promyelocytic leukemia HL-60 cells and murine leukemia L1210 cells with galangin followed by addition of CDDP 40 min later led to a suppression of drug cytotoxicity and reduction of apoptotic cell death, suggesting that galangin might exert negative effect on CDDP-induced therapeutic activity [84, 86]. At that, posttreatment of HL-60 cells with galangin did not significantly affect the efficacy of chemotherapeutic drug [86] (Table 6.6 and Table 6.7). Antagonistic action on CDDP chemotherapeutic efficacy was observed also in the case of dietary component, flavonol *kaempferol*, that significantly reduced the cytotoxicity of CDDP in human glioblastoma cell line T98G. Multidrug resistance (MDR) phenomenon of these cells is associated with overexpression of MRPs, whereas chronic exposure to kaempferol decreased MRP2 protein while oppositely increasing MRP1 and glutathione S-transferase (GST) level. Reduction of CDDP cytotoxicity is probably associated with increased metabolization of CDDP by GST and with efflux of respective conjugates by MRP1 from the glioma cells [109]. On the contrary, in CDDP-resistant human ovarian cancer OVCAR-3 cells, combined treatment of kaempferol and CDDP suppressed MRP6 and cMyc expression, prevented the removal of drug from the cells leading to significant cooperative interaction in inducing apoptosis and inhibiting ovarian cancer cell viability. Thus, kaempferol deserves further investigation for possible application in combined chemotherapeutic regimens for treatment of CDDP-resistant ovarian tumors [110] (Table 6.6). This situation is in turn different from the behavior of flavonol *morin* in human ovarian cancer cells that exerted dose- and schedule-dependent action in CDDP-resistant SKOV-3 and CDDP-sensitive TOV-21G cells. At low doses of morin, simultaneous treatment with CDDP led to additive to synergistic cytotoxicity, while combination with high doses of morin and high doses of CDDP resulted in antagonistic outcome in SKOV-3 cells. Antagonistic response revealed also in preincubation of ovarian cancer cells with morin for 24 hours, followed by treatment with high doses of CDDP. In TOV-21G cells, antagonistic effects appeared, when high CDDP doses were simultaneously combined with morin or when cells were pretreated with morin before subsequent coincubation with both agents [71] (Table 6.6). In SKOV-3 line, flavonol sugar conjugate, *hyperoside* or quercetin 3-galactoside, sensitized ovarian cancer cells to CDDP treatment. Resistance to CDDP can be partially related to drug induced overexpression of progesterone receptor membrane component (PGRMC)1 in ovarian cancer cells that promotes autophagy, activates CYP enzymes, accelerates drug efflux and enhances cell survival and invasion, thereby reducing the effect of drug treatment. Combination of CDDP and hyperoside blocked cell proliferation, induced autophagy and subsequently evoked mitochondrial apoptotic cell death. Thus, hyperoside functioned as a complementary agent for treatment of ovarian cancer patients with CDDP chemotherapy [111] (Table 6.6). Human ovarian cancer cells OVCAR-3 were sensitized to CDDP treatment also by another glycosidic quercetin derivative, *spiraeoside* or quercetin 4`-glucoside, significantly reducing cell viability with combined treatment [112] (Table 6.6). However, quercetin sugar conjugate *rutin* or quercetin 3-rutinoside did not affect the CDDP cytotoxic action in either human ovarian cancer cell line OVCA 433 or primary malignant ovarian and endometrial cells [90] (Table 6.6). *Avicularin* or quercetin 3-arabinofuranoside markedly sensitized drug-resistant human gastric cancer SGC-7901/DDP cells to CDDP cytotoxicity, decreased tumor cell proliferation and enhanced apoptosis. Moreover, this combination also led to reduced tumor growth in SGC-7901/DDP bearing mice, suggesting a novel combinational therapeutic approach for treatment of patients suffering from drug-resistant stomach cancer [56] (Table 6.6 and Table 6.7).

Thus, the inclusion of structurally different flavonols and their glycosides in CDDP chemotherapeutic regimens can lead to completely different results, whereas besides sensitization of various cancer cells to CDDP treatment also opposite effects have been described, requiring great caution in consumption of flavonol-rich dietary supplements or food items during administration of CDDP in clinical settings.

Among flavanols (catechins), epigallocatechin 3-gallate (EGCG) as the major polyphenol in green tea, has been most often studied in combination with CDDP against various tumor types (Table 6.6 and Table 6.7). *EGCG* significantly increased CDDP-induced cytotoxicity in human lung cancer cell line A549 by inducing mitochondrial apoptotic pathway [113]. The chemosensitizing potential of EGCG to CDDP therapy was associated with abrogation of the hepatoma-derived growth factor (HDGF). HDGF is often overexpressed in several tumor types being related to increased migration, invasion, survival and resistance of malignant cells to therapy and representing an important prognostic marker that correlates with advanced stages and poor outcome in liver and esophageal cancers. Thus, decrease in this growth factor can serve as a novel strategy to improve clinical management of lung adenocarcinoma, and cotreatment with EGCG and CDDP might provide an attractive therapeutic combination [113]. In CDDP-resistant A549 cells, A549/DDP, combined treatment with EGCG and CDDP resulted in inhibition of cancer cell proliferation, cell cycle arrest in G1 phase, enhanced apoptosis and thereby reversal of drug resistance. These effects were accompanied by suppression of activities of DNA methyltransferase (DNMT) and histone deacetylase (HDAC) and restoration of expression of several methylation-silenced key genes, targeting thus the cancer epigenome. Moreover, combined treatment with EGCG and CDDP reversed drug resistance also in the respective *in vivo* model, leading to inhibition of xenograft tumor growth in nude mice [114]. Furthermore, EGCG treatment also decreased microvessel density (MVD) and angiopoietin (Ang)-2 levels and improved oxygenation in tumor tissue of A549 bearing mice, modifying microvasculature and microenvironment and leading to suppression of tumor growth when combined with CDDP [115]. To overcome bioavailability issues related to oral administration of flavonoids, combination of nanoencapsulated EGCG and CDDP has been investigated. Encapsulating EGCG in biodegradable poly(lactide-co-glycolic acid) (PLGA) nanoparticles increased antitumor potential of CDDP in A549 cells, whereas this chemosensitizing effect was superior compared to bulk EGCG. Such combined treatment inhibited NF-κB activation and suppressed expression of its downstream target genes involved in proliferation, angiogenesis and metastasis; also, generation of ROS was increased and apoptotic response was augmented [116, 117]. In addition, EGCG upregulated and affected intracellular localization of copper transporter 1 (CTR1) that transports CDDP, thereby increasing drug accumulation and DNA-platinum adduct levels in several human lung cancer cells, such as H1299, H460, A549 and its CDDP-resistant subline A549/DDP [79]. CTR1 is an important regulator of the efficacy of platinum drugs and its overexpression can sensitize cells to CDDP by increasing drug uptake. Moreover, EGCG stimulated CTR1 expression and drug absorption also in tumor tissues of A549 bearing mice. As a result, CDDP-induced cell growth inhibition and apoptotic death were promoted by EGCG both *in vitro* and *in vivo*, suggesting that EGCG could be considered as an effective adjuvant agent to combat CDDP resistance in treatment of some types of non-small cell lung tumors. CTR1 was shown to be directly regulated by hsa-miR-98-5p/NEAT1 axis [79]. EGCG-induced silencing of hsa-miR-98-5p increased p53 and led to enhanced CDDP efficacy in A549 and LTEP-α-2 cells as well as A549 bearing mice; but still not in NCI-H460 cells, where EGCG attenuated the chemotherapeutic efficacy of CDDP and promoted cellular proliferation. In NCI-H460 cells, hsa-miR-98-5p was upregulated by EGCG, suggesting that hsa-miR-98-5p might be a potential target for CDDP therapy and highlighting the possibility of antagonistic interaction between EGCG and CDDP in treatment of certain types of non-small cell lung cancer [75]. Such controversial results certainly need further preclinical investigations but also warn lung cancer patients against intake of EGCG-containing dietary supplements on their own during the active treatment phase with CDDP. Somewhat contrary results have been demonstrated also for other types of malignancies cotreated with EGCG and CDDP. In the case of ovarian cancer, the trend of combinational treatment of EGCG and CDDP depended on sequence of addition of these agents. In human ovarian cancer cell line A2780 and its CDDP-resistant sublines A2780cisR and A2780ZD0473R, preincubation of cells with EGCG followed by treatment with CDDP led to antagonistic responses and this attenuation of drug cytotoxicity could be related to antioxidant properties of EGCG and decreased ROS levels. On the contrary, addition of CDDP before EGCG caused synergistic outcomes through augmentation of oxidative stress, greatly increased cellular drug accumulation and binding of CDDP to DNA. With this synergistic scheme cell killing effect was achieved at much lower CDDP doses as compared to monotherapy, allowing to reduce the extent of toxic side effects. Co-administration of CDDP and EGCG produced only weak synergism in both drug-sensitive and drug-resistant lines [58,

118]. Potentiation of CDDP cytotoxicity by EGCG has been observed also in other human ovarian cancer cell lines. In three lines with different degrees of CDDP sensitivity, i.e., SKOV3, relatively resistant CAOV3 and highly resistant C200 cells, addition of EGCG increased CDDP potency by three- to sixfold by accentuating oxidative stress to damage DNA and suppress the growth of ovarian cancer cells [78]. Also, in OVCAR3 and SKOV3 cell lines, EGCG inhibited CDDP-induced rapid degradation of CTR1 leading to increased cellular drug accumulation, drug-DNA adducts level and sensitivity of ovarian cancer cells to CDDP treatment. The combination of EGCG and CDDP promoted apoptotic cell death. Similarly, CTR1 expression was upregulated by EGCG also in OVCAR3 xenograft nude mice model with suppressing the tumor growth by combined treatment with CDDP, suggesting that properly administered EGCG can be an important adjuvant for CDDP chemotherapy against ovarian tumors [70]. In other gynecological tumors, human cervical cancer cells, EGCG potentiated CDDP anticancer responses, irrespective of the HPV subtype in these cells. In both HeLa (HPV18) and SiHa (HPV16) cells, the combined treatment of EGCG and CDDP enhanced cell growth inhibition and mitochondrial apoptosis by producing ROS and suppressing activation of protein kinase B (Akt) and NF-κB survival signaling; thus, potentially improving the therapeutic outcome of CDDP against cervical cancer [119]. Moreover, loading of EGCG into biodegradable PLGA-based nanoparticles further enhanced the antitumor potential of CDDP in HeLa cells as compared to bulk doses of EGCG, due to sustained and long-term delivery of nanoformulation [116, 117]. EGCG also increased CDDP-induced cytotoxicity in human TN breast cancer cells MDA-MB231 and MDA-MB231 tumor xenografts in mice resulting in greater tumor growth reduction compared to treatment with CDDP alone [120]. Also, in mice bearing murine mammary adenocarcinoma cells (Ehrlich`s ascites carcinoma, EAC), combined treatment with CDDP and nanoencapsulated EGCG decreased tumor volume and increased life span of rodents [116]. In addition, CDDP-induced apoptosis was promoted by EGCG also in human prostate cancer PC3 cells and therefore, administration of EGCG with CDDP to prostate cancer patients might represent an efficient adjuvant therapy for treatment of prostate tumors [46]. In human colorectal adenocarcinoma cell lines DLD-1 and HT-29, treatment with EGCG plus CDDP exhibited synergistic effects on inhibition of cell proliferation and induction of cell death through the autophagy related pathway [121]. However, the outcome of combined treatment of malignant biliary tract cells with combination of EGCG and CDDP showed both synergistic (BDC, GBC, TFK-1, MzChA-2 and MzChA-1 lines) as well as antagonistic effects (CCSW-1 and EGI-1 lines). These results demonstrate that the cytotoxic action of EGCG and CDDP combined treatments of gallbladder and bile duct cancers is highly dependent on molecular characteristics of tumor cells. The cellular mechanisms underlying these different activities need further studies [122]. Somewhat more data are available about the mechanism of sensitization of human head and neck squamous carcinoma cells to CDDP cytotoxicity by cotreatment with EGCG. In cancer stem cells (CSCs) isolated from a patient with head and neck squamous carcinoma, EGCG augmented CDDP-induced efficacy by inhibiting MRP2 (ABCC2) and BCRP (ABCG2) transporters, thereby reducing resistance of cells to CDDP therapy. In addition, cotreatment of EGCG and CDDP suppressed tumor formation of CSCs in a xenograft mice model. As CSCs are considered as a potential root for tumor recurrence and metastasis and are remarkably resistant to conventional chemotherapeutics, EGCG in combination with CDDP can be used for clinical management of head and neck squamous carcinomas [123]. Beneficial therapeutic outcome in combination of EGCG and CDDP was observed also in human glioma cell lines 1321N1 and U87-MG by inhibiting telomerase expression that causes shortening of telomeres to a critical length resulting in genome instability and activating apoptotic pathway; thereby tackling drug resistance phenomenon in glioma tissues [124]. In rat leiomyosarcoma cells, only preincubation with EGCG before treatment with CDDP led to an increased cytotoxicity and apoptosis, while simultaneous treatment and addition of EGCG subsequent to CDDP did not significantly alter the efficacy of CDDP alone [66]. EGCG also potentiated the inhibitory effects of CDDP in murine melanoma B16-FL6 bearing mice and suppressed melanoma growth [104]. Positive cooperation and increase in anticancer potential were observed also in human acute monocytic leukemia THP-1 cells when CDDP was combined with nanoencapsulated EGCG [116, 117] (Table 6.6 and Table 6.7).

Thus, EGCG can influence numerous targets and multiple cellular pathways in combination with CDDP, modulating both the drug transport across the cell membrane as well as the level of drug binding to DNA in various cancer types. Outcomes of such combined treatments might not be always positively cooperative, i.e., additive or synergistic, as EGCG may play opposite roles either by exhibiting antioxidant and free radical scavenging properties and protecting cancer cells against CDDP-induced death, or by increasing cytotoxic action of drug. The behavior of EGCG in combination with CDDP obviously depends on the sequenced schedule and dosage regimens, besides molecular characteristics of malignant cells. Particular caution should be exercised by patients suffering from ovarian cancer, bile duct carcinoma or non-small cell lung cancer when receiving CDDP treatment.

Only a few studies have been performed using other flavanols, i.e., catechin and epicatechin, in combination treatment with CDDP. *Catechin* augmented CDDP-induced decrease in survival of human TN breast cancer MDA-MB-231 cells and inhibited activation of DNA damage repair mechanisms when administered with platinum drug, showing a potential therapeutic benefit to breast cancer patients receiving CDDP therapy [87] (Table 6.6). *Epicatechin* synergistically inhibited cell growth and promoted CDDP-induced apoptosis in human lung adenocarcinoma cell line A549 [69] (Table 6.6) and might prove to be an adjuvant in CDDP treatments against lung cancer, if further cell culture works and animal studies will confirm this finding.

Structurally diverse isoflavones and their methylated derivatives have been studied in combination with CDDP in various types of tumor cells showing different impact on therapeutic outcome. Most on these studies have been focused on the chemomodulating action of genistein (Table 6.6 and Table 6.7). Combination of dietary *genistein* and CDDP induced significantly greater growth inhibition and enhanced apoptosis in human lung adenocarcinoma A549 cells compared to CDDP monotherapy. Such cotreatment inhibited constitutive activation of Akt and phosphoinositide 3-kinase (PI3K) conferring to augmented cytotoxic response. In addition, combined treatment increased also tumor growth suppression *in vivo* xenograft model of A549 cells in mice leading to significantly smaller tumors [125]. Enhanced growth inhibition and apoptotic cell death by combined treatment with CDDP plus EGCG were detected also in other human non-small cell lung cancer lines, such as H460 [62] and NCI-H596 [126]. The latter line strongly expresses epidermal growth factor receptor (EGFR) and as genistein is known as a tyrosine kinase inhibitor its chemosensitizing action towards CDDP treatment could be regulated by inhibition of EGFR phosphorylation in NCI-H596 cells. Indeed, efficacy of CDDP was not altered by genistein in NCI-H358 cells with only weak or undetectable expression of EGFR [126]. Thus, inclusion of genistein in CDDP treatment regimens might be a potential therapeutic approach for management of EGFR-positive non-small cell lung tumors reducing the inherent resistance of cancer cells to this platinum drug. Genistein also augmented the CDDP cytotoxicity in several human ovarian carcinoma cell lines, such as 2008 and its CDDP-resistant subline C13*, by stimulating intracellular drug accumulation through passive diffusion of plasma membrane [127]. In CDDP-sensitive A2780 cell line and its CDDP-resistant clone C200, pretreatment with genistein led to potentiation of CDDP-induced cell viability reduction and apoptosis promotion. This was accompanied by inactivation of NF-κB DNA binding activity and downregulation of several antiapoptotic survival factors [128]. Although pretreatment with genistein could overcome CDDP resistance in ovarian tumors, this action seems to depend on the phenotypic behavior of certain ovarian cancer cells. In fact, genistein reversed resistance to CDDP in 2008 C13 and CP70 cell lines but not in OVCAR 8 cells, suggesting some selectivity in chemosensitization of malignant ovarian cells by this dietary isoflavone [73]. In human breast tumors, the action of genistein on CDDP efficacy depended on the ratio of expression of two estrogen receptor (ER) subtypes, ERα and ERβ. In ERα-expressing MCF-7 cells, 1 and 10 μM genistein counteracted the antitumor efficacy of CDDP, antagonized drug-induced growth inhibitory activity, increased cellular viability and suppressed apoptosis [129]. Genistein provoked the levels of antioxidant enzymes in MCF-7 cells and thereby reduced the production of ROS, contributing at least partially to the attenuation of chemotherapeutic efficacy of CDDP [130]. However, in predominantly ERβ-expressing T47D cells, combined treatment with genistein and CDDP did not alter the antitumor activity of antineoplastic drug alone [130]. Therefore, in women diagnosed with breast tumors whose cancer cells have high ERα/ERβ ratio, the intake of genisteincontaining food products or dietary supplements may be counterproductive for chemotherapeutic treatment with CDDP. On contrary, in human prostate cancer PC-3 cells, pretreatment with genistein followed by addition of CDDP resulted in synergistic increase in antiproliferative and proapoptotic effects compared to drug alone, associated with suppression of CDDP-induced NF-κB activity [62]. Genistein pretreatment was able to chemosensitize also human gastric cancer MGC-803 cells to CDDP, inhibiting BCRP (ABCG2) expression and extracellular signal-regulated kinase (ERK) 1/2 activity [131]. In human pancreatic cancer cell line BxPC-3, pretreatment with genistein before addition of CDDP led to a synergistic antitumor response and apoptotic cell death by blocking NF-κB activation stimulated by CDDP and reducing cancer cell resistance to chemotherapeutic drug [62, 132]. Similarly, in human hepatocellular carcinoma HCCLM3 cells, combined treatment with genistein and CDDP exhibited significantly greater antiproliferative activities and mitigated both endogenous as well as CDDP-induced matrix metalloproteinase (MMP)-2 upregulation conferring suppression of metastatic spread. Indeed, cotreatment of HCCLM3 tumor bearing mice with genistein and CDDP restrained tumor recurrence and pulmonary metastasis after curative hepatectomy, being of potential clinical importance [133]. Such additive to synergistic combinations of genistein and CDDP suggest that dietary genistein might prove to be a potent adjunctive agent to CDDP chemotherapy, allowing to reduce the recommended drug dosage with better antitumor activities in cancer cells and thereby overcoming the issue of devastating side effects induced by high doses of CDDP. However, in human colon cancer cell line HT-29, 10 μM genistein counteracted the anticancer activity of CDDP, suppressed the ability of drug to induce apoptosis and stimulated cancer cell proliferation. Although the exact molecular mechanisms of this antagonistic action need further studies, colon cancer patients should avoid consuming diets and dietary supplements rich in genistein during treatment with CDDP [129]. Likewise, in human medulloblastoma cell line D283 Med, low physiological concentrations of soy-derived genistein (10 nM) reduced sensitivity of malignant cells towards cytotoxicity of CDDP, suggesting that preventing exposure to genistein may benefit responses of medulloblastoma patients to chemotherapeutic treatment. Phytoestrogen genistein, similarly to estradiol, exerted cytoprotective action on medulloblastoma cells and thereby increased tumor survival and progression [134]. Responses of medulloblastoma cells to genistein may be heterogenous, as remarkably higher doses of genistein (6 μM) enhanced antiproliferative and cytotoxic action of CDDP in some other human medulloblastoma lines, including CRL-8805, HTB-186 and MED-1 cells. These potentiating effects were apparently not mediated through apoptotic cell death [135]. Augmentation of CDDP-induced cell growth inhibition and proapoptotic action by genistein was observed also in several human melanoma cell lines, such as A101D, HM3KO, MeWo, p22 and p39, suggesting that inclusion of genistein in CDDP treatment regimens may enhance the chemosensitivity of melanoma patients [136] (Table 6.6 and Table 6.7).

Although soy isoflavone genistein seems to be a promising candidate agent for combination with CDDP to reinforce antitumor activities of CDDP in several tumor types, including malignancies in lung, ovary, prostate, stomach, pancreas and liver; consumption of genistein may also be counterproductive in patients with breast, colon and brain cancers, antagonizing the chemotherapeutic efficacy of CDDP. These data suggest that diets rich in phytoestrogen genistein should be consumed only with a particular caution by the patients with breast and colon cancers or medulloblastoma during the active treatment period with CDDP.

Similar to genistein, low physiological levels (10 nM) of another soy isoflavone *daidzein* and the bacterial metabolite of daidzein, *equol*, decreased sensitivity of human medulloblastoma D283 Med cells towards anticancer activity of CDDP. Such general cytoprotective action of soy isoflavones increased resistance of medulloblastoma cells to this platinum drug, meaning that more aggressive chemotherapeutic interventions would be required to achieve desired therapeutic response in patients consuming products rich in genistein, daidzein or equol [134] (Table 6.6). On contrary, another isoflavone, *orobol*, enhanced the sensitivity of human ovarian cancer cell line 2008 and its CDDP-resistant subline 2008/C13*5.25 (C13) to CDDP. This mechanism did not involve classical pathways like altering intracellular drug accumulation or glutathione content, but still significantly enhanced mitochondrial apoptosis in CDDP-treated cells [137, 138] (Table 6.6). O-methylated derivative of isoflavone, *formononetin*, did not affect anticancer efficacy of CDDP in different human cervical cancer cell lines, CaSKi, HeLa and SiHa [60] (Table 6.6). However, another methylated isoflavone, *calycosin*, reinforced the CDDP-induced cell growth inhibition and antiproliferative action in several human gastric cancer cell lines, SGC7901, BGC823 and NCI-N87, by inhibiting the activation of Akt pathway. At that, cotreatment with calycosin and CDDP induced cell cycle arrest in G1 phase, promoted apoptotic death, and suppressed invasion and migration of malignant cells. Thus, combined treatment of gastric cancer cells with calycosin and CDDP might lead to better therapeutic effects in lower drug doses [139] (Table 6.6).

Based on the current preclinical data, structurally different isoflavones augment anticancer action of CDDP in different ovarian cancer cells, both CDDP-sensitive and CDDP-resistant, but also in malignant cells of gastric tumors. Nonetheless, children with medulloblastoma should be cautious in exposing to soy isoflavones that reduce the sensitivity of these brain tumors to cytotoxic chemotherapy with CDDP, thereby requiring more aggressive treatment to achieve the therapeutic effect.

Various structurally different dietary flavones and their methylated and glycosidic derivatives have been studied in combination with CDDP on diverse types of malignant cells, derived both from solid tumors as well as hematological cancers. Naturally abundant flavone *apigenin* influenced CDDP-induced cytotoxicity in human cancer cells in a p53-dependent manner, increasing antiproliferative and proapoptotic action in wild-type p53-expressing breast cancer MCF-7, colorectal cancer HCT 116, lung cancer A549

Effects of Plant Flavonoids on Chemotherapeutic Efficacy of Cancer Drugs 189

and cervical cancer HeLa cells, but not in p53-null H1299 cells. This mechanism involved elevated accumulation of p53 and induction of p53-regulated proapoptotic gene expression, whereas activation of Erk/MAPK was responsible for induced p53 stabilization [53]. Cytotoxic activity of CDDP was augmented by apigenin also in human pancreatic cancer BxPC-3 cells [140] and human head and neck squamous cell carcinoma SCC25 cells [141]. In human laryngeal carcinoma Hep-2 cells, cotreatment with apigenin and CDDP suppressed glucose transporter (GLUT)-1 protein level and PI3K/Akt pathway, leading to an increase in cell growth inhibition and circumventing drug resistance phenotype. Insensitivity of Hep-2 cells to CDDP treatment may be related to overexpression of GLUT-1, a hypoxic marker that plays an important role in glucose metabolism in tumors and increases malignant cell turnover; whereas the level of GLUT-1 is regulated by multiple cellular signaling pathways, including PI3K/Akt cascade [55]. Combined treatment with apigenin and CDDP significantly enhanced the drug cytotoxicity and proapoptotic action also in CSCs subset derived from human prostate cancer PC3 cells. This potentiation was associated with inhibition of NF-κB expression and suppression of PI3K and Akt phosphorylation levels. Moreover, apigenin remarkably enhanced the CDDP-induced inhibitory effects on cancer stem cell migration [54]. However, apigenin did not show any significant effect on CDDP cytotoxicity in human ovarian cancer OVCAR-3 cells [112] and oppositely decreased the CDDP anticancer action in murine leukemia cell line L1210 [84] (Table 6.6). The only study performed with animal model showed that combined treatment of murine melanoma B16-BL6 bearing mice with apigenin and CDDP led to positive cooperation and enhanced drug-induced suppression of tumor growth [104] (Table 6.7). Another widespread natural flavone, *luteolin*, enhanced the therapeutic potential of CDDP and chemosensitized human malignant cells in p53-dependent manner. Luteolin expedited and reinforced CDDP-induced apoptosis in wild-type p53-expressing colorectal cancer HCT116 and liver cancer HepG2 cells, but not in mutant p53-expressing colorectal cancer HT29 and liver cancer Hep3B cells. In HCT116 cells, treatment with luteolin activated JNK, and JNK then stabilized p53 protein via phosphorylation and elevated its level, further leading to mitochondrial apoptotic cell death. Moreover, *in vivo* nude mice model bearing HCT116 tumor also confirmed the enhancement of CDDP therapeutic activity by luteolin via upregulation of p53 protein [142]. Thus, luteolin may act as a potent chemosensitizer, especially in tumors with wild-type p53. In two other human colorectal cancer cell lines, oxaliplatin (OXA)-resistant HCT-116 (HCT116-OX) and OXA-resistant SW620 (SW620-OX) cells, combined treatment with luteolin and CDDP reversed multidrug resistance and resulted in synergistic anticancer response. This chemosensitizing effect was accompanied by suppression of overactivated nuclear factor (erythroid-derived 2)-like 2 (Nrf2) pathway by inclusion of luteolin [143]. Luteolin significantly increased anticancer efficacy of CDDP also in human gastric cancer AGS cells [144] and human pancreatic cancer BxPC-3 cells [140]. In CDDP-resistant human ovarian cancer

CAOV3/DDP cells, luteolin enhanced antiproliferative and proapoptotic activities of CDDP. Combined treatment also inhibited invasion and migration of ovarian cancer cells stronger than either agent alone. In addition, luteolin potentiated CDDP-induced decrease in tumor growth in CAOV3/DDP bearing mice, appeared as remarkably reduced tumor volume and weight [80]. However, in another CDDP-resistant human ovarian cancer cell line, OVCAR-3, luteolin did not affect the chemotherapeutic activity of this platinum drug [112]. Besides influencing the CDDP therapeutic efficacy in various human malignant cells, luteolin augmented antiproliferative and cytotoxic properties of CDDP also in canine osteosarcoma cell lines D17 and DSN [145], and murine leukemia cell line L1210 [84]. Thus, luteolin exerts potential chemosensitizing properties for various cancer types preventing tumor progression when combined with CDDP (Table 6.6 and Table 6.7). Flavone *chrysin* potentiated antiproliferative and proapoptotic activities of CDDP in human glioma U87 cells [146], human lung adenocarcinoma A549 cells [147] and human liver cancer HepG2 cells [57]. In HepG2 cells, combined treatment with chrysin and CDDP activated ERK1/2 leading to increased phosphorylation and accumulation of p53 protein, thereby promoting both extrinsic and intrinsic apoptotic cell death [57]. In A549 cells, potentiation of CDDP cytotoxicity by chrysin was associated with cooperative prooxidant action exacerbating drug-induced mitochondrial dysfunction, whereas glutathione (GSH) as an important antioxidant defense was depleted [147]. Therefore, this combination may be a solution to the clinical treatment of CDDP-resistant tumors. However, chrysin had no effect on CDDP cytotoxicity in human promyelocytic leukemia HL-60 cells [86] and in murine leukemia L1210, this natural flavone even decreased the anticancer action of CDDP [84]. To overcome the low bioavailability of chrysin, both chrysin and CDDP were coencapsulated into multilayer nanoparticles (MLNPs) resulting in superior cytotoxic potential in human oral cancer KB cells. This potentiation was achieved through increased production of ROS, mitochondrial dysfunction and apoptotic cell death. Moreover, in 7,12-dimethylbenz[a] anthracene (DMBA)-induced buccal pouch carcinoma in hamster, treatment with dual agents loaded MLNPs led to a significant regression of tumor volume and decrease in tumor incidence [148] (Table 6.6 and Table 6.7). Natural flavone *baicalein* also increased CDDP sensitivity in human non-small cell lung cancer A549 and H460 cells via downregulation of miR-424-3p and targeting the phosphatase and tensin homolog (PTEN)/PI3K/Akt pathway. In fact, this flavone upregulated PTEN and suppressed the PI3K/Akt signaling leading to a greater inhibition of cell viability when combined with CDDP [149]. In A549 cells, cotreatment with baicalein and CDDP was effective in improvement of apoptotic rate, and suppressed also the secretion of proinflammatory cytokines interleukin-6 (IL-6) and tumor necrosis factor-α (TNF-α) which are considered as endogenous tumor promoters [48]. In CDDP-resistant A549 cells, A549/CDDP, baicalein reversed drug resistance through inhibition of PI3K/Akt/NF-κB pathway, promoted apoptosis, and converted CDDP-induced EMT to mesenchymal-epithelial transition (MET) thereby downregulating cell invasion and migration [150]. Moreover, in A549 xenograft model in mice, the tumor weights were significantly lower when cotreated with baicalein and CDDP [149]; and similar results were observed also in A549/CDDP bearing mice, where tumor volumes were remarkably decreased by combined treatment as compared to CDDP monotherapy [150]. In addition, baicalein increased CDDP cytotoxicity also in human cervical cancer HeLa cells transfected with connexin 26 (Cx26), but this effect required the presence of functional gap junctions (GJs) composed of Cx26 between the densely located cells. Inclusion of baicalein promoted tumoricidal action of CDDP through enhancing GJ intercellular communication (GJIC) in conditions permissive of junction contacts, i.e., in high-density cultures but not in low-density cultures [49]. Although these data convincingly show that baicalein has the potential to become a safe and proper chemoadjuvant combined with CDDP in the treatment of lung and cervical tumors, this plant-derived flavone contrariwise prevented CDDP-induced loss of cell viability and apoptosis in human glioma A172 cells. At that, baicalein suppressed CDDP-caused mitochondrial depolarization, cytochrome c release into the cytosol and activation of caspases, exerting protective effects against antitumor and proapoptotic action of CDDP [151]. Therefore, exposure to baicalein should be avoided during the CDDP chemotherapy of glioma patients. Possible effect of another flavone, *scutellarein*, on cytotoxicity of CDDP has been studied only in human ovarian cancer cell line OVCAR-3, where this natural compound increased drug induced reduction of cellular viability. Although the cellular mechanism of this positive cooperation is still not clear, it did not directly correlate with antioxidant-prooxidant properties of flavone [112] (Table 6.6 and Table 6.7).

Various structural derivatives of flavones have been described, whereas mono- and polymethylated flavones are common in the nature. Monomethylated *wogonin* significantly sensitized chemoresistant human head and neck cancer cell lines AMC-HN4-cisR and AMC-HN9-cisR to CDDP, increasing expression of proapoptotic proteins. The underlying molecular mechanism behind this potentiation involved targeting of Nrf2-mediated oxidative stress response. In addition, combined treatment with wogonin and CDDP suppressed tumor growth also in nude mice injected with AMC-HN4-cisR or AMC-HN9-cisR cells [68]. As CDDP is currently a first-line chemotherapeutic drug for treatment of aggressive head and neck tumors, its combination with wogonin might be effective in clinical settings to reduce drug dosage, decrease toxic side effects and overcome resistance phenomenon. Suppression of Nrf2 and subsequent enhancement of oxidative stress were observed also in human hepatocellular carcinoma HepG2 cells cotreated with wogonin and CDDP, leading to increased cytotoxic effects [152]. Intracellular accumulation of ROS (H_2O_2) was triggered also in human cervical cancer cell line HeLa and non-small cell lung cancer cell line A549 cotreated with wogonin and CDDP, substantially contributing to potent augmentation of drug induced apoptosis by wogonin [72]. These results provide new evidence supporting the use of wogonin in combination with CDDP chemotherapy in clinical settings to attain better efficacy at lower drug doses with fewer adverse side effects. However, in another study with A549 cells, wogonin was shown to have no effect on CDDP-caused apoptosis [153]. This discrepancy in results might proceed from the different incubation times used in respective *in vitro* studies (72 vs 24 hours cotreatment). Nevertheless, wogonin was ineffective to impact CDDP-induced cytotoxicity also in human ovarian cancer cell line OVCAR-3 [112], and human leukemia cell lines HL-60 and Jurkat [154]. Furthermore, although in different human gastric cancer cell lines, BGC-823, HGC-27, MGC-803 and MKN-45, combination of wogonin and CDDP synergistically suppressed cell growth and enhanced apoptotic cell death, *in vivo* conditions combined treatment with wogonin and CDDP synergistically decreased the survival of mice bearing BGC-823 and MKN-45 xenografts showing that these agents are actually not proper partners in treatment of stomach cancer [155]. Different effects of wogonin in diverse cancer cells cotreated with CDDP may reflect differences in signaling pathways involved in action of wogonin and CDDP in these cells (Table 6.6 and Table 6.7). Polymethylated flavone *tangeretin* with five methoxy groups in its structural backbone enhanced antitumor efficacy of CDDP in CDDP-resistant human ovarian cancer cell lines A2780/CP70 and 2008/C13. Pretreatment with tangeretin followed by addition of CDDP synergistically inhibited malignant cell proliferation, induced cell cycle arrest at G2/M phase and activated apoptosis via downregulation of PI3K/Akt pathway and its downstream substrates, NF-κB and glycogen synthase kinase (GSK)-3β level. Posttreatment with tangeretin after incubation with CDDP led to additive antitumor effects. Thus, combination of tangeretin with CDDP might provide a new approach in overcoming drug resistance and effective treatment of ovarian tumors [81] (Table 6.6). Another natural pentamethoxyflavone, *3`,4`,5`,5,7-pentamethoxyflavone (PMF)*, sensitized CDDP-resistant human lung cancer A549/CDDP cells to CDDP and promoted apoptotic cell death by potently suppressing Nrf2 protein level and reducing its downstream genes. These data suggest that PMF might be a natural agent to reverse chemoresistance to CDDP in lung cancer treatment [156] (Table 6.6). Polymethylated flavone with six methoxy groups in flavonoid skeleton, *nobiletin*, exhibited schedule-dependent effects in human gastric cancer cell lines MKN-45 and TMK-1. Pretreatment of cells with nobiletin 24 hours prior to addition of CDDP led to a synergistic anticancer response, while CDDP followed by nobiletin revealed additive action. On contrary, simultaneous treatment of gastric cancer cells with nobiletin and CDDP showed antagonistic antitumor effects, suggesting that patients with stomach tumors should be cautious when consuming nobiletin containing food products during the active treatment phase with CDDP [157] (Table 6.6).

The effects of two flavone sugar conjugates on the cytotoxic action of CDDP have also been studied. *Baicalin* or baicalein 7-O-glucuronide revealed dosage- and time-dependent effects when combined with CDDP in human lung cancer cell line A549 and its CDDP-resistant subline A549/DDP. At 24 hours cotreatment, baicalin antagonized antitumor activities of CDDP; however, at 48 hours, addition of baicalin resulted in additive to synergistic increase in drug-induced antiproliferative effects, whereas CDDP concentration also played an important role. A549/DDP cells had significantly higher expression of microtubule affinity-regulating kinase 2 (MARK2) and phosphorylated Akt, baicalin suppressed these levels and inhibited cell proliferation and invasion, still only at appropriately chosen dosages and incubation times. In proper conditions, baicalin can increase the sensitivity of both drug-sensitive and drug-resistant lung cancer cells to CDDP; in improper conditions, baicalin can still counteract the cytotoxic action of CDDP [40] (Table 6.6). *Scutellarin* or scutellarein 7-O-glucuronide greatly enhanced the responses of human ovarian cancer OVCAR-3 cells [112] and human prostate cancer PC3 cells to CDDP-induced cytotoxicity [77]. In PC3 cells, a significant increase in the frequency of DNA damage was observed in combined treatment of scutellarin and CDDP compared to monotherapy with this widely used chemotherapeutic agent [77] (Table 6.6). Drug-induced DNA lesions can activate the phosphorylation of checkpoint kinases (Chks) 1 and 2 representing hallmarks of DNA damage response and initiating DNA crosslink repair mechanisms. Cotreatment of human breast cancer MDA-MB-231 cells and human lung cancer A549 cells with CDDP and a natural flavone derivative *protoapigenone* led to increased antitumor effects by suppressing the activation of Chk1 and Fanconi anemia group D2 (FANCD2) protein. However, in a tumor xenograft nude mice model with MDA-MB-231 cells, protoapigenone was still unable to affect CDDP sensitivity [158] (Table 6.6 and Table 6.7).

Thus, various flavones and their methylated and glycosidic derivatives can enhance the antitumor activities of CDDP in different tumor cells providing possibilities to develop novel therapeutic strategies against diverse malignant disorders and reduce the serious side effects of CDDP. Certain combinations can still be antagonistic in specific cancer cells and therefore, intake of flavones during CDDP chemotherapy must be well-informed and scientifically evident. For instance, consumption of baicalein containing dietary supplements should be avoided by glioma patients who are receiving chemotherapy with CDDP. However, based on the rather extensive preclinical knowledge available so far, no contradictory data and often additive to synergistic cooperation have been described in combined administration of CDDP and luteolin in different tumor types, suggesting the possible safety of consuming the food products rich in luteolin during active treatment phase with CDDP. In the future, luteolin might be applied as a potential universal chemosensitizer in chemotherapy with CDDP in clinical settings.

Diverse flavanones have also been tested in combination with CDDP in several tumor cells. *Naringenin* enhanced the sensitivity of human breast cancer HTB26 cells and human colorectal cancer SW1116 cells to CDDP-induced cytotoxicity [10] (Table 6.6). *Liquiritigenin* combined with CDDP reduced viability of murine melanoma B16F10 cells and suppressed cell migration and invasion, by downregulating protein expression of MMP-2 and MMP-9 and inhibiting PI3K/Akt signaling pathway. Moreover, this combination also suppressed lung metastasis in xenograft mice model injected with B16F10 cells, whereas the content of MMP-2 and MMP-9 in serum was significantly lower in those mice treated with both agents compared to their counterparts receiving CDDP monotherapy. Liquiritigenin can therefore be an important adjuvant agent in CDDP chemotherapy against melanoma [159] (Table 6.6 and Table 6.7). Methylated flavanone *alpinetin* chemosensitized human hepatic cancer HepG2 cells towards CDDP [52] and reversed drug resistance in CDDP-resistant human lung cancer A549/CDDP cells [160], suggesting that alpinetin is worth further studies as a promising chemoadjuvant for CDDP therapy. At that, alpinetin induced a significant downregulation of MRP1, MRP5 and P-gp protein levels in A549/CDDP cells. In addition, treatment of A549/CDDP bearing mice with combination of alpinetin and CDDP resulted in remarkably smaller tumors, thereby inhibiting the progression of lung cancer [160] (Table 6.6 and Table 6.7). Although another methylated flavanone, *5,7,4`-trihydroxy-8-methoxyflavanone* potentiated CDDP-induced decrease in viability of human ovarian cancer OVCAR-3 cells, *6-methoxynaringenin* or 5,7,4`-trihydroxy-6-methoxyflavanone was unable to affect the viability of these cells [112] (Table 6.6). Sensitivity of malignant gynecological cells, i.e., human ovarian cancer OVCA 433 cells and primary ovarian and endometrial cancer cells, towards antitumor action of CDDP was not affected also by flavanone sugar conjugate *hesperidin* or hesperetin 7-rutinoside [90, 91] (Table 6.6).

Thus, although flavanones potentiate the chemosensitivity of malignant cells to CDDP in a cancer type dependent manner, no antagonistic effects between different flavanones and CDDP have been described so far, suggesting that food products rich in flavanones could be consumed during chemotherapeutic treatment with CDDP.

Milk thistle flavonolignan *silibinin* synergistically enhanced the antitumor responses of CDDP in different human breast cancer cells. Cotreatment of estrogen-dependent MCF-7 cells with silibinin and CDDP led to increased antiproliferative and proapoptotic effects [161, 162]. In addition, silibinin reinforced cytotoxic potency of CDDP also in estrogen-independent breast cancer MDA-MB468 cells [162] and doxorubicin (DOX)-resistant MDA-MB-435/DOX cells [163]. In human ovarian cancer, silibinin potentiated the effect of CDDP inhibiting the growth of both A2780 cells as well as CDDP-resistant A2780/CDDP cells [164, 165]. Moreover, bioavailable phospholipid complex of silibinin, silipide (IdB 1016), synergistically decreased the tumor weight and size in A2780 bearing mice suggesting that further clinical trials are needed to verify the potential therapeutic benefit of silibinin in combination with CDDP against ovarian cancer [165]. Silibinin reinforced CDDP antitumor activities also in prostate cancer cells. In human advanced hormone refractory prostate cancer cell line DU145, combination of silibinin and CDDP led to a significant increase in cell growth inhibition, G2/M phase cell cycle arrest and apoptotic cell death as compared to single treatment with CDDP. These data can open new avenues for better treatment of metastatic prostate tumors [166].

Synergistic antiproliferative effects were observed also in human esophageal squamous cell carcinoma KYSE270 cells when cotreated with silibinin and CDDP. In addition, KYSE270 tumor xenografts in nude mice treated with a combination of silibinin and CDDP were remarkably smaller than those in rodents receiving CDDP monotreatment, supporting the application of silibinin as a promising complement to CDDP chemotherapy in treatment of esophageal cancer [65]. However, silibinin did not impact the cytotoxic action of CDDP in human non-small cell lung cancer H69 cells and human multidrug resistant small cell lung cancer VPA17 cells [167] (Table 6.6 and Table 6.7).

Silibinin revealed remarkable augmentation of CDDP cytotoxicity in several human cancer types, including breast, ovarian, prostate and esophageal tumor cells. To date, no contradictory effects in combination of silibinin and CDDP have been described. Therefore, silibinin could be a novel valuable adjuvant in CDDP chemotherapy in clinical settings, with possible therapeutic benefits on patient`s survival and their quality of life.

The possible action of several chalcones on the antitumor activity of CDDP has also been studied. *Butein* enhanced the growth inhibitory and proapoptotic effects of CDDP in human cervical cancer HeLa cells. Combination of butein and CDDP resulted in G1 phase cell cycle arrest, suppressed activation of Akt and ERK/p38 MAPK pathways, and promoted the nuclear translocation and expression of the tumor suppressor protein forkhead box O3a (FoxO3a). Moreover, combined treatment with both agents remarkably inhibited tumor growth and increased FoxO3a level also in mice bearing HeLa tumor xenografts [168] (Table 6.6 and Table 6.7). Another chalcone, *isoliquiritigenin*, behaved as a potent chemosensitizer to CDDP in CSCs derived from human oral squamous cell carcinoma lines OECM1 and SAS. At that, isoliquiritigenin potentiated downregulation of BCRP (ABCG2) expression and reduced colony forming and invasion abilities of malignant cells. Cotreatment with this chalcone also led to reduced levels of GRP78 protein [169]. However, in human bladder cancer T24 cells, the effect of isoliquiritigenin on CDDP cytotoxicity essentially depended on concentration of chalcone. Pretreatment of cells with low doses of isoliquiritigenin (5 µM) caused antagonistic effects in combination with CDDP, while higher chalcone doses (15 µM and 25 µM) synergistically augmented the cell death induced by CDDP [51] (Table 6.6). All the results available to date about the role of chalcones in treatment of lung cancer cells with CDDP confirm positive cooperative action making malignant cells more susceptible to CDDP treatment. *Phloretin* increased CDDP-induced antiproliferative, proapoptotic, antiinvasive and antimigratory properties in human lung cancer cell lines A549, Calu-1, H520 and H838 [170]. *4-Methoxychalcone* exacerbated cytotoxicity of CDDP in human lung cancer A549 cells by stimulating generation of oxidative stress via suppression of constitutively activated Nrf2 signaling-mediated antioxidant responses. At that, PI3K/Akt

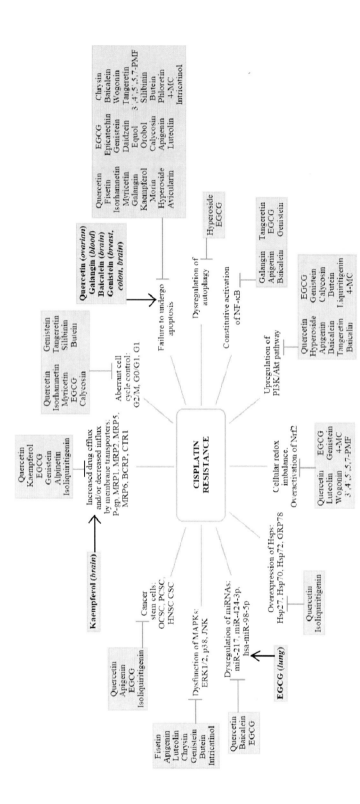

Figure 6.3. Major cellular mechanisms of cisplatin resistance and possibilities to intervene with flavonoids (Akt, protein kinase B; BCRP, breast cancer resistance protein; CSC, cancer stem cell; CTR1, copper transporter 1; ERK, extracellular signal-regulated kinase; GRP, glucose-regulated protein; HNSC, head and neck squamous carcinoma; Hsp, heat shock protein; JNK, c-Jun N-terminal kinase; MAPK, mitogen-activated protein kinase; miRNA, microRNA; MC, methoxychalcone; MRP, multidrug resistance-associated protein; NF-κB, nuclear factor-κB; Nrf2, nuclear factor (erythroid-derived 2)-like 2; OCSC, oral CSC; P-gp, P-glycoprotein; PCSC, prostate CSC; PI3K, phosphoinositide 3-kinase; PMF, pentamethoxyflavone).

pathway played an important role in regulation of Nrf2 activity [83]. 2`,5`-*Dihydroxychalcone* also acted as a potent chemosensitizer to CDDP in A549 cells by inducing GSH depletion and mitochondrial dysfunction [147]. Therefore, chalcone derivatives might prove to be important adjuvants in CDDP chemotherapy in treatment of non-small cell lung cancer (Table 6.6). The effect of *licochalcone A* was studied in combination with CDDP in murine colon cancer CT-26 cells inoculated mice, but in these *in vivo* conditions orally administered licochalcone A exerted no significant impact on CDDP-induced therapeutic efficacy [63] (Table 6.7).

Homoisoflavonoid *intricatinol* augmented proapoptotic and antimigratory activities of CDDP in human non-small cell lung cancer A549 cells. These effects were accompanied by promotion of p53 and p38 MAPK expression [42] (Table 6.6). On contrary, the only prenylated flavonoid studied in combination with CDDP so far, *isoxanthohumol*, exerted antagonistic efficacy in both human melanoma A375 cells as well as murine melanoma B16 cells when cotreated with isoxanthohumol and CDDP, suggesting that caution must be exercised by melanoma patients when consuming products rich in isoxanthohumol during the active treatment phase with CDDP [171] (Table 6.6).

Altogether, dietary flavonoids affect the important biological activities related to cancer chemotherapy, modulating the sensitivity of malignant cells to CDDP in different ways. Combined treatment of certain flavonoids and CDDP might be of therapeutic benefit for various cancer types, allowing to use lower dosages of this anticancer drug while protecting the kidneys against damage. If certain combinations will be efficient also in vivo experiments and further clinical trials, they can provide important means of overcoming drug resistance in clinical settings and development of novel treatment schemes for different cancer types. In this view, combinations between luteolin and CDDP or silibinin and CDDP or certain flavanones and CDDP are of particular interest. However, some antagonistic combinations still indicate the necessity to be cautious in the voluntary and uninformed consumption of flavonoids by cancer patients during CDDP chemotherapy, suggesting that combinations of flavonoids and CDDP must be scientifically fine-tuned to receive desired therapeutic benefit. Our current knowledge about the effects of different plant flavonoids on resistance mechanisms of CDDP is summarized in Figure 6.3.

According to the current experimental findings it is recommended for cancer patients *not to consume* dietary products or dietary supplements rich in following plant flavonoids during the active chemotherapeutic treatment phase with **cisplatin**:

- **morin** in ovarian cancer
- **EGCG** in ovarian cancer (*pretreatment with flavonoid*)
- **quercetin** in ovarian cancer (*simultaneous administration*)
- **genistein** in estrogen receptor-positive breast cancer
- **EGCG** in non-small cell lung cancer

- **baicalin** in non-small cell lung cancer
- **nobiletin** in gastric cancer (*simultaneous administration*)
- **genistein** in colon cancer
- **EGCG** in biliary tract carcinoma
- **isoliquiritigenin** in bladder cancer
- **baicalein** in glioma
- **genistein** in medulloblastoma
- **daidzein** in medulloblastoma
- **equol** in medulloblastoma
- **kaempferol** in glioblastoma
- **isoxanthohumol** in melanoma
- **apigenin** in leukemia
- **chrysin** in leukemia
- **galangin** in leukemia (*pretreatment with flavonoid*)

6.1.2.2. Carboplatin (CBP)

Carboplatin (CBP) is another platinum anticancer agent that acts through induction of DNA damage [172]. Its chemical structure is very similar to that of CDDP and these drugs have demonstrated more or less equal efficacy in most (but not all) malignancies [173]. CBP has been used for treatment of ovarian and lung tumors and cancers of the upper aerodigestive tract [1, 174]. Although it is less toxic to kidneys than CDDP, hematological adverse effects like myelosuppression are more common and also peripheral nerve toxicity and ototoxicity limit sufficient clinical application of CBP [2, 174]. Therefore, development of chemosensitizers for CBP treatment is necessary.

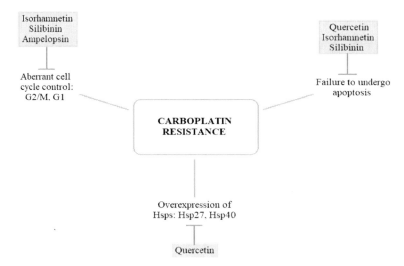

Figure 6.4. Modulation of carboplatin resistance by plant-derived natural flavonoids (Hsp, heat shock protein).

Table 6.8. Effects of flavonoids on anticancer action of carboplatin (CBP) *in vitro* conditions

Drug	Flavonoid	Biological system	Direction of combination	Effects	Ref.
CBP, 6.25-100 µg/ml	Ampelopsin sodium, 6.25-100 µg/ml (=Dihydromyricetin)	SPC-A1 human non-small cell **lung** cancer cell line	↑	Synergism in cytotoxicity. Increase in G1 phase cell cycle arrest by upregulating p21 and downregulating CDK2	[174]
CBP, 0.5 µM	Isorhamnetin, 25 µM	A549 human non-small cell **lung** cancer cell line	↑	Potentiation of CBP-induced cell growth inhibition, increase in apoptosis ($\Delta\Psi$m disruption, caspases-3/-9 activation, PARP cleavage), aberrant microtubule disruption, increase in G2/M phase cell cycle arrest, inhibition of migration	[107]
CBP, 0.1-100 µM	Naringenin, 1 mM	HTB26 human **breast** cancer cell line	↑	Increase in CBP-induced cytotoxicity	[10]
CBP, 0.1-100 µM	Naringenin, 1 mM	SW1116 human **colorectal** cancer cell line	↑	Increase in CBP-induced cytotoxicity	[10]
CBP	Nobiletin	A549 human non-small cell **lung** cancer cell line	↑	Additive effect on cell proliferation inhibition (CI~1)	[175]
CBP	Nobiletin	H460 human non-small cell **lung** cancer cell line	↑	Additive effect on cell proliferation inhibition (CI~1)	[175]
CBP, 125 µM	Quercetin, 50 µM	Hep3B human **hepatocellular** carcinoma cell line	↑	Potentiation of CBP-induced apoptosis (increase in caspase-3) by inhibiting Hsp27 and Hsp40 levels	[172]
CBP, 100 µM	Quercetin, 50 µM	HepG2 human **hepatocellular** carcinoma cell line	↑	Potentiation of CBP-induced apoptosis (increase in caspase-3) by inhibiting Hsp27 and Hsp40 levels	[172]
CBP, 20 µg/ml	Silibinin, 50, 75, 100 µM	DU145 human advanced **prostate** carcinoma cell line	↑	Increase in CBP-induced cell growth inhibition, G2/M phase cell cycle arrest (decrease in cdc2, cyclin B1, cdc25C; increase in Chk1, wee1) and apoptosis (cleavage of caspases-3/-9/-7 and PARP, cyt c release)	[166]
CBP, 2-20 µg/ml	Silibinin 25-100 µM	MCF-7 human estrogen-dependent **breast** cancer cell line	↑	Synergism in cell growth inhibition (CI<1), increase in apoptosis	[162]
CBP, 2-20 µg/ml	Silibinin, 25-100 uM	MDA-MB-468 human estrogen-independent **breast** cancer cell line	↑	Synergism in cell growth inhibition (CI<1)	[162]

CDK, cyclin-dependent kinase; Chk1, checkpoint kinase 1; CI, combination index; cyt c, cytochrome c; Hsp, heat shock protein; PARP, poly (ADP-ribose) polymerase; $\Delta\Psi$m, mitochondrial membrane potential.

Molecular targets and cellular pathways through which flavonoids intervene in the resistance mechanisms of CBP are depicted in Figure 6.4. Dietary flavonol *quercetin* potentiated the proapoptotic action of CBP via suppression of drug-induced expression of Hsp27 and Hsp40 in human hepatoma Hep3B and HepG2 cells [172]. *Isorhamnetin* or 3`-methylquercetin augmented growth inhibitory and apoptosis inducing effects of CBP in human non-small cell lung cancer A549 cells. Combination of isorhamnetin with CBP increased the number of cells in G2/M phase and triggered microtubule disruption more pronouncedly than single drug treatment. In addition, combined treatment also inhibited the migratory potential of malignant cells [107]. Inhibition of proliferation of human non-small cell lung cancer A549 and H460 cells was enhanced also using the combination of polymethylated flavone *nobiletin* and CBP as compared to monotherapy with the platinum drug [175]. In human non-small cell lung cancer SPC-A1 cells, combined treatment of natural plant-derived flavanonol *ampelopsin* sodium and CBP exhibited substantially higher cytotoxic effects than each agent alone. This action was accompanied with increased arrest of cells in G1 phase [174]. Flavanone *naringenin* increased the sensitivity of human colorectal cancer SW1116 cells and human breast cancer HTB26 cells to CBP leading to significantly stronger cytotoxic responses [10]. The growth of human breast cancer MCF-7 and MDA-MB-468 cells was synergistically inhibited also by cotreatment with flavonolignan *silibinin* and CBP, whereas this potentiating action was independent on the expression of estrogen receptors in these cells [162]. In human advanced prostate carcinoma cell line DU145, combination of silibinin and CBP resulted in a significantly enhanced rate of growth inhibition, stronger G2/M phase cell cycle arrest and apoptotic cell death [166] (Table 6.8).

It is important to highlight that to date only potentiating effects (with no contradictory antagonistic results) have been described in cotreating various malignant cells with structurally different flavonoids and CBP. Although the amount of studies is not very high and no investigations with experimental animals have still been performed, current preclinical data indicate that combination of flavonoids and CBP might prove to be a rational chemotherapeutic treatment approach for clinical management of diverse tumors, including lung, colorectal, liver, breast and prostate cancers, allowing to reduce drug dosages and thereby also the extent of toxic side effects. Further exploration in this field, both in vitro and in vivo preclinical studies as well as clinical trials, are urgently needed. However, based on existing data, consuming food products rich in flavonoids is not contraindicated during active treatment phase with CBP.

6.1.2.3. Nedaplatin (NDP)

Nedaplatin (NDP) is a second-generation platinum compound with wide spectrum antitumor applications. This drug was approved for sale in Japan in 1995 and has been used for treatment of head and neck, esophageal, lung, cervical and ovarian cancers. However, the repeated dosage of NDP causes several adverse reactions, such as nausea, vomiting and nephrotoxicity, besides drug resistance, highlighting the necessity towards strategies for increasing sensitivity and reducing side effects of this platinum agent [45].

Ampelopsin or dihydromyricetin synergistically enhanced NDP chemotherapeutic efficacy in human hepatocellular carcinoma cell lines QGY7701 and SMMC7721. Combined treatment with ampelopsin and NDP augmented mitochondrial dysfunction, promoted growth inhibition and apoptotic cell death as compared to treatment with drug alone, highlighting ampelopsin as a potential adjuvant for chemotherapeutic regimens with NDP [45] (Table 6.9). However, further studies with more flavonoids are needed to identify the most proper plant-derived complements for treatment of diverse tumors with NDP and also to determine the possible contradicted combinations.

6.1.2.4. Oxaliplatin (OXA)

Oxaliplatin (OXA) is a third-generation platinum-based chemotherapeutic agent approved for the treatment of colorectal cancer by the FDA in 2002 [176]. OXA is currently the mainstay of chemotherapeutic regimens for colorectal cancers, both as an adjuvant treatment as well as in the case of metastatic disease, being used alone or in combination with other conventional chemotherapeutic agents like 5-fluorouracil and folinic acid [143, 176-179]. This platinum drug is expected to bind with DNA to form mainly intrastrand adducts which suppress DNA synthesis and repair, contributing to cytotoxic and antitumor responses [143, 176, 178, 179]. However, the clinical use of OXA is limited by toxic side effects, including acute or chronic peripheral neuropathy, nausea and vomiting, and by the acquired drug resistance [176, 177, 179, 180]. Resistance to OXA mainly involves the decreased drug influx, improved DNA damage repair and enhanced detoxification mechanisms [179]. Therefore, identification of interventions to reverse resistance to OXA and sensitize malignant cells to this platinum compound is important in development of novel successful treatment strategies.

Possibilities for modulation of OXA resistance by different flavonoids are summarized in Figure 6.5. Abundant dietary flavonol *quercetin* exerted an additive increase in antitumor activity of OXA when two agents were combined in human ovarian cancer cell line A2780. Moreover, in CDDP-resistant subline A2780cisR, quercetin could synergistically sensitize malignant cells to OXA, whereas the synergism was greatest when quercetin was added 2 hours before OXA. Preincubation with quercetin could serve to stimulate ovarian tumor cells for enhanced drug uptake and/or decreased efflux. If these results will be further confirmed *in vivo* conditions, they could open new options for treatment of ovarian cancer patients resistant to conventional chemotherapeutics [43]. Cytotoxic responses to OXA were augmented also by green tea catechin *EGCG* in both A2780 and A2780cisR cells [176]. In addition, EGCG was effective in potentiating OXA cytotoxicity in human colorectal cancer DLD-1 and HT-29 cells. Cotreatment of these cells with EGCG and OXA led to more potent inhibition of cellular proliferation and survival than treatment with drug alone. At that, EGCG augmented the effect of OXA-induced autophagic cell death as characterized by the accumulation of acidic vesicular organelles (AVOs), a marker of autophagy [121]. In another human colorectal cancer cell line SW480, flavone *luteolin* augmented antitumor and proapoptotic properties of OXA. Currently, the exact mechanisms regulating the cellular uptake and efflux of this platinum drug are not completely known, whereas it has been proposed that a member of solute

Table 6.9. Effects of flavonoids on anticancer action of nedaplatin (NDP) and oxaliplatin (OXA) *in vitro* conditions

Drug	Flavonoid	Biological system	Direction of combination	Effects	Ref.
NDP, 10 μg/ml	Dihydromyricetin, 100 μM	QGY7701 human **hepatocellular** carcinoma cell line	↑	Synergism in inhibition of proliferation, suppression of colony formation. Promotion of apoptosis, activation of p53/Bcl-2 pathway (increase in Bak, Bax, Bad; decrease in Bcl-2; activation of p53)	[45]
NDP, 15 μg/ml	Dihydromyricetin, 100 μM	SMMC7721 human **hepatocellular** carcinoma cell line	↑	Synergism in inhibition of proliferation, suppression of colony formation. Promotion of apoptosis, activation of p53/Bcl-2 pathway (increase in Bak, Bax, Bad; decrease in Bcl-2; activation of p53)	[45]
OXA, 0.1 μM	Apigenin, 11-19 μM	BxPC-3 human **pancreatic** cancer cell line	↑	Increase in cell growth inhibitory potential of OXA	[140]
OXA, 6.25-200 μg/ml	Dihydromyricetin, 100 μM	HCT116 human **colorectal** carcinoma cell line	~	No effect on OXA-induced cytotoxicity	[177]
OXA, 6.25-200 μg/ml	Dihydromyricetin, 100 μM	HCT116/L-OHP human **colorectal** carcinoma cell line, OXA-resistant	↑	Reversal of OXA resistance, increase in OXA-induced apoptosis. Inhibition of MRP2 expression and promoter activity regulated by Nrf2 pathway	[177]
OXA, 2.5-20 μM	EGCG, 25, 50, 100 μM	DLD-1 human **colorectal** adenocarcinoma cell line	↑	Synergism in cytotoxicity (CI<1). Potentiation of autophagy induction (accumulation of LC3-II, increase in AVOs, formation of autophagosome)	[121]
OXA, 2.5-20 μM	EGCG, 25, 50, 100 μM	HT-29 human **colorectal** adenocarcinoma cell line	↑	Synergism in cytotoxicity (CI<1). Potentiation of autophagy induction (accumulation of LC3-II, increase in AVOs, formation of autophagosome)	[121]
OXA	EGCG	A2780 human **ovarian** cancer cell line	↑	Synergistic response	[176]
OXA	EGCG	A2780cisR human **ovarian** cancer cell line, CDDP-resistant	↑	Synergistic response	[176]
OXA, 50-200 μM	Luteolin, 5 μM	HCT116-OX human **colorectal** cancer cell line, OXA-resistant	↑	Synergism in anticancer activity (CI<1), 2-fold decrease in OXA IC_{50}. Inhibition of Nrf2 pathway	[143]
OXA, 0.1-100 μM	Luteolin, 5, 10, 20 μM	SW480 human **colorectal** cancer cell line	↑	Augmentation of OXA antitumor activity, increase in apoptosis. Potentiation uptake and intracellular accumulation of OXA through OCTN2	[178]
OXA, 50-200 μM	Luteolin, 5 μM	SW620-OX human **colorectal** cancer cell line, OXA-resistant	↑	Synergism in anticancer activity (CI<1), 2.6-fold decrease in OXA IC_{50}. Inhibition of Nrf2 pathway	[143]
OXA, 0-100 μM	Luteolin, 5 μM	A549 human non-small cell **lung** cancer cell line	↑	Synergism in sensitization to OXA (CI<1). Inhibition of Nrf2	[181]

Drug	Flavonoid	Biological system	Direction of combination	Effects	Ref.
OXA, 0.1 µM	Luteolin, 11-19 µM	BxPC-3 human **pancreatic** cancer cell line	↑	Increase in cell growth inhibitory potential of OXA	[140]
OXA, 5 µM	Nobiletin, 100, 200 µM	HT29 human **colorectal** cancer cell line	↑	Increase in OXA-induced cytotoxicity and apoptosis (increase in Bax, cleaved caspase-3; decrease in Bcl-2). Downregulation of PI3K/Akt/mTOR pathways	[179]
OXA, 5 µM	Nobiletin, 100, 200 µM	SW480 human **colorectal** cancer cell line	↑	Increase in OXA-induced cytotoxicity and apoptosis (increase in Bax, cleaved caspase-3; decrease in Bcl-2). Downregulation of PI3K/Akt/mTOR pathways	[179]
OXA, 0.16-2.62 µM	Quercetin, 9.08-145.22 µM	A2780 human **ovarian** cancer cell line	↑	Mostly additive increase in antitumor activity (CI 0.91-1.12)	[43]
OXA, 0.59-9.41 µM	Quercetin, 10.38-166.10 µM	A2780cisR human **ovarian** cancer cell line, CDDP-resistant	↑	Synergism in antitumor activity (CI 0.36-0.68)	[43]
OXA, 10 µM	Wogonin, 50 µM	BGC-823 human **gastric** cancer cell line	↑	Increase in OXA-induced cytotoxicity and apoptosis (decrease in $\Delta\Psi m$). Increase in JNK phosphorylation, decrease in ULK1 phosphorylation, elevation of autophagy, exacerbation of nitrosative stress	[180]

Akt, protein kinase B; AVO, acidic vesicular organelle; Bad, Bcl-2-associated death promoter; Bak, Bcl-2 homologous antagonist/killer; Bax, Bcl-2-associated X protein; Bcl-2, B-cell lymphoma 2; CI, combination index; JNK, c-Jun N-terminal kinase; MRP, multidrug resistance-associated protein; mTOR, mammalian target of rapamycin; Nrf2, nuclear factor (erythroid-derived 2)-like 2; OCTN2, organic cation/carnitine transporter 2; PI3K, phosphoinositide 3-kinase; ULK, Unc-51 like autophagy activating kinase; $\Delta\Psi m$, mitochondrial membrane potential.

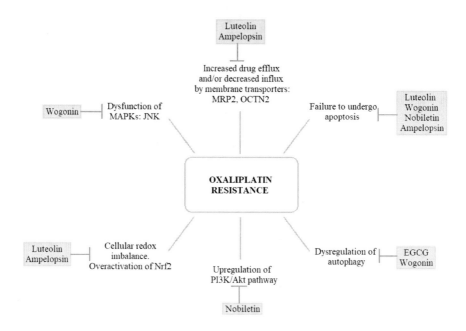

Figure 6.5. Modulation of oxaliplatin resistance by plant-derived natural flavonoids (Akt, protein kinase B; JNK, c-Jun N-terminal kinase; MAPK, mitogen-activated protein kinase; MRP, multidrug resistance-associated protein; Nrf2, nuclear factor (erythroid-derived 2)-like 2; OCTN2, organic cation/carnitine transporter 2; PI3K, phosphoinositide 3-kinase).

carrier superfamily, organic cation/carnitine transporter 2 (OCTN2), can control uptake and intracellular accumulation of OXA. It was demonstrated that luteolin upregulated expression, binding affinity and transport capacity of OCTN2 towards OXA, thereby increasing intracellular drug concentration and subsequent cytotoxic action [178]. In two OXA-resistant human colorectal cancer cell lines, HCT116-OX and SW620-OX, luteolin reversed multidrug resistance by inhibiting Nrf2 pathway [143]. Sensitization of human non-small cell lung cancer A549 cells to OXA also involved suppression of constitutively active Nrf2 levels by luteolin [181]. In addition, pretreatment with luteolin enhanced OXA-induced cell growth inhibition also in human pancreatic cancer cell line BxPC-3 [140]; suggesting that luteolin could be applied as a valuable natural sensitizer in OXA chemotherapy against different cancer types, including colorectal, lung and pancreatic tumors. Another common flavone, *apigenin*, also sensitized BxPC-3 cells to antiproliferative activity of OXA [140]. Monomethylated flavone *wogonin* reinforced the cytotoxic action of OXA in human gastric cancer BGC-823 cells via increasing mitochondrial apoptosis and autophagic death due to exacerbation of nitrosative stress. Moreover, combined treatment with wogonin and OXA resulted in a stronger tumor growth inhibition in zebrafish xenograft model of BGC-823 [180]. Polymethylated flavone *nobiletin* enhanced OXA-induced antiproliferative and proapoptotic activities in human colorectal cancer HT29 and SW480 cells through downregulation of PI3K/Akt/mTOR signaling pathway [179]. Last but not least, flavanonol *ampelopsin* or dihydromyricetin chemosensitized OXA-resistant human colorectal cancer HCT116/L-OHP cells to OXA by augmenting apoptotic cell death. These effects were mediated via substantial suppression of MRP2 expression level and function, closely accompanied by decreased nuclear translocation of Nrf2. However, combination of ampelopsin and OXA was still ineffective in altering drug cytotoxicity in parent HCT116 cells [177] (Table 6.9).

Inclusion of flavonoids in the chemotherapeutic regimen with OXA might offer a means to overcome drug resistance. At that, only additive to synergistic (and not antagonistic) cytotoxic responses have been found in combined treatment of different malignant cells with flavonoids and OXA; suggesting that based on the current preclinical knowledge, flavonoids-containing food items might not be contravened in patients receiving chemotherapeutic treatment with OXA. Moreover, in the future, certain flavonoids could be used in combined treatment regimens with OXA in clinical settings against different tumors, allowing to reduce the drug dosage and prevent OXA-induced neurotoxic reactions.

Among platinum compounds, cisplatin is the most often studied drug in combination with different flavonoids. Numerous investigations on combinations of flavonoids and cisplatin have revealed both synergistic, additive as well as antagonistic effects in diverse cancer cells indicating that caution is required to exercise by patients when consuming food products or dietary supplements rich in certain flavonoids during the active treatment phase with cisplatin. To date, no contraindicative combinations have been described for carboplatin, oxaliplatin and nedaplatin with flavonoids in various types of malignant cells. Therefore, several flavonoids reveal the potential for further therapeutic development.

6.1.3. Topoisomerase Inhibitors

Topoisomerase (Topo) inhibitors form a major class of chemotherapeutic agents that are in frequent clinical use for the therapeutic treatment of various malignancies [182]. Topo I and II enzymes generally act in concert to wind or unwind DNA strands and relieve the tension in the double helix, allowing replication and transcription to occur [183, 184]. Topo enzymes bind to DNA and introduce intermediated breaks, transient single strand breaks by Topo I and transient double strand breaks by Topo II [185]. At the end of the cell cycle processes, the DNA backbone is normally rejoined again. However, Topo inhibitors block the religation step and impede DNA repair mechanisms so that DNA strand breaks can harm the genome integrity, eventually leading to apoptotic cell death. Commonly applied Topo II inhibitors anthracycline antibiotics, including doxorubicin, daunorubicin, epirubicin and pirarubicin, are basically derived from the fungus *Streptococcus peucetius*. Besides blocking Topo II enzyme, these drugs act also through production of ROS and inducing oxidative stress, thereby causing many serious side effects to normal healthy tissues. In addition, the clinical use of Topo inhibitors is limited also by the development of resistance in malignant cells [2]. To overcome these drawbacks, novel safe compounds with chemosensitizing properties, preferably derived from natural sources, are highly needed allowing to achieve therapeutic effects at lower drug doses with fewer side effects and better tolerability to cancer patients.

6.1.3.1. Topoisomerase I Inhibitors

Camptothecin (CPT)

Camptothecin (CPT) is an alkaloidal anticancer drug that was originally isolated from the fruit and bark of the Chinese tree *Camptotheca acuminata* in 1966 [186]. CPT interacts with Topo I and DNA to stabilize complexes that prevent resealing to Topo I-induced DNA single strand breaks, further lead to formation of double strand breaks within DNA synthesis and ultimately cause apoptotic cell death [187]. Although CPT is in clinical use against various tumors, its application is limited by a very low solubility and toxic side effects, including bone marrow suppression and hemorrhagic cystitis [183, 186-188]. In addition, several cellular mechanisms confer tumor cell resistance to this drug [186]. Better understanding of the molecular mechanisms related to CPT action could probably lead to improved therapeutic outcomes.

Although cotreatment of human lung cancer A549 cells with monomethylated flavone *wogonin* and CPT did not affect the CPT-induced cytotoxicity [153], inclusion of flavanone *naringenin* in CPT treatment regimens significantly increased antitumor responses of CPT in human breast cancer cell line HTB26 and human colorectal cancer cell line SW1116 [10] (Table 6.10). Thus, naringenin might enhance the sensitivity of colorectal and breast cancer cells to Topo I inhibitor CPT.

Hydroxycamptothecin (HCPT)

10-Hydroxycamptothecin (HCPT) as a CPT analogue is also a naturally occurring alkaloid. This Topo I inhibitor has potent cytotoxic effects on a variety of malignancies, including bladder and gastric cancer, hepatoma and leukemia [189, 190]. Apoptotic death and cycle arrest of tumor cells are induced by formation of a ternary complex with DNA and Topo I, preventing DNA religation and converting single strand breaks into double strand breaks [152, 190]. Similar to CPT, poor aqueous solubility essentially limits the clinical use of HCPT [189], suggesting that identification of safe compounds with chemosensitizing properties towards this drug could substantially improve the therapeutic applications and clinical responses.

Table 6.10. Effects of flavonoids on anticancer action of camptothecins *in vitro* conditions

Drug	Flavonoid	Biological system	Direction of combination	Effects	Ref.
CPT, 0.1 nM-1mM	Naringenin, 1 mM	HTB26 human **breast** cancer cell line	↑	Increase in CPT-induced cytotoxicity	[10]
CPT, 0.1 nM-1mM	Naringenin, 1 mM	SW1116 human **colorectal** cancer cell line	↑	Increase in CPT-induced cytotoxicity	[10]
CPT	Wogonin	A549 human **lung** cancer cell line	~	No effect on CPT-induced cytotoxicity	[153]
HCPT, 0.39-12.5 μM	Baicalein, 6.25, 12.5 μM	MCF7 human **breast** cancer cell line	↑	Synergism in cell viability inhibition (CI<1)	[189]
HCPT, 0.78-25 μM	Baicalein, 15.625, 31.25, 62.5 μM	SMMC7721 human **hepatocellular** carcinoma cell line	↑	Synergism in cell viability inhibition (CI<1)	[189]
HCPT, 0.78-25 μM	Baicalein, 15.625 μM	BGC823 human **gastric** carcinoma cell line	↑	Synergism in cell viability inhibition (CI<1), increase in HCPT-induced apoptosis (cleavage of caspases-3/-9, PARP1; increase in Bax/Bcl-2 ratio, loss of $\Delta\Psi m$), upregulation of p53 and p21. Increase in G1 and G2 phases cell cycle arrest, exacerbation of DNA damage. Increase in HCPT-induced Topo I inhibition	[189]
HCPT, 1 μM	Genistein, 10 μM	J82 human **bladder** cancer cell line	↑	Increase in HCPT-induced cell viability inhibition	[190]
HCPT, 1 μM	Genistein, 10 μM	T24 human **bladder** cancer cell line	↑	Increase in HCPT-induced cell viability inhibition	[190]
HCPT, 1, 2, 5 μM	Genistein, 3, 10, 20 μM	TCCSUP human **bladder** cancer cell line	↑	Increase in HCPT-induced cell viability inhibition, G2/M phase cell cycle arrest and apoptosis. Induction of DSBs leading to synergistic activation of ATM kinase and attenuation of NEMO/NF-κB/IKK/caspase signaling	[190]
HCPT, 1 μM	Genistein, 10 μM	TSGH8301 human **bladder** cancer cell line	↑	Increase in HCPT-induced cell viability inhibition	[190]
HCPT, 25-100 μg/ml	Wogonin, 20-60 μM	HepG2 human **hepatocellular** carcinoma cell line, wild-type p53	↑	Increase in HCPT-induced cytotoxicity. Suppression of Nrf2	[152]
CPT-11	Genistein	OAW-42 human **ovarian** adenocarcinoma cell line	↑	Synergism in antiproliferation (CI<1). Partial inhibition of CPT-11-induced G2/M phase cell cycle arrest, increase in apoptosis (PARP cleavage)	[183]
CPT-11	Genistein	HeLa human **cervical** cancer cell line	↑	Synergism in antiproliferation (CI<1). Partial inhibition of CPT-11-induced G2/M phase cell cycle arrest, increase in apoptosis (PARP cleavage), decrease in CDK1 phosphorylation	[183]
CPT-11, 0-50 μM	Silibinin, 50 μM	LN229 human **glioma** cell line, mutant p53	~	No effect on CPT-11-induced cytotoxicity	[28]
SN-38, 0-100 ng/ml	(+)-Catechin, 3 μM	K562/BCRP human **leukemia** cell line, expressing BCRP not P-gp or MRP1	~	No reversal of (BCRP-mediated) SN-38 resistance	[197]
SN-38, 0-100 ng/ml	Acacetin, 1, 3, 10 μM	K562/BCRP human **leukemia** cell line, expressing BCRP not P-gp or MRP1	↑	Reversal of (BCRP-mediated) resistance; 15.2-fold decrease in SN-38 IC_{50} at 1 μM acacetin, 21.4-fold at 3 μM acacetin. No suppression of BCRP expression, inhibition of BCRP function	[197]

Table 6.10. (Continued)

Drug	Flavonoid	Biological system	Direction of combination	Effects	Ref.
SN-38, 0-100 ng/ml	Apigenin, 3 μM	K562/BCRP human **leukemia** cell line, expressing BCRP not P-gp or MRP1	↑	Reversal of (BCRP-mediated) resistance to SN-38	[197]
SN-38, 0-100 ng/ml	Astragalin, 3 μM	K562/BCRP human **leukemia** cell line, expressing BCRP not P-gp or MRP1	~	No reversal of (BCRP-mediated) SN-38 resistance	[197]
SN-38, 0-100 ng/ml	Chrysin, 3 μM	K562/BCRP human **leukemia** cell line, expressing BCRP not P-gp or MRP1	↑	Reversal of (BCRP-mediated) resistance to SN-38	[197]
SN-38, 0-100 ng/ml	Diosmetin, 3 μM	K562/BCRP human **leukemia** cell line, expressing BCRP not P-gp or MRP1	↑	Reversal of (BCRP-mediated) resistance to SN-38	[197]
SN-38, 0-100 ng/ml	Diosmin, 3 μM	K562/BCRP human **leukemia** cell line, expressing BCRP not P-gp or MRP1	~	No reversal of (BCRP-mediated) SN-38 resistance	[197]
SN-38, 0-100 ng/ml	Eriodictyol, 3 μM	K562/BCRP human **leukemia** cell line, expressing BCRP not P-gp or MRP1	~	No reversal of (BCRP-mediated) SN-38 resistance	[197]
SN-38, 0-100 ng/ml	Fisetin, 3 μM	K562/BCRP human **leukemia** cell line, expressing BCRP not P-gp or MRP1	~	No reversal of (BCRP-mediated) SN-38 resistance	[197]
SN-38, 0-100 ng/ml	Galangin, 3 μM	K562/BCRP human **leukemia** cell line, expressing BCRP not P-gp or MRP1	↑	Reversal of (BCRP-mediated) resistance to SN-38	[197]
SN-38, 0-100 ng/ml	Genistein, 1, 3, 10 μM	K562 human **leukemia** cells, no expressing BCRP, P-gp or MRP1	~	No reversal of (BCRP-mediated) SN-38 resistance	[197]
SN-38, 0-100 ng/ml	Genistein, 1, 3, 10 μM	K562/BCRP human **leukemia** cell line, expressing BCRP not P-gp or MRP1	↑	Reversal of (BCRP-mediated) resistance; 7.23-fold decrease in SN-38 IC_{50} at 3 μM genistein, 16.4-fold at 10 μM genistein. No suppression of BCRP expression, inhibition of BCRP function	[197]
SN-38, 0-100 ng/ml	Hesperetin, 3 μM	K562/BCRP human **leukemia** cell line, expressing BCRP not P-gp or MRP1	↑	Reversal of (BCRP-mediated) resistance to SN-38	[197]
SN-38, 0-100 ng/ml	Kaempferide, 3 μM	K562/BCRP human **leukemia** cell line, expressing BCRP not P-gp or MRP1	↑	Reversal of (BCRP-mediated) resistance to SN-38	[197]
SN-38, 0-100 ng/ml	Kaempferol, 1, 3, 10 μM	K562/BCRP human **leukemia** cell line, expressing BCRP not P-gp or MRP1	↑	Reversal of (BCRP-mediated) resistance; 9.96-fold decrease in SN-38 IC_{50} at 1 μM kaempferol, 21.5-fold at 3 μM kaempferol	[197]
SN-38, 0-100 ng/ml	Kaempferol-7-O-neohesperidoside, 3 μM	K562/BCRP human **leukemia** cell line, expressing BCRP not P-gp or MRP1	~	No reversal of (BCRP-mediated) SN-38 resistance	[197]
SN-38, 0-100 ng/ml	Luteolin, 3 μM	K562/BCRP human **leukemia** cell line, expressing BCRP not P-gp or MRP1	↑	Reversal of (BCRP-mediated) resistance to SN-38	[197]
SN-38, 0-100 ng/ml	Luteolin-4`-O-glucoside, 3, 10 μM	K562/BCRP human **leukemia** cell line, expressing BCRP not P-gp or MRP1	↑	Reversal of (BCRP-mediated) resistance to SN-38	[197]

Drug	Flavonoid	Biological system	Direction of combination	Effects	Ref.
SN-38, 0-100 ng/ml	Myricetin, 3 μM	K562/BCRP human **leukemia** cell line, expressing BCRP not P-gp or MRP1	~	No reversal of (BCRP-mediated) SN-38 resistance	[197]
SN-38, 0-100 ng/ml	Naringenin, 1, 3, 10 μM	K562 human **leukemia** cells, no expressing BCRP, P-gp or MRP1	~	No reversal of (BCRP-mediated) SN-38 resistance	[197]
SN-38, 0-100 ng/ml	Naringenin, 1, 3, 10 μM	K562/BCRP human **leukemia** cell line, expressing BCRP not P-gp or MRP1	↑	Reversal of (BCRP-mediated) resistance; 5.94-fold decrease in SN-38 IC_{50} at 3 μM naringenin, 15.2-fold at 10 μM naringenin. No suppression of BCRP expression, inhibition of BCRP function	[197]
SN-38, 0-100 ng/ml	Peltatoside, 3 μM	K562/BCRP human **leukemia** cell line, expressing BCRP not P-gp or MRP1	~	No reversal of (BCRP-mediated) SN-38 resistance	[197]
SN-38, 0-100 ng/ml	Prunin, 3, 10 μM	K562/BCRP human **leukemia** cell line, expressing BCRP not P-gp or MRP1	↑	Reversal of (BCRP-mediated) resistance; 5.7-fold decrease in SN-38 IC_{50} at 3 μM prunin, 14.7-fold at 10 μM prunin	[197]
SN-38, 0-100 ng/ml	Quercetin, 3 μM	K562/BCRP human **leukemia** cell line, expressing BCRP not P-gp or MRP1	~	No reversal of (BCRP-mediated) SN-38 resistance	[197]
SN-38, 5 nM	Quercetin, 12.5 μM	AGS human **gastric** adenocarcinoma cell line	↑	Increase in SN-38-induced cell survival inhibition and apoptosis. Modulation of GSK-3β/β-catenin signaling	[192]
SN-38, 0-100 ng/ml	Rhoifolin, 3 μM	K562/BCRP human **leukemia** cell line, expressing BCRP not P-gp or MRP1	~	No reversal of (BCRP-mediated) SN-38 resistance	[197]
SN-38, 0-100 ng/ml	Rutin, 3 μM	K562/BCRP human **leukemia** cell line, expressing BCRP not P-gp or MRP1	~	No reversal of (BCRP-mediated) SN-38 resistance	[197]
SN-38, 0-100 ng/ml	Silibinin, 3 μM	K562/BCRP human **leukemia** cell line, expressing BCRP not P-gp or MRP1	~	No reversal of (BCRP-mediated) SN-38 resistance	[197]
TPT, 25 μM	Chrysin, 250 μM	Caco-2 human **colorectal** cancer cell line	↓	Inhibition of TPT-induced apoptosis (decrease in caspases-3/-8). Increase in transporters expression (P-gp, MRP-2, BCRP), stabilization of cytosolic β-catenin	[200]
TPT	Genistein	OAW-42 human **ovarian** adenocarcinoma cell line	↑	Synergism in antiproliferation (CI<1)	[183]
TPT, 0.5-10 μM	Genistein, 30 μM	LNCaP human **prostate** cancer cell line	↑	Increase in reducing cell viability, promotion of apoptosis (activation of caspases-9/-3), generation of ROS	[188]
TPT	Genistein	HeLa human **cervical** cancer cell line	↑	Synergism in antiproliferation (CI<1)	[183]
TPT, 0.5 ng/ml-100 μg/ml	Quercetin, 0.62 μM	MCF-7 human **breast** cancer cell line, ER-positive, P-gp-negative	↑	1.4-fold increase in TPT-induced cytotoxicity	[198]
TPT, 0.5 ng/ml-100 μg/ml	Quercetin, 0.62 μM	MDA-MB-231 human **breast** cancer cell line, ER-negative, P-gp-negative	↑	1.3-fold increase in TPT-induced cytotoxicity	[198]

ATM, ataxia telangiectasia mutated; Bax, Bcl-2-associated X protein; Bcl-2, B-cell lymphoma 2; BCRP, breast cancer resistance protein; CDK, cyclin-dependent kinase; CI, combination index; DSB, double-stranded DNA break; ER, estrogen receptor; GSK, glycogen synthase kinase; IKK, IκB kinase; MRP, multidrug resistance-associated protein; NF-κB, nuclear factor-κB; Nrf2, nuclear factor (erythroid-derived 2)-like 2; PARP, poly (ADP-ribose) polymerase; P-gp, P-glycoprotein; ROS, reactive oxygen species; Topo, topoisomerase; ΔΨm, mitochondrial membrane potential.

Table 6.11. Effects of flavonoids on anticancer action of camptothecins *in vivo* conditions

Drug	Flavonoid	Biological system	Direction of combination	Effects	Ref.
HCPT, 3 mg/kg, s.c., every two days	Baicalein, 5 mg/kg, s.c., every two days	BGC823 human **gastric** cancer cells injected s.c. into axilla of 4-5w old female athymic nude mice	↑	Increase in HCPT-induced tumor growth repression	[189]
HCPT, 3 µg/ml, transperitoneally	Genistein, 1 g/kg diet, orally with food	TCCSUP human **bladder** cancer cells inoculated s.c. into the flanks of 10w old female SCID nude mice	↑	Increase in tumor growth inhibition. Attenuation of HCPT-induced NF-κB activation, decrease in IKK1/2 activation, increase in IκBα phosphorylation. Cleavage of caspases-3/-9 and PARP	[190]
CPT-11, 50 mg/kg, i.p., on days 1-9	Hesperetin, 20 or 100 mg/kg, oral gavage, daily	CT-26 murine **colon** cancer cells injected s.c. into the posterior mid-dorsum of 6-8w old female Balb/cJ mice	↑	Potentiation of tumor growth inhibition. Increase in apoptosis, suppression of STAT3 activity, recruitment of tumoricidal macrophages into the tumor microenvironment	[191]
CPT-11, 50 mg/kg, on days 1, 13, 19	Naringin, 100 mg/kg, on days 3-5	EAC murine **mammary** adenocarcinoma cells injected i.p. into 2 months old male Swiss albino mice	↑	Increase in antitumor activity, inhibition of tumor growth, decrease in the number of tumor cells in peritoneal cavity. Increase in lifespan of mice	[196]
CPT-11, 50 mg/kg. on days 1, 13, 19	Quercetin, 100 mg/kg, on days 3-5	EAC murine **mammary** adenocarcinoma cells injected i.p. into 2 months old male Swiss albino mice	↑	Increase in antitumor activity, inhibition of tumor growth, decrease in the number of tumor cells in peritoneal cavity. Increase in lifespan of mice	[196]
CPT-11, 10 mg/kg, i.p., weekly	Quercetin 20 mg/kg, i.p., thrice weekly	AGS human **gastric** cancer cells injected into the right flank region of female BALB/c nude mice	↑	Inhibition of growth, decrease in tumor sizes. Decrease in the levels of VEGF-R2, VEGF-A and COX-2, reduction of percentage of TEMs, restoration of E-cadherin expression	[192]

COX, cyclooxygenase; EAC, Ehrlich ascites carcinoma; IKK, IκB kinase; IκBα, nuclear factor of kappa light polypeptide gene enhancer in B-cells inhibitor, alpha; NF-κB, nuclear factor-κB; PARP, poly (ADP-ribose) polymerase; STAT3, signal transducer and activator of transcription 3; TEM, Tie2-expressing monocyte; VEGF, vascular endothelial growth factor; VEGF-R, VEGF receptor.

Natural flavone *baicalein* synergistically sensitized human gastric cancer BGC823, human breast cancer MCF7 and human hepatocellular carcinoma SMMC7721 cells to antitumor action of HCPT. In BGC823 cells, cotreatment with baicalein and HCPT exacerbated repression of Topo I activity and drug-induced DNA damage, augmented mitochondrial apoptosis and induced cell cycle arrest in G1 and G2 phases through upregulation of p53. In addition, combined treatment with baicalein and HCPT enhanced tumor growth suppression in BGC823 xenografts bearing mice as compared to single drug treated experimental rodents [189]. Monomethylated flavone *wogonin* potentiated HCPT cytotoxicity in human hepatocellular carcinoma HepG2 cells by blocking the translocation of Nrf2 into nucleus [152]. In several human bladder cancer cell lines (TCCSUP, J82, T24 and TSGH8301), soy isoflavone *genistein* sensitized cells towards growth inhibitory and antiproliferative properties of HCPT. At that, in TCCSUP cells, pretreatment with genistein before addition of HCPT induced more DNA double strand breaks and delayed DNA damage repair process, augmenting G2/M phase cell cycle arrest and apoptosis. These effects were accompanied by substantial attenuation of drug-induced activation of antiapoptotic NF-κB signaling pathway. Moreover, in TCCSUP bladder tumor xenograft model of mice, combined treatment with genistein and HCPT suppressed the tumor growth more strongly than treatment with drug alone, counteracting the protective effects of NF-κB against cell death [190] (Table 6.10 and Table 6.11). These data show that certain flavonoids may serve as non-toxic adjuvants to suppress the catalytic activity of Topo I in HCPT treatment regimens, thereby improving the chemotherapeutic efficacy and broaden clinical application possibilities of this antineoplastic agent.

Irinotecan (CPT-11) and Its Active Metabolite (SN-38)

Several dose-limiting adverse side effects of CPT have initiated numerous studies to find novel camptothecins with higher antitumor efficacy and lower toxicity. Irinotecan (CPT-11) is a semisynthetic analog of CPT considered as a pro-drug, hydrolysis of which by human liver carboxylesterase produces the active metabolite SN-38 [186, 191, 192]. SN-38 potently interacts with Topo I and DNA to stabilize this covalent complex, generate permanent DNA strand breaks, and lead to cell cycle arrest and apoptosis [187, 192-194]. The use of CPT-11 was approved by the FDA in 1996 and since then, this Topo I inhibitor has been widely used against numerous solid tumors and hematological malignancies in both children and adults [186, 191, 195]. Today, CPT-11 is approved for the treatment of advanced colon cancer and gastric cancer, but has also shown some activity against metastatic breast cancer in clinical trials [187, 191, 194]. However, the administration of CPT-11 is accompanied by acquisition of resistance related to several cellular mechanisms, including overexpression of BCRP (ABCG2) [186]. In addition, in clinical practice, high doses of CPT-11 may cause adverse side effects, such as gastrointestinal toxicity (nausea, vomiting, diarrhea, abdominal cramps) and

212 *Katrin Sak*

hematological toxicity (myelosuppression) [192, 196]. Development of strategies to optimize the antitumor efficacy of CPT-11 while reducing its adverse reactions by inclusion of novel safe compounds in the combinatorial treatment regimens is a highly attractive approach for improvement of therapeutic outcome.

Abundant dietary flavonol *quercetin* potentiated SN-38-induced inhibition of cell viability and increase in apoptosis in human gastric cancer AGS cells via modulating GSK-3β/β-catenin signaling (Table 6.10). Combined treatment with quercetin and CPT-11 exerted a stronger tumor growth inhibition in AGS xenograft mouse model as compared to single treatment with the drug. This *in vivo* inhibitory action was accompanied by the decrease in expression of cyclooxygenase-2 (COX-2), EMT-associated markers and angiogenesis-related factors like vascular endothelial growth factor (VEGF) and percentage of Tie2-expressing monocytes (TEM), suggesting that inclusion of quercetin in CPT-11 treatment schemes could reinforce antimetastatic potential [192]. Quercetin increased antitumor activity of CPT-11 also in Ehrlich ascites tumor-bearing mice, reducing the number of tumor cells in peritoneal cavity and prolonging the lifespan of experimental animals. Similar effects were observed also by combining CPT-11 and glycosidic flavanone, *naringin* or naringenin 7-O-neohesperidoside, in Ehrlich ascites carcinoma-bearing mice [196]. Another citrus flavanone, *hesperetin*, potentiated the ability of CPT-11 to inhibit tumor growth and induce apoptosis by reducing STAT3 activity and recruiting tumoricidal macrophages into the tumor microenvironment in murine colon cancer CT-26 bearing mice [191] (Table 6.11). Addition of soy isoflavone *genistein* synergistically enhanced antiproliferative action of CPT-11 in human ovarian cancer OAW-42 cells and human cervical cancer HeLa cells, causing abrogation of the G2/M checkpoint control and promoting apoptotic cell death [183]. However, flavonolignan *silibinin* did not affect the CPT-11-induced cytotoxicity in human glioma cell line LN229 [28]. The effect of various flavonoids on antitumor activity of SN-38 was tested also in BCRP-expressing human leukemia K562/BCRP cells. As flavonols *galangin, kaempferol* and *kaempferide*; flavones *apigenin, chrysin, luteolin, acacetin, diosmetin* and *luteolin 4`-O-glucoside*; flavanones hesperetin, *naringenin* and *prunin*; and isoflavone genistein reversed BCRP-mediated resistance by inhibiting BCRP function, several other flavonoids were unable to modulate SN-38 chemotherapeutic efficacy [197] (Table 6.10). Thus, several structurally different flavonoids, among others quercetin, hesperetin, naringin and genistein, may improve the efficacy of SN-38 (*in vitro*)/CPT-11 (*in vivo*) in different malignant models thereby suppressing the progression of respective tumors. To date, no contraindicative combinations of flavonoids with CPT-11 have been detected in any studied malignant models, suggesting that intake of flavonoid-rich food products during the active treatment phase with CPT-11 might be rather beneficial.

Topotecan (TPT)

Topotecan (TPT) is another semisynthetic derivative of CPT that induces apoptosis in malignant cells through inhibition of Topo I. TPT interposes itself between Topo I and DNA, destabilizes genetic material, leads to irreversible DNA double stand breaks, induces cell cycle arrest and eventually cell death [188, 198]. In addition, antitumor action of TPT may be related also to induction of oxidative stress by enhancing the levels of ROS and nitrite in malignant cells [188, 198, 199]. TPT is primarily used for secondary treatment of ovarian, cervical and small cell lung cancers, being limited to patients with recurring tumors and/or those whose malignancies have progressed under standard chemotherapeutic treatments [188, 198]. Similar to other CPT analogs, the most common side effects of TPT include myelosuppression (neutropenia, thrombocytopenia), thereby suppressing immune functions resulting in an increase in susceptibility to infections [188, 199].

Dietary flavonol *quercetin*, at only 0.62 µM concentration, markedly enhanced TPT cytotoxic efficacy in both estrogen receptor-positive human breast cancer MCF-7 cells as well as estrogen receptor-negative human breast cancer MDA-MB-231 cells. At that, quercetin did not change the TPT-induced generation of ROS and nitrite levels [198]. Likewise, soy isoflavone *genistein* synergistically increased antiproliferative action of TPT in human ovarian cancer OAW-42 cells and human cervical cancer HeLa cells [183]. In human hormone-sensitive prostate cancer LNCaP cells, combined treatment with genistein and TPT led to augmentation of cell viability reduction and mitochondrial apoptosis through increase in ROS production [188]; suggesting that intake of genistein containing products during chemotherapeutic treatment with CPT analogs, including TPT, might strengthen the drug efficacy and be beneficial for patients suffering from different hormone-dependent malignancies (ovarian, cervical, prostate tumors). Nevertheless, in contrast to these potentiating effects, flavone *chrysin* almost completely inhibited TPT-induced apoptosis in human colorectal carcinoma Caco-2 cells by stabilizing cytosolic β-catenin. This inhibitory action involved transport-independent functions of ABC transporters, as despite upregulation of P-gp, MRP-2 and BCRP expression, their activity was still inhibited by chrysin leading to intracellular accumulation of TPT [200]. These data indicate that consumption of chrysin containing food items and dietary supplements might be contraindicated to colorectal cancer patients who are receiving TPT-based chemotherapy (Table 6.10).

> According to the current experimental findings it is recommended for cancer patients *not to consume* dietary products or dietary supplements rich in following plant flavonoids during the active chemotherapeutic treatment phase with **topotecan**:
> - **chrysin** in colorectal cancer

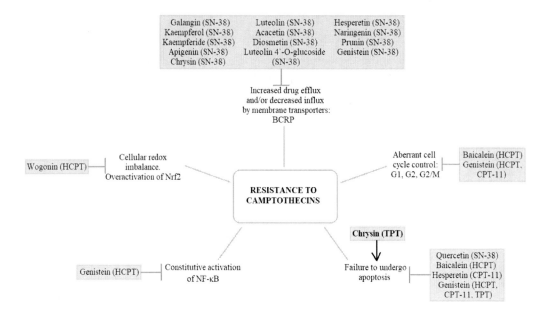

Figure 6.6. Modulation of resistance mechanisms of camptothecins by plant-derived natural flavonoids (BCRP, breast cancer resistance protein; CTP-11, irinotecan; GSK, glycogen synthase kinase; HCPT, hydrocamptothecin; NF-κB, nuclear factor-κB; Nrf2, nuclear factor (erythroid-derived 2)-like 2; SN-38, active metabolite of CPT-11; TPT, topotecan).

Possibilities for modulation of resistance of tumor cells to camptothecins are summarized in Figure 6.6. Different flavonoids possess the ability to augment the antitumor activities of CPT and its analogs in several malignancies, including brain, lung, gastric, colorectal, liver, bladder, breast, ovarian, cervical and prostate cancers as well as certain types of leukemia. If these effects will be confirmed in further preclinical studies and clinical trials, inclusion of specific flavonoids in chemotherapeutic regimens with camptothecins might be potentially useful in clinical management of different cancer types leading to improvement of patient outcomes. The only currently known contraindicative combination, i.e., combination of chrysin and TPT, still gives a warning signal to colorectal cancer patients to avoid intake of chrysin during the active chemotherapeutic treatment phase with TPT.

6.1.3.2. Topoisomerase II Inhibitors

Etoposide (VP-16)

Etoposide (VP-16) belongs to the group of drugs known as podophyllotoxin derivatives [201]. VP-16 is a Topo II inhibitor that prevents religation of the DNA strands by forming a ternary complex with Topo II enzyme and DNA leading to breaks in DNA strands to further arrest the cell cycle and promote apoptosis in malignant cells [72, 152, 153, 201-204]. VP-16 is approved for the treatment of small cell lung cancer and testicular cancer, but has been used also against lymphomas (Hodgkin lymphoma and

Effects of Plant Flavonoids on Chemotherapeutic Efficacy of Cancer Drugs 215

non-Hodgkin lymphoma), leukemias (acute myelogenous leukemia and acute lymphocytic leukemia) and some types of solid tumors [201, 202, 204]. However, the clinical use of VP-16 is limited by its very low oral bioavailability and is also related to severe adverse reactions, such as myelosuppression and formation of secondary malignancies [154, 201, 202, 204, 205]. Therefore, identification of novel safe adjuvants which would allow to reduce the needful drug dosages is important to achieve desired therapeutic responses and improve clinical outcome.

Modes to intervene in resistance mechanisms of VP-16 in diverse malignant cells by various plant-derived flavonoids are depicted in Figure 6.7. Inclusion of naturally ubiquitous flavonol *quercetin* in VP-16 treatment led to synergistic anticancer effects in several human lymphoid and myeloid leukemia cell lines (acute lymphoblastic leukemia CCRF-CEM cells, T-cell leukemia Jurkat cells, myelogenous leukemia KG-1a cells and acute monocytic leukemia THP-1 cells). This action was accompanied by downregulation of GSH levels and increase in DNA damage, driving apoptosis and cell cycle arrest at S and/or G2/M phases [206]. Although quercetin did not affect VP-16 antiproliferative potential in human primary endometrial and ovarian cancer cells [90]; coencapsulation of quercetin and VP-16 in PLGA nanoparticles led to enhancement of bioavailability and sensitized human breast cancer MCF-7 cells to VP-16 cytotoxicity, by inhibiting P-gp expression at the cell surface and thereby reducing drug efflux [201]. Thus, quercetin can augment the cytotoxic action of VP-16 in several ways, including facilitation of the entry of drug into tumor cells via suppression of P-gp that is a major route of VP-16 excretion from the cells. Another flavonol *fisetin* enhanced antiproliferative properties of VP-16 in human osteosarcoma cell lines MG-63 and Saos-2, associated with the cell cycle arrest in G2 phase [205]. Monomethylated flavonol *rhamnetin* or 7-methoxyquercetin augmented VP-16 growth inhibitory activity in human hepatocellular carcinoma HepG2 cells and its multidrug resistant (MDR) subline HepG2/ADR. This potentiating effect of rhamnetin was related to enhancement of miR-34a level and subsequent decrease in Notch-1 expression. Attenuation of MDR by rhamnetin in hepatocellular carcinoma cells might contribute to more efficient strategies for the treatment of liver cancer in the future [207] (Table 6.12).

Dietary flavone *apigenin* enhanced VP-16 activity in several human lymphoid leukemia cell lines (CCRF-CEM and Jurkat) and myeloid leukemia cell lines (KG-1a and THP-1) in additive to synergistic manner, reducing GSH levels and increasing DNA damage, resulting in cell cycle arrest at S and/or G2/M phases and apoptosis. Therefore, combination of apigenin and VP-16 can provide a new promising therapeutic approach for the treatment of certain types of leukemias [206]. In addition, apigenin increased VP-16-induced apoptosis also in human neuroblastoma IMR32 cells through complete restoration of nuclear localization of p53 [208]. Monomethylated flavone *wogonin*

216   *Katrin Sak*

Table 6.12. Effects of flavonoids on anticancer action of etoposide (VP-16) *in vitro* conditions

Drug	Flavonoid	Biological system	Direction of combination	Effects	Ref.
VP-16	Apigenin	CCRF-CEM human acute lymphoblastic **leukemia** cell line, p53-null	↑	Additive anticancer effect; induction of apoptosis (activation of caspases-3/-8/-9), increase in S and G2/M phase cell cycle arrest. Decrease in GSH, increase in DNA damage	[206]
VP-16	Apigenin	Jurkat human peripheral blood T-cell **leukemia** cell line, p53-null	↑	Additive anticancer effect; induction of apoptosis (activation of caspases-3/-8/-9), increase in S phase cell cycle arrest. Decrease in GSH, increase in DNA damage	[206]
VP-16	Apigenin	KG-1a human myelogenous **leukemia** cell line, p53-null	↑	Additive anticancer effect; induction of apoptosis (activation of caspases-3/-8/-9), increase in S and G2/M phase cell cycle arrest. Decrease in GSH, increase in DNA damage	[206]
VP-16	Apigenin	THP-1 human acute monocytic **leukemia** cell line, p53-null	↑	Synergistic anticancer effect; induction of apoptosis (activation of caspases-3/-8/-9), increase in S and G2/M phase cell cycle arrest. Decrease in GSH, increase in DNA damage	[206]
VP-16, 10 μM	Apigenin, 40 μM	IMR32 human **neuroblastoma** cell line	↑	Increase in apoptosis (increase in Bax). Inhibition of phosphorylation and restoration of p53 nuclear localization	[208]
VP-16, 5 μg/ml	Deguelin, 10, 100 nM	HL60PT human **leukemia** cell line	~	No effect on VP-16-induced cytotoxicity	[211]
VP-16, 5 μg/ml	Deguelin, 10, 100 nM	U937 human **leukemia** cell line	↑	Increase in VP-16-induced apoptosis. Downregulation of Akt phosphorylation	[211]
VP-16, 0.1 μM	EGCG, 10 μM	MDA-MB-231 human **breast** cancer cell line	↑	Reduction of colony number and size. Prevention of formation of inhibitory GRP78-caspase-7-complex, increase in VP-16-induced apoptosis (activation of caspase-7)	[209]
VP-16, 0.1 μM	EGCG, 10 μM	T-47D human **breast** cancer cell line	↑	Reduction of colony number and size. Prevention of formation of inhibitory GRP78-caspase-7-complex, increase in VP-16-induced apoptosis (activation of caspase-7)	[209]
VP-16, 50 μM	EGCG, 100 μM	HT-29 human **colon** cancer cell line	↑	Increase in VP-16-induced cell growth inhibition and apoptosis	[210]
VP-16, 0.5-4 μM	Fisetin, 18-36 μM	MG-63 human **osteosarcoma** cell line	↑	Dose-dependent effect: strongest antiproliferation with 36 μM fisetin and 0.5 μM VP-16 (CI 0.59). Increase in cells in G2 phase, decrease in G1 phase. Decrease in cyclin B1/E1 and Cdk1/2 levels	[205]
VP-16, 1, 1.5, 2.2 μM	Fisetin, 12.1, 31.6, 45.5 μM	Saos-2 human **osteosarcoma** cell line, p53-null	↑	Dose-dependent effect: strongest antiproliferation with 45.5 μM fisetin and 1 μM VP-16 (CI 1.11). Increase in cells in G2 phase, decrease in G1 phase. Decrease in cyclin E1 level	[205]
VP-16, 0-10 μg/ml	Genistein, 3, 10 μM	KB/MRP human **epidermoid** carcinoma cell line, expressing MRP1 not BCRP or P-gp	~	No reversal of (MRP-1-mediated) VP-16 resistance	[197]
VP-16, 0-10 μg/ml	Genistein, 3, 10 μM	KB-3-1 human **epidermoid** carcinoma cell line, no expressing BCRP, P-gp or MRP1	~	No reversal of VP-16 resistance	[197]

Drug	Flavonoid	Biological system	Direction of combination	Effects	Ref.
VP-16, 0.25 μg/ml	Genistein, 25 μg/ml	NCI-H358 human non-small cell **lung** cancer cell line	~	No effect on VP-16 anticancer activity	[126]
VP-16, 5 μg/ml	Genistein, 40 μg/ml	NCI-H596 human non-small cell **lung** cancer cell line	↑	Increase in proliferation suppression. Inhibition of EGFR phosphorylation, induction of apoptosis (PARP cleavage)	[126]
VP-16, 6.5 μM	Hesperetin, 281 μM	U2OS human **osteosarcoma** cell line	↑	Additivity in cell growth inhibition. Increase in G2 phase cell cycle arrest	[203]
VP-16, 0.1 nM-1 mM	Naringenin, 1 mM	HTB26 human **breast** cancer cell line	↑	Increase in VP-16-induced cytotoxicity	[10]
VP-16, 0.1 nM-1 mM	Naringenin, 1 mM	SW1116 human **colorectal** cancer cell line	↑	Increase in VP-16-induced cytotoxicity	[10]
VP-16, 0-10 μg/ml	Naringenin, 3, 10 μM	KB/MRP human **epidermoid** carcinoma cell line, expressing MRP1 not BCRP or P-gp	~	No reversal of (MRP1-mediated) VP-16 resistance	[197]
VP-16, 0-10 μg/ml	Naringenin, 3, 10 μM	KB-3-1 human **epidermoid** carcinoma cell line, no expressing BCRP, P-gp or MRP1	~	No reversal of VP-16 resistance	[197]
VP-16	Quercetin	CCRF-CEM human acute lymphoblastic **leukemia** cell line, p53-null	↑	Synergistic anticancer effect; induction of apoptosis (activation of caspases-3/-8/-9), increase in S and G2/M phase cell cycle arrest. Decrease in GSH, increase in DNA damage	[206]
VP-16	Quercetin	Jurkat human peripheral **blood** T-cell leukemia cell line, p53-null	↑	Synergistic anticancer effect; induction of apoptosis (activation of caspases-3/-8/-9), increase in G2/M phase cell cycle arrest. Decrease in GSH, increase in DNA damage	[206]
VP-16	Quercetin	KG-1a human myelogenous **leukemia** cell line, p53-null	↑	Synergistic anticancer effect; induction of apoptosis (activation of caspases-3/-8/-9). Decrease in GSH, increase in DNA damage	[206]
VP-16	Quercetin	THP-1 human acute monocytic **leukemia** cell line, p53-null	↑	Synergistic anticancer effect; induction of apoptosis (activation of caspases-3/-8/-9), increase in S and G2/M phase cell cycle arrest. Decrease in GSH, increase in DNA damage	[206]
VP-16, in dual-loaded PLGA NPs	Quercetin, in dual-loaded PLGA-NPs	MCF-7 human **breast** adenocarcinoma cell line	↑	Increase in VP-16-induced cytotoxicity. Inhibition of P-gp, decrease in VP-16 efflux, increase in VP-16 uptake	[201]
VP-16, 0.01-0.05 μg/ml	Quercetin, 0.1, 1 μM	Primary **endometrial** cancer cells	~	No increase in VP-16-induced antiproliferative activity	[90]
VP-16, 0.01-0.05 μg/ml	Quercetin, 0.1, 1 μM	Primary **ovarian** cancer cells	~	No increase in VP-16-induced antiproliferative activity	[90]
VP-16, 0.003-3 μM	Rhamnetin, 3 μM	HepG2 human **hepatocellular** carcinoma cell line	↑	Increase in VP-16-induced growth inhibition. Enhancement of anchorage-independent cell growth, increase in S phase cell cycle arrest. Suppression of miR-34a-mediated Notch-1	[207]
VP-16, 0.003-3 μM	Rhamnetin, 3 μM	HepG2/ADR, human **hepatocellular** carcinoma cell line, DOX-resistant, MDR features	↑	Increase in sensitivity, decrease in VP-16 IC_{50}	[207]
VP-16, 0-50 μM	Silibinin, 50 μM	LN229 human **glioma** cell line, mutant p53	↑	Additive effect on VP-16-induced cytotoxicity	[28]
VP-16, 1.5-24 μM	Silibinin, 12.5-200 μM	H69 human small-cell **lung** carcinoma cell line	~	No effect on VP-16-induced cytotoxicity	[167]
VP-16, 1.5-24 μM	Silibinin, 12.5-200 μM	VPA17 human small-cell **lung** carcinoma cell line, VP-16-resistant H69 cells, overexpressing P-gp	↑	Synergism in cytotoxicity (CI<1), decrease in VP-16 IC_{50}. Reversal of MDR	[167]
VP-16, 5 μM	Wogonin, 5-30 μM	HL-60 human **leukemia** cell line	↑	Potentiation of VP-16-induced apoptosis. Inhibition of P-gp, increase in VP-16 cellular content	[204]

Table 6.12. (Continued)

Drug	Flavonoid	Biological system	Direction of combination	Effects	Ref.
VP-16, 5 μM	Wogonin, 10 μM	HL-60 human **leukemia** cell line	↑	Potentiation of VP-16-induced apoptosis	[154]
VP-16, 1, 10 μM	Wogonin, 10 μM	HL-60 human **leukemia** cell line	↑	Potentiation of VP-16-induced cytotoxicity. Slight increase in VP-16 intracellular content	[153]
VP-16, 5 μM	Wogonin, 10 μM	Jurkat human **leukemia** cell line	↑	About 4-fold increase in VP-16-induced apoptosis (caspase activation)	[154]
VP-16, 1, 10 μM	Wogonin, 10 μM	Jurkat human **leukemia** cell line	↑	Potentiation of VP-16-induced cytotoxicity and apoptosis. Increase in VP-16 intracellular content	[153]
VP-16, 25-100 μg/ml	Wogonin, 20, 40, 60 μM	HepG2 human **hepatocellular** carcinoma cell line, wild-type p53	↑	Increase in VP-16-induced cytotoxicity. Suppression of Nrf2	[152]
VP-16, 5 μM	Wogonin, 10 μM	A549 human non-small cell **lung** cancer cell line	↑	Increase in VP-16-induced cell death	[154]
VP-16, 1, 10 μM	Wogonin, 25 μM	A549 human **lung** cancer cell line	↑	Weak potentiation of VP-16-induced cytotoxicity	[153]
VP-16, 5 μM	Wogonin, 10 μM	NCI-H226 human non-small cell **lung** cancer cell line	↑	Increase in VP-16-induced cell death	[154]
VP-16, 10, 100 μM	Wogonin, 25 μM	NCI-H226 human **lung** cancer cell line	↑	Weak potentiation of VP-16-induced cytotoxicity	[153]

Akt, protein kinase B; Bax, Bcl-2-associated X protein; Cdk, cyclin-dependent kinase; CI, combination index; EGFR, epidermal growth factor receptor; GRP, glucose-regulated protein; GSH, glutathione; MDR, multidrug resistance; miR, microRNA; MRP, multidrug resistance-associated protein; Nrf2, nuclear factor (erythroid-derived 2)-like 2; PARP, poly (ADP-ribose) polymerase; P-gp, P-glycoprotein.

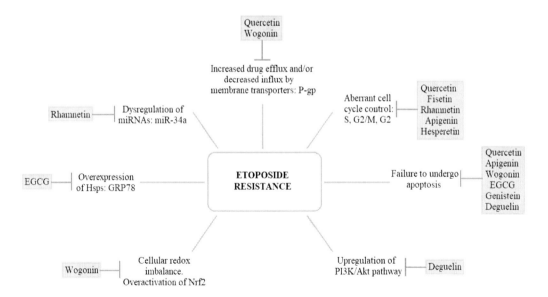

Figure 6.7. Possibilities to intervene in etoposide resistance with flavonoids (Akt, protein kinase B; GRP, glucose-regulated protein; Hsp, heat shock protein; miR, microRNA; Nrf2, nuclear factor (erythroid-derived 2)-like 2; P-gp, P-glycoprotein; PI3K, phosphoinositide 3-kinase).

sensitized human leukemia HL-60 cells to VP-16-induced apoptosis, suppressing P-gp function and increasing intracellular drug accumulation [153, 154, 204]. Similar potentiation of proapoptotic properties of VP-16 was observed also in another human leukemia cell line Jurkat in the presence of wogonin [153, 154]. In addition, wogonin augmented VP-16-induced cytotoxicity in human non-small cell lung cancer cell lines A549 and NCI-H226 [153, 154], and in human hepatocellular carcinoma cell line HepG2 [152]. In HepG2 cells, wogonin sensitized malignant cells to VP-16 via blocking of the translocation of Nrf2 into nucleus and regulating downstream target genes, including MRP transporter genes [152]. These findings indicate that wogonin could be used as a chemotherapeutic adjuvant to increase the pharmacological action of VP-16 against leukemia cells but also lung and liver tumor cells, thereby ameliorating adverse reactions related to the clinical use of this antineoplastic agent (Table 6.12).

The major green tea flavanol *EGCG* directly interacted with GRP78 and prevented the formation of antiapoptotic complex between GRP78 and caspase-7, thereby promoting VP-16-induced apoptosis in human breast cancer cell lines MDA-MB-231 and T47D [209]. EGCG potentiated cell growth inhibitory and proapoptotic effects of VP-16 also in human colon cancer HT-29 cells [210]. EGCG could thus chemosensitize certain breast and colon tumor cells towards VP-16 (Table 6.12). The only *in vivo* study performed so far revealed augmentation of antileukemic properties of VP-16 in the presence of *epicatechin* in Brown Norway rats with acute myeloid leukemia. At that, epicatechin increased drug-induced oxidative stress, and enhanced proapoptotic action of VP-16 in the spleen and bone marrow of rats [202].

Cotreatment of human osteosarcoma U2OS cells with flavanone *hesperetin* and VP-16 revealed additive effects in cell growth inhibition and caused cell cycle arrest at G2 phase [203]. Another flavanone *naringenin* markedly increased VP-16-induced cytotoxicity in human breast cancer HTB26 cells and human colorectal cancer SW1116 cells [10], but did not affect resistance to VP-16 in human epidermoid carcinoma cell line KB-3-1 and its MRP1-transfected subline KB/MRP [197]. The sensitivity of these two human epidermoid carcinoma lines to anticancer action of VP-16 was not altered also by soy isoflavone *genistein* [197]. However, genistein as a general tyrosine kinase inhibitor, enhanced antiproliferative and proapoptotic activities of VP-16 in human non-small cell lung cancer NCI-H596 cells that strongly express EGFR, but not in NCI-H358 cells with only weak level of EGFR, suggesting that inhibition of EGFR phosphorylation is one of the potential mechanisms to chemosensitize malignant cells towards VP-16 [126]. Although flavonolignan *silibinin* exerted no effects on the VP-16-induced cytotoxicity in human small-cell lung carcinoma H69 cells, pretreatment of VP-16-resistant H69 cells, VPA17, with silibinin prior to addition of VP-16 led to synergistic anticancer responses and reversal of resistance phenotype [167]. In addition, silibinin potentiated the antitumor activity of VP-16 also in human glioma LN229 cells [28]. The only studied rotenoid, *deguelin*, suppressed PI3K/Akt signaling pathway in human leukemia cell line U937 and sensitized these cells to VP-16-induced apoptosis, even at very low 10 nM concentration. As parental line HL60PT does not possess an active PI3K/Akt pathway, cytotoxic action of VP-16 in these cells was not affected by deguelin. Thus, decrease in Akt phosphorylation is an important step in chemosensitization of leukemia cells towards VP-

220   *Katrin Sak*

16, whereas PI3K inhibitor deguelin might be of clinical benefit as a potent chemotherapeutic adjuvant in treatment of leukemia patients in the future [211] (Table 6.12).

To date, no contraindicative combinations with flavonoids and VP-16 have been described suggesting that based on the current knowledge, intake of flavonoids is not contravened for patients who are receiving treatment with VP-16. Although more preclinical studies and also clinical trials are needed, several investigated flavonoids might prove to be potential novel candidates for natural non-toxic adjuvants in VP-16 chemotherapeutic treatment of both leukemias and some solid tumors (including poorly treatable osteosarcoma) to lower the drug dosage and reduce severe adverse reactions related to clinical use of VP-16. Development of such combinatorial strategies might lead to better therapeutic responses, improve quality of life of patients and prolong their survival.

Doxorubicin (DOX)

Doxorubicin (DOX) is a naturally occurring anthracycline antibiotic that is produced by a variant of *Streptomyeces peucetius* (*var. caesius*) [212-214]. DOX was first discovered in the 1960s as a promising therapeutic option in the treatment of acute leukemia and lymphoma [215]. This first-generation anthracycline has been one of the most frequently used anticancer drugs and is still an important cornerstone in the treatment of various types of solid tumors and hematological malignancies [216-218]. It has many clinical indications in oncology in adults, but is also commonly used for the treatment of a variety of childhood cancers [219]. DOX has been administered for a broad spectrum of malignancies, including lung, breast, ovarian, prostate, gastric, colon, liver, pancreatic and thyroid cancers, neuroblastoma, soft tissue sarcoma, multiple myeloma, leukemia, lymphoma and melanoma [62, 164, 185, 212, 213, 215, 220-234]. DOX is a Topo II inhibitor that accumulates in the nucleus where it interacts with DNA by intercalation between DNA base pairs on the double helix and inhibits the progression of Topo II, an enzyme responsible for DNA helix conformation and stability. Stabilized ternary complex of DOX, Topo II and DNA prevents religation of the DNA strands and induces permanent DNA damage [184, 185, 203, 220, 222, 228, 235-239]. Therefore, treatment with DOX can lead to inhibition of cell proliferation, G2/M phase cell cycle arrest and apoptotic death of tumor cells, mostly via mitochondrial pathway but also through death receptor signaling [139, 185, 222, 223, 229, 239-241]. In addition, cytotoxic action of DOX is partly associated also with production of ROS (hydroxyl radicals) and induction of oxidative stress [109, 216, 221, 236, 238, 239, 242]. However, besides malignant cells, DOX can induce serious oxidative DNA damage also in non-tumoral cells, resulting in severe adverse reactions and impairing the functions of heart, liver, kidney, brain and immune system [185, 214, 216, 234]. Indeed, despite strong antitumor efficacy and potency, the clinical use of DOX is severely hindered because of cumulative toxicity, low water solubility, poor drug delivery to the tumor site throughout the body and development of multidrug resistance (MDR) [212-214, 217, 219-221, 223, 226, 229, 232, 243-245]. Several MRPs are involved in elimination of DOX metabolites from the cells, including P-gp, MRP1, MRP2 and BCRP; however, different tested compounds have revealed only poor efficiency in prevention from MDR [219, 236, 242]. In addition, nanotechnological approaches have been used to improve the targeting of drug to malignant cells, encapsulating DOX in different nanocarriers [214, 219, 224]. As a result, Doxil® as the first cancer nanomedicine approved by the US FDA was prepared [220]. However, administration of DOX is still related to severe systemic toxicity and several undesirable adverse effects, including cardiotoxicity, hepatotoxicity, nephrotoxicity, myelosuppression, hypertension and stomatitis [216, 218, 220, 224, 234, 246]. Among these health problems, the major limiting factor of DOX therapeutic potential is cardiotoxicity manifesting in the worst circumstances even in its most severe form of fatal congestive heart failure. This irreversible life-threatening damage on myocardial cells may occur either during the administration of DOX therapy or months to many years after the termination of treatment with DOX, whereas the severity of condition is potentiated when the drug doses are increased [212, 214, 215, 219, 228, 238, 247]. Comprehensive studies have shown that the risk of development of congestive heart failure is even more than 25% when the cumulative doses reach to 550 mg/m^2, whereas the associated fatality rate is about 30-50% [215]. Therefore, a lifetime cumulative dose limit of 450-550 mg/mg^2 has been established [232]. The current major focus of DOX research is to find alternative strategies to minimize DOX toxicity on normal healthy tissues and improve therapeutic efficacy [212, 238]. These approaches involve intense cardiac monitoring, application of new anthracycline analogs with lower cardiotoxicity, and introduction of novel non-toxic cardioprotective agents in the treatment regimens with DOX [215]. Although in the past 40 years numerous agents have been explored to ameliorate serious cardiotoxicity caused by DOX, only the compound dexrazoxane is used as a cardioprotective agent in clinical settings. Nevertheless, this compound can compromise the antineoplastic activity of DOX and increase the latent risk for development of acute myeloid leukemia and other malignancies, especially in pediatric cancer patients [215]. Therefore, identification of novel safe adjuvant compounds which are able to sensitize DOX-based chemotherapy, allow to reduce drug dosages without attenuating therapeutic potential, and thereby mitigate life-threatening side effects is urgently needed.

Table 6.13. Effects of flavonoids on anticancer action of doxorubicin (DOX) *in vitro* conditions

Drug	Flavonoid	Biological system	Direction of combination	Effects	Ref.
DOX, 10 nM	Acacetin, 25 μM	A549 human non-small cell **lung** cancer cell line	↑	Synergism in cytotoxicity (CI<1), inhibition of colony forming ability. Increase in G2/M phase cell cycle arrest (decrease in CDC2). Decrease in DOX efflux, increase in DOX cellular accumulation, downregulation of MDR1	[212]
DOX, 25 nM	Acacetin, 25 μM	H1299 human non-small cell **lung** cancer cell line	↑	Synergism in cytotoxicity (CI<1). Increase in intracellular DOX accumulation	[212]
DOX	Alopecurone B, 10 μM	MG-63-DOX human **osteosarcoma** cell line, MDR, DOX-resistant	↑	14.35-fold decrease in DOX IC_{50}, reversal of MDR. Increase in DOX-induced apoptosis, inhibition of P-gp via NF-κB signaling, increase in DOX cellular accumulation	[235]
DOX	Apigenin	CCRF-CEM human acute lymphoblastic **leukemia** cell line, p53-null	↑	Synergistic anticancer effect; induction of apoptosis (activation of caspases-3/-8/-9), increase in S and G2/M phase cell cycle arrest. Decrease in GSH, increase in DNA damage	[206]
DOX	Apigenin	Jurkat human peripheral **blood** T-cell leukemia cell line, p53-null	↑	Synergistic anticancer effect; induction of apoptosis (activation of caspases-3/-8/-9), increase in G2/M phase cell cycle arrest. Decrease in GSH, increase in DNA damage	[206]
DOX	Apigenin	KG-1a human myelogenous **leukemia** cell line, p53-null	↑	Additive anticancer effect; induction of apoptosis (activation of caspases-3/-8/-9). Decrease in GSH, increase in DNA damage	[206]
DOX	Apigenin	THP-1 human acute monocytic **leukemia** cell line, p53-null	↑	Synergistic anticancer effect; induction of apoptosis (activation of caspases-3/-8/-9), increase in S and G2/M phase cell cycle arrest. Decrease in GSH, increase in DNA damage	[206]
DOX, 10, 40 nM	Apigenin, 5, 10 μM	L1210 murine **leukemia** cell line	↓	Decrease in DOX-induced cytotoxicity. Shift from G2/M to S phase arrest of cell cycle	[84]
DOX	Apigenin, μM level	HCC1806 human **breast** cancer cell line, ER-negative, PR-negative, p53-deficient	↑	Potentiation of DOX-induced growth inhibition, induction of apoptosis	[266]
DOX	Apigenin, μM level	HCC70 human **breast** cancer cell line, ER-positive, PR-negative, wild-type p53	↑	Potentiation of DOX-induced growth inhibition, induction of apoptosis	[266]
DOX	Apigenin, μM level	MDA-MB-157 human **breast** cancer cell line, ER-negative, PR-negative, p53-deficient	↑	Potentiation of DOX-induced growth inhibition, induction of apoptosis	[266]
DOX	Apigenin, μM level	MDA-MB-468 human **breast** cancer cell line, ER-negative, PR-negative, mutant p53	↑	Potentiation of DOX-induced growth inhibition, induction of apoptosis	[266]

Drug	Flavonoid	Biological system	Direction of combination	Effects	Ref.
DOX, 0-8 μM	Apigenin	BEL-7402/ADM human **hepatocellular** carcinoma cell line, DOX-resistant	↑	Increase in sensitivity to DOX. Inhibition of miR-520b/ATG7-related autophagy	[268]
DOX, 0.5-8 μM	Apigenin, 10 μM	BEL-7402/ADM human **hepatocellular** carcinoma cell line, DOX-resistant	↑	3.41-fold decrease in DOX IC_{50}. Potentiation of apoptosis, increase in DOX cellular accumulation. Reduction of Nrf2 expression through downregulation of PI3K/Akt pathway	[267]
DOX, 2, 8 μM	Apigenin, 10 μM	MES-SA/Dx5 human **uterine** sarcoma cell line, DOX-resistant, overexpressing P-gp	↑	Increase in DOX-induced cytotoxicity. Enhancement of DOX cellular accumulation. Decrease in GSH content, increase in ROS production	[263]
DOX, in HA-decorated dual-loaded NLCs	Baicalein, in HA-decorated dual-loaded NLCs	MCF-7/ADR human **breast** cancer cell line, DOX-resistant	↑	Synergism in cytotoxicity	[213]
DOX, 5-40 μM	Baicalin, 5, 10 μM	HL-60/ADM human acute myeloid **leukemia** cell line, DOX-resistant	↑	1.89-fold decrease in DOX IC_{50} at 5 μM, 3.02-fold at 10 μM baicalin. Inhibition of PI3K/Akt pathway, downregulation of MRP1 and LRP, increase in DOX cellular concentration	[278]
DOX, 2.5-40 μM	Barbigerone, 0.5-4 μM	MCF-7 human **breast** cancer cell line	~	No effect on DOX-induced cytotoxicity	[293]
DOX, 2.5-160 μM	Barbigerone, 0.5-4 μM	MCF-7/ADR human **breast** cancer cell line, DOX-resistant	↑	Increase in DOX cytotoxicity, reversal of MDR. Increase in DOX uptake, decrease in efflux, relocalization of DOX to nuclei. Inhibition of P-gp (ATPase) activity	[293]
DOX, 0-300 μM	Biochanin A, 100 μM	MDA435/LCC6 human **breast** cancer cell line, E2-independent, moderate expression P-gp, no MRP1	↑	Increase in DOX-induced cytotoxicity, 10.3-fold decrease in DOX IC_{50}. Inhibition of P-gp-mediated DOX efflux	[264]
DOX, 0-300 μM	Biochanin A, 100 μM	MDA435/LCC6MDR1 human **breast** cancer cell line, E2-independent, MDR, P-gp-positive, no MRP1	↑	Increase in DOX-induced cytotoxicity, 37.83-fold decrease in DOX IC_{50}. Inhibition of P-gp-mediated DOX efflux	[264]
DOX, 0.1-100 μM	Biochanin A, 1-100 μM	ColoR human **colorectal** adenocarcinoma cell line, DOX-resistant COLO205 cells	↑	Increase in sensitivity to DOX	[290]
DOX, 5-10 μM, co-encapsulated into liposomes	Biochanin A, 20-80 μM, co-encapsulated into liposomes	ColoR human **colorectal** adenocarcinoma cell line, DOX-resistant COLO205 cells	↑	Increase in sensitivity to DOX, reversal of resistance. Increase in DOX cellular uptake	[290]
DOX, 50 μg/ml	Calycosin, 10 μg/ml	BGC823 human **gastric** cancer cell line	↑	Increase in DOX antiproliferative effect. Suppression of migration potential	[139]
DOX, 50 μg/ml	Calycosin, 10 μg/ml	NCI-N87 human **gastric** cancer cell line	↑	Increase in DOX antiproliferative effect. Suppression of migration potential	[139]
DOX, 50 μg/ml	Calycosin, 10 μg/ml	SGC7901 human **gastric** cancer cell line	↑	Increase in DOX antiproliferative effect. Suppression of migration potential	[139]
DOX, 1-8 μM	(+)-Catechin, 5 μM	HCT-8 human **colorectal** adenocarcinoma cell line	~	No effect on DOX anticancer efficacy	[216]

Table 6.13. (Continued)

Drug	Flavonoid	Biological system	Direction of combination	Effects	Ref.
DOX, 10 nM-2 μM	Catechin, 3 μg/ml, in NGO Dex-CT nanohybrids	BE(2)C human neuroblastoma cell line	↑	Synergism in growth inhibition (CI<0.9)	[285]
DOX, 1-200 μM	Catechin, 3 μg/ml, in NGO Dex-CT nanohybrids	BE(2)C/ADR human neuroblastoma cell line, DOX-resistant	↑	Synergism in growth inhibition (CI<0.5), reversal of DOX resistance. Decrease in P-gp expression	[285]
DOX, 10, 40 nM	Chrysin, 5, 10 μM	L1210 murine leukemia cell line	→	Decrease in DOX-induced cytotoxicity. Shift from G2/M to S phase arrest of cell cycle	[84]
DOX, 3.25-120 μM	Chrysin, 10 μM	MCF7/ADM human breast cancer cell line, DOX-resistant	↑	Sensitization of cells to DOX	[271]
DOX, 0.5-8 μM	Chrysin, 10 μM	BEL-7402/ADM human hepatocellular carcinoma cell line, DOX-resistant cells	↑	Increase in DOX cytotoxicity, reversal of resistance. Increase in DOX cellular accumulation, downregulation of Nrf2 through inhibiting PI3K/Akt and ERK pathway	[271]
DOX, 0.025-2 μM	Chrysin, 5-30 μM	A549 human non-small cell lung cancer cell line	↑	Synergism in DOX-induced cytotoxicity (CI<1), partly through chrysin-mediated intracellular GSH depletion	[242]
DOX, 0.025-2 μM	Chrysin, 5-30 μM	H157 human non-small cell lung cancer cell line	↑	Synergism in DOX-induced cytotoxicity (CI<1), partly through chrysin-mediated intracellular GSH depletion	[242]
DOX, 0.025-2 μM	Chrysin, 5-30 μM	H1975 human non-small cell lung cancer cell line	↑	Synergism in DOX-induced cytotoxicity (CI<1), partly through chrysin-mediated intracellular GSH depletion	[242]
DOX, 0.02-2.5 μM	Chrysin, 5 μM	H23 human non-small cell lung cancer cell line	↑	Overcoming IL-6-induced chemoresistance. Inhibition of IL-6-induced AKR1C1/1C2 expression	[270]
DOX, 0.025-2 μM	Chrysin, 5-30 μM	H460 human non-small cell lung cancer cell line	↑	Synergism in DOX-induced cytotoxicity (CI<1), partly through chrysin-mediated intracellular GSH depletion	[242]
DOX	CJY, 1-10 μM	K562 human myelogenous leukemia cell line	~	No effect on DOX-induced cytotoxicity	[292]
DOX	CJY, 1-10 μM	K562/DOX human myelogenous leukemia cell line, DOX-resistant	↑	Reversal of resistance to DOX. Elevation of DOX-induced apoptosis, increase in G2/M phase cell cycle arrest. Increase in DOX cellular accumulation	[292]
DOX, 1 μM	Deguelin, 5 μM	A549 human lung cancer cell line, wild-type p53	↑	Increase in sensitivity to DOX. Concurrent PUMA induction through both p53-dependent and -independent pathways by DOX and deguelin, respectively, promotion of apoptosis (increase in caspase-3)	[305]
DOX, 1 μM	Deguelin, 5 μM	H1299 human lung cancer cell line, mutant p53	↑	Increase in sensitivity to DOX. Concurrent PUMA induction through both p53-dependent and -independent pathways by DOX and deguelin, respectively, promotion of apoptosis (increase in caspase-3)	[305]

Drug	Flavonoid	Biological system	Direction of combination	Effects	Ref.
DOX, 1, 2.5, 5 μM	Deguelin, 25 μM	MIA PaCa-2 human **pancreatic** cancer cell line	↑	Increase in DOX-induced cytotoxicity, inhibition of colony formation. Augmentation of apoptosis (cleavage of caspase-3 and PARP) by suppression of DOX-induced autophagy	[306]
DOX, 1, 2.5, 5 μM	Deguelin, 25 μM	Panc-1 human **pancreatic** cancer cell line	↑	Increase in DOX-induced cytotoxicity, inhibition of colony formation. Augmentation of apoptosis (cleavage of caspase-3 and PARP) by suppression of DOX-induced autophagy	[306]
DOX, 0.25-4 μM	Dihydromyricetin, 12.5, 25 μM	HL-60 human **leukemia** cell line, p53-null	~	No effect on DOX-induced cell growth inhibition	[215]
DOX, 0.25-4 μM	Dihydromyricetin, 12.5, 25 μM	K-562 human **leukemia** cell line, mutant p53	~	No effect on DOX-induced cell growth inhibition	[215]
DOX, 0.25-4 μM	Dihydromyricetin, 12.5, 25 μM	U937 human **leukemia** cell line, wild-type p53	↑	Increase in DOX-induced cytotoxicity and apoptosis (decrease in $\Delta\Psi m$, upregulation of Bax, downregulation of Bcl-2, caspase-3 cleavage), accumulation of p53	[215]
DOX, 1, 2, 4 μM	Dihydromyricetin, 25 μM	A2780/DOX human **ovarian** cancer cell line, DOX-resistant, wild-type p53	↑	Sensitization of cells to DOX, increase in DOX-induced apoptosis (PARP cleavage). p53-mediated downregulation of survivin	[303]
DOX, 0-8 μg/ml	DMC, 4, 8 μM	BEL-7402/5-FU human **hepatocellular** carcinoma cell line, 5-FU-resistant	↑	1.71-fold increase in sensitivity to DOX at 4 μM, 2.35-fold at 8 μM DMC. Partial reversal of MDR	[299]
DOX, 0-5 μg/ml	DMC, 5 μM	KB-3-1 human **oral** epidermoid carcinoma cell line	~	No effect on DOX-induced cytotoxicity or intracellular DOX concentration	[298]
DOX, 0-20 μg/ml	DMC, 5 μM	KB-A1 human **oral** epidermoid carcinoma cell line, DOX-resistant, overexpressing P-gp	↑	Potentiation of DOX-induced cytotoxicity, 3.9-fold decrease in DOX IC_{50}, reversal of MDR phenotype. Increase in intracellular DOX accumulation, downregulation of MDR1 (P-gp) gene expression	[298]
DOX, 0.0001-100 μM	ECG, 1, 5, 10 μM	MCF-7/ADR human **breast** cancer cell line, DOX-resistant	↑	1.4-fold decrease in DOX resistance at 1 μM, 2.3-fold at 5 μM, 8.6-fold at 10 μM ECG	[255]
DOX, 1-8 μM	ECG, 5 μM	HCT-8 human **colorectal** adenocarcinoma cell line	~	No effect on DOX antiproliferative activity	[216]
DOX	ECG, 60 μg/ml	BEL-7404 human **hepatocellular** carcinoma cell line	↑	Increase in DOX-induced cytotoxicity, 2.76-fold decrease in DOX IC_{50}	[184]
DOX	ECG, 60 μg/ml	BEL-7404/DOX human **hepatocellular** carcinoma cell line, DOX-resistant	↑	Increase in DOX-induced cytotoxicity, 15.7-fold decrease in DOX IC_{50}. Downregulation of MDR1 gene expression, suppression of P-gp pump function, increase in DOX cellular concentration	[184]

Table 6.13. (Continued)

Drug	Flavonoid	Biological system	Direction of combination	Effects	Ref.
DOX, 0,0001-100 μM	ECG, 1, 5, 10 μM	KBCH^{R}8-5 human **oral** carcinoma cell line, overexpressing P-gp, MDR KB 3-1 cells	↑	1.4-fold decrease in DOX resistance at 1 μM, 2.3-fold at 5 μM, 7-fold at 10 μM ECG. Increase in DOX-induced G2/M phase cell cycle arrest and apoptosis, downregulation of P-gp by targeting Wnt/β-catenin signaling	[255]
DOX, 5 μg/ml	EGC, 10 μg/ml	S180-dox murine **sarcoma** cell line, DOX-resistant	↑~	Sensitization of cells to DOX when pretreated with EGCG for 24h. No effect with simultaneous treatment	[236]
DOX,1.5 μg/ml	EGC, 5 μg/ml	SW620-dox human **colon** carcinoma cell line, DOX-resistant	↑~	Sensitization of cells to DOX when pretreated with EGCG for 24h. No effect with simultaneous treatment	[236]
DOX, 1-8 μM	EGC, 5 μM	HCT-8 human **colorectal** adenocarcinoma cell line	~	No effect on DOX antiproliferative activity	[216]
DOX, 5 μg/ml	EGCG, 20 μg/ml	S180-dox murine **sarcoma** cell line, DOX-resistant	↑~	Sensitization of cells to DOX when pretreated with EGCG for 24h. No effect with simultaneous treatment	[236]
DOX, 0.5-100 μg/ml, co-loaded in PIC micelles	EGCG, co-loaded in PIC micelles	MCF-7/Adr human **breast** carcinoma cell line, DOX-resistant	↑	Reversal of MDR, increase in cytotoxicity. Inhibition of DOX efflux, enhancement of DOX accumulation	[214]
DOX, 1.5 μg/ml	EGCG, 10 μg/ml	SW620-dox human **colon** carcinoma cell line, DOX-resistant	↑~	Sensitization of cells to DOX when pretreated with EGCG for 24h. No effect with simultaneous treatment	[236]
DOX, 1-8 μM	EGCG, 5 μM	HCT-8 human **colorectal** adenocarcinoma cell line	~	No effect on DOX-induced antiproliferative activity	[216]
DOX, 0.2 μg/ml	EGCG, 5, 25 μg/ml	Eca109/ABCG2 human **esophageal** squamous cell carcinoma cell line, ABCG2 gene-transfected	↑	Reversal of DOX resistance. Decrease in ABCG2 expression, increase in DOX cellular concentration. Increase in DOX-induced apoptosis (decrease in $\Delta\Psi m$)	[282]
DOX	EGCG, 14 μg/ml	BEL-7404 human **hepatocellular** carcinoma cell line	↑	Increase in DOX-induced cytotoxicity, 2.76-fold decrease in DOX IC$_{50}$	[184]
DOX	EGCG, 10 μM	BEL-7404 human **hepatocellular** carcinoma cell line	~	No effect on DOX-induced cytotoxicity	[284]
DOX	EGCG, 14 μg/ml	BEL-7404/DOX human **hepatocellular** carcinoma cell line, DOX-resistant	↑	Increase in DOX-induced cytotoxicity, 19-fold decrease in DOX IC$_{50}$. Downregulation of MDR1 gene expression, suppression of P-gp pump function, increase in DOX cellular concentration	[184]
DOX	EGCG, 10 μM	BEL-7404/DOX human **hepatocellular** cancer cell line, DOX-resistant	↑	Reversal of DOX resistance, 5.49-fold decrease in DOX IC$_{50}$. Increase in apoptosis, decrease in HIF-1α and MDR1/P-gp expression	[284]
DOX, 0.725-10 μM	EGCG, 2.5-40 μg/ml	Hep3B human **hepatocellular** carcinoma cell line	↑	Synergism in DOX anticancer activity (CI<1). Increase in apoptosis, inhibition of DOX-induced autophagy	[221]

Drug	Flavonoid	Biological system	Direction of combination	Effects	Ref.
DOX, 0.0625-1 μM	EGCG, 5-80 μg/ml	HepG2 human **hepatocellular** carcinoma cell line	↑	Synergism in DOX anticancer activity (CI<1)	[221]
DOX	EGCG, 10 μg/ml	KB-3-1 human **oral** epidermoid carcinoma cell line	~	No effect on DOX cytotoxicity	[279]
DOX, 0-20 μg/ml	EGCG, 10 μg/ml	KB-3-1 human **oral** epidermoid carcinoma cell line	~	No effect on DOX-induced cytotoxicity	[243]
DOX	EGCG, 10 μg/ml	KB-3-1 human **oral** epidermoid carcinoma cell line	~	No effect on DOX-induced cytotoxicity	[280]
DOX, 0-20 μg/ml	EGCG, 20 μM	KB-A1 human **oral** carcinoma cell line, MDR KB-3-1 cells, overexpressing P-gp	↑	Reversal of MDR, 2.3-fold decrease in DOX IC_{50}. Increase in DOX cellular accumulation	[281]
DOX	EGCG, 10 μg/ml	KB-A-1 human **oral** epidermoid carcinoma cell line, MDR KB-3-1 cells, overexpressing MDR1	↑	Reversal of MDR, 2.5-fold increase in DOX cytotoxicity. Increase in DOX cellular accumulation through increase in DOX influx and decrease in DOX efflux, inhibition of P-gp ATPase activity and downregulation of MDR1 gene expression	[279]
DOX, 0-20 μg/ml	EGCG, 10 μg/ml	KB-A-1 human **oral** epidermoid carcinoma cell line, MDR KB-3-1 cells	↑	Reversal of MDR, 2.5-fold increase in DOX cytotoxicity	[243]
DOX	EGCG, 10 μg/ml	KB-A-1 human **oral** epidermoid carcinoma cell line, MDR KB-3-1 cells	↑	Reversal of MDR, 2.5-fold decrease in DOX IC_{50}. Lowering DOX-induced ROS level	[280]
DOX	EGCG, 10 μg/ml	KB-A-1 human **oral** epidermoid carcinoma cell line, DOX-resistant	↑	Reversal of MDR, 4.4-fold decrease in DOX IC_{50}. Increase in DOX cellular concentration	[244]
DOX, 2 nM	EGCG, 20 μM	IBC-10a human **prostate** cancer cell line	↑	Almost complete inhibition of cell growth	[283]
DOX, in EGCG/ GLT-DOX-coated AuNPs	EGCG, in EGCG/ GLT-DOX-coated AuNPs	PC-3 human highly metastatic **prostate** cancer cell line, DOX-resistant	↑	Increase in proliferation inhibition. Increase in DOX uptake via Lam 67R receptor-mediated endocytosis, increase in DOX cellular accumulation	[220]
DOX, 2 nM	EGCG, 10-60 μM	PC-3ML human **prostate** cancer cell line	↑	Potentiation of cell growth inhibition, suppression of colony formation. Increase in DOX retention	[283]
DOX	EGCG, ethylated (Y6), 10, 15 μM	BEL-7404 human **hepatocellular** cancer cell line	~	No effect on DOX-induced cytotoxicity	[284]
DOX	EGCG, ethylated (Y6), 10, 15 μM	BEL-7404/DOX human **hepatocellular** cancer cell line, DOX-resistant	↑	Reversal of DOX resistance; 7.7-fold decrease in DOX IC_{50} at 10 μM, 10.1-fold at 15 μM Y6). Increase in apoptosis, decrease in HIF-1α and MDR1/P-gp expression	[284]
DOX, 1-8 μM	Epicatechin, 5 μM	HCT-8 human **colorectal** adenocarcinoma cell line	~	No effect on DOX antiproliferative activity	[216]
DOX, 1 μM	Eupatorin, 100 μM	HT-29 human **colon** cancer cell line	↑	Increase in antiproliferative action, potentiation of DOX-induced apoptosis (increase in Bax/Bcl-2 ratio, caspase-3, PARP cleavage), increase in ROS production	[245]

Table 6.13. (Continued)

Drug	Flavonoid	Biological system	Direction of combination	Effects	Ref.
DOX, 1 μM	Eupatorin, 100 μM	SW948 human **colon** cancer cell line	↑	Increase in antiproliferative action, potentiation of DOX-induced apoptosis (increase in Bax/Bcl-2 ratio, caspase-3, PARP cleavage), increase in ROS production	[245]
DOX, 10 nM	Fisetin, 10 μM	A549 human non-small cell **lung** cancer cell line	↓	Antagonism in cytotoxic activity	[212]
DOX, 25 nM	Fisetin, 10 μM	H1299 human non-small cell **lung** cancer cell line	↓↑	Time-dependent mechanism: antagonism in cytotoxic activity at 48h coincubation, synergism at 72h	[212]
DOX, 300 nM	Fisetin, 25 μM	H1299 human **lung** adenocarcinoma cell line	↑	Increase in DOX-induced cytotoxicity	[105]
DOX, 2, 8 μM	Fisetin, 10 μM	MES-SA/Dx5 human **uterine** sarcoma cell line, DOX resistant, overexpressing P-gp	↑	Increase in DOX-induced cytotoxicity. Increase in DOX cellular accumulation, reduction of ROS	[263]
DOX	Formononetin, 100 μM	T98G human **glioma** cell line	↑	Increase in DOX-induced cytotoxicity	[291]
DOX	Formononetin, 100 μM	U215MG human **glioma** cell line	↑	Increase in DOX-induced cytotoxicity	[291]
DOX	Formononetin, 100 μM	U87MG human **glioma** cell line	↑	Increase in DOX-induced cytotoxicity. Reversal of EMT (decrease in vimentin, increase in E-cadherin) through suppression of HDAC5	[291]
DOX, 0.25-3 μM	Galangin, 50 μM	HCT-15 human **colon** carcinoma cell line, expressing P-gp	↓	Decrease in DOX-induced cytotoxicity, doubling of DOX IC_{50}. Increase in DOX efflux, inhibition of DOX accumulation	[261]
DOX, 10, 40 nM	Galangin, 5, 10 μM	L1210 murine **leukemia** cell line	↓	Decrease in DOX-induced cytotoxicity. Shift from G2/M to S phase arrest of cell cycle	[84]
DOX, 5-100 μM	Genistein, 25, 50 μM	MCF-7 human **mammary** tumor cell line, ER-positive	↓~	Decrease in sensitivity to DOX, promotion of resistance at 50 μM genistein. No effect at 25 μM genistein	[287]
DOX	Genistein	MCF-7/WT human **breast** cancer cell line, ER-positive	↓↑	Moderate synergism in proliferation inhibition (at molar ratio 1:4000, DOX:GEN). Antagonism at low f_a values	[288]
DOX, 0.07-70 μM	Genistein, 30 μM	MCF-7/Adr human **breast** cancer cell line, DOX-resistant	↑	Synergism in DOX-induced cytotoxicity. Increase in DOX-induced G2/M phase cell cycle arrest and apoptosis, P-gp-independent increase in DOX cellular accumulation, suppression of HER2/neu expression	[223]
DOX	Genistein	MCF-7/ADR^R human **breast** cancer cell line, ER-negative, MDR, DOX-resistant	↑	Additivity in proliferation inhibition (at molar ratio 1:4, DOX:GEN)	[288]
DOX, 50 ng/ml	Genistein, 30 μM	MDA-MB-231 human **breast** cancer cell line	↑	Synergism in cell growth inhibition (CI 0.57). Increase in apoptosis	[62]
DOX, 5-100 μM	Genistein, 25, 50 μM	MDA-MB-231 human **mammary** tumor cell line, ER-negative	↑	Increase in sensitivity to DOX	[287]

Drug	Flavonoid	Biological system	Direction of combination	Effects	Ref.
DOX	Genistein	MDA-231 human **breast** cancer cell line, ER-negative	↑	Synergism in proliferation inhibition (at molar ratio 1:4000, DOX:GEN)	[288]
DOX, 0.1 µM	Genistein, 5 µM	MDA-MB-453 human **breast** cancer cell line, overexpressing HER-2, mutant p53	↑	Increase in DOX-induced cytotoxicity, increase in necrotic-like cell death. Inactivation of HER-2 and Akt	[289]
DOX, 0.0625 µg/ml	Genistein, 25 µg/ml	NCI-H358 human non-small cell **lung** cancer cell line	~	No effect on DOX-induced cytotoxicity	[126]
DOX, 0.5 µg/ml	Genistein, 40 µg/ml	NCI-H596 human non-small cell **lung** cancer cell line	↑	Increase in DOX antiproliferative effect. Inhibition of EGFR phosphorylation, induction of apoptosis (PARP cleavage)	[126]
DOX, 0.125 µM	Hesperetin, 281 µM	U2OS human **osteosarcoma** cell line	↓	Antagonism in cell growth inhibition. Increase in S-phase cell cycle arrest	[203]
DOX, 500 nM	Hesperidin, 10-100 µM	Ramos human Burkitt`s **lymphoma** cell line, mutant p53	↑	Potentiation of DOX-induced growth inhibition. Induction of apoptosis, suppression of DOX-induced IκB phosphorylation and NF-κB activation	[286]
DOX	Icariin, 1, 5, 10 µM	MG-63/DOX human **osteosarcoma** cell line, DOX-resistant	↑	Reversal of MDR, increase in DOX cytotoxicity	[301]
DOX	Icariin, 1, 5, 10 µM	MG-63/DOX human **osteosarcoma** cell line, DOX-resistant	↑	Reversal of MDR, decrease in DOX IC_{50}. Increase in DOX cellular accumulation and retention, increase in DOX-induced apoptosis (cleavage of caspases-9/-3 and PARP) by blocking of PI3K/Akt pathway, downregulation of MDR1	[302]
DOX	Icariside II, 1, 5, 10 µM	MG-63/DOX human **osteosarcoma** cell line, DOX-resistant	↑	Reversal of MDR, increase in DOX-induced cytotoxicity	[301]
DOX	Icaritin, 1, 5, 10 µM	MG-63/DOX human **osteosarcoma** cell line, DOX-resistant	↑	Increase in DOX-induced cytotoxicity. Increase in DOX cellular accumulation. Reversal of MDR1- and MRP1-mediated MDR by inhibition of STAT3 phosphorylation. Increase in DOX-induced apoptosis	[301]
DOX	Icaritin, 1, 15, 30 µM	HepG2/ADR human **hepatocellular** carcinoma cell line, MDR, DOX-resistant	↑	Reversal of MDR, 1.65-fold decrease in DOX IC_{50} at 1 µM, 2.50-fold at 15 µM, 7.18-fold at 30 µM icaritin. Increase in DOX cellular accumulation, downregulation of MDR1 gene and P-gp protein expression	[226]
DOX, 1 µM	Isorhamnetin, 10 µM	AGS human **gastric** cancer cell line	↑	1.89-fold increase in DOX-induced cytotoxicity	[265]
DOX, 0.04-1 µM	Isoxanthohumol, 5.75-23 µM	A375 human **melanoma** cell line	↓	Antagonism in DOX efficacy	[171]
DOX, 0.04-1 µM	Isoxanthohumol, 5.75-23 µM	B16 murine **melanoma** cell line	↓	Antagonism in DOX efficacy	[171]
DOX	Kaempferol, 20 µM	T98G human **glioblastoma** cell line, overexpressing MRPs and BCRP, not P-gp	~	No effect on DOX-induced cytotoxicity. Increase in MRP1 and GST-π, decrease in MRP2 protein; increase in GST activity	[109]

Table 6.13. (Continued)

Drug	Flavonoid	Biological system	Direction of combination	Effects	Ref.
DOX, 0.25-3 μM	Kaempferol, 50 μM	HCT-15 human **colon** carcinoma cell line, expressing P-gp	↓	Decrease in DOX-induced cytotoxicity. Increase in DOX efflux, inhibition of DOX cellular accumulation	[261]
DOX, 10, 40 nM	Luteolin, 5, 10 μM	L1210 murine **leukemia** cell line	↓	Decrease in DOX-induced cytotoxicity. Shift from G2/M to S phase arrest of cell cycle	[84]
DOX, 5-100 μM	Luteolin, 100 μM	U2OS human **osteosarcoma** cell line	↑	Potentiation of cell growth inhibition. Increase in DOX-induced autophagy (upregulation of beclin1, conversion of LC3-I to LC3-II)	[247]
DOX, 1.7 μM	Luteolin, 10 μM	MCF-7 human **breast** cancer cell line, ER-positive	↓	Attenuation of DOX-induced cytotoxicity. Reduction of DOX-induced ROS generation (attenuation of DOX-induced mitochondrial damage), increase in Bcl-2	[238]
DOX	Luteolin, loaded in phytosomes	MDA-MB-231 human **breast** carcinoma cell line	↑	Increase in growth inhibition. Inhibition of Nrf2	[269]
DOX, 2, 2.4 μM	Luteolin, 10 μM	MDA-MB-453 human **breast** cancer cell line, ER-negative	↓	Attenuation of DOX-induced cytotoxicity	[238]
DOX, 1-10 μg/ml	Luteolin, 5 μM	HCT116-OX human **colorectal** cancer cell line, OXA-resistant	↑	Synergism in anticancer activity (CI<1), 2-fold decrease in DOX IC_{50}. Inhibition of Nrf2 pathway	[143]
DOX, 1-10 μg/ml	Luteolin, 5 μM	SW620-OX human **colorectal** cancer cell line, OXA-resistant	↑	Synergism in anticancer activity (CI<1), 2.48-fold decrease in DOX IC_{50}. Inhibition of Nrf2 pathway	[143]
DOX, 0-3 μg/ml	Luteolin, 5 μM	A549 human non-small cell **lung** cancer cell line	↑	Synergism in sensitization to DOX (CI<1), decrease in DOX IC_{50}. Inhibition of Nrf2	[181]
DOX	Luteolin	AGS human **gastric** cancer cell line	~	No sensitization of DOX treatment	[144]
DOX, 0-300 μM	Morin, 100 μM	MDA435/LCC6MDR1 human **breast** cancer cell line, E2-independent, P-gp-positive, no MRP1	~	No effect on DOX-induced cytotoxicity. Inhibition of P-gp-mediated DOX efflux	[264]
DOX, 2 μM	Myricetin, 1.56-12.5 μM	SCC 84 human **head and neck** squamous cell carcinoma cell line, HPV-negative	~	Resistance to DOX in both presence and absence of myricetin	[108]
DOX, 2 μM	Myricetin, 1.56-12.5 μM	UMSCC 29 human **head and neck** squamous cell carcinoma cell line, HPV-negative	~	Resistance to DOX in both presence and absence of myricetin	[108]
DOX, 2 μM	Myricetin, 1.56-12.5 μM	UMSCC 47 human **head and neck** squamous cell carcinoma cell line, HPV-positive	↑	Increase in cell death, sensitization of HPV-positive cells to DOX-triggered apoptosis	[108]
DOX, 2 μM	Myricetin, 1.56-12.5 μM	UM-SCC47-TC-Clone 3 human **head and neck** squamous cell carcinoma cell line, HPV-positive	↑	Increase in cell death, sensitization of HPV-positive cells to DOX-triggered apoptosis	[108]

Drug	Flavonoid	Biological system	Direction of combination	Effects	Ref.
DOX, 2 μM	Myricetin, 1.56-12.5 μM	UPCI-SCC90-UP-Clone 35 human **head and neck** squamous cell carcinoma cell line, HPV-positive	↑	Increase in cell death, sensitization of HPV-positive cells to DOX-triggered apoptosis	[108]
DOX, 2.5-10 μM	Myricetin, 100 μM	SiHa human **cervical** carcinoma cell line, HPV-positive	↑	Sensitization of HPV-positive cells to DOX. Reactivation of E6-compromised apoptotic pathway (increase in p53 and caspases-3/-7 activity)	[108]
DOX, 0.1 nM-1 mM	Naringenin, 1 mM	HTB26 human **breast** cancer cell line	↑	Increase in DOX-induced cytotoxicity	[10]
DOX, 0-2 μM	Naringenin, 100 μM	MCF-7 human **breast** carcinoma cell line, expressing MRP1 and MRP2, not MDR1/P-gp	↑	Increase in DOX-induced cell growth inhibition, 2-fold decrease in DOX IC$_{50}$. Increase in DOX cellular accumulation through inhibiting efflux	[217]
DOX, 0-2 μM	Naringenin, 100 μM	MCF-7/DOX human **breast** carcinoma cell line, DOX-resistant, expressing MRP1, MRP2, overexpressing MDR1/P-gp	~	No effect on DOX-induced cell growth inhibition	[217]
DOX, 0.1 nM-1 mM	Naringenin, 1 mM	SW1116 human **colorectal** cancer cell line	↑	Increase in DOX-induced cytotoxicity	[10]
DOX, 0-2 μM	Naringenin, 100 μM	HepG2 human **hepatocellular** carcinoma cell line, expressing MRP1, MRP2, MDR1/P-gp	~	No effect on DOX-induced cell growth inhibition	[217]
DOX, 0-2 μM	Naringenin, 100 μM	A549 human non-small cell **lung** carcinoma cell line, expressing MRP1 and MRP2, not MDR1/P-gp	↑	Increase in DOX-induced cell growth inhibition, 2.24-fold decrease in DOX IC$_{50}$. Increase in DOX cellular accumulation through inhibiting efflux. Increase in DOX-induced apoptosis	[217]
DOX, 200 nM	Nobiletin, 5, 10, 15 μM	MCF-7 human **breast** cancer cell line, wild-type p53	↑	Increase in DOX-induced cytotoxicity, G2/M phase cell cycle arrest and apoptosis	[277]
DOX, 7.5 nM	Nobiletin, 5, 10, 15 μM	T47D human **breast** cancer cell line, mutant p53	~	No effect on DOX-induced cytotoxicity	[277]
DOX	Nobiletin, 0.5-9 μM	A549/T human non-small cell **lung** cancer cell line, PTX-resistant, overexpressing ABCB1	↑	Sensitization to DOX, decrease in DOX IC$_{50}$	[276]
DOX	Nobiletin, 0.5-9 μM	A2780 human **ovarian** cancer cell line	~	No effect on DOX anticancer activity	[276]
DOX	Nobiletin, 0.5-9 μM	A2780/T human **ovarian** cancer cell line, PTX-resistant, overexpressing ABCB1	↑	Sensitization to DOX; decrease in DOX IC$_{50}$. Intracellular accumulation of DOX	[276]
DOX, 0-10 μM	Oroxylin A, 15, 30, 60 μM	K562/ADM human chronic myeloid **leukemia** cell line, DOX-resistant	↑	1.56-fold increase in sensitivity to DOX at 15 μM, 4.29-fold at 30 μM, 17.99-fold at 60 μM oroxylin A; decrease in colonies number and size. Increase in DOX-induced apoptosis, decrease in CXCR4 level and related PI3K/Akt/NF-κB pathway	[275]
DOX, 0-300 μM	Phloretin, 100 μM	MDA435/LCC6MDR1 human **breast** cancer cell line, E2-independent, MDR, P-gp positive, no MRP1	~	No effect on DOX-induced cytotoxicity. Inhibition of P-gp-mediated DOX efflux	[264]

Table 6.13. (Continued)

Drug	Flavonoid	Biological system	Direction of combination	Effects	Ref.
DOX	Quercetin	CCRF-CEM human acute lymphoblastic **leukemia** cell line, p53-null	↑	Synergistic anticancer effect; induction of apoptosis (activation of caspases-3/-8/-9), increase in S phase cell cycle arrest. Decrease in GSH, increase in DNA damage	[206]
DOX	Quercetin	Jurkat human peripheral blood T cell **leukemia** cell line, p53-null	↑	Synergistic anticancer effect; induction of apoptosis (activation of caspases-3/-8/-9), increase in G2/M phase cell cycle arrest. Decrease in GSH, increase in DNA damage	[206]
DOX, 12 μg/ml	Quercetin, 25-125 μg/ml	K562/ADR human **leukemia** cell line, MDR	↑	Synergism in cell proliferation inhibition. Promotion of apoptosis via extrinsic and intrinsic pathways (ΔΨm loss, activation of caspases-8/-9/-3, decrease in Bcl-2, Bcl-xL; increase in Bim, Bad, Bax), regulation of MAPK/ERK/JNK signaling, downregulation of P-gp	[262]
DOX	Quercetin	KG-1a human acute myelogenous **leukemia** cell line, p53-null	↑	Synergistic anticancer effect; induction of apoptosis (activation of caspases-3/-8/-9), Decrease in GSH, increase in DNA damage	[206]
DOX, 10, 40 nM	Quercetin, 5, 10 μM	L1210 murine **leukemia** cell line	↓	Decrease in DOX-induced cytotoxicity. Shift from G2/M to S phase arrest of cell cycle	[84]
DOX	Quercetin	THP-1 human acute monocytic **leukemia** cell line, p53-null	↑	Synergistic anticancer effect; induction of apoptosis (activation of caspases-3/-8/-9), increase in S and G2/M phase cell cycle arrest. Decrease in GSH, increase in DNA damage	[206]
DOX, 0.01-1000 nM	Quercetin, 15 μM	6647 human Ewing's **sarcoma** cell line	↑	13.43-fold decrease in DOX IC_{50}. Inhibition of HSPs	[260]
DOX, 0.01-1000 nM	Quercetin, 15 μM	PDE02 human Ewing's **sarcoma** cell line	↑	1.82-fold decrease in DOX IC_{50}. Inhibition of HSPs	[260]
DOX, 0.01-1000 nM	Quercetin, 15 μM	TC106 human Ewing's **sarcoma** cell line	↑	44-fold decrease in DOX IC_{50}. Inhibition of HSPs	[260]
DOX, 0.01-2 μM	Quercetin, 10-100 μM	4T1 murine **breast** cancer cell line	↑	Slight effect on DOX-induced cytotoxicity under normoxia, significant increase under hypoxia; reversal of hypoxia-conferred resistance to DOX. Synergistic promotion of DOX-induced apoptosis, induction of HIF-1α degradation under hypoxia	[246]
DOX, 0.25-2 μM	Quercetin, 0.7 μM	BCSCs from MCF-7 and MDA-MB-231 human **breast** cancer cell lines	↑	Synergism in elimination of BCSCs	[227]
DOX, 4.3 μg/ml	Quercetin, 5-50 μg/ml	MCF7 human **breast** carcinoma cell line	↑	Increase in DOX-induced cytotoxicity	[218]
DOX, 0.25-2 μM	Quercetin, 0.7 μM	MCF-7 human **breast** cancer cell line	↑	Increase in DOX-induced cytotoxicity and apoptosis. Promotion of DOX accumulation through downregulation of P-gp, BCRP and MRP1	[227]

Drug	Flavonoid	Biological system	Direction of combination	Effects	Ref.
DOX, 1.5-4 μg/ml	Quercetin, 0.7 μM	MCF-7 human **breast** cancer cell line	↑	1.49-fold increase in DOX-induced cytotoxicity. Promotion of DOX accumulation, inhibition of HIF-1α and P-gp expression. Decrease in invasion	[248]
DOX, 1.5-4 μg/ml	Quercetin, 0.7 μM	MCF-7 human **breast** cancer cell line	↑	1.38-fold increase in DOX-induced cytotoxicity. Upregulation of PTEN, downregulation of p-Akt, increase in apoptosis and necrosis, inhibition of invasion	[249]
DOX, 10 nM	Quercetin, 10 μM	MCF-7 human **breast** cancer cell line	↗	No effect on DOX-induced cytotoxicity	[185]
DOX, 0.01-1 μg/ml	Quercetin, 1, 10 μM	MCF-7 human **breast** cancer cell line, no P-gp	↗	No effect on DOX-induced growth inhibition	[252]
DOX, 1 μM	Quercetin, 100 μM	MCF-7 human **breast** cancer cell line	↑	Increase in apoptosis and G0/G1 phase cell cycle arrest	[228]
DOX	Quercetin	MCF-7 human **breast** cancer cell line	↗	No effect on DOX-induced cytotoxicity	[253]
DOX, 1-10 μg/ml	Quercetin, 0.7 μM	MCF-7 human **breast** cancer cell line	↑	1.38-fold increase in DOX antitumor effect, increase in apoptosis. Elimination of BCSCs (CD44$^+$/CD24$^{-/low}$). Increase in DOX cellular accumulation	[250]
DOX	Quercetin	MCF-7 human **breast** cancer cell line	↗	No effect on DOX-induced cytotoxicity	[254]
DOX, 0.001 μM	Quercetin, 75 μM, as nano-quercetin (phytosomes)	MCF-7 human **breast** cancer cell line	↑	Sensitization to DOX, decrease in DOX IC$_{50}$. Decrease in NQO1 and MRP1 expression	[251]
DOX	Quercetin	MCF-7/ADR human **breast** cancer cell line, DOX-resistant, overexpressing P-gp	↑	1.43-fold decrease in DOX IC$_{50}$. Inhibition of P-gp, decrease in DOX efflux. Significant reduction in DOX resistance with biotin-decorated combined NPs	[254]
DOX	Quercetin	MCF-7/adr human **breast** cancer cell line, MDR	↑	Reversal of MDR, increase in DOX-induced cytotoxicity. Inhibition of P-gp, increase in uptake and accumulation of cytoplasmic DOX	[253]
DOX, in BPL NPs	Quercetin, in BPL NPs	MCF-7/adr human **breast** cancer cell line, MDR	↑	Increase in cytotoxicity. Decrease in P-gp, increase in uptake and accumulation of DOX in cytoplasm	[253]
DOX, 0.0001-100 μM	Quercetin, 1, 5, 10 μM	MCF-7/ADR human **breast** cancer cell line, DOX-resistant	↑	Reversal of resistance; 1.5-fold decrease in DOX IC$_{50}$ at 1 μM, 2.5-fold at 5 μM, 7.8-fold at 10 μM quercetin	[255]
DOX, 1-10 μg/ml	Quercetin, 1, 5, 10 μM	MCF-7 ADRr human **breast** cancer cell line, DOX-resistant, MDR, expressing P-gp	↑	Reversal of DOX resistance, decrease in DOX IC$_{50}$. Inhibition of P-gp expression and efflux activity	[252]
DOX, 1.5-4 μg/ml	Quercetin, 0.7 μM	MCF-7/dox human **breast** cancer cell line	↑	1.98-fold increase in DOX-induced cytotoxicity. Promotion of DOX cellular accumulation, inhibition of HIF-1α and P-gp expression. Decrease in invasion	[248]
DOX, 1-10 μg/ml	Quercetin, 0.7 μM	MCF-7/Dox human **breast** cancer cell line, DOX-resistant	↑	Reversal of MDR, 1.73-fold increase in DOX antitumor effect, increase in apoptosis. Downregulation of P-gp, increase in DOX cellular accumulation. Elimination of BCSCs (CD44$^+$/CD24$^{-/low}$). Inhibition of YB-1 nuclear translocation	[250]

Table 6.13. (Continued)

Drug	Flavonoid	Biological system	Direction of combination	Effects	Ref.
DOX, 2-12 μg/ml	Quercetin, 0.7 μM	MCF-7/dox human **breast** cancer cell line	↑	1.73-fold increase in DOX-induced cytotoxicity. Upregulation of PTEN, downregulation of p-Akt, increase in apoptosis and necrosis, inhibition of invasion	[249]
DOX, 10-100 μg/ml, loaded into PSi NPs	3-Aminopropoxy-linked quercetin, conjugated onto PSi NPs	MCF-7 human **breast** cancer cell line	↑	Synergism in cytotoxic effect. Extensive uptake of NPs, increase in DOX cellular concentration	[256]
DOX, 10-100 μg/ml, loaded into PSi NPs	3-Aminopropoxy-linked quercetin, conjugated onto PSi NPs	MCF-7/DOX^R human **breast** cancer cell line, DOX-resistant	↑	Synergism in cytotoxic effect. Extensive uptake of NPs, increase in DOX cellular concentration	[256]
DOX, 0.25-2 μM	Quercetin, 0.7 μM	MDA-MB-231 human **breast** cancer cell line	↑	Increase in DOX-induced cytotoxicity and apoptosis. Promotion of DOX accumulation through downregulation of P-gp, BCRP and MRP1	[227]
DOX, 10 nM	Quercetin, 10 μM	MDA-MB-231 human **breast** cancer cell line	↑	Increase in DOX-induced cytotoxicity. Suppression of cell migration, induction of cell polynucleation	[185]
DOX, 0.25-3 μM	Quercetin, 50 μM	HCT-15 human **colon** carcinoma cell line, expressing P-gp	↓	Decrease in DOX-induced cytotoxicity. Increase in DOX efflux, inhibition of DOX accumulation	[261]
DOX, 0.001-0.05 μg/ml	Quercetin, 0.1 and 1 μM	Primary **endometrial** cancer cells	~	No effect on DOX-induced antiproliferative activity	[90]
DOX, 0.2-125 μg/ml	Quercetin, 40, 80, 160 μM	BEL/5-FU human **hepatocellular** carcinoma cell line, MDR, DOX-resistant	↑	1.33-fold increase in sensitivity to DOX at 40 μM, 1.78-fold at 80 μM, 2.79-fold at 160 μM quercetin. Downregulation of ABCB1, ABCC1 and ABCC2; increase in DOX accumulation. Decrease in FZD7 and β-catenin expression	[38]
DOX, 4.2 μg/ml	Quercetin, 5-50 μg/ml	HepG2 human **liver** carcinoma cell line	↑	Increase in DOX-induced cytotoxicity	[218]
DOX, 0-10 μM	Quercetin, 20 μM	QGY7701 human **hepatoma** cell line	↑	Increase in DOX-induced cytotoxicity, 2.3-fold decrease in DOX IC_{50}. Potentiation of DOX-mediated apoptosis (activation of caspases-9/3, PARP cleavage)	[258]
DOX, 0-10 μM	Quercetin, 20 μM	SMMC7721 human **hepatoma** cell line	↑	Increase in DOX-induced cytotoxicity, 2.3-fold decrease in DOX IC_{50}. p53-dependent enhancement of DOX-mediated apoptosis (ΔΨm loss, cyt c release, activation of caspases-9/3, PARP cleavage, decrease in Bcl-xl, increase in Bax and PUMA)	[258]
DOX, 1-200 μg/ml, in silica-coated luminomagnetic BTN-conjugated NPs	Quercetin, 1-200 μg/ml, in silica-coated luminomagnetic BTN-conjugated NPs	A549 human **lung** carcinoma cell line	↑	Sensitization of cells to DOX, increase in apoptosis and G2/M phase cell cycle arrest	[259]

Drug	Flavonoid	Biological system	Direction of combination	Effects	Ref.
DOX, 1-200 µg/ml, in silica-coated luminomagnetic BTN-conjugated NPs	Quercetin, 1-200 µg/ml, in silica-coated luminomagnetic BTN-conjugated NPs	A549/DOX human **lung** carcinoma cell line, DOX-resistant	↑	Potentiation of DOX efficacy, increase in apoptosis and G2/M phase cell cycle arrest	[259]
DOX, 0.0001-100 µM	Quercetin, 1, 5, 10 µM	KBCH^{R}8-5 human **oral** carcinoma cell line, MDR KB 3-1 cells, overexpressing P-gp	↑	1.75-fold decrease in DOX IC$_{50}$ at 1 µM, 7-fold at 5 µM, 11.7-fold at 10 µM quercetin. Increase in DOX-induced G2/M phase cell cycle arrest and apoptosis. Downregulation of P-gp by targeting Wnt/β-catenin signaling	[255]
DOX, 0.01-1000 nM	Quercetin, 15 µM	AF8 human **neuroblastoma** cell line	↑	873.3-fold decrease in DOX IC$_{50}$. Inhibition of HSPs	[260]
DOX, 0.01-1000 nM	Quercetin, 15 µM	IMR-5 human **neuroblastoma** cell line	↑	156.8-fold decrease in DOX IC$_{50}$. Inhibition of HSPs	[260]
DOX, 0.01-1000 nM	Quercetin, 15 µM	SJ-N-KP human **neuroblastoma** cell line	↑	230-fold decrease in DOX IC$_{50}$. Inhibition of HSPs, increase in DOX-induced apoptosis	[260]
DOX, 0.001-0.05 µg/ml	Quercetin, 0.1, 1 µM	Primary **ovarian** cancer cells	~	No effect on DOX antiproliferative activity	[90]
DOX, 5.4 µg/ml	Quercetin, 5-50 µg/ml	PC3 human **prostate** carcinoma cell line	↑	Increase in DOX-induced cytotoxicity	[218]
DOX, 0.5 µM	Quercetin, 25, 50 µM	CYR61-AGS human **gastric** adenocarcinoma cell line, overexpressing CYR61	↑	Synergism in cytotoxicity (CI 0.18-0.34), increase in apoptosis	[257]
DOX, co-loaded in HA-modified SiLN	Quercetin, co-loaded in HA-modified SiLN	SGC7901/ADR human **gastric** cancer cell line, DOX-resistant	↑	Synergism in cytotoxicity (CI 0.19), increase in apoptosis (increase in caspase-3), decrease in P-gp. Selective uptake of NPs via HA-mediated endocytosis and increased DOX retention	[231]
DOX, 6.4 µg/ml	Quercetin, 5-50 µg/ml	HeLa human **cervical** carcinoma cell line	↑	Increase in DOX-induced cytotoxicity	[218]
DOX, 0.003-3 µM	Rhamnetin, 3 µM	HepG2/ADR human **hepatocellular** carcinoma cell line, MDR, DOX resistant	↑	Increase in sensitivity to DOX, decrease in DOX IC$_{50}$	[207]
DOX, 1-10 µg/ml	Rutin, 10 µM	MCF-7 ADRr human **breast** cancer cell line, MDR, DOX-resistant, expressing P-gp	~	No effect on DOX-induced growth inhibition	[252]
DOX, 0.0001-100 µM	Rutin, 1, 5, 10 µM	MCF-7/ADR human **breast** cancer cell line, DOX-resistant	↑	Increase in DOX efficacy; 1.3-fold decrease in DOX IC$_{50}$ at 1 µM, 1.9-fold at 5 µM, 5.4-fold at 10 µM rutin	[255]
DOX, 0.0001-100 µM	Rutin, 1, 5, 10 µM	KBCH^{R}8-5 human **oral** carcinoma cell line, MDR KB 3-1 cells, overexpressing P-gp	↑	1.2-fold decrease in DOX IC$_{50}$ at 1 µM, 2.3-fold at 5 µM, 10-fold at 10 µM rutin. Increase in DOX-induced G2/M phase cell cycle arrest and apoptosis. Downregulation of P-gp by targeting Wnt/β-catenin signaling	[255]
DOX, 1 µM	Salvigenin, 150 µM	HT-29 human **colon** cancer cell line	↑	Increase in DOX-induced antiproliferative effect and mitochondrial apoptosis (increase in Bax/Bcl-2 ratio, caspase-3, PARP cleavage), increase in ROS	[245]
DOX, 1 µM	Salvigenin, 150 µM	SW948 human **colon** cancer cell line	↑	Increase in DOX-induced antiproliferative effect and mitochondrial apoptosis (increase in Bax/Bcl-2 ratio, caspase-3, PARP cleavage), increase in ROS	[245]

Table 6.13. (Continued)

Drug	Flavonoid	Biological system	Direction of combination	Effects	Ref.
DOX, 200 nM	Silibinin, 200 μM	Karpas 299 human anaplastic lymphoma kinase-positive anaplastic large cell **lymphoma** cell line	↑	Increase in DOX-induced growth inhibition	[297]
DOX, 200 nM	Silibinin, 200 μM	SupM2 human anaplastic lymphoma kinase-positive anaplastic large cell **lymphoma** cell line	↑	Increase in DOX-induced growth inhibition. Augmentation of sensitivity in particular of a small cell subset expressing transcriptional activity of Sox2 (Sox2^{active} cells)	[297]
DOX, 10-75 nM	Silibinin, 25-100 μM	MCF-7 human E2-dependent **breast** carcinoma cell line	↑	Synergism in cell growth inhibition (CI 0.35 at 100 μM silibinin plus 25 nM DOX). Increase in apoptosis	[162]
DOX, 0.1-10 μg/ml	Silibinin, 0.1 μM	MCF-7 DOXr human **breast** cancer cell line, DOX-resistant	↑	Potentiation of DOX-induced cell growth inhibition, synergistic antiproliferative effect (CI<1)	[164]
DOX, 0.25 μg/ml	Silibinin, 200 μM	MDA-MB-435 human **breast** cancer cell line	↑	Synergism in decrease in cell viability (CI 0.68). Increase in apoptosis. Suppression of STAT3, AKT and ERK pathways	[163]
DOX, 5-40 μg/ml	Silibinin, 200 μM	MDA-MB-435/DOX human **breast** cancer cell line, DOX-resistant	↑	Synergism in cell viability inhibition (CI 0.69). 7.1-fold decrease in DOX IC$_{50}$. Suppression of STAT3, AKT and ERK pathways	[163]
DOX, 10-75 nM	Silibinin, 25-100 μM	MDA-MB468 human E2-independent **breast** carcinoma cell line	↑	Synergism in cell growth inhibition (CI 0.45 at 100 μM silibinin plus 25 nM DOX). Increase in apoptosis	[162]
DOX, 1-10 μM	Silibinin, 5-50 μM	LoVo DOX human **colorectal** adenocarcinoma cell line, DOX-resistant	↑	Overcoming DOX resistance, synergistic increase in DOX efficacy (CI 0.41-0.81). Reduction of glucose uptake linked to lower GLUT1 expression	[295]
DOX, 10, 25 nM	Silibinin, 50, 100 μM	HEPG2 human **liver** cancer cell line	↑	Synergistic increase in cell growth inhibition, apoptosis and G2/M phase cell cycle arrest (inhibition of cdc2/p34 kinase, downregulation cdc25C, cyclin B1)	[296]
DOX, 25 nM	Silibinin, 60 μM	A549 human non-small cell **lung** carcinoma cell line	↑	Increase in DOX-induced cell growth inhibition and apoptosis. Inhibition of DOX-induced NF-κB activation, decrease in COX-2	[233]
DOX, 0.15-2.4 μM	Silibinin, 12.5-200 μM	H69 human small-cell **lung** carcinoma cell line	~	No effect on DOX cytotoxicity	[167]
DOX, 0.15-2.4 μM	Silibinin, 12.5-200 μM	VPA17 human small-cell **lung** carcinoma cell line, VP-16-resistant H69 cells, DOX-resistant, overexpressing P-gp	↑	Reversal of MDR, synergism in DOX cytotoxicity (CI<1)	[167]
DOX, 25 nM	Silibinin, 100 μM	DU145 human advanced **prostate** cancer cell line	↑	Synergism in cell growth inhibition (CI 0.235-0.587). Increase in apoptosis and G2/M phase cell cycle arrest (inhibition of cdc25C, cdc2/p34, cyclin B1 proteins and cdc2/p34 kinase activity)	[294]
DOX, 15 nM	Silibinin, 25 μM	LNCaP human androgen-dependent **prostate** carcinoma cell line	↑	Increase in cell growth inhibition (CI 0.929-1.13)	[294]

Drug	Flavonoid	Biological system	Direction of combination	Effects	Ref.
DOX, 0.0001-100 μM	Tamarixetin, 1, 5, 10 μM	MCF-7/ADR human **breast** cancer cell line, DOX-resistant	↑	Increase in DOX efficacy; 1.2-fold decrease in DOX IC_{50} at 1 μM, 1.7-fold at 5 μM, 3.4-fold at 10 μM tamarixetin	[255]
DOX, 0.0001-100 μM	Tamarixetin, 1, 5, 10 μM	$KBCH^R$8-5 human **oral** carcinoma cell line, MDR KB 3-1 cells, overexpressing P-gp	↑	1.2-fold decrease in DOX IC_{50} at 1 μM, 1.7-fold at 5 μM, 3.4-fold at 10 μM tamarixetin. Increase in DOX-induced G2/M phase cell cycle arrest and apoptosis. Downregulation of P-gp by targeting Wnt/β-catenin signaling	[255]
DOX, 10 nM	Taxifolin, 80, 100 μM	HeLaS3 human **cervical** carcinoma cell line	~	No effect on DOX-induced cell viability inhibition	[304]
DOX, 1000 nM	Taxifolin, 80, 100 μM	KB-vin human **cervical** cancer cell line, MDR	↑	Synergism in cell viability reduction (CI 0.36 at 100 μM, CI 0.55 at 80 μM taxifolin). Increase in DOX-induced apoptosis, decrease in ABCB1 expression and P-gp efflux function	[304]
DOX, 10 μM	Wogonin, 40 μM	K562/A02 human chronic myelogenous **leukemia** cell line, DOX-resistant	↑	Decrease in colony formation ability. Inhibition of Nrf2 signaling via Stat3/NF-κB inactivation	[272]
DOX, 0-1 μg/ml	Wogonin	Bcap-37 human **breast** cancer cell line	↑	Increase in DOX-induced cytotoxicity. Suppression of IGF-1R expression and phosphorylation of AKT	[274]
DOX, 0-1 μg/ml	Wogonin	MCF-7 human **breast** cancer cell line	↑	Increase in DOX-induced cytotoxicity. Suppression of IGF-1R expression and phosphorylation of AKT	[274]
DOX	Wogonin, 20, 40, 60 μM	MCF-7/DOX human **breast** cancer cell line, DOX-induced MDR	↑	1.24-fold increase in sensitivity to DOX at 20 μM, 1.93-fold at 40 μM, 3.24-fold at 60 μM wogonin; increase in apoptosis. Suppression of Nrf2	[273]
DOX, 10, 200 μM	Wogonin, 25 μM	A549 human **lung** cancer cell line	~	No effect on DOX-induced cytotoxicity	[153]
DOX, 0.02-2.5 μM	Wogonin, 5 μM	H23 human **lung** cancer cell line	↑	Overcoming of IL-6-induced chemoresistance, inhibition of IL-6-induced AKR1C1/1C2 expression	[270]

ABC, ATP-binding cassette; AKR, aldo-keto reductase; Akt, protein kinase B; ATG, autophagy-related; AuNP, gold NP; Bad, Bcl-2-associated death promoter; Bax, Bcl-2-associated X protein; Bcl-2, B-cell lymphoma 2; Bcl-xL, B-cell lymphoma-extra large; BCRP, breast cancer resistance protein; BCSC, breast cancer stem cell; Bim, Bcl-2-like protein 11; BPL, biotin-modified PEGylated liposomes; BTN, biotin; CDC, cell division cycle; CI, combination index; COX, cyclooxygenase; CXCR, chemokine receptor; CYR61, cysteine-rich angiogenic induces 61; cyt c, cytochrome c; Dex-CT, dextran-catechin; DMC, 2`,4`-dihydroxy-6`-methoxy-3`,5`-dimethylchalcone; E2, estradiol; EGFR, epidermal growth factor receptor; EMT, epithelial-mesenchymal transition; ER, estrogen receptor; ERK, extracellular signal-regulated kinase; f_a, fraction affected; FZD7, Frizzled homolog protein 7; GLUT, glucose transporter; GSH, glutathione; GST, glutathione S-transferase; HA, hyaluronic acid; HDAC, histone deacetylase; HER2 (erbB2), human epidermal growth factor receptor 2; HIF-1α, hypoxia-inducible factor 1α; HPV, human papillomavirus; Hsp, heat shock protein; IGF-1R, insulin like growth factor 1 receptor; IL, interleukin; IκB, nuclear factor of kappa light polypeptide gene enhancer in B-cells inhibitor; JNK, c-Jun N-terminal kinase; Lam, laminin; LRP, lung resistance protein; MAPK, mitogen-activated protein kinase; MDR, multidrug resistance; miR, microRNA; MRP, multidrug resistance-associated protein; NF-κB, nuclear factor-κB; NGO, nanographene oxide; NP, nanoparticle; NQO, NAD(P)H:quinone oxidoreductase; Nrf2, nuclear factor (erythroid-derived 2)-like 2; PARP, poly (ADP-ribose) polymerase; P-gp, P-glycoprotein; PI3K, phosphoinositide 3-kinase; PIC, polyion complex; PR, progesterone receptor; PSi, porous silicon; PTEN, phosphatase and tensin homolog; PUMA, p53 upregulated modulator of apoptosis; ROS, reactive oxygen species; SiLN, silica nanoparticle; Sox2, sex-determining region Y-Box; STAT3, signal transducer and activator of transcription 3; wt, wild type; YB-1, Y-box binding protein 1; ΔΨm, mitochondrial membrane potential.

Table 6.14. Effects of flavonoids on anticancer action of anthracyclines (DOX, DNR, EPI) *in vivo* conditions

Drug	Flavonoid	Biological system	Direction of combination	Effects	Ref.
DOX, 3 mg/kg, i.p., every 3 days for 7 doses	Apigenin, 50 mg/kg, i.p., every 3 days for 7 doses	BEL-7402 human **hepatocellular** carcinoma cells injected into subdermal space on the right flanks of male BALB/c nude mice	↑	Increase in growth inhibition, decrease in tumor weight. Potentiation of proliferation reduction, induction of apoptosis, inhibition of Nrf2 expression	[267]
DOX, i.v., in HA-decorated dual-loaded NLCs	Baicalein, i.v., in HA-decorated dual-loaded NLCs	MCF-7/ADR human **breast** cancer cells inoculated into the right armpit of 4-6w old Kunming mice	↑	Synergism in tumor growth inhibition	[213]
DOX, 5 mg/kg, i.v., once every two days	Barbigerone, 5 mg/kg, i.v., once every two days, 1h before DOX	MCF-7/ADR human **breast** cancer cells injected into the right flank of 5-7w old athymic nude BALB/c mice	↑	Restoration of DOX antitumor activity, suppression of tumor growth	[293]
DOX, 1 mg/kg, i.p., every two days for 10 days	Deguelin, 2 mg/kg, i.p., every two days for 10 days	A549 human **lung** cancer cells injected s.c. into the flanks of 5-6w old nude mice	↑	Increase in sensitivity to DOX, suppression of tumor volume. Increase in PUMA expression, stimulation of cell death (activation of caspase-3)	[305]
DOX, 2 mg/kg, i.g., 2-3 times a week	Dihydromyricetin, 50 mg/kg, i.p., 2-3 times a week	U937 human **leukemia** cells injected into the armpit of BALB/C mice	↑	Potentiation of DOX-induced tumor growth inhibition rate. Cleavage of caspase-3 and PARP in tumor tissue, accumulation of p53	[215]
DOX, 2 mg/kg, i.p., on days 2, 4, 6, 8	DMC, 20 or 40 mg/kg, i.p., on days 1-9	KB-A1 human **oral** cancer cells injected s.c. into right flank of mouse; dissection of tumors after 3 weeks, s.c. injection into the right flank of 4-6w old athymic male nude mice	↑	Increase in tumor growth inhibition rate, decrease in tumor weight	[298]
DOX, 2 mg/kg, i.p., every 4 days	EGCG, 40, 80 or 160 mg/kg, i.g., every day	BEL-7404/DOX human **hepatocellular** carcinoma cells transplanted s.c. on the right axilla of 4-5w old male and female BALB/c nu/nu mice	↑	Increase in tumor inhibition rate, decrease in tumor dimensions. Increase in DOX cellular accumulation, suppression of P-gp pump function, downregulation of MDR1 and HIF-1α	[184]
DOX, 2 mg/kg, i.p., every 4 days	EGCG, 50 mg/kg, i.g., every day	Hep3B human **hepatocellular** cells inoculated s.c. into the right side fossa axillaries of male nude mice	↑	Increase in inhibition of tumor size and weight, increase in apoptosis. Inhibition of autophagy (suppression of LC3, Atg5, beclin1)	[221]
DOX, 2 mg/kg, i.p., on days 2, 4, 6, 8	EGCG, 40 mg/kg, i.p., on days 1-9	KB-A1 human **oral** cancer cells implanted s.c. into nude mice	↑	Reversal of MDR, increase in DOX-induced tumor growth inhibition. Increase in DOX concentration in tumors	[281]
DOX, 2 mg/kg, i.p., on days 2, 4, 6, 8; 5h after EGCG	EGCG, 20 or 40 mg/kg, i.p., on days 1-9	KB-A-1 human **oral** cancer cells injected s.c. into the right flank of 4-6w old athymic male BALB/c nu/nu nude mice	↑	Reversal of DOX resistance, decrease in tumor mass and weight. Increase in DOX concentration in tumors, promotion of apoptosis	[240]
DOX, 0.14 mg/kg, i.p., every 2 days	EGCG, 228 mg/kg, i.p., every 2 days	PC-3ML human **prostate** cancer cells injected i.p. in 5-6w old male CB17-SCID mice	↑	Blocking of tumor growth, decrease in tumor size and incidence of recurrence. Promotion of DOX retention by tumors. Increase in survival rates of mice	[283]
DOX, 0.07 mg/kg, i.p., biweekly for 2 months	EGCG, 57 mg/kg, i.p., biweekly for 2 months	CD44[hi] tumor initiating cells from PCa-20a human **prostate** cancer cells injected i.p. into 6w old male NOD-SCID mice	↑	Eradication of established tumors derived from CD44[hi] tumor initiating cells	[283]

Drug	Flavonoid	Biological system	Direction of combination	Effects	Ref.
DOX, 5 mg/kg, i.v., in polypeptide NPs	Genistein, 0.45 mg/mouse, p.o., every other day	RM-1 murine **prostate** cancer cells injected s.c. into the armpit of the right anterior limb of 5-6w old C57BL/6 male mice	↑	Restraint of tumor growth. Amplifying ROS production, increase in oxidative damage, decrease in damage repair through decrease in APE1 level. Inhibition of distant metastasis	[224]
DOX, 2 mg/kg, i.p., for 2 weeks	Hesperidin, 100 mg/kg, orally, every other day for 2 weeks	EAC murine **mammary** adenocarcinoma cells injected i.p. into female Swiss albino mice	↑	Prolongation of life span of mice related to decrease in ascitic volume and number of viable tumor cells, increase in number of dead tumor cells. Stimulation of caspase-3 and Bax; downregulation of Bcl-2 gene	[225]
DOX, 5 mg/kg/week, i.v., for 2 weeks	Isoliquiritigenin, 200 µg/kg, i.p., daily for 15 days	MPC-11 murine **myeloma** cells injected s.c. into the right flank of male BALB/C mice	↑	Increase in DOX antimyeloma activity, augmentation of therapeutic potential	[300]
DOX, 5 mg/kg, on days 7, 14, 21	Naringenin, 50 mg/kg, orally, daily for 3 weeks	LLC murine Lewis **lung** carcinoma cells injected s.c. in the right flank of 6-8w old C57B1/6 female mice	↑	Increase in DOX-induced antitumor effect, decrease in tumor growth	[217]
DOX, 4 mg/kg	Oroxylin A, 80 mg/kg	K562/ADM human **leukemia** cells injected via tail vein into 5-6w old female BALB/c nude mice	↑	Reduction of tumor progression, decrease in number of CD13+ leukemia cells in blood and spleen. Decrease in CXCR4, PI3K, pAkt	[275]
DOX, 5 mg/kg, i.v., on days 1, 8, 15	Quercetin, 100 mg/kg, orally, daily for 3 weeks	4T1 murine **breast** cancer cells injected into the second mammary fat pad of 7-8w old female BALB/c mice	↑	Increase in DOX antitumor effect, prolongation of life span of mice. Decrease in metastatic nodes in lung	[246]
DOX, 5 mg/kg, intratumorally, on days 1, 8, 15	Quercetin, 100 mg/kg, dietary, added to the chow	4T1 murine **breast** cancer cells injected into the second mammary fat pad of 7-8w old female BALB/c mice	↑	Synergism in cancer rejection, decrease in tumor volume, increase in tumor-free survival of mice. Promotion of immunosurveillance and induction of persistent T-cell tumor-specific responses; more necrotic tumors with no metastatic spread in lungs. Increase in intratumoral DOX	[230]
DOX, 5 mg/kg, through tail vein, every 3 days for 13 days, in BPL NPs	Quercetin, through tail vein, every 3 days for 13 days, in BPL NPs	MCF-7/adr human **breast** cancer cells injected s.c. into the upper back area of female nude mice	↑	Increase in DOX antitumor efficacy, induction of apoptosis. Inhibition of P-gp activity, increase in DOX cellular uptake and accumulation	[253]
DOX, 5 mg/kg, i.v., 7 doses	Quercetin, i.v., 7 doses	MCF-7/ADR human **breast** cancer cells injected s.c. into the right axilla of 6w old female BALB/c nude mice	~↑	No effect on tumor volume. Decrease in tumor volume and weight with biotin-decorated combined NPs showing highest tumor accumulation of DOX	[254]
DOX, 4 mg/kg, i.p., weekly for 3 weeks	Quercetin, 100 mg/kg, i.p., thrice a week for 3 weeks	SMMC7721 human **liver** cancer cells injected s.c. into the right supra scapula region of 4-6w old female nude athymic BALB/c nu/nu mice	↑	Decrease in tumor growth, volume and weight. Decrease in Ki67-positive tumor cells; increase in p53, decrease in Bcl-xl	[258]
DOX, 5 mg/kg, i.v., every 2 days for 14 days, co-loaded in HA-modified SiLN	Quercetin, 5 mg/kg, i.v., every 2 days for 14 days, co-loaded in HA-modified SiLN	SGC7901/ADR human **gastric** cancer cells inoculated s.c. into the left flank of 5w old male BALB/c nude mice	↑	Increase in antitumor efficacy. Increase in caspase-3, decrease in P-gp	[231]
DOX, 2 mg/kg, i.p., weekly for 5 weeks	Silibinin, 1.9 mg/kg, i.p., weekly for 5 weeks	Morris **hepatoma** (MH)-3924A rat hepatocellular carcinoma cells injected s.c. in syngeneic ACI rats; livers implanted with portion of tumors to rats	↑	Increase in tumor growth reduction	[296]

Table 6.14. (Continued)

Drug	Flavonoid	Biological system	Direction of combination	Effects	Ref.
DOX, 4 mg/kg, i.p., on days 1, 8, 15, 22	Silibinin, 200 mg/kg, by oral gavage, 5 days in week for 33 days	A549 human **lung** cancer cells injected s.c. into right flank of athymic BALB/c nu/nu male nude mice	↑	Increase in DOX antitumor efficacy, decrease in tumor weight. Potentiation of DOX-induced inhibition of PCNA and MVD, increase in apoptosis	[233]
DOX, 4 mg/kg, i.v., twice a week	Wogonin, 40 mg/kg, i.v., once every other day	K562/A02 **leukemia** cells injected via tail vein into 5-6w old NOD/SCID immunodeficient mice	↑	Potentiation of DOX-induced antileukemic effect, reduction of CD13$^+$ leukemia cells in bone marrow, spleen and peripheral blood. Suppression of Nrf2 signaling by Stat3/NF-κB inactivation	[272]
DNR, 1 mg/kg, i.p., on days 1, 3, 5, 7, 9, 11, 13, 5h after EGCG	EGCG, 40 mg/kg, i.p., on days 1-14	Hep3B human **hepatocellular** carcinoma cells injected s.c. into the right flank of athymic female nude mice	~	No effect on DNR antitumor activity	[311]
DNR, 1 mg/kg, i.p., on days 1, 3, 5, 7, 9, 11, 13, 5h after EGCG	EGCG, 40 mg/kg, i.p., on days 1-14	SMMC7721 human **hepatocellular** carcinoma cells injected s.c. into the right flank of athymic female nude mice	↑	Increase in DNR antitumor effect, decrease in tumor weight	[311]
EPI, 2.5 mg/kg/week, i.p., for 4 weeks	Isoliquiritigenin, 50 mg/kg/day, oral gavage	CSCs sorted from MDA-MB-231 human **breast** cancer cells implanted into the mammary glands of 4w old female NOD/SCID mice	↑	Chemosensitization of CSCs, suppression of tumor growth. Decrease in Ki67, inhibition of GRP78/β-catenin signaling	[319]
EPI, 2.5 mg/kg/week, i.p.	Isoliquiritigenin, 50 mg/kg/day, i.p.	MCF-7/ADR human **breast** cancer cells injected into the fourth mammary gland fat pad of 4-5w old female NOD/SCID mice	↑	Sensitization of tumors to EPI, decrease in tumor volume. Inhibition of miR-25 accompanied by increase in LC3-II, ULK1, BECN1 and decrease in ABCG2	[318]

ABC, ATP-binding cassette; Akt, protein kinase B; APE1, apurinic/apyrimidinic endonuclease 1; Bax, Bcl-2-associated X protein; Bcl-2, B-cell lymphoma 2; Bcl-xl, B-cell lymphoma-extra large; BECN, beclin; BPL, biotin-modified PEGylated liposomes; CSC, cancer stem cell; CXCR, chemokine receptor; DMC, 2`,4`-dihydroxy-6`-methoxy-3`,5`-dimethylchalcone; GRP, glucose-regulated protein; HA, hyaluronic acid; HIF-1α, hypoxia-inducible factor 1α; MDR, multidrug resistance; miR, microRNA; MVD, microvessel density; NF-κB, nuclear factor-κB; NP, nanoparticle; Nrf2, nuclear factor (erythroid-derived 2)-like 2; PARP, poly (ADP-ribose) polymerase; PCNA, proliferating cell nuclear antigen; P-gp, P-glycoprotein; PI3K, phosphoinositide 3-kinase; PUMA, p53 upregulated modulator of apoptosis; ROS, reactive oxygen species; SiLN, silica nanoparticle; STAT3, signal transducer and activator of transcription 3; ULK, Unc-51 like autophagy activating kinase.

Numerous different plant-based flavonoids have been studied in combination with DOX in various preclinical malignant models, both in cancer cell lines as well as xenografted animals (Table 6.13 and Table 6.14). At that, the most investigated phytochemical is abundant food flavonol quercetin. Combined treatment of human breast cancer MCF-7 and MDA-MB-231 cells with low dose of *quercetin* (0.7 μM) and DOX enhanced intracellular drug accumulation through downregulation of the expression of P-gp, MRP1 and BCRP transporters and led to significant increase in DOX-induced cytotoxicity and apoptosis. These effects were specific for tumor cells as the drug cytotoxicity was not enhanced in normal mammary cells and myocardial cells. Moreover, this treatment combination was more effective in elimination of breast cancer stem cells (BCSCs) as compared to single treatment with the drug [227]. In highly aggressive estrogen-independent breast cancer MDA-MB-231 cells, quercetin enhanced chemosensitivity to DOX by diminishing also tumor cell migration [185]. Several additional studies demonstrated potentiating effects of DOX cytotoxicity by quercetin in less aggressive estrogen-dependent MCF-7 cells [218, 228, 248-251]. Quercetin, at only 0.7 μM concentration, augmented antiproliferative and antiinvasive properties of DOX in this tumor cell line by suppressing the expression of hypoxia-inducible factor (HIF)-1α and P-gp, and increasing intracellular accumulation of drug. Similar effects were observed also in DOX-resistant MCF-7 cells, MCF-7/dox [248]. Combined treatment with quercetin and doxorubicin increased also apoptosis via suppression of Akt signaling pathway in both MCF-7 and MCF-7/dox cells [249]. Moreover, quercetin significantly synergized with DOX in eliminating BCSCs in MCF-7 and MCF-7/dox cells, and reversed MDR in drug resistant line [250]. In addition, combined treatment with high doses of quercetin (100 μM) and DOX blocked MCF-7 cells in G0/G1 phase of the cell cycle and induced apoptotic death [228]. Nanoencapsulated quercetin (phytosomes) sensitized MCF-7 cells to DOX reducing expression levels of several Nrf2-target genes, including NAD(P)H:quinone oxidoreductase 1 (NQO1) and MRP1 [251]. However, some other studies did not display the chemosensitizing effects of quercetin in MCF-7 cells, revealing ineffectiveness in modifying the DOX-induced cytotoxicity in these parental estrogen-dependent breast cancer cells, probably because of the low expression level of P-gp [185, 252-254]. In DOX-resistant MCF-7 cells (MCF-7 ADRr), quercetin reversed drug resistance and potentiated growth inhibitory activities of DOX by inhibiting P-gp expression and suppressing efflux activity of this membrane transporter [252, 255]. This augmentation was even stronger when both quercetin and DOX were nanoencapsulated into biotin-decorated drug delivery systems in increasing the cytotoxicity against MCF-7/adr cells. At this, the presence of biotin on the surface of nanoparticles played an essential role for efficient cellular uptake of DOX due to receptor-mediated endocytosis. These findings were confirmed in MCF-7/adr bearing nude mice models, where nanoencapsulated quercetin and DOX exhibited the highest antitumor effects with the smallest tumors, achieved by inhibiting P-gp activity and increasing DOX intratumoral accumulation. It is therefore feasible that these dual-loaded nanopreparations could further reduce cardiotoxicity related to the clinical application of DOX [253, 254]. In addition, dual loading of DOX and 3-aminopropoxy-linked quercetin in porous silicon-based nanoparticles resulted in a synergism in antiproliferation and cytotoxicity in both normal MCF-7 cells as well as its DOX-resistant line MCF-7/DOX[R] [256]. Quercetin potentiated the cytotoxic activity of DOX also in murine breast cancer cell line 4T1. This action was regulated in a hypoxia-dependent way, as therapeutic efficacy of DOX was only slightly affected by quercetin under normoxia while being substantially reinforced under hypoxia by suppressing intratumoral HIF-1α. The results obtained using an implant mouse model of 4T1 breast tumor were consistent with *in vitro* findings, confirming the ability of quercetin to enhance antitumor efficacy of DOX in breast cancer models. Moreover, the lifespan of mice treated with combination of quercetin and DOX was significantly prolonged and the pulmonary metastasis was suppressed as compared to their single drug treated counterparts [246]. Besides reduction of initial tumor volumes and prolonging tumor-free survival in immunocompetent mice bearing 4T1 tumors, combination of dietary quercetin and intratumoral DOX also promoted system immunosurveillance inducing persistent T-cell tumor-specific responses [230]. Although quercetin did not affect DOX-induced antiproliferative activity in human primary endometrial and ovarian cancer cells [90], this ubiquitous dietary flavonol increased DOX cytotoxicity in human cervical carcinoma HeLa cells and human prostate carcinoma PC3 cells [218]. In MDR human oral carcinoma KBCH[R]8-5 cells, quercetin reversed drug resistance and enhanced DOX-induced G2/M phase cell cycle arrest and apoptosis through downregulating P-gp overexpression by modulating Wnt/β-catenin signaling [255]. Combination of quercetin and DOX revealed a strong synergism in cytotoxic and apoptotic activities in human gastric adenocarcinoma AGS cells overexpressing cysteine-rich angiogenic inducer 61 (CYR61), CYR61-AGS. As CYR61 might be implicated in MDR through upregulation of MRP1 in gastric cancer cells, inclusion of quercetin to DOX treatment schemes contributed to reversal of this resistance phenomenon [257]. In another DOX-resistant human gastric cancer cell line, SGC7901/ADR, coencapsulation of quercetin and DOX in hyaluronic acid (HA)-modified silica nanoparticles led to selective uptake via HA-mediated endocytosis and increased intracellular retention of DOX, leading to synergistic proapoptotic effects. This action was accompanied by decrease in P-gp level in cell surface. Moreover, *in vivo* assays in SGC7901/ADR tumor bearing mice revealed significantly increased antitumor efficacy of combined treatment with nanoencapsulated quercetin and DOX compared to treatment with DOX monodelivery system. Such superior therapeutic activity was related to selective tumor targeting, as HA moiety could recognize the CD44 receptors overexpressed on gastric cancer cells [231]. Quercetin potentiated DOX-induced cytotoxicity also in different liver cancer cell lines. In human hepatocellular carcinoma BEL/5-FU cells, combined treatment with quercetin and DOX suppressed both function and expression of P-gp (ABCB1), MRP1 (ABCC1) and MRP2 (ABCC2) efflux pumps, thereby increasing the sensitivity of cells towards DOX [38]. DOX cytotoxicity was enhanced by quercetin also in human liver carcinoma HepG2 cells [218]. In human hepatoma cell lines QGY7701 and SMMC7721, quercetin potentiated DOX-induced cytotoxicity and p53-dependent mitochondrial apoptosis. Combined treatment of quercetin and DOX reduced also the tumor growth in SMMC7721 bearing mice [258]. In human lung carcinoma cell line A549 and its DOX-resistant subline A549/DOX, conjugation of quercetin and DOX to the surface of multifunctional nanoparticles resulted in augmentation of proapoptotic and antiproliferative properties of DOX, with an increase in G2/M phase cell cycle arrest [259]. Furthermore, quercetin intensely strengthened the chemotherapeutic efficacy of DOX in several human neuroblastoma cell lines (AF8, IMR-5 and SJ-N-KP) and moderately also in human Ewing`s sarcoma cell lines (6647, PDE02 and TC106), by inhibiting the expression of a number of Hsps. Following treatment with DOX, much higher Hsps levels were observed in neuroblastoma cells than Ewing`s sarcoma cells, explaining the much stronger DOX sensitization of neuroblastoma cells by quercetin [260]. On the contrary to above presented findings, quercetin still antagonized DOX-induced cytotoxicity in human colon carcinoma HCT-15 cells, by stimulating drug efflux probably via P-gp-mediated mechanism and reducing DOX intracellular concentration. Such cytoprotective effect of quercetin against DOX-induced growth inhibition suggests that colon cancer patients should avoid consuming quercetin containing food products and dietary supplements when they are receiving DOX chemotherapy, with the aim not to impair the drug therapeutic efficacy [261]. Lastly, current data about the role of quercetin in DOX treatment regimens against hematological malignancies are somewhat controversial. As quercetin decreased DOX-induced cytotoxicity by inducing cells to shift from G2/M to S phase of the cell cycle in murine leukemia L1210 cells [84], this dietary flavonol rather potentiated DOX-induced cytotoxicity in different human leukemia cell lines. In MDR human leukemia K562/ADR cells, combined treatment with quercetin and DOX synergistically promoted antiproliferative and proapoptotic properties of DOX through regulation of MAPK/ERK/JNK signaling and reduction of P-gp expression [262]. In several other human lymphoid and myeloid leukemia cell lines (CCRF-CEM, Jurkat, KG-1a and THP-1), cotreatment with quercetin and DOX led to synergistic downregulation of glutathione levels, increase in DNA damage, and induction of apoptosis and S and/or G2/M phase cell cycle arrest [206] (Table 6.13 and Table 6.14).

Thus, inclusion of quercetin in DOX treatment protocols could potentiate the antitumor efficacy of DOX at lower doses and thereby attenuate the toxic side effects of it in certain types of cancer cells, including breast, gastric, liver and lung tumors. This chemosensitizing action can be even more prevalent in highly aggressive and/or drug-resistant cells, providing a novel therapeutic regimen to treat some malignancies. Although quercetin might prove to be a potent adjuvant agent for DOX chemotherapy against certain types of tumors, few exceptions with opposite results have still been described. These data suggest that caution is required when cancer patients decide to consume food items rich in quercetin on their own initiative during the active treatment phase with DOX. In fact, based on the current preclinical findings, patients suffering from colon tumors or leukemia should be advised to avoid the intake of quercetin containing products in the period of receiving DOX chemotherapy. It is obvious that specific effects of quercetin on DOX cytotoxicity depend on cancer types and specific molecular characteristics of malignant cells.

Several other flavonols have also been studied in combination with DOX in preclinical cancer models. *Myricetin* sensitized HPV-positive (but not HPV-negative) human head and neck squamous carcinoma cells and human cervical cancer SiHa cells to cytotoxic responses of DOX, by interacting and suppressing the ability of E6 to bind to E6AP, a protein that is involved in p53 degradation. Resultant increase in p53 level enhanced apoptotic death. As high-risk E6 proteins subvert both intrinsic and extrinsic programmed cell death pathways, the ability of DOX to activate apoptosis is impeded in HPV-associated malignancies. Restoration of missing signaling molecules and chemosensitization of HPV-positive malignant cells to DOX by myricetin might be of clinical relevance, especially considering the relative resistance of cervical tumors to standard chemotherapeutic treatments [108]. *Fisetin* augmented cytotoxic action of DOX in drug-resistant human uterine sarcoma MES-SA/Dx5 cells via enhancement of drug retention inside the cells [263]. However, cotreatment of human non-small cell lung cancer A549 and H1299 cells with fisetin and DOX revealed time-dependent effects and led to antagonistic antitumor responses [212]; in spite of the fact that pretreatment of H1299 cells with fisetin for 6 hours before addition of drug still potentiated the DOX-induced cytotoxicity [105]. These data suggest that patients suffering from lung adenocarcinoma should avoid the consumption of fisetin containing products during the active treatment phase with DOX, with the aim not to attenuate the chemotherapeutic efficacy. Patients suffering from leukemia or colon carcinoma should also be advised to avoid the exposure to galangin. Flavonol *galangin* decreased cytotoxic potential of DOX in murine leukemia L1210 cells, causing cells to shift from G2/M to S phase of the cell cycle [84]. In human colon carcinoma HCT-15 cells, galangin stimulated drug efflux and inhibited accumulation of DOX inside the tumor cells, probably through a P-gp-mediated mechanism, conferring decreased cytotoxicity of DOX. Moreover, similar protection against DOX-induced cell growth inhibition was observed also in the presence of another dietary flavonol, *kaempferol* [261]. In human glioblastoma cell line T98G, cytotoxicity of DOX was not affected by kaempferol, although GST activity and MRP1 expression were increased [109]. DOX cytotoxicity was not influenced also by flavonol *morin* in human breast cancer cell line MDA435/LCC6MDR1, despite suppression of P-gp-mediated cellular drug efflux [264]. Methylated flavonol derivative *rhamnetin* or 7-methylquercetin increased the susceptibility of multidrug resistant human hepatocellular carcinoma HepG2/ADR cells to anticancer action of DOX [207]. Cytotoxicity of DOX was upregulated also by *isorhamnetin* or 3`-methylquercetin in human gastric cancer AGS cells [265]. *Tamarixetin* or 4`-methylquercetin decreased DOX resistance in drug-resistant human breast cancer MCF-7/ADR cells and human oral carcinoma KBCH^{R}8-5 cells. In the latest cell line, pretreatment with tamarixetin suppressed P-gp overexpression, induced DOX-mediated arrest at G2/M phase of the cell cycle and increased apoptosis. Moreover, glycosidic flavonol *rutin* or quercetin 3-O-rutinoside was even stronger chemosensitizer to DOX in these MDR cells than tamarixetin [255]. However, cotreatment of MCF-7 ADRr cells with rutin and DOX did still not affect the growth inhibitory action of DOX [252] (Table 6.13).

Certain flavonols and their analogs might serve as important chemoadjuvants for DOX therapeutic protocols against several cancers. In fact, combination of myricetin and DOX certainly needs further studies to develop more effective treatment options for HPV-positive cervical and oral tumors. However, patients with lung or colon cancer or leukemia must be very cautious in consuming food products or dietary supplements containing flavonols, i.e., fisetin, galangin or kaempferol, during chemotherapeutic treatment with DOX. At that, a special caution must be exercised in exposure to flavonol galangin, for which only antagonistic effects have been described in preclinical combinational studies with DOX.

The possible effects of structurally different flavones and their derivatives on therapeutic efficacy of DOX have also been investigated in diverse preclinical cancer models, both in malignant cell lines as well as xenografted tumor animals (Table 6.13 and Table 6.14). Common dietary flavone *apigenin* potentiated growth inhibitory and proapoptotic properties of DOX in different human breast cancer cell lines, i.e., estrogen receptor (ER)-positive/progesterone receptor (PR)-negative HCC70 cells and ER-negative/PR-negative lines MDA-MB-468, HCC1806 and MDA-MB-157, suggesting that apigenin could increase responsiveness of breast cancer patients to DOX antitumor effects even in the case of more aggressive hormone-independent tumor forms [266]. In addition, apigenin intensified DOX sensitivity in drug-resistant human uterine sarcoma cell line MES-SA/Dx5 through upregulation of DOX retention inside the cells, decrease in intracellular GSH content and increase in ROS generation [263]. In DOX-resistant human hepatocellular carcinoma BEL-7402/ADM cells, apigenin significantly increased intracellular drug accumulation and DOX-induced cytotoxic and proapoptotic responses. These effects were achieved via downregulation of PI3K/Akt signaling pathway and subsequent decrease in Nrf2 expression, further leading to reduction of downstream target genes [267]. In addition, apigenin substantially induced miR-520b expression and inhibited autophagy, thereby contributing to sensitizing BEL-7402/ADM cells to DOX [268]. Moreover, coadministration of apigenin and DOX to BEL-7402 bearing mice resulted in stronger suppression of tumor growth than observed with DOX monotreatment, again inhibiting Nrf2 levels in tumor tissues and increasing the proportion of apoptotic cells [267]. These findings show that dietary apigenin could be used as an effective adjuvant to chemosensitize liver cancer cells towards DOX treatment, revealing an important potential of this flavone for further therapeutic development [267, 268]. In several human lymphoid and myeloid leukemia cell lines, i.e., CCRF-CEM, Jurkat, KG-1a and THP-1, combined treatment with apigenin and DOX induced additive to synergistic increase in apoptosis and S and/or G2/M phase cell cycle arrest, through reduction of intracellular GSH levels and elevation of DNA damage [206]. However, in murine leukemia L1210 cells, apigenin and two other dietary flavones *luteolin* and chrysin antagonized DOX-induced cytotoxicity and caused cells to shift from G2/M to S phase of the cell cycle [84]. Moreover, luteolin diminished DOX-evoked cytotoxicity and enhanced cellular viability also in human ER-positive breast cancer MCF-7 cells and ER-negative breast cancer MDA-MB-453 cells. In MCF-7 cells, these cytoprotective effects were accompanied by decrease in DOX-induced ROS production and attenuation of mitochondrial damage, indicating that suppression of pharmacological action of DOX might be due to the antioxidant properties of luteolin [238]. However, in another human breast cancer cell line, MDA-MB-231, luteolin loaded in phytosomes as a potential nanodelivery system still augmented DOX-induced growth inhibition through suppression of Nrf2 signaling pathway and its downstream target genes [269]. Although luteolin did not affect antitumor efficacy of DOX in human gastric cancer AGS cells [144], this flavone synergistically increased cytotoxic action of DOX in two oxaliplatin (OXA)-resistant human colorectal cancer cell lines, HCT116-OX and SW620-OX, by inhibiting Nrf2 pathway [143]. Similarly, luteolin was able to chemosensitize human non-small cell lung cancer A549 cells to DOX, via reduction of Nrf2 expression and downregulation of respective target genes [181]. Therefore, luteolin might prove to be an important natural sensitizer for DOX chemotherapy in specific cancer types and cells through inhibition of Nrf2 signaling pathway, especially for tumors with constitutively active Nrf2. In human osteosarcoma cell line U2OS, luteolin also enhanced growth inhibitory activity of DOX, but this effect was mediated by increasing DOX-elicited autophagy [247]. Combined treatment of several human non-small cell lung cancer cell lines, i.e., A549, H157, H1975 and H460, with flavone *chrysin* and DOX led to a long-term depletion of intracellular GSH level and synergistically potentiated DOX-induced cytotoxicity [242]. In another human non-small cell lung cancer cell line, H23, chrysin suppressed expression of aldo-keto reductases (AKRs) induced by proinflammatory mediators like interleukin-6 (IL-6), thereby reducing IL-6-provoked chemoresistance phenotype. Overexpression of a member of AKR superfamily, dihydrodiol dehydrogenase (DDH), has previously been associated with chronic inflammatory conditions; besides progression, drug resistance and poor prognosis of human non-small cell lung cancer [270]. Therefore, further studies are certainly needed to determine the possibilities for clinical application of chrysin as an adjunct in the DOX treatment of chemoresistant non-small cell lung cancers. Inclusion of chrysin in DOX treatment protocols led to reversal of resistance also in human DOX-resistant hepatocellular carcinoma BEL-7402/ADM cells. These cells were distinguished by remarkably higher levels of Nrf2 compared to parent BEL-7402 cells, whereas pretreatment with chrysin resulted in downregulation of Nrf2 signaling through inhibition of PI3K/Akt and ERK pathways and sensitization of BEL-7402/ADM cells to therapeutic efficacy of DOX. Similar chemosensitizing mechanisms were initiated by chrysin apparently also in DOX-resistant human breast cancer MCF7/ADM cells [271]. Coencapsulation of flavone *baicalein* and DOX in HA-decorated nanostructured lipid carriers revealed synergistic anticancer responses both in DOX-resistant human breast cancer MCF-7/ADR cells as well as MCF-7/ADR tumors bearing mice, leading to considerably smaller tumors [213] (Table 6.13 and Table 6.14).

Studies with several natural monomethylated and polymethylated flavones demonstrated potentiating activity on DOX cytotoxicity in different malignant cells. Monomethylated flavone *wogonin* reversed DOX resistance in human chronic myelogenous leukemia K562/A02 cells by inactivating NF-κB and suppressing Nrf2 transcription. These results were confirmed also *in vivo* conditions, showing that wogonin potentiated DOX inhibitory effects on leukemia development in K562/A02 bearing mice by suppressing NF-κB/Nrf2 pathway. This was accompanied by attenuation of leukemic cell infiltration of the spleen and liver [272]. Wogonin inhibited Nrf2 signaling pathway also in DOX-resistant human breast cancer MCF-7/DOX cells, thereby increasing the sensitivity of cells to cytotoxic and proapoptotic activities of DOX [273]. In two other human breast cancer cell lines, Bcap-37 and MCF-7, combined treatment with wogonin and DOX enhanced therapeutic efficacy through downregulation of insulin like growth factor 1 receptor (IGF-1R) and inhibition of Akt signaling pathway, suggesting that inclusion of wogonin in DOX treatment protocols might confer improved antitumor activities in fighting against breast tumors [274]. Although wogonin had no effects on antitumor action of DOX in human lung cancer A549 cells [153], this flavone still contributed to overcoming of IL-6-induced DOX resistance in human non-small cell lung cancer H23 cells, suggesting that chemosensitizing activities of wogonin largely depend on the molecular characteristics of tumoral lung cells and involve multiple cellular mechanisms. In H23 cells, wogonin inhibited IL-6-induced AKRs overexpression and thereby attenuated inflammation-associated resistance to DOX [270]. Another monomethylated flavone, *acacetin* or 4`-methoxyapigenin, showed synergistic anticancer responses in combination with DOX in human non-small cell lung cancer A549 and H1299 cells. Such augmentation of DOX cytotoxicity involved increase in drug retention inside the cells through downregulation of P-gp (MDR1) transporter. In A549 line, combined treatment with acacetin and DOX induced a strong G2/M phase cell cycle arrest, repressed clonogenic potential and proliferation of cells [212]. *Oroxylin A* or 6-methoxybaicalein remarkably increased the sensitivity of DOX-resistant human chronic myeloid leukemia K562/ADM cells to DOX. This action was mediated by reducing the

248   *Katrin Sak*

expression of chemokine receptor 4 (CXCR4) and inhibiting PI3K/Akt/NF-κB pathway, eventually inducing apoptotic cell death. CXCR4 has been shown to be an important factor for survival and drug resistance of leukemic cells. The ligand of this receptor, CXCL12, is constitutively secreted by bone marrow stromal cells and regulates survival, proliferation and migration of leukemic cells. Targeting the leukemia microenvironment and suppression of CXCR4 could confer overcoming resistance to conventional chemotherapeutic drugs. Overexpression of CXCR4, upregulation of its downstream PI3K/Akt signaling and promoting nuclear translocation of NF-κB all contributed to resistance of K562 cells towards pharmacological action of DOX, whereas oroxylin A reversed these effects and resulted in apoptotic death. Moreover, oroxylin A inhibited CXCL12/CXCR4 pathway also *in vivo* in K562/ADM bearing mice, leading to a significant decrease in CD13$^+$ leukemic cells in the blood and spleen, besides suppression of Akt activation and CXCR4 expression in malignant cells derived from bone marrow. Therefore, oroxylin A might serve as a valuable adjuvant for treatment of myelogenous leukemias with DOX to circumvent CXCR4-associated chemoresistance [275]. Two trimethylated flavones, i.e., *eupatorin* and *salvigenin*, potentiated mitochondrial apoptotic cascade through increased production of ROS in combination with DOX in human colon cancer HT-29 and SW948 cells [245]. Hexamethoxyflavone *nobiletin* sensitized P-gp-overexpressing paclitaxel (PTX)-resistant human non-small cell lung cancer A549/T cells and human ovarian cancer A2780/T cells to DOX by increasing intracellular drug accumulation through inhibition of transporter function of P-gp (ABCB1), while not affecting intracellular levels and therapeutic potential of DOX in parental A2780 cells. Therefore, nobiletin might be a good candidate for further studies on reversal of P-gp-mediated drug resistance in combinational cancer chemotherapy [276]. In human breast cancer cells, nobiletin increased DOX cytotoxicity at least partly on p53-dependent manner. In wild-type p53-expressing MCF-7 cells, nobiletin potentiated antiproliferative and proapoptotic action of DOX; while in T47D cells with mutant p53, this polymethylated flavone did not affect DOX-induced cytotoxicity [277]. The only glycosylated flavone studied so far, i.e., *baicalin* or baicalein 7-O-glucuronide, increased intracellular accumulation of DOX and augmented drug therapeutic efficacy in DOX-resistant human acute myeloid leukemia HL-60/ADM cells. At that, potentiation of drug cytotoxicity and reversal of DOX resistance were achieved by suppression of PI3K/Akt pathway and downstream MDR-related genes, including MRP1 and lung resistance protein (LRP), suggesting that this glycosidic flavone might be a potential complement agent for therapeutic treatment of resistant leukemias with DOX-based regimens. Further clinical validation of these findings is currently on the table [278] (Table 6.13 and Table 6.14).

The above-described data convincingly indicate that certain flavones and their methylated derivatives can be valuable chemoadjuvants for DOX treatment of different tumors, allowing to achieve therapeutical effectiveness at lower drug doses and thereby reduce the extent of toxicity on normal healthy cells, including life-threatening cardiotoxicity. Specific synergistic combinations certainly need further therapeutic development to enhance clinical outcome and improve quality of life of patients. However, a few opposite findings still point to the need to be careful with the intake of plant-derived flavones during the active treatment phase with DOX chemotherapy, preventing the exposure to specific compounds (apigenin, luteolin, chrysin) in case of certain cancers (leukemia, breast cancer). Consumption of flavones without a special knowledge about the possible coeffects with DOX in malignant cells can be risky and, in some cases, even harmful.

Studies with structurally different green tea flavanols have shown predominantly potentiating effects on DOX cytotoxicity in diverse malignant cells (Table 6.13 and Table 6.14). The major green tea catechin, *EGCG*, could reverse the multidrug resistance phenotype in human oral carcinoma cell line KB-A1, that is a P-gp-overexpressing subline of KB-3-1 cells. This chemosensitization was associated with suppression of MDR1 gene expression and/or inhibition of ATPase activity of P-gp, leading to increase in DOX concentration inside the cells [243, 244, 279-281]. Modulation of DOX-generated oxidative stress by EGCG could also contribute to reversal of MDR [280]. Moreover, EGCG was able to increase intratumoral DOX concentration also in mice xenografts of resistant KB-A1 cells, accompanied by enhancement of DOX efficacy in promoting apoptosis and inhibiting tumor growth [240, 281]. However, EGCG did not reveal any modulating effects on DOX-induced cytotoxicity in parental drug-sensitive oral carcinoma KB-3-1 cells with no P-gp expression on cell surface [243, 279, 280]. In human esophageal squamous cell carcinoma Eca109 cells transfected with ABCG2 gene, Eca109/ABCG2, combined treatment with EGCG and DOX led to increased intracellular drug concentration through reduction of ABCG2 expression, followed by enhanced apoptosis rate compared to DOX monotreatment [282]. EGCG was able to inhibit drug efflux and effectively reverse MDR also in DOX-resistant human breast cancer MCF-7/Adr cells. In fact, co-loading EGCG and DOX into polyion complex (PIC) micelles sensitized resistant cells to DOX [214]. A novel nanocomplex of EGCG and DOX, i.e., assembled gold nanoparticles (AuNPs), significantly inhibited proliferation of highly metastatic human prostate cancer PC-3 cells. As EGCG can specifically bind to the laminin (Lam) receptor overexpressed in some tumor cells, including malignant prostate cells, cellular uptake of DOX was enhanced by Lam 67R receptor-mediated endocytosis leading to intracellular drug accumulation [220]. In two human prostate cancer lines, highly metastatic PC-3ML cells and primary prostate cancer IBC-10a cells, EGCG potentiated DOX-induced inhibition of cell growth and colony formation. In addition, *in vivo* conditions, EGCG sensitized PC-3ML xenografts bearing mice to DOX treatment, accompanied by enhanced intratumoral drug retention, blocking of tumor growth and recurrence, and increasing overall survival rates of experimental animals. Moreover, combined treatment with EGCG and DOX was able to eradicate established tumors even in mice injected with CD44^{hi} tumor-initiating cells that were isolated from human prostate cancer PCa-20a cells. Based on these promising *in vitro* and *in vivo* findings, application of EGCG as a novel potent adjuvant for DOX chemotherapy might be of clinical significance in the treatment of highly aggressive, metastatic tumors or primary prostate tumors. At that, therapeutically effective doses of DOX were significantly (tenfold) lowered compared to concentrations required in DOX monotherapy to block the tumor growth [283]. EGCG can be a valuable adjuvant of DOX chemotherapy also in the treatment of hepatocellular carcinomas. In two human liver cancer cell lines, Hep3B and HepG2, cotreatment with EGCG and DOX synergistically promoted inhibition of cell growth and viability. In Hep3B cells, presence of EGCG completely inhibited DOX-induced autophagy and augmented apoptotic cell death. In Hep3B xenograft tumor model, combined treatment with EGCG and DOX led to increased reduction of tumor growth, with decrease in expression of autophagic hallmarks and enhanced proportion of apoptotic cells. As DOX-induced autophagy served as a self-protective mechanism to escape from drug cytotoxicity in liver cancer cells, inhibition of autophagy by EGCG led to chemosensitization of tumor cells towards DOX antineoplastic action [221]. EGCG and another dietary flavanol *epicatechin 3-gallate (ECG)* significantly augmented antiproliferative properties of DOX also in DOX-resistant human hepatocellular carcinoma BEL-7404/DOX cells, by increasing drug concentration inside the cells through downregulation of gene expression and efflux activity of P-gp transporter. At that, EGCG was somewhat more effective than ECG in reversing drug resistance, whereas some increase in DOX cytotoxicity was detected also in parental BEL-7404 cells. Moreover, combined administration of EGCG and DOX resulted in a substantial inhibition of hepatoma growth in BEL-7404/DOX bearing mice, as compared to treatment with drug alone. This *in vivo* anticancer action was accompanied by suppression of MDR1 expression, inhibition of P-gp pump function and enhancement of drug accumulation in tumoral tissues, consistent with *in vitro* results [184]. Furthermore, besides EGCG, its chemically modified ethylated derivative, Y6, being essentially more stable than parent EGCG, improved also the chemosensitizing potential in drug-resistant BEL-7404/DOX cells through inhibition of cellular proliferation and inducing apoptotic death. These mechanisms were likely to be related to the decline in expression of HIF-1α and MDR1 proteins [284]. Thus, it is evident that EGCG can impact the therapeutic efficacy of DOX by modulating several cellular signaling pathways in different liver cancer cells, resulting in increase in antitumor activities. Regarding the unsatisfying efficacy of current liver cancer therapies, application of EGCG as a novel chemosensitizer in DOX treatment regimens might be of clinical relevance and certainly needs further investigations. Besides hepatocellular carcinoma cells, natural flavanol ECG increased susceptibility to DOX-induced cytotoxicity also in DOX-resistant human breast cancer MCF-7/ADR cells and human oral carcinoma KBCH^{R}8-5 cells. In the latest cells, ECG enhanced DOX-mediated G2/M phase cell cycle arrest and promoted apoptotic death by downregulating P-gp (ABCB1) overexpression through modulating Wnt/β-catenin signaling [255]. In DOX-resistant human colon carcinoma SW620-dox cells and murine sarcoma S180-dox cells, EGCG and another flavanol *epigallocatechin (EGC)* augmented DOX-induced cytotoxic responses only in the case of pretreatment with flavanols for 24 hours prior to addition of DOX, but not with simultaneous treatment [236]. Similar results were found also in human colorectal adenocarcinoma HCT-8 cells, where cotreatment with DOX and different flavanols (EGCG, EGC, ECG, *epicatechin* or catechin) did not affect the antiproliferative activity observed with drug alone [216]. Lastly, flavanol *catechin* loaded into dextran-catechin (Dex-CT) conjugate and used for coating of nanographene oxide (NGO) nanocarrier revealed a synergistic activity with DOX in human neuroblastoma cell line BE(2)C and its DOX-resistant subline BE(2)C/ADR. In the respective resistant cells, catechin decreased P-gp expression and reversed DOX chemoresistant phenotype [285] (Table 6.13 and Table 6.14).

To date, only beneficial interactions have been reported between different flavanols and DOX, with no contraindicative effects found in diverse malignant cells. Chemosensitization of tumors to DOX treatment by EGCG and other catechins was especially notable in drug resistant cancers, suggesting that inclusion of these natural compounds in DOX treatment protocols could effectively address the limitations of chemotherapy, including DOX-induced cardiotoxicity. In fact, combined application of EGCG and DOX might be of special interest for development of improved treatment options for clinical management of prostate and liver tumors, among other common malignancies. The currently available data allow to suppose that consumption of flavanols, including drinking of green tea or intake of EGCG-containing dietary supplements, is not contravened, but even recommended, during the active chemotherapeutic treatment phase with DOX. Further animal studies and clinical trials must be performed to prove (or disprove) this statement, currently based only on preclinical findings.

Chemotherapeutic efficacy of DOX has been studied also in combination with a few most common dietary flavanones (Table 6.13 and Table 6.14). *Naringenin* enhanced the sensitivity of both human colorectal cancer SW1116 cells and human breast cancer HTB26 cells to DOX, compared to single treatment with the drug [10]. In addition, naringenin increased cell growth inhibitory and proapoptotic potential of DOX also in human non-small cell lung cancer A549 cells and human breast cancer MCF-7 cells, but not in human hepatocellular carcinoma HepG2 cells and DOX-resistant breast cancer MCF-7/DOX cells. Such cancer cell type-dependent activity pattern indicated a selective modulation of drug efflux pathways by naringenin. In fact, this dietary flavanone increased the intracellular DOX accumulation via suppression of drug efflux in the cells expressing MRP1 and MRP2 transporters, but not P-gp. This means that naringenin might be useful to reduce the development of chemoresistance in P-gp non-expressing tumors, modulating selectively the functions of MRP proteins. Naringenin potentiated antitumor action of DOX also in murine Lewis lung carcinoma LLC cells bearing mice, resulting in significantly decreased tumor growth and substantially smaller tumors [217]. However, another common dietary flavanone, *hesperetin*, showed antagonistic antitumor action in combination with DOX in human osteosarcoma U2OS cells. This antagonism was associated with increase in S phase arrest of the cell cycle [203]. The only studied glycosylated flavanone, *hesperidin* or hesperetin 7-rutinoside, sensitized human Ramos Burkitt's lymphoma cells to DOX-induced growth inhibition and apoptosis through suppression of both constitutive and DOX-mediated NF-κB activation [286]. Hesperidin potentiated the antitumor activities of DOX also in Ehrlich ascites carcinoma (EAC) bearing mice. At that, combined treatment of xenograft mice led to decrease in ascitic volume and the number of viable cells, besides prolongation of the lifespan of mice [225] (Table 6.13 and Table 6.14).

Common dietary flavanone naringenin can behave as a cancer type-dependent chemosensitizer to DOX antineoplastic effects, acting selectively in tumors with drug resistance modulated by MRPs while being inactive in targeting P-gp function. Therefore, in certain cases, the combination of naringenin with other flavonoids that modulate P-gp functions may be necessary to achieve the highest chemosensitizing potential to DOX anticancer responses. Such complex combinations are still not explored to date, but might probably open new avenues in combinational chemotherapy with adjuvant natural non-toxic agents. However, it must be always kept in mind that specific antagonistic combinations can reduce or even abolish the therapeutic efficacy of DOX. One such contraindicated flavanone in DOX chemotherapy against osteosarcoma is hesperetin, suggesting that patients suffering from bone cancer should avoid exposure to citrus products rich in hesperetin during the active treatment phase with DOX.

The possible role of soy isoflavones and their derivatives on antitumor action of DOX has also been studied in different preclinical cancer models, both in malignant cell lines as well as xenografted animals (Table 6.13 and Table 6.14). As genistein is a well-known phytoestrogen, its action in hormone-dependent malignancies has been of great interest; however, data about possible coeffects with conventional chemotherapeutics like DOX are still rather scarce. Exposure to *genistein* has been demonstrated to antagonize DOX cytotoxicity and further promote chemoresistance to DOX treatment in human estrogen receptor (ER)-positive breast cancer MCF-7 cells, whereas this effect depended somewhat also on the concentration ratio of both agents [287, 288]. However, in DOX-resistant MCF-7/ADR[R] cells that is an ER-negative subline, combined treatment with genistein and DOX led to enhanced inhibition of cellular proliferation as compared to the drug alone [288]. Similarly, in another DOX-resistant subline, MCF-7/Adr, genistein and DOX revealed synergistic cytotoxic responses associated with increased intracellular drug accumulation, cell cycle arrest at the G2/M phase and apoptotic death, besides suppression of human epidermal growth factor receptor 2 (HER2/neu) expression [223]. In addition, genistein made human ER-negative breast cancer cells MDA-MB-231 and

MDA-231 more sensitive to DOX treatment, with synergistic potentiation of cell growth inhibition [62, 287, 288]. In HER2-overexpressing human breast cancer MDA-MB-453 cells, genistein enhanced DOX cytotoxicity by inducing necrotic-like cell death, but not apoptosis, through the inactivation of HER-2 and Akt [289]. The possible therapeutic value of these findings certainly requires further investigations, but still warn that patients with hormone-positive breast tumors should abstain from intake of food items rich in genistein during their chemotherapeutic treatment with DOX. Genistein modulated DOX cytotoxicity also in human non-small cell lung cancer cells, whereas this effect was dependent on the expression of epidermal growth factor receptor (EGFR) on cell membrane. In fact, in NCI-H596 cells with strong expression of EGFR, genistein as a general tyrosine kinase inhibitor suppressed EGFR and led to increase in antiproliferative and proapoptotic activities of DOX. However, in NCI-H358 cells with only weak expression of EGFR, genistein did not affect DOX-induced cytotoxicity [126]. Moreover, in murine prostate cancer RM-1 cells bearing mice, administration of genistein in combination with nanoencapsulated DOX (DOX-NPs) resulted in amplification of ROS-induced oxidative damage and reduction of oxidative DNA repair, by downregulating expression of the oxidative DNA repair enzyme apurinic/apyrimidinic endonuclease 1 (APE1). Hence, the tumor growth and also distant metastasis of prostate cancer cells were significantly suppressed [224]. A methylated genistein derivative, *biochanin A* or 4`-methylgenistein, potentiated DOX-induced cytotoxicity in estradiol-independent human breast cancer cell line MDA435/LCC6 and its multidrug resistant subline MDA435/LCC6MDR1, consistent with inhibition of P-gp-mediated drug efflux [264]. Also, biochanin A was able to sensitize DOX-resistant human colorectal adenocarcinoma ColoR cells to antitumor action of DOX, whereas coencapsulation of both agents into liposomes further increased drug uptake and inhibition of cell viability [290]. Another natural methylated isoflavone, *formononetin* or 4`-methyldaidzein, enhanced DOX cytotoxicity in several human glioma cells, i.e., T98G, U215MG and U87MG. In the latest line, cotreatment with formononetin and DOX significantly downregulated drug-induced expression of histone deacetylase 5 (HDAC5) and reversed epithelial-mesenchymal transition (EMT), thus contributing to improved therapeutic efficacy of DOX-based chemotherapy against gliomas [291]. Augmentation of antiproliferative and antimigratory properties of DOX was observed also in combined treatment of several human gastric cancer cell lines (BGC823, NCI-N87 and SGC7901) with dietary methylated isoflavone *calycosin* and DOX. Hence, combination of calycosin and DOX could result in better therapeutic effects at markedly lower drug concentrations [139]. Isoflavone derivative *CJY* potentiated DOX-induced cytotoxicity in drug-resistant human myelogenous leukemia K562/DOX cells, but not in parental K562 cells. At that, reversal of resistance was related to increase in intracellular drug accumulation, G2/M phase cell cycle arrest and apoptotic cell death [292]. Pyranoisoflavone *barbigerone* augmented DOX cytotoxicity in DOX-resistant human breast cancer MCF-7/ADR cells with no modulation of drug activity in parental MCF-7 cells. This potentiation was achieved through decrease in efflux and increase in intracellular concentration of DOX by suppressing P-gp ATPase activity. Moreover, combined administration of barbigerone and DOX to MCF-7/ADR bearing mice significantly inhibited the tumor growth, despite the fact that treatment of xenografted mice with DOX alone revealed no substantial effect on tumor growth [293] (Table 6.13 and Table 6.14).

Isoflavones can modulate the antitumor action of DOX in several ways, acting on diverse molecular targets and regulating different signaling pathways in a variety of malignant cells. Thus, introduction of certain isoflavones or their derivatives into DOX chemotherapeutic protocols could increase anticancer activities with fewer toxic side effects to normal healthy cells. However, among other things, effects of isoflavones as common dietary phytoestrogens on DOX cytotoxicity depend also on the presence of estrogen receptors in target tumoral cells. Therefore, patients with hormone-dependent cancers (breast tumors) should be particularly cautious in consuming isoflavones (genistein) containing food products or dietary supplements when they are receiving chemotherapeutic treatment with DOX; based on a couple of preclinical studies, this combination can be antagonistic.

Combined effects of milk thistle flavonolignan silibinin and DOX have also been studied in different preclinical cancer models (Table 6.13 and Table 6.14). *Silibinin* synergistically increased DOX-induced growth inhibitory and proapoptotic activities in both human estrogen-dependent breast cancer MCF-7 cells as well as estrogen-independent breast cancer MDA-MB468 cells [162]. Silibinin synergistically potentiated DOX-induced cell growth inhibition also in DOX-resistant MCF-7 cells, MCF-7 DOXr [164]. In estrogen-independent human breast cancer cell line MDA-MB-435 and its DOX-resistant subline, MDA-MB-435/DOX, silibinin and DOX synergistically inhibited cell viability and promoted apoptotic death through suppression of STAT3, ERK and Akt oncogenic pathways [163]. These findings clearly suggest that potentiation of DOX antitumor activities by silibinin is independent on the expression of estrogen receptors in breast cancer cells, providing thus a valuable and universal adjuvant agent for DOX-based chemotherapy against different types of breast tumors. Silibinin increased DOX-induced cell growth inhibition also in human androgen-dependent prostate carcinoma LNCaP cells and human advanced prostate cancer DU145 cells. This effect was more prominent in advanced prostate cancer DU145 cells revealing a strong synergistic potentiation that was associated with G2/M phase arrest in cell cycle progression and apoptotic cell death; providing thus an attractive option to lower drug dosages and thereby reduce DOX-caused life-threatening toxicities in the treatment of metastatic prostate tumors [294]. In DOX-resistant human colorectal adenocarcinoma cell line LoVo DOX, silibinin reversed resistance phenotype and led to a synergistic increase in therapeutic efficacy of DOX. This effect was accompanied by reduction of glucose uptake after silibinin treatment, as this flavonolignan decreased the expression of glucose transporter 1 (GLUT1), leading to modulation of glucose metabolism in malignant cells [295]. Growth of human liver cancer HEPG2 cells was also synergistically decreased by combination treatment with silibinin and DOX, attributed to the cell cycle arrest at G2/M phase and increase in apoptotic cell death. Moreover, in an orthotopic rat model of liver cancer, combined treatment with silibinin and DOX significantly slowed the tumor progression as compared to individual treatment with the drug [296]. Although silibinin did not affect DOX cytotoxicity in parental human small-cell lung carcinoma H69 cells, this natural flavonolignan synergistically enhanced antitumor action of DOX and reversed resistance phenotype in multidrug resistant subline of H69, VPA17 [167]. In addition, in human non-small cell lung cancer A549 cells, silibinin augmented cell growth inhibitory and proapoptotic activities of DOX via almost complete suppression of DOX-induced NF-κB activation and reduction of cyclooxygenase (COX)-2 levels. Moreover, silibinin enhanced the therapeutic efficacy of DOX also *in vivo* conditions in suppressing A549 tumor xenograft growth in athymic nude mice, decreasing proliferation index and microvessel density while increasing the proportion of apoptotic cells [233]. Last but not least, silibinin augmented DOX chemosensitivity also in human anaplastic lymphoma kinase (ALK)-positive anaplastic large cell lymphoma cell lines Karpas 299 and SupM2, particularly in a small subset of cells expressing the embryonic stem cell marker Sox2 [297] (Table 6.13 and Table 6.14).

The current findings have demonstrated only beneficial (mostly synergistic) cooperation between silibinin and DOX in different preclinical cancer models, suggesting that intake of silibinin containing products is not contravened, but could be even advisable, for cancer patients under active chemotherapeutic treatment with DOX; of course, if confirmed in further studies. More research is urgently needed to evolve current promising preclinical results to clinically applicable therapeutic strategies, particularly in the treatment of breast and prostate tumors.

Numerous structurally different analogs of flavonoids have been tested in combination with DOX in a variety of preclinical cancer models revealing diverse results (Table 6.13 and Table 6.14). Although chalcone *phloretin* inhibited P-gp-mediated DOX efflux in multidrug resistant human breast cancer MDA435/LCC6MDR1 cells, this natural compound did still not affect the cytotoxic responses induced by DOX [264]. Natural chalcone derivative *2`,4`-dihydroxy-6`-methoxy-3`,5`-dimethylchalcone (DMC)* had no obvious effects on DOX cytotoxicity in parent human oral carcinoma KB-3-1 cells, but potentiated anticancer action of DOX in the respective DOX-resistant KB-A1 cells through downregulation of P-gp and increase in intracellular drug accumulation. Combined treatment with DMC and DOX significantly inhibited tumor growth also in KB-A1 bearing mice as demonstrated by a considerable decrease in xenograft weights [298]. In addition, DMC was able, at least partially, to reverse DOX resistance also in human hepatocellular carcinoma BEL-7402/5-FU cells [299]. Another chalcone

256   *Katrin Sak*

isoliquiritigenin enhanced DOX-induced antimyeloma activity in murine myeloma MPC-11 bearing mice [300] (Table 6.13 and Table 6.14).

Prenylated flavonoid *isoxanthohumol* clearly antagonized DOX efficacy in both invasive human melanoma A375 cells as well as nonmetastatic murine melanoma B16 cells [171], suggesting that isoxanthohumol may counteract antimelanoma activities of DOX and promote tumor development. Nevertheless, another prenylated flavonoid, *icaritin*, potentiated DOX cytotoxicity in DOX-resistant human hepatocellular carcinoma HepG2/ADR cells, by enhancing the accumulation of DOX inside the cells through downregulation of P-gp expression [226]. Icaritin strengthened DOX-induced cytotoxicity also in DOX-resistant human osteosarcoma MG-63/DOX cells. This effect was associated with decrease in the mRNA and protein levels of P-gp (MDR1) and MRP1 by inhibition of STAT3 pathway, ultimately leading to augmentation of DOX-induced apoptosis [301]. Similarly, two glycosylated icaritin derivatives, *icariin* and *icariside II*, also reversed drug resistance and increased DOX cytotoxicity in MG-63/DOX cells [301]. Moreover, icariin downregulated P-gp (MDR1) expression, enhanced DOX accumulation and retention inside the MG-63/DOX cells and increased apoptotic cell death, by inhibiting PI3K/Akt signaling pathway [302]. Thus, icaritin and its glycosides are able to effectively reverse multidrug resistance phenomenon and thereby represent potential candidates for adjunctive agents for DOX chemotherapy in the treatment of osteosarcoma (Table 6.13).

Flavanonol *ampelopsin* or dihydromyricetin sensitized DOX-resistant human ovarian cancer A2780/DOX cells to proapoptotic action of DOX via activation of p53 and subsequent downregulation of survivin expression [303]. These data indicate that the status of functional p53 might be an important factor determining the susceptibility of malignant ovarian cells to ampelopsin. The same was true also in human leukemia cells, where pretreatment with ampelopsin augmented proapoptotic activities of DOX in U937 cells with wild-type p53, but not in mutant p53 expressing K-562 cells and p53-null HL-60 cells. Moreover, ampelopsin potentiated DOX-induced tumor growth inhibition also in U937 bearing mice, by inducing p53 accumulation and increasing apoptotic death within cancerous tissue [215]. Another studied flavanonol, *taxifolin*, sensitized multidrug resistant human cervical cancer KB-vin cells towards DOX-induced cell viability reduction and apoptosis via suppression of P-gp expression and efflux function, while revealing no effect on DOX cytotoxicity in drug-sensitive human cervical cancer HeLaS3 cells [304]. Rotenoid *deguelin* enhanced the chemotherapeutic efficacy of DOX both *in vitro* in two human lung cancer cell lines, A549 with wild-type p53 and H1299 with mutant p53, as well as *in vivo* in A549 bearing mice. This potentiation was associated with induction of the p53 upregulated modulator of apoptosis (PUMA) independently on p53 through inhibition of PI3K/Akt pathway, leading to mitochondrial apoptotic cell death. As resistance to DOX can be partly raised via p53 mutation, inclusion of deguelin in DOX treatment protocols could contribute to enhancing PUMA through p53-

independent pathway to overcome resistance phenotype and improve therapeutic outcome in lung cancer treatment [305]. Furthermore, in human pancreatic cancer cell lines MIA PaCa-2 and Panc-1, deguelin was able to markedly potentiate apoptotic cell death by suppression of DOX-induced protective autophagy. Therefore, combination of deguelin and DOX may have the potential to be developed into a novel therapeutic strategy for the treatment of highly lethal pancreatic cancer in the future [306]. Last but not least, flavonostilbene *alopecurone B* reversed multidrug resistance phenotype in DOX-resistant human osteosarcoma MG-63-DOX cells, reinforcing DOX-induced apoptosis. This potentiation was associated with increase in intracellular DOX accumulation through inhibition of expression and function of P-gp, by suppressing NF-κB signaling pathway [235] (Table 6.13 and Table 6.14).

The results representing the different possibilities to intervene in DOX resistance by various natural flavonoids are summarized in Figure 6.8. Several structurally different flavonoids can chemosensitize diverse cancer cells towards antineoplastic action of DOX allowing to lower drug doses and reduce the extent of toxic side effects, including fatal cardiotoxicity. Therefore, application of DOX in combination with specific flavonoids can bring along an important breakthrough in traditional DOX chemotherapy enhancing cytotoxic efficacy, while concurrently improving quality of life of patients. Nevertheless, it must be always beard in mind that some flavonoids can antagonize the cytotoxic responses of DOX against certain types of malignancies, indicating that patients should be advised about these contraindicative combinations to be able to avoid them. Intake of flavonoid rich food items or dietary supplements by cancer patients must be well-informed and evidence-based.

According to the current experimental findings it is recommended for cancer patients *not to consume* dietary products or dietary supplements rich in following plant flavonoids during the active chemotherapeutic treatment phase with **doxorubicin**:

- **quercetin** in colon carcinoma
- **galangin** in colon carcinoma
- **kaempferol** in colon carcinoma
- **luteolin** in estrogen receptor-positive and estrogen receptor-negative breast cancer
- **genistein** in estrogen receptor-positive breast cancer
- **fisetin** in non-small cell lung cancer (*simultaneous administration*)
- **hesperetin** in osteosarcoma
- **isoxanthohumol** in melanoma
- **quercetin** in leukemia
- **galangin** in leukemia
- **apigenin** in leukemia
- **luteolin** in leukemia
- **chrysin** in leukemia

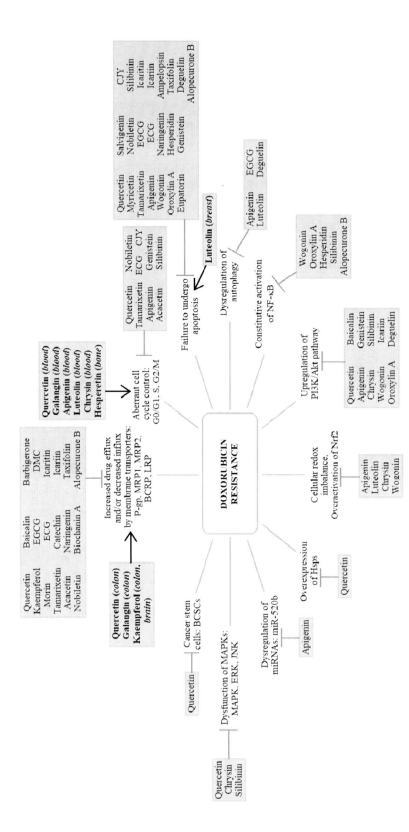

Figure 6.8. Major cellular mechanisms of doxorubicin resistance and possibilities to intervene with flavonoids (Akt, protein kinase B; BCRP, breast cancer resistance protein; BCSC, breast cancer stem cell; DMC, 2',4'-dihydroxy-6'-methoxy-3',5'-dimethylchalcone; ERK, extracellular signal-regulated kinase; Hsp, heat shock protein; JNK, c-Jun N-terminal kinase; LRP, lung resistance protein; MAPK, mitogen-activated protein kinase; miR, microRNA; MRP, multidrug resistance-associated protein; NF-κB, nuclear factor-κB; Nrf2, nuclear factor (erythroid-derived 2)-like 2; P-gp, P-glycoprotein; PI3K, phosphoinositide 3-kinase).

Daunorubicin (DNR)

Table 6.15. Effects of flavonoids on anticancer action of daunorubicin (DNR) *in vitro* conditions

Drug	Flavonoid	Biological system	Direction of combination	Effects	Ref.
DNR, 0.2-30 μM	4`,7-DMF, 10, 20 μM	CCRF-CEM human acute lymphoblastic **leukemia** cell line	~	No effect on DNR cytotoxicity	[312]
DNR, 0.2-30 μM	4`,7-Dimethoxyisoflavone, 10, 20 μM	CEM/VBL$_{100}$ human acute lymphoblastic **leukemia** cell line, VBL-resistant, overexpressing P-gp	↓	Decrease in DNR-induced cytotoxicity, increase in DNR IC$_{50}$. Activation of DNR-stimulated P-gp ATPase activity, decrease in DNR cellular accumulation	[312]
DNR, 0.2-30 μM	Baptigenin Ψ, 10, 20 μM	CEM/VBL$_{100}$ human acute lymphoblastic **leukemia** cell line, VBL-resistant, overexpressing P-gp	↓	Decrease in DNR-induced cytotoxicity, increase in DNR IC$_{50}$. Activation of DNR-stimulated P-gp ATPase activity, decrease in DNR cellular accumulation	[312]
DNR, 0.2-30 μM	Biochanin A, 10, 20 μM	CEM/VBL$_{100}$ human acute lymphoblastic **leukemia** cell line, VBL-resistant, overexpressing P-gp	↓	Decrease in DNR-induced cytotoxicity, increase in DNR IC$_{50}$. Decrease in DNR cellular accumulation	[312]
DNR, 0.2-30 μM	Chrysin, 10, 20 μM	CEM/VBL$_{100}$ human acute lymphoblastic **leukemia** cell line, VBL-resistant, overexpressing P-gp	↓	Decrease in DNR-induced cytotoxicity, increase in DNR IC$_{50}$. Decrease in DNR cellular accumulation	[312]
DNR, 0.4 μM	ECG, 20 μM	HepG2 human **hepatocellular** carcinoma cell line, CBR1 high expression	↑	Increase in DNR-induced cell growth inhibition. Suppression of CBR1 activity	[311]
DNR, 0.1 μM	ECG, 20 μM	SMMC7721 human **hepatocellular** carcinoma cell line, CBR1 high expression	↑	Increase in DNR-induced cell growth inhibition. Suppression of CBR1 activity	[311]
DNR, 0.4 μM	EGC, 20 μM	HepG2 human **hepatocellular** carcinoma cell line, CBR1 high expression	~	No effect on DNR-mediated cell growth inhibition	[311]
DNR, 0.1 μM	EGC, 20 μM	SMMC7721 human **hepatocellular** carcinoma cell line, CBR1 high expression	~	No effect on DNR-mediated cell growth inhibition	[311]
DNR, 300 nM	EGCG with peracetate protecting groups (Pro-EGCG), 20 μM	Jurkat human T-cell **leukemia** cell line	↑	Sensitization to DNR, increase in cell death	[308]
DNR, 100 nM	EGCG	K562 human chronic myelogenous **leukemia** cell line	~	No effect on DNR cytotoxicity	[308]
DNR, 100 nM	EGCG with peracetate protecting groups (Pro-EGCG), 20 μM	K562 human chronic myelogenous **leukemia** cell line	↑	Sensitization to DNR, increase in cell death (increase in caspase-3 activity, PARP cleavage). Decrease in Bcr-Abl protein levels	[308]
DNR, 0.2 μM	EGCG, 10, 20 μM	Hep3B human **hepatocellular** carcinoma cell line, CBR1 low expression	~	No effect on DNR-mediated cell growth inhibition	[311]
DNR, 0.4 μM	EGCG, 10, 20 μM	HepG2 human **hepatocellular** carcinoma cell line, CBR1 high expression	↑	Increase in DNR-induced growth inhibition, G2/M phase cell cycle arrest and apoptosis. Inhibition of CBR1 activity, decrease in DNR reduction	[311]

Table 6.15. (Continued)

Drug	Flavonoid	Biological system	Direction of combination	Effects	Ref.
DNR, 0.1 µM	EGCG, 10, 20 µM	SMMC7721 human **hepatocellular** carcinoma cell line, CBR1 high expression	↑	Increase in DNR-induced growth inhibition, G2/M phase cell cycle arrest and apoptosis. Inhibition of CBR1 activity, decrease in DNR reduction	[311]
DNR, 0.4 µM	Epicatechin, 20 µM	HepG2 human **hepatocellular** carcinoma cell line, CBR1 high expression	~	No effect on DNR-mediated cell growth inhibition	[311]
DNR, 0.1 µM	Epicatechin, 20 µM	SMMC7721 human **hepatocellular** carcinoma cell line, CBR1 high expression	~	No effect on DNR-mediated cell growth inhibition	[311]
DNR, 0.01 µM	Flavokawain B, 3 µM	CEM1 human acute lymphoblastic **leukemia** cell line	~	No effect on DNR-induced cell viability reduction	[307]
DNR, 0.15 µM	Flavokawain B, 10 µM	HL-60 human acute promyelocytic **leukemia** cell line, mutant TP53	↑	Additive effect on cell viability reduction. Increase in NF-κB activation	[307]
DNR, 0.05 µM	Flavokawain B, 12 µM	K562 human chronic myelogenous **leukemia** cell line	~	No effect on DNR-induced cell viability reduction	[307]
DNR, 0.005 µM	Flavokawain B, 2 µM	MOLT4 human acute lymphoblastic **leukemia** cell line	~	No effect on DNR-induced cell viability reduction	[307]
DNR, 0.2-30 µM	Flavone, 10, 20 µM	CCRF-CEM human acute lymphoblastic **leukemia** cell line	~	No effect on DNR cytotoxicity	[312]
DNR, 0.2-30 µM	Flavone, 10, 20 µM	CEM/VBL$_{100}$ human acute lymphoblastic **leukemia** cell line, VBL-resistant, overexpressing P-gp	↓	Decrease in DNR-induced cytotoxicity, increase in DNR IC$_{50}$. Activation of DNR-stimulated P-gp ATPase activity, decrease in DNR cellular accumulation	[312]
DNR, 0.002-2 µg/ml	Genistein, 5, 25 µM	Bone marrow and peripheral blood samples from childhood acute lymphoblastic **leukemia** patients	↓	Increase in resistance to DNR (1.8-fold increase in resistance at 25 µM genistein)	[313]
DNR	Nobiletin, 0.5-9 µM	A549/T human non-small cell **lung** cancer cell line, PTX-resistant, overexpressing ABCB1	↑	Sensitization to DNR, decrease in DNR IC$_{50}$	[276]
DNR	Nobiletin, 0.5-9 µM	A2780/T human **ovarian** cancer cell line, PTX-resistant, overexpressing ABCB1	↑	Sensitization to DNR, decrease in DNR IC$_{50}$	[276]
DNR, 0.043, 0.43, 4.3 µM	Quercetin, 3, 6, 12 µM	EPG85-257P human **gastric** cancer cell line	↑	Increase in cytotoxicity and apoptosis	[309]
DNR, 0.043, 0.43, 4.3 µM	Quercetin, 3, 6, 12 µM	EPG85-257RDB human **gastric** cancer cell line, DNR-resistant, overexpressing P-gp and its gene ABCB1	↑	Reversal of DNR resistance, increase in apoptosis. Decrease in P-gp, downregulation of ABCB1 expression	[309]

ABC, ATP-binding cassette; Abl, Abelson murine leukemia viral oncogene homolog; Bcr, breakpoint cluster region; CBR, carbonyl reductase; DMF, dimethoxyflavone; NF-κB, nuclear factor-κB; PARP, poly (ADP-ribose) polymerase; P-gp, P-glycoprotein.

Daunorubicin (DNR) is a first-generation anthracycline, originally isolated from *Streptomyces peucetius* [219, 307]. DNR is authorized in the treatment of several types of leukemias and lymphomas, being a standard chemotherapy for patients with acute myeloid leukemia [1, 307, 308]. As a Topo II inhibitor, DNR intercalates into DNA sequence and interacts with Topo II, thereby inducing distortion of the double helix and stabilizing Topo II-DNA complex, preventing religation and further inhibiting DNA synthesis and repair [307-310]. Cytotoxic action of DNR has been associated also with generation of ROS and subsequent lipid peroxidation [307, 310]. However, similar to treatment with DOX, administration of DNR is also associated with severe cardiac damage manifesting as chronic cardiomyopathy and congestive heart failure even years after termination of the treatment; besides other common side effects related to DNR therapy, including bone marrow suppression and thrombosis [310, 311]. Moreover, intrinsic or acquired resistance of malignant cells to DNR also contributes to limited clinical use of this Topo II inhibitor [311].

Our current preclinical knowledge about the possible role of flavonoids on the therapeutic efficacy of DNR is much more scarce as compared to DOX (Table 6.14 and Table 6.15). It is well known that human carbonyl reductase 1 (CBR1) converts DNR into the alcohol metabolite daunorubicinol (DNROL) with substantially reduced antitumor activities, limiting the clinical use of this anthracycline. Moreover, DNROL has been shown to be responsible for the severe cardiotoxicity of DNR. Therefore, suppression of CBR1 enzyme can increase the therapeutic efficacy and decrease resistance to DNR treatment, concurrently reducing the drug-induced cardiotoxic adverse reactions [311]. The major green tea flavanol *EGCG* has been shown to be a promising CBR1 inhibitor. In fact, EGCG directly interacted with CBR1, inhibited its enzymatic activity and enhanced DNR-induced growth inhibition in human hepatocellular carcinoma SMMC7721 cells with high expression of CBR1 enzyme. Such chemosensitization was accompanied by increase in cells in the G2/M phase of the cell cycle and promotion of apoptotic death. Similar effects were observed in another liver cancer cell line HepG2 that also expresses high levels of CBR1, but not in Hep3B cells with low CBR1 expression level. An essential criterion for activity of flavanols was found to be the presence of gallate moiety in their backbone. Indeed, similarly to EGCG, also *epicatechin 3-gallate (ECG)* inhibited CBR1 activity and increased DNR-induced cytotoxicity in both SMMC7721 and HepG2 cells, whereas *epigallocatechin (EGC)* and *epicatechin (EC)* with no gallate group in their structure did not affect the growth inhibitory potential of DNR. *In vivo* experiments with athymic nude mice further confirmed the *in vitro* results, as EGCG augmented antitumor effects of DNR in SMMC7721 xenografts, but not in Hep3B xenografts. Thus, EGCG might serve as a novel attractive adjuvant agent for DNR chemotherapy in the treatment of liver cancer in the future, by suppressing the CBR1-mediated intracellular drug metabolism and thereby lowering the extent of toxic side effects on normal healthy tissues [311]. Although EGCG did not affect the antitumor activities of DNR in human chronic myelogenous leukemia K562 cells, its more bioavailable analog with peracetate protecting groups, i.e., Pro-EGCG, revealed a significant potentiation of DNR-induced cell death in both K562 cells as well as human T-cell leukemia Jurkat cells. Furthermore, in K562 cells, elevation of apoptotic indices was associated with a decrease in Bcr-Abl oncoprotein levels [308]. Abundant dietary plant flavonol *quercetin* increased DNR cytotoxicity and promoted apoptosis in human gastric cancer EPG85-257P cells. In the respective DNR-resistant subline, EPG85-257RDB, quercetin reversed resistance to DNR treatment through downregulation of expression and function of P-gp [309]. Resistance to DNR was decreased also by polymethylated citrus flavone *nobiletin* in paclitaxel (PTX)-resistant human non-small cell lung cancer A549/T cells and human ovarian cancer A2780/T cells, probably through inhibition of P-gp (ABCB1) transporter activity and subsequent increase in intracellular drug accumulation [276]. However, in P-gp-overexpressing vinblastine (VBL)-resistant human acute lymphoblastic leukemia CEM/VBL$_{100}$ cells, several natural flavones (*flavone, chrysin*) and isoflavones (*biochanin A, baptigenin Ψ and 4`,7-dimethoxyisoflavone*) antagonized anticancer action of DNR, by reducing drug accumulation inside the cells and significantly decreasing the cytotoxicity to DNR, around two- to threefold. These effects were associated with increases in DNR-stimulated P-gp ATPase activity. In parental CCRF-CEM cells, neither flavone nor *4`,7-dimethoxyflavone (4`,7-DMF)* was able to impact DNR transport or cytotoxicity. These data demonstrate that inclusion of certain flavones and isoflavones in DNR treatment protocols against acute lymphoblastic leukemia might undesirably promote the development of resistance to antileukemic action of DNR and should be definitely prevented [312]. Moreover, the common dietary isoflavone, *genistein*, was also shown to increase the resistance to DNR in bone marrow and peripheral blood samples isolated from childhood acute lymphoblastic leukemia patients, further confirming the contraindication of isoflavones during the DNR chemotherapy [313]. The only studied chalcone so far, *flavokawain B*, did not significantly affect DNR-induced cytotoxic responses in human acute lymphoblastic leukemia cell lines CEM1 and MOLT4 or human chronic myelogenous leukemia cell line K562, but still led to an additive activity in reducing viability of human acute promyelocytic leukemia HL-60 cells [307] (Table 6.14 and Table 6.15).

Currently available preclinical data about combined effects of different flavonoids with DNR in several malignant model systems have revealed rather varied results (Figure 6.9). Whereas drinking of green tea or intake of gallate moiety-containing flavanol supplements might be beneficial for patients with liver cancer who are receiving chemotherapeutic treatment with DNR, leukemia patients under DNR therapy should be especially cautious in consuming products rich in flavonoids. In particular, based on so far reported experimental findings, patients suffering from acute lymphoblastic leukemia should abstain from consumption of any soy isoflavones during the active treatment phase with DNR. With no doubt, further studies are urgently needed to prove the current findings and provide more information.

Effects of Plant Flavonoids on Chemotherapeutic Efficacy of Cancer Drugs 263

According to the current experimental findings it is recommended for cancer patients *not to consume* dietary products or dietary supplements rich in following plant flavonoids during the active chemotherapeutic treatment phase with **daunorubicin**:
- **flavone** in acute lymphoblastic leukemia
- **chrysin** in acute lymphoblastic leukemia
- **genistein** in acute lymphoblastic leukemia
- **biochanin A** in acute lymphoblastic leukemia
- **baptigenin Ψ** in acute lymphoblastic leukemia
- **4`,7-dimethoxyisoflavone** in acute lymphoblastic leukemia

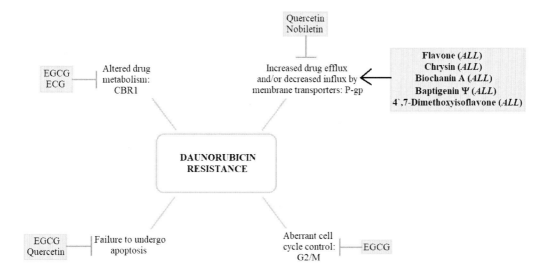

Figure 6.9. Modulation of daunorubicin resistance by plant flavonoids (ALL, acute lymphoblastic leukemia; CBR, carbonyl reductase; P-gp, P-glycoprotein).

Epirubicin (EPI)

Epirubicin (EPI) is a second-generation anthracycline with a wide range of indications that has been used for the treatment of breast, ovarian, esophageal, gastric, pancreatic, liver and lung cancers, sarcomas and lymphomas [1, 219, 314].

Interactions of flavonoids and EPI have been studied in some preclinical cancer models but these data are still rather few (Table 6.14 and Table 6.16). Natural isoflavone *8-hydroxydaidzein*, a product of daidzein biotransformation, synergistically intensified EPI-induced chemotherapeutic potency in human colon adenocarcinoma Caco-2 cells. This potentiation was associated with ROS-dependent suppression of MDR transporters, i.e., P-gp, MRP1 and MRP2, followed by increase in intracellular drug accumulation, and enhancement of both mitochondrial and death receptor-mediated apoptotic cell death. Thus, 8-hydroxydaidzein has the potential to reduce EPI dosage and corresponding adverse reactions, as well as improve therapeutic effects [315]. Methylated isoflavone *formononetin* augmented EPI cytotoxicity in human cervical cancer HeLa cells, also increasing intracellular drug retention through reversal of EPI-induced MRP1 and MRP2 expression, and significantly enhancing ROS-mediated intrinsic and extrinsic apoptosis [316]. Formononetin synergistically potentiated EPI-induced anticancer action also in human breast cancer MDA-MB-231 cells, but not in murine T-cell lymphoma L5718 cells [317]. Another methylated isoflavone, *afrormosin*, enhanced antiproliferative properties of EPI in MDA-MB-231 cells, still in an additive manner [317]. Combined treatment of L5718 cells with isoflavone *rotenone* and EPI also led to additive cytotoxic effects [317]. Chalcone *isoliquiritigenin* sensitized drug-resistant human breast cancer MCF-7/ADR cells to EPI, inducing G2/M phase cell cycle arrest and autophagic cell death, but not apoptosis, by inhibiting miR-25. Furthermore, isoliquiritigenin promoted degradation of BCRP transporter protein primarily via the autophagy-lysosome pathway, resulting in an elevation of drug influx in the cells. In addition, this natural chalcone chemosensitized EPI antitumor activities also in MCF-7/ADR bearing mice, reducing miR-25 expression, triggering autophagy and downregulating BCRP (ABCG2) [318]. Inclusion of isoliquiritigenin in EPI treatment schemes synergistically inhibited proliferation also in several other human breast cancer cell lines, i.e., estrogen receptor-positive MCF-7 cells, and triple negative (TN) BT-549 and MDA-MB-231 cells, whereas inhibitory effects were much stronger in TN tumor cells. Moreover, this chalcone enhanced antitumor action of EPI also in cancer stem cells (CSCs) isolated from MCF-7 and MDA-MB-231 cells by suppressing β-catenin/ABCG2 signaling pathway via direct targeting of GRP78. These *in vitro* findings were further confirmed by *in vivo* results, exhibiting enhanced tumor growth inhibition by combined treatment of MDA-MB-231 CSCs xenografts; demonstrating that isoliquiritigenin might be developed to a novel potential chemosensitizing agent for epirubicin therapy against breast tumors, particularly basal-like breast tumors [319]. Prenylated flavonoid *icaritin* synergistically augmented antiproliferative properties of EPI in human bladder cancer cell lines BT5637 and T24, by inhibiting EPI-induced autophagy; thereby providing a potent adjuvant compound for EPI chemotherapy for the treatment of bladder cancers [320]. Natural flavone *baicalein* reversed resistance and promoted cytotoxic and proapoptotic responses of EPI in multidrug resistant human hepatocellular carcinoma Bel7402/5-FU cells. These effects were accompanied by decrease in EPI efflux from the cells and increase in EPI intracellular accumulation, by downregulating expression and function of P-gp [314]. Several other flavonoids, such as *kaempferol* and *robinin*, enhanced antitumor activity of EPI in human breast cancer MDA-MB-231 cells, whereas *EGC* and *amorphigenin* did not affect EPI-induced cytotoxicity. Combined treatment of murine T-cell lymphoma L5718 cells with *chrysin* and EPI or amorphigenin and EPI revealed synergistic antiproliferative effects [317] (Table 6.14 and Table 6.16).

Effects of Plant Flavonoids on Chemotherapeutic Efficacy of Cancer Drugs 265

Table 6.16. Effects of flavonoids on anticancer action
of epirubicin (EPI) *in vitro* conditions

Drug	Flavonoid	Biological system	Direction of combination	Effects	Ref.
EPI, 0.1 ng/ml-100 mg/ml	8-Hydroxydaidzein, 25 μM	Caco-2 human **colon** adenocarcinoma cell line	↑	Synergistic increase in EPI cytotoxicity (11.88-fold, CI 0.28). Circumvention of MDR through ROS-dependent inhibition of efflux transporters (P-gp, MRP1, MRP2) and increase in EPI cellular accumulation. p53-mediated activation of extrinsic and mitochondrial apoptosis (decrease in ΔΨm; increase in p53, Bax/Bcl-2 ratio, caspases-3/-8/-9)	[315]
EPI	Afrormosin	MDA-MB-231 human **breast** cancer cell line	↑	Additive effect with EPI	[317]
EPI	Amorphigenin	L5718 murine T-cell **lymphoma** cell line	↑	Synergistic increase in EPI efficacy	[317]
EPI	Amorphigenin	MDA-MB-231 human **breast** cancer cell line	~	No interaction with EPI	[317]
EPI, 5-80 μg/ml	Baicalein, 5, 10 μg/ml	Bel7402/5-FU human **hepatocellular** carcinoma cell line, MDR, EPI-resistant	↑	Increase in EPI-induced cytotoxicity and apoptosis, 2.08-fold decrease in EPI IC_{50} at 10 μg/ml baicalein. Reduction of EPI efflux, increase in EPI cellular accumulation	[314]
EPI	Chrysin	L5718 murine T-cell **lymphoma** cell line	↑	Synergistic increase in EPI effect	[317]
EPI	EGC	MDA-MB-231 human **breast** cancer cell line	~	No interaction with EPI	[317]
EPI	Formononetin	L5718 murine T-cell **lymphoma** cell line	~	No interaction with EPI	[317]
EPI	Formononetin	MDA-MB-231 human **breast** cancer cell line	↑	Synergistic increase in EPI effect	[317]
EPI, 0.1 nM-100 μM	Formononetin, 25 μM	HeLa human **cervical** cancer cell line	↑	Increase in EPI cytotoxicity. ROS-mediated inhibition of MRP1 and MRP2, increase in EPI uptake. Activation of mitochondrial and DR-mediated apoptosis (loss of ΔΨm, increase in Bax/Bcl-2 ratio, activation of caspases-9/-8/-3)	[316]
EPI, 0-50 μg/ml	Icaritin, 0-50 μM	BT5637 human **bladder** cancer cell line	↑	Synergism in cell proliferation suppression (CI 0.53), decrease in EPI IC_{50}. Inhibition of EPI-induced autophagy	[320]
EPI, 0-50 μg/ml	Icaritin, 0-50 μM	T24 human **bladder** cancer cell line	↑	Synergism in cell proliferation suppression (CI 0.56), decrease in EPI IC_{50}. Inhibition of EPI-induced autophagy	[320]
EPI, 0.375 μg/ml	Isoliquiritigenin, 25 μM	BT-549 human TN **breast** cancer cell line	↑	Synergism in cell proliferation inhibition	[319]
EPI, 0.375 μg/ml	Isoliquiritigenin, 25 μM	CSCs sorted from MCF-7 human **breast** cancer cell line, CD44+CD23-/low	↑	Synergism in CSCs subpopulation decrease, increase in chemosensitivity	[319]
EPI, 0.375 μg/ml	Isoliquiritigenin, 25 μM	CSCs sorted from MDA-MB-231 human TN **breast** cancer cell line, CD44+CD23-/low	↑	Synergism in CSCs subpopulation decrease, increase in chemosensitivity. Suppression of β-catenin/ABCG2 signaling via direct targeting of GRP78	[319]
EPI, 0.375 μg/ml	Isoliquiritigenin, 25 μM	MCF-7 human **breast** cancer cell line, ER-positive	↑	Synergism in cell proliferation inhibition	[319]

Table 6.16. (Continued)

Drug	Flavonoid	Biological system	Direction of combination	Effects	Ref.
EPI, 0.5 µg/ml	Isoliquiritigenin, 20-100 µM	MCF-7/ADR human **breast** cancer cell line	↑	Sensitization of cells to EPI, inhibition of colony number. Increase in G2/M phase cell cycle arrest, inhibition of miR-25 leading to upregulation of ULK1 and induction of autophagy, ultimately resulting in accelerated ABCG2 degradation via lysosome pathway and promotion of EPI cellular concentration	[318]
EPI, 0.375 µg/ml	Isoliquiritigenin, 25 µM	MDA-MB-231 human TN **breast** cancer cell line	↑	Synergism in cell proliferation inhibition, increase in colony growth reduction	[319]
EPI	Kaempferol	MDA-MB-231 human **breast** cancer cell line	↑	Synergistic increase in EPI efficacy	[317]
EPI	Robinin	MDA-MB-231 human **breast** cancer cell line	↑	Additive effect with EPI	[317]
EPI	Rotenone	L5718 murine T-cell **lymphoma** cell line	↑	Additive effect with EPI	[317]

ABC, ATP-binding cassette; Bax, Bcl-2-associated X protein; Bcl-2, B-cell lymphoma 2; CI, combination index; CSC, cancer stem cell; DR, death receptor; ER, estrogen receptor; GRP, glucose-regulated protein; MDR, multidrug resistance; miR, microRNA; MRP, multidrug resistance-associated protein; P-gp, P-glycoprotein; ROS, reactive oxygen species; TN, triple negative; ULK, Unc-51 like autophagy activating kinase; ΔΨm, mitochondrial membrane potential.

All currently available experimental data indicate positive cooperation between flavonoids and EPI with no contraindicative findings described so far in any studied preclinical cancer models (Figure 6.10). However, the current knowledge is scarce and the possible effects of several most common dietary flavonoids on antitumor action of EPI are still unexplored.

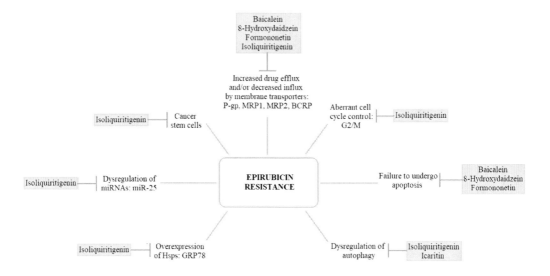

Figure 6.10. Modulation of epirubicin resistance by plant flavonoids (BCRP, breast cancer resistance protein; GRP, glucose-regulated protein; miR, microRNA; MRP, multidrug resistance-associated protein; P-gp P-glycoprotein).

Pirarubicin (THP)

Pirarubicin (THP) is a second-generation anthracycline [219].

The only so far explored interaction with natural flavonoids, i.e., combination of common dietary flavonol *quercetin* and THP, revealed antagonistic effects in CDDP-resistant clone of human ovarian cancer cell line ov2008. In this subline C13*, cotreatment of cells with quercetin and THP attenuated therapeutic efficacy of THP and promoted cell survival, independent on administered quercetin doses (10-100 μM). This undesired increase in drug resistance was related to suppression of intracellular ROS level by quercetin, thereby reducing ROS-induced oxidative damage on malignant ovarian cells [95]. Thus, quercetin supplementation may be contraindicated for ovarian cancer patients who are receiving chemotherapy with THP.

According to the current experimental findings it is recommended for cancer patients *not to consume* dietary products or dietary supplements rich in following plant flavonoids during the active chemotherapeutic treatment phase with **pirarubicin**:

- **quercetin** in ovarian cancer

Mitoxantrone (MX)

Mitoxantrone (MX) is an anthracenedione that is structurally similar to anthracyclines and also interacts with Topo II and causes DNA damage [2, 219, 321, 322]. MX is indicated for the treatment of metastatic breast cancer, acute myeloid leukemia and non-Hodgkin lymphoma; but has also shown activity against advanced hormone-resistant prostate tumor, and liver, lung and bladder cancers [1, 2, 182, 322]. Compared to anthracyclines, MX is considerably less toxic and therefore better tolerable for patients, reducing the risks of cardiotoxicity; however, high-dose regimens induce genetic damage in normal healthy cells, which might further lead to secondary malignancies [1, 182, 322]. Drug resistance represents another major drawback of using MX, being associated with overexpression of efflux transporters, especially BCRP [182, 322].

Combination of natural flavonoids and MX has revealed positive cooperation in different cancer cell lines. To date, no *in vivo* animal experiments have still been performed to prove the *in vitro* results (Table 6.17). Flavonolignan *silibinin* was shown to synergistically increase cell growth inhibitory and proapoptotic activities of MX in different human prostate cancer cell lines, i.e., LNCaP, DU145 and PC-3 [321]. Common natural anthocyanidin *malvidin* enhanced MX-induced cell viability reduction and apoptosis in human hepatocellular carcinoma HepG2 cells, whereas another anthocyanidin, *pelargonidin*, was almost inactive in affecting MX cytotoxicity [182]. An abundant dietary flavonol *fisetin* had no significant effects on the antitumor action of MX in human non-small cell lung cancer A549 cells [323]. Numerous structurally different flavonoids (flavones *apigenin*, *chrysin*, *8-methylflavone* and *5,7-dimethoxyflavone*;

flavonols *kaempferol* and *kaempferide*; flavanones *hesperetin* and *naringenin*; isoflavones *genistein* and *biochanin A*) reversed resistance and augmented MX cytotoxicity in BCRP overexpressing human breast cancer MCF-7 MX100 cells [322, 324]. These effects were associated with decrease in MX efflux from the cells, followed by increase in intracellular drug accumulation through inhibition of BCRP [324]. As chrysin and biochanin A enhanced the therapeutic efficacy of MX also in MCF-7 cells to some small extent; apigenin, kaempferol and genistein remained inactive in influencing MX cytotoxicity in these parental breast cancer cells with very low expression level of BCRP [324]. Moreover, low micromolar concentrations of flavone *acacetin*, flavonol kaempferol, flavanones naringenin and *prunin* (or naringenin 7-glucoside) and isoflavone genistein were shown to reduce BCRP function, reverse drug resistance and potentiate anticancer action of MX in BCRP-transduced human leukemia K562/BCRP cells, but not in parental K562 cells with no BCRP expression [197] (Table 6.17). These data indicate that certain flavonoids might be used as chemosensitizing agents in MX chemotherapy, being of potential clinical significance.

Table 6.17. Effects of flavonoids on anticancer action of mitoxantrone (MX)
***in vitro* conditions**

Drug	Flavonoid	Biological system	Direction of combination	Effects	Ref.
MX, 0.1-1000 µM	5,7-DMF, 2.5, 5 µM	MCF-7/MX100 human **breast** cancer cell line, overexpressing BCRP	↑	Reversal of BCRP-mediated resistance, increase in MX cytotoxicity. Increase in MX cellular accumulation	[322]
MX, 0.1-1000 µM	8-Methylflavone, 2.5, 5 µM	MCF-7/MX100 human **breast** cancer cell line, overexpressing BCRP	↑	Reversal of BCRP-mediated resistance, increase in MX cytotoxicity. Increase in MX cellular accumulation	[322]
MX, 0-10 ng/ml	Acacetin, 1, 3, 10 µM	K562/BCRP human **leukemia** cell line, expressing BCRP, no P-gp or MRP1	↑	Reversal of (BCRP-mediated) resistance; 9.89-fold decrease in MX IC_{50} at 1 µM, 9.71-fold at 3 µM acacetin. Inhibition of BCRP function	[197]
MX, 0.05-1000 µM	Apigenin, 10, 50 µM	MCF-7 human **breast** cancer cell line; very low BCRP, no P-gp or MRP1 expression	~	No effect on MX cytotoxicity	[324]
MX, 0.05-1000 µM	Apigenin, 5, 10, 50 µM	MCF-7 MX100 human **breast** cancer cell line, overexpressing BCRP, no P-gp or MRP1	↑	Potentiation of MX cytotoxicity, decrease in MX IC_{50}. Increase in MX accumulation through complete inhibition of BCRP	[324]
MX, 0.05-1000 µM	Biochanin A, 10, 50 µM	MCF-7 human **breast** cancer cell line; very low BCRP, no P-gp or MRP1 expression	↑	Increase in MX cytotoxicity. Inhibition of small amount of BCRP	[324]
MX, 0.05-1000 µM	Biochanin A, 2.5-50 µM	MCF-7 MX100 human **breast** cancer cell line, overexpressing BCRP, no P-gp or MRP1	↑	Potentiation of MX cytotoxicity, decrease in MX IC_{50}. Increase in MX accumulation through complete inhibition of BCRP	[324]
MX, 0.1-1000 µM	Biochanin A, 2.5, 5 µM	MCF-7/MX100 human **breast** cancer cell line, overexpressing BCRP	↑	Reversal of BCRP-mediated resistance, increase in MX cytotoxicity. Increase in MX cellular accumulation	[322]
MX, 0.05-1000 µM	Chrysin, 50 µM	MCF-7 human **breast** cancer cell line; very low BCRP, no P-gp or MRP1 expression	↑	Increase in MX cytotoxicity. Inhibition of small amount of BCRP	[324]
MX, 0.05-1000 µM	Chrysin, 2.5-50 µM	MCF-7 MX100 human **breast** cancer cell line, overexpressing BCRP, no P-gp or MRP1	↑	Potentiation of MX cytotoxicity, decrease in MX IC_{50}. Increase in MX accumulation through complete inhibition of BCRP	[324]

Effects of Plant Flavonoids on Chemotherapeutic Efficacy of Cancer Drugs   269

Drug	Flavonoid	Biological system	Direction of combination	Effects	Ref.
MX	Fisetin, 10-50 μM	A549 human non-small cell **lung** cancer cell line, wild-type p53	~	No effect on MX-induced cytotoxicity	[323]
MX, 0-10 ng/ml	Genistein, 1, 3, 10 μM	K562 human **leukemia** cell line, expressing no BCRP, P-gp or MRP1	~	No reversal of (BCRP-mediated) MX resistance	[197]
MX, 0-10 ng/ml	Genistein, 1, 3, 10 μM	K562/BCRP human **leukemia** cell line, expressing BCRP, no P-gp or MRP1	↑	Reversal of (BCRP-mediated) resistance; 6.28-fold decrease in MX IC_{50} at 3 μM, 11.7-fold at 10 μM genistein. Inhibition of BCRP function	[197]
MX, 0.05-1000 μM	Genistein, 50 μM	MCF-7 human **breast** cancer cell line; very low BCRP, no P-gp or MRP1 expression	~	No effect on MX cytotoxicity	[324]
MX, 0.05-1000 μM	Genistein, 5, 10, 50 μM	MCF-7 MX100 human **breast** cancer cell line, overexpressing BCRP, no P-gp or MRP1	↑	Potentiation of MX cytotoxicity, decrease in MX IC_{50}. Increase in MX accumulation through complete inhibition of BCRP	[324]
MX, 0.05-1000 μM	Hesperetin, 5, 10, 50 μM	MCF-7 MX100 human **breast** cancer cell line, overexpressing BCRP, no P-gp or MRP1	↑	Potentiation of MX cytotoxicity, decrease in MX IC_{50}. Increase in MX accumulation through complete inhibition of BCRP	[324]
MX, 0.1-1000 μM	Kaempferide, 2.5, 5 μM	MCF-7/MX100 human **breast** cancer cell line, overexpressing BCRP	↑	Reversal of BCRP-mediated resistance, increase in MX cytotoxicity. Increase in MX cellular accumulation	[322]
MX, 0-10 ng/ml	Kaempferol, 1, 3, 10 μM	K562/BCRP human **leukemia** cell line, expressing BCRP, no P-gp or MRP1	↑	Reversal of (BCRP-mediated) resistance; 10.6-fold decrease in MX IC_{50} at 1 μM, 14.2-fold at 3 μM kaempferol	[197]
MX, 0.05-1000 μM	Kaempferol, 50 μM	MCF-7 human **breast** cancer cell line; very low BCRP, no P-gp or MRP1 expression	~	No effect on MX-induced cytotoxicity	[324]
MX, 0.05-1000 μM	Kaempferol, 5, 10, 50 μM	MCF-7 MX100 human **breast** cancer cell line, overexpressing BCRP, no P-gp or MRP1	↑	Potentiation of MX cytotoxicity, decrease in MX IC_{50}. Increase in MX accumulation through complete inhibition of BCRP	[324]
MX, 1 μM	Malvidin, 40, 80 μM	HepG2 human **hepatocellular** carcinoma cell line	↑	Increase in cell viability reduction and apoptosis induction	[182]
MX, 0-10 ng/ml	Naringenin, 1, 3, 10 μM	K562 human **leukemia** cell line, expressing no BCRP, P-gp or MRP1	~	No effect on (BCRP-mediated) MX resistance	[197]
MX, 0-10 ng/ml	Naringenin, 1, 3, 10 μM	K562/BCRP human **leukemia** cell line, expressing BCRP, no P-gp or MRP1	↑	Reversal of (BCRP-mediated) resistance; 3.42-fold decrease in MX IC_{50} at 3 μM, 10.6-fold at 10 μM naringenin. Inhibition of BCRP function	[197]
MX, 0.05-1000 μM	Naringenin, 5, 10, 50 μM	MCF-7 MX100 human **breast** cancer cell line, overexpressing BCRP, no P-gp or MRP1	↑	Potentiation of MX cytotoxicity, decrease in MX IC_{50}. Increase in MX accumulation through complete inhibition of BCRP	[324]
MX, 1 μM	Pelargonidin, 40, 80 μM	HepG2 human **hepatocellular** carcinoma cell line	~	No effect on MX-induced cytotoxicity	[182]
MX, 0-10 ng/ml	Prunin, 3, 10 μM	K562/BCRP human **leukemia** cell line, expressing BCRP, no P-gp or MRP1	↑	Reversal of (BCRP-mediated) resistance; 5.17-fold decrease in MX IC_{50} at 3 μM, 9.44-fold at 10 μM prunin	[197]
MX, 25-200 nM	Silibinin, 10, 20, 40 μM	DU145 human **prostate** cancer cell line, mutant p53	↑	Synergism in cell viability reduction (CI 0.515-0.929). Increase in apoptosis (increase in caspases-3/-7)	[321]
MX, 25-200 nM	Silibinin, 10, 20, 40 μM	LNCaP human **prostate** cancer cell line, wild-type p53	↑	Synergism in cell viability reduction (CI 0.521-0.967). Increase in apoptosis (increase in caspases-3/-7)	[321]
MX, 50-200 nM	Silibinin, 10, 20, 40 μM	PC-3 human **prostate** cancer cell line, mutant p53	↑	Synergism in cell viability reduction. Increase in apoptosis (increase in caspases-3/-7)	[321]

BCRP, breast cancer resistance protein; DMF, dimethoxyflavone; MRP, multidrug resistance-associated protein; P-gp, P-glycoprotein.

Although so far reported findings demonstrate positive (or no) cooperation between flavonoids and MX in several human cancer cell lines, there is no doubt that more data, including in vivo results, are highly needed about the role of natural flavonoids on antitumor action of MX.

Dactinomycin (ACT)

Dactinomycin (ACT) is another chemotherapeutic agent interacting with Topo II and inducing DNA damage. ACT has been used for the treatment of a number of malignancies, including sarcomas, trophoblastic neoplasms, and testicular and ovarian cancers. The only study devoted to investigation of effects of flavonoids on antitumor activity of ACT was focused on the green tea flavanol *EGCG* that was shown to be able to potentiate ACT cytotoxicity in human placenta choriocarcinoma JAR cells. Combined treatment with EGCG and ACT decreased cell proliferation and promoted non-mitochondrial apoptosis more intensively than treatment with the drug alone, suggesting that EGCG could help to overcome resistance phenomenon in the treatment of choriocarcinoma by ACT chemotherapy, improving clinical outcome and increasing survival of patients [325].

To date, doxorubicin is the most commonly studied Topo inhibitor in combination with various natural flavonoids in different preclinical malignant models. Specific combinations with strong synergy in antitumor activities certainly need further therapeutic development probably leading to novel treatment strategies with lower drug dosages and fewer side effects. However, it is also evident that in the future, patients should be advised concerning the possible antagonistic combinations to be able to avoid the consumption of plant-based food products and dietary supplements rich in the respective flavonoids. Currently, no contraindicative combinations can be found for chemotherapeutic treatment with epirubicin, mitoxantrone and dactinomycin, but the amount of studies with these antineoplastic agents is also much smaller than in the case of doxorubicin. Therefore, more investigations on the possible interactions of dietary flavonoids with different Topo inhibitors are urgently needed, both in cancer cell lines as well as in vivo animal models before initiating clinical trials, to enhance current therapeutic efficacy and improve quality of life of patients.

6.2. ANTIMETABOLITES

Antimetabolites are a relatively large group of chemotherapeutic agents which interfere with DNA synthesis, impair division of rapidly proliferating malignant cells and inhibit tumor growth. Cytotoxic action of these drugs involves either incorporation of chemically altered nucleotides in DNA replication machinery or by deleting the supply of deoxynucleotides needed for DNA synthesis and cell proliferation. This class of

Effects of Plant Flavonoids on Chemotherapeutic Efficacy of Cancer Drugs 271

antineoplastic agents comprises pyrimidine antagonists, antifolates and purine nucleoside analogs. Like most cytotoxic chemotherapeutic agents, also antimetabolites are toxic to normal healthy cells, especially those in gastrointestinal tract and bone marrow, inducing severe undesired side effects.

6.2.1. 5-Fluorouracil (5-FU)

5-Fluorouracil (5-FU) is a pyrimidine antimetabolite which has been widely used for the treatment of many human tumor types for years [172, 326-329]. This antineoplastic agent was first introduced in 1957 and is still a key systemic chemotherapy against several malignancies in clinical practice [330]. 5-FU is commonly used for patients with head and neck cancer, tumors of the aerodigestive tract, breast, esophageal, gastric, colorectal, liver, pancreatic and gallbladder tumors, and skin cancer [56, 65, 139, 141, 328, 331-336]. 5-FU is known to suppress the growth of tumor cells and promote apoptotic death. Its anticancer action is exerted through inhibition of thymidylate synthase and incorporation of 5-FU metabolites into RNA and DNA, disrupting normal RNA processing and blocking DNA synthesis, leading to lethal DNA damage [327, 330, 333, 337]. 5-FU may be first converted to fluorouridine monophosphate (FUMP) and further to fluorouridine triphosphate (FUTP) that incorporates into RNA and induces RNA damage. FUMP may be converted also to fluorodeoxyuridine monophosphate (FdUMP) that intervenes in thymidylate synthase (TS) function. TS plays a central role in DNA synthesis in the reductive methylation of deoxyuridine monophosphate (dUMP) to deoxythymidine monophosphate (dTMP), using 5,10-methylenetetrahydrofolate (MTHF) as a cofactor and forming a covalent ternary complex with dUMP and MTHF. FdUMP competes with dUMP in joining this ternary complex, impedes transference of methyl group and formation of dTMP, thereby blocking DNA synthesis [327, 330, 338]. However, when 5-FU enters the *in vivo* system, the majority of the drug, i.e., over 80% of administered drug, is degraded to inactive dihydrofluorouracil (DHFU) by the rate-limiting enzyme dihydropyrimidine dehydrogenase (DPD) [327, 330, 338]. Although DPD is present mainly in the liver in healthy humans, this enzyme is expressed also in a variety of tumor tissues, including breast, cervical, esophageal, gastric, colorectal, hepatic, pancreatic, renal, bladder and prostate cancers [330]. The activity of DPD in malignant cells is a critical factor for therapeutic efficacy of 5-FU, as enzymatic inactivation of this antimetabolite represents a possible mechanism of drug resistance. Therefore, optimization of 5-FU dosage should be apparently possible based on individual`s DPD activity while minimizing systemic toxicity [327, 330]. Moreover, extensive efforts have been made to find inhibitors for DPD enzyme, thereby improving antitumor efficacy of 5-FU [327]. Besides drug resistance, clinical application of 5-FU has been limited also by undesired adverse reactions. 5-FU may cause damaging effects not only to malignant cells but also to normal tissues, inducing hematological toxicity and gastrointestinal problems [56, 139, 326, 329, 333, 335, 339]. Therefore, development of new therapeutic strategies is highly needed to enhance 5-FU antitumor efficacy and minimize adverse side effects in patients suffering from different solid tumors, combining 5-FU chemotherapeutic treatment with novel safe adjuvant agents, preferably obtained from natural products.

The role of plant-derived flavonoids on the therapeutic efficacy of 5-FU has been studied in different preclinical cancer models, both *in vitro* cancer cell lines as well as *in vivo* tumor xenografts in mice (Table 6.18 and Table 6.19). Abundant dietary flavonol *quercetin* was shown to reveal antagonistic activity towards antineoplastic effects of 5-FU in CDDP-resistant subline of human ovarian cancer ov2008 cells, C13*, particularly at low quercetin concentrations at 20 µM and below. This cytoprotective action was probably associated with suppression of intracellular level of ROS and attenuation of ROS-induced oxidative damage to malignant cells. Therefore, quercetin supplementation in ovarian cancer patients during 5-FU chemotherapy might be opposing to drug cytotoxicity and should be avoided [95]. However, quercetin augmented 5-FU-triggered cell growth inhibition and apoptosis in human esophageal cancer cell lines, EC9706 and Eca109, by suppressing drug-induced NF-κB activation [340]. Addition of quercetin synergistically enhanced cytotoxic and proapoptotic responses of 5-FU also in human gastric cancer AGS cells overexpressing cysteine-rich angiogenic inducer 61 (CYR61), CYR61-AGS. CYR61 as a potential regulator implicated in multidrug resistance phenomenon was highly expressed in more advanced gastric adenocarcinoma specimens, whereas its overexpression in gastric cancer cell line was associated with increased motility and invasion of malignant cells [257]. In addition, antitumor effects of 5-FU were increased by quercetin in microsatellite instable (MSI) human colon carcinoma cell line CO115. Potentiation of apoptosis in these wild-type p53 harboring cells was mediated through p53-dependent activation of mitochondrial apoptotic pathway. However, some additive increase in apoptotic death was detected also in mutated p53 expressing HCT15 colon cancer cells by cotreatment with quercetin and 5-FU [341]. In human colorectal carcinoma HCT116 cells with wild-type p53, inclusion of quercetin in 5-FU treatment protocols revealed bimodal effects. On one hand, this flavonol was able to enhance 5-FU-induced suppression of colony formation ability in long term assays; on the other hand, quercetin still reversed G1/S phase cell cycle arrest detected after drug treatment and reduced 5-FU-induced upregulation of p53 and its target proteins p21 and Bax. Furthermore, at lower physiologically achievable quercetin concentrations (3-6 µM) inhibition of clonogenicity was dependent on p53 expression, whereas this flavonol even supported the clonogenicity in p53-null HCT116 cells treated with 5-FU. Therefore, antagonistic effects with 5-FU may be of pharmacological significance and coadministration of quercetin and 5-FU should be avoided by colorectal cancer patients [342]. In several human hepatocellular carcinoma cell lines, i.e., Hep3B, HepG2 and

SMCC-7721, quercetin increased cell viability inhibitory and proapoptotic activities of 5-FU [172, 343], through suppression of Hsp27 and Hsp40 levels in Hep3B and HepG2 cells [172]. Moreover, combined treatment with quercetin and 5-FU revealed superior inhibition of tumor growth also in HepG2 bearing mice compared to treatment with the drug alone [343]. In 5-FU-resistant human hepatocellular carcinoma BEL/5-FU cells, quercetin was able to reverse resistance to 5-FU by downregulating expression and activities of P-gp (ABCB1), MRP1 (ABCC1) and MRP2 (ABCC2) efflux pumps through inhibition of Wnt/β-catenin pathway [38]. Therefore, based on the currently available preclinical data, interactions between quercetin and 5-FU might be dependent on cancer type and molecular characteristics of specific malignant cells, being not always additive or synergistic but revealing in certain cases also undesired antagonism, calling for caution by cancer patients. Another dietary flavonol, *myricetin*, potentiated antiproliferative and proapoptotic properties of 5-FU in human esophageal cancer EC9706 cells, increasing cell cycle arrest at G0/G1 phase and delaying the progression of the cell cycle. In addition, combined treatment with myricetin and 5-FU significantly reduced growth speed of tumor xenografts in EC9706 bearing mice as compared to 5-FU monotreatment [329]. Common natural flavonol *fisetin* strengthened chemosensitivity towards 5-FU in human triple-negative (TN) breast cancer cell lines MDA-MB-231 and MDA-MB-468 [5]. Methylated flavonol *isorhamnetin* augmented 5-FU-induced cytotoxicity in human gastric cancer AGC cells [265]. Gastric cancer cells were chemosensitized towards antitumor efficacy of 5-FU also by glycosidic flavonols avicularin or quercetin 3-O-α-arabinofuranoside and rutin derivative troxerutin. *Avicularin* markedly enhanced 5-FU cytotoxicity in drug resistant human gastric cancer SGC-7901/5-Fu cells [56]; whereas *troxerutin* potentiated 5-FU-induced anticlonogenic, proapoptotic and antimigratory activities in both human gastric cancer cell line SGC7901 as well as its drug resistant subline SGC7901/5-FU [328]. Enhancement of apoptotic death of these drug resistant cells was achieved through suppression of STAT3/NF-κB pathway by combined treatment with troxerutin and 5-FU. Moreover, troxerutin enhanced 5-FU-induced tumor growth inhibition also in SGC7901/5-FU bearing mice by inhibiting NF-κB and Bcl-2 signaling pathways, suggesting that troxerutin might be a therapeutically valuable adjuvant agent for 5-FU chemotherapy against gastric tumors [328] (Table 6.18 and Table 6.19).

Although the major green tea flavanol, *EGCG*, increased 5-FU-induced apoptotic rate in human TN breast cancer MDA-MB231 cells at shorter incubation times (48 and 72 hours), cotreatment of cells with EGCG and 5-FU for longer periods (96 hours) led to a considerable decrease in apoptotic cell death as compared to 5-FU single therapy. These findings suggest that EGCG can exert protective action with respect to 5-FU cytotoxicity at later time points and highlight the necessity to be cautious in consuming EGCG containing products by breast cancer patients under 5-FU chemotherapy [120]. However,

Table 6.18. Effects of flavonoids on anticancer action of 5-fluorouracil (5-FU) *in vitro* conditions

Drug	Flavonoid	Biological system	Direction of combination	Effects	Ref.
5-FU, 0-0.5 mg/ml	DMC, 4, 8 μM	BEL-7402/5-FU human **hepatocellular** carcinoma cell line, 5-FU-resistant	↑	3.68-fold increase in sensitivity to 5-FU at 4 μM, 4.70-fold at 8 μM DMC; promotion of apoptosis. Increase in 5-FU cellular concentration, downregulation of MRP1 and GST-π	[299]
5-FU, 0-800 μg/ml	DMC, 5, 10 μM	BEL-7402/5-FU human **hepatocellular** carcinoma cell line, 5-FU-resistant	↑	Reversal of resistance; 2.02-fold decrease in 5-FU IC_{50} at 5 μM, 3.77-fold at 10 μM DMC. Suppression of Nrf2/ARE pathway leading to decrease in GSH content and GST activity, thereby inhibiting MRP1-mediated 5-FU efflux	[356]
5-FU, 90 μM	Apigenin, 5-100 μM	MDA-MB-453 human **breast** cancer cell line, overexpressing ErbB2, 5-FU-resistant	↑	Increase in cell growth inhibition and apoptosis (activation of caspase-3) via downregulation of ErbB2 expression and Akt signaling	[331]
5-FU, 10-100 μM	Apigenin, 5 μM	SCC25 human **head and neck** squamous cell carcinoma cell line	↑	Synergism in cell proliferation inhibition (CI<1), increase in 5-FU-induced cytotoxicity	[141]
5-FU, 100, 300, 500 μg/ml	Apigenin, 5-30 μM	BEL-7402 human **hepatocellular** carcinoma cell line	↑	Synergism in cytotoxicity. Increase in ROS production and apoptosis (decrease in ΔΨm, Bcl-2; activation of caspase-3, PARP)	[345]
5-FU, 100, 300, 500 μg/ml	Apigenin, 5-30 μM	SK-Hep-1 human **hepatocellular** carcinoma cell line	↑	Synergism in cytotoxicity. Increase in ROS production and apoptosis (decrease in ΔΨm, Bcl-2; activation of caspase-3, PARP)	[345]
5-FU, 50 μM	Apigenin, 11-19 μM	BxPC-3 human **pancreatic** cancer cell line	↑	Increase in cell growth inhibition	[140]
5-FU, 1.25-80 μM	Avicularin, 10 μM	SGC-7901/5-Fu human **gastric** cancer cell line, 5-FU-resistant	↑	Sensitization to 5-FU cytotoxicity, decrease in colony formation ability	[56]
5-FU, 50-800 μg/ml	Baicalein, 5, 10 μg/ml	Bel7402/5-FU human **hepatocellular** carcinoma cell line, MDR, 5-FU-resistant	↑	4.31-fold decrease in 5-FU IC_{50} at 10 μg/ml baicalein. Reduction of 5-FU efflux, increase in 5-FU cellular accumulation. Promotion of 5-FU-induced apoptosis	[314]
5-FU, 125-2000 μM	Baicalein, 10, 20, 40 μM	AGS human **gastric** cancer cell line	↑	Sensitization to 5-FU under hypoxia, reversal of hypoxia-induced resistance. Inhibition of glycolysis via regulation of PTEN/Akt/HIF-1α signaling, decrease in glycolysis-associated enzymes (HK2, LDHA, PDK1)	[346]
5-FU, 200 μg/ml	Calycosin, 10 μg/ml	BGC823 human **gastric** cancer cell line	↑	Increase in 5-FU-induced cell proliferation inhibition. Promotion of 5-FU-induced suppression of migration	[139]
5-FU, 200 μg/ml	Calycosin, 10 μg/ml	NCI-N87 human **gastric** cancer cell line	↑	Increase in 5-FU-induced cell proliferation inhibition. Promotion of 5-FU-induced suppression of migration	[139]
5-FU, 200 μg/ml	Calycosin, 10 μg/ml	SGC7901 human **gastric** cancer cell line	↑	Increase in 5-FU-induced cell proliferation inhibition. Promotion of 5-FU-induced suppression of migration	[139]

Drug	Flavonoid	Biological system	Direction of combination	Effects	Ref.
5-FU, 40 μM	EGC, 1 μM	Mz-ChA-1 human **cholangiocarcinoma** cell line from metastatic gallbladder cancer	~	No effect on 5-FU-induced cytotoxicity	[37]
5-FU, 40 μM	EGCG, 1 μM	Mz-ChA-1 human **cholangiocarcinoma** cell line from metastatic gallbladder cancer	↑	Increase in 5-FU-induced cytotoxicity and apoptosis	[37]
5-FU, 0.1-10 μg/ml	EGCG, 0.1 μg/ml	BIU-87 human **bladder** cancer cell line	~	No effect on 5-FU-induced cytotoxicity	[333]
5-FU, 10, 25, 50 μM	EGCG, 50 μM	MDA-MB231 human TN **breast** cancer cell line	↓↑	Decrease in 5-FU-induced apoptosis at later time points (96h; increase in apoptotic rate at 48h and 72h)	[120]
5-FU, 50 μM	EGCG, 100 μM	HT-29 human **colon** cancer cell line	↑	Increase in 5-FU-induced cell growth inhibition and apoptosis	[210]
5-FU, 0.1-10 μg/ml	EGCG, 0.1 μg/ml	SW480 human **colon** cancer cell line	~	No effect on 5-FU-induced cytotoxicity	[333]
5-FU, 50 μM	EGCG, 10 μM	Caco-2 human **colorectal** cancer cell line	↑	Increase in cell growth inhibition	[334]
5-FU, 0.003-30 μg/ml	EGCG, 0.1 μg/ml	YCU-H891 human **head and neck** cancer cell line from hypopharynx	↑	45-fold increase in 5-FU-induced growth inhibition, increase in colony formation inhibition	[344]
5-FU, 0.003-30 μg/ml	EGCG, 0.1 μg/ml	YCU-N861 human **head and neck** cancer cell line from nasopharynx	↑	3.6-fold increase in 5-FU-induced growth inhibition, increase in colony formation inhibition	[344]
5-FU, 30 μM	EGCG, 10, 25, 50 μM	Hep3B human **hepatocellular** carcinoma cell line	↑	Synergism in antitumor effect. Activation of AMPK, abrogation of COX-2 expression, suppression of PGE2 secretion, inactivation of Akt pathway	[332]
5-FU, 0.1-10 μg/ml	EGCG, 0.1 μg/ml	BGC823 human **gastric** cancer cell line	~	No effect on 5-FU-induced cytotoxicity	[333]
5-FU, 6.25-200 μM	Fisetin, 25 μM	MDA-MB-231 human TN **breast** cancer cell line, p53-deficient	↑	Increase in 5-FU-induced cytotoxicity	[5]
5-FU, 6.25-200 μM	Fisetin, 25 μM	MDA-MB-468 human TN **breast** cancer cell line, p53-deficient	↑	Increase in 5-FU-induced cytotoxicity	[5]
5-FU, 50 μM	Genistein, 100 μM	MCF-7 human **breast** cancer cell line, 5-FU-resistant	↑	Decrease in cell viability, no effect of 5-FU alone	[335]
5-FU, 50 μM	Genistein, 50, 100, 200 μM	HT-29 human **colon** cancer cell line, 5-FU-resistant	↑	Synergism in cell viability reduction. Generation of ROS, activation of AMPK, abolishment of 5-FU-caused upregulation of COX-2 expression and PGE2 secretion. Upregulation of p53, p21, Bax; decrease in 5-FU-induced induction of Glut-1, induction of apoptosis (PARP cleavage)	[335]
5-FU, 100 μM	Genistein, 100 μM	MIA PaCa-2 human **pancreatic** cancer cell line	↑	Increase in 5-FU-induced cytotoxicity, apoptosis (decrease in Bcl-2, increase in caspase-3, PARP cleavage) and autophagy (increase in LC3-II, beclin-1)	[352]
5-FU, 0.5-2 μg/ml	Genistein, 15 μM	MGC-803 human **gastric** cancer cell line	↑	Decrease in resistance to 5-FU. Inhibition of ABCG2 expression and ERK1/2 activity	[131]
5-FU, 50 μM	Genistein, 100 μM	HeLa human **cervical** cancer cell line, 5-FU-resistant	↑	Decrease in cell viability, no effect of 5-FU alone	[335]

Table 6.18. (Continued)

Drug	Flavonoid	Biological system	Direction of combination	Effects	Ref.
5-FU, 1 μM	Hispidulin, 12.5 μM	GBC-SD human **gallbladder** carcinoma cell line	↑	Increase in 5-FU antitumor effect. Downregulation of P-gp through repression of HIF-1α	[349]
5-FU, 10 μM	Icariin, 20 μM	HCT116 human **colorectal** cancer cell line	↑	Increase in 5-FU-induced growth inhibition and apoptosis (increase in Bax, cleavage of caspases-8/-9/-3 and PARP; decrease in Bcl-xL), suppression of 5-FU-induced NF-κB activation, downregulation of cyclin D1	[336]
5-FU, 10 μM	Icariin, 20 μM	HT29 human **colorectal** cancer cell line	↑	Increase in 5-FU-induced growth inhibition and apoptosis (increase in Bax, cleavage of caspases-8/-9/-3 and PARP; decrease in Bcl-xL), suppression of 5-FU-induced NF-κB activation, downregulation of cyclin D1	[336]
5-FU, 0.625 μg/ml	Isoliquiritigenin, 25 μM	BT-549 human TN **breast** cancer cell line	↑	Synergism in cell proliferation inhibition	[319]
5-FU, 0.625 μg/ml	Isoliquiritigenin, 25 μM	MCF-7 human **breast** cancer cell line, ER-positive	↑	Synergism in cell proliferation inhibition	[319]
5-FU, 0.625 μg/ml	Isoliquiritigenin, 25 μM	MDA-MB-231 human TN **breast** cancer cell line	↑	Synergism in cell proliferation inhibition	[319]
5-FU, 60 μM	Isorhamnetin, 10 μM	AGS human **gastric** cancer cell line	↑	1.63-fold increase in 5-FU-induced cytotoxicity	[265]
5-FU, 15.625 μg/ml	Licochalcone A, 25 μM	MKN-45 human **gastric** cancer cell line	↑	Inhibition of cell proliferation, increase in apoptosis (increase in caspase-3, PARP cleavage, p53)	[355]
5-FU, 15.625 μg/ml	Licochalcone A, 25 μM	SGC7901 human **gastric** cancer cell line	↑	Inhibition of cell proliferation. Increase in G0/G1 phase cell cycle arrest and apoptosis (increase in Bax, caspase-3, PARP cleavage, p53)	[355]
5-FU, 1 μM	Luteolin, 12 μM	CO115 human **colon** carcinoma-derived cell line, MSI, wild-type p53	↑	Increase in 5-FU-induced apoptosis	[341]
5-FU, 100 μM	Luteolin, 12 μM	HCT15 human **colon** carcinoma-derived cell line, MSI, mutant p53	↑	Increase in 5-FU-induced apoptosis	[341]
5-FU	Luteolin	Bel7402 human **hepatocellular** carcinoma cell line	↑	Synergism in antiproliferative effect (CI<1). Increase in apoptosis (loss of ΔΨm, increase in caspases-3/-7, Bax/Bcl-2 ratio, p53, PARP cleavage). Increase in G1 and G2 phase cell cycle arrest. Regulation of 5-FU metabolism (decrease in DPD, increase in TS levels)	[338]
5-FU	Luteolin	HepG2 human **hepatocellular** carcinoma cell line	↑	Synergism in antiproliferative effect (CI<1). Increase in apoptosis (loss of ΔΨm, increase in caspases-3/-7, Bax/Bcl-2 ratio, p53, PARP cleavage). Increase in G1 and G2 phase cell cycle arrest. Regulation of 5-FU metabolism (decrease in DPD, increase in TS levels)	[338]
5-FU, 50 μM	Luteolin, 11-19 μM	BxPC-3 human **pancreatic** cancer cell line	↑	Increase in cell growth inhibition	[140]

Drug	Flavonoid	Biological system	Direction of combination	Effects	Ref.
5-FU	Luteolin	AGS human **gastric** cancer cell line	~	No sensitization to 5-FU	[144]
5-FU, 20-320 μM	Myricetin, 25, 50, 100 μM	EC9706 human **esophageal** squamous carcinoma cell line	↑	Increase in antiproliferative effect, inhibition of clonogenic survival. Increase in apoptosis and G0/G1 phase cell cycle arrest (decrease in survivin, cyclin D1, Bcl-2; increase in caspase-3, p53)	[329]
5-FU, 0.1 nM-1 mM	Naringenin, 1 mM	HTB26 human **breast** cancer cell line	↑	Increase in 5-FU-induced cytotoxicity	[10]
5-FU, 0.1 nM-1 mM	Naringenin, 1 mM	SW1116 human **colorectal** cancer cell line	↑	Increase in 5-FU-induced cytotoxicity	[10]
5-FU	Nobiletin, 0.5-9 μM	A549/T human non-small cell **lung** cancer cell line, PTX-resistant, overexpressing ABCB1	↑	Sensitization to 5-FU, decrease in 5-FU IC_{50}	[276]
5-FU	Nobiletin, 0.5-9 μM	A2780/T human **ovarian** cancer cell line, PTX-resistant, overexpressing ABCB1	↑	Sensitization to 5-FU, decrease in 5-FU IC_{50}	[276]
5-FU, 10 μM	Nobiletin, 10 μM	SNU-16 human **gastric** cancer cell line, mutant p53	↑	Synergism in cell viability inhibition (CI 0.38). Induction of apoptosis by modulating different pathways: increase in p53 by 5-FU, increase in p21$^{WAF1/CIP1}$ by nobiletin	[350]
5-FU, 1 mM	Oroxylin A, 200 μM	HT-29 human **colon** cancer cell line	↑	Synergism in cell proliferation inhibition. Decrease in COX-2 expression, increase in apoptosis (decrease in Bcl-2; increase in p53, Bax, caspase-3, PARP cleavage)	[347]
5-FU	Oroxylin A, 30, 60, 90 μM	BEL7402/5-FU human **hepatocellular** carcinoma cell line, MDR, 5-FU-resistant	↑	Reversal of MDR; 3.41-fold increase in sensitivity to 5-FU at 30 μM, 3.95-fold at 60 μM, 4.69-fold at 90 μM oroxylin A. Increase in 5-FU-induced apoptosis. Inhibition of P-gp and downregulation of MDR1 through inhibiting NF-κB signaling	[348]
5-FU	Oroxylin A	HepG2 human **hepatocellular** carcinoma cell line	↑	Increase in 5-FU-induced growth inhibition and apoptosis (decrease in Bcl-2, activation of caspase-3, PARP cleavage). Decrease in 5-FU-induced TS and DPD mRNA levels; decrease in COX-2, increase in p53	[327]
5-FU, 40 μM	Puerarin, 400 μM	Eca-109 human **esophageal** cancer cell line	↑	Increase in 5-FU-induced growth inhibition and apoptosis	[353]
5-FU, 80-240 μM	Puerarin, 1600-2400 μM	BGC-823 human **gastric** cancer cell line	↑	Synergism in growth inhibition (CI<1). Increase in apoptosis (increase in Bax, decrease in Bcl-2)	[326]
5-FU, 1 μM	Quercetin, 12 μM	CO115 human **colon** carcinoma-derived cell line, MSI, wild-type p53	↑	Potentiation of apoptosis through p53 signaling (increase in cleavage of caspases-3/-9, PARP; decrease in Bcl-2)	[341]
5-FU, 100 μM	Quercetin, 12 μM	HCT15 human **colon** carcinoma-derived cell line, MSI, mutant p53	↑	Additive induction of apoptosis	[341]
5-FU, 0.6 μM	Quercetin, 12.5-50 μM	HCT116 human **colorectal** carcinoma cell line, wild-type p53	↑↓	Bimodal effect: Inhibition of clonogenicity (long term effect). Reversal of 5-FU-induced G1/S phase cell cycle arrest, inhibition of 5-FU-induced p53, p21, Bax and survivin expression (short term effect). At lower doses of quercetin (3.1, 6.25 μM), the effect is dependent on p53 expression	[342]

Table 6.18. (Continued)

Drug	Flavonoid	Biological system	Direction of combination	Effects	Ref.
5-FU, 0.2 mM	Quercetin, 100 μM	EC9706 human **esophageal** cancer cell line	↑	Increase in 5-FU-induced cytotoxicity and apoptosis. Inhibition of 5-FU-induced NF-κB activation	[340]
5-FU, 0.2 mM	Quercetin, 100 μM	Eca109 human **esophageal** cancer cell line	↑	Increase in 5-FU-induced cytotoxicity and apoptosis. Inhibition of 5-FU-induced NF-κB activation	[340]
5-FU, 0.2-125 μg/ml	Quercetin, 40, 80, 160 μM	BEL/5-FU human **hepatocellular** carcinoma cell line, MDR, 5-FU-resistant	↑	1.63-fold increase in sensitivity to 5-FU at 40 μM, 2.03-fold at 80 μM, 3.41-fold at 160 μM quercetin. Inhibition of ABCB1, ABCC1, ABCC2, FZD7, β-catenin expression	[38]
5-FU, 100 μM	Quercetin, 50 μM	Hep3B human **hepatoma** cell line	↑	Potentiation of 5-FU-induced apoptosis (increase in caspase-3) by inhibiting Hsp27 and Hsp40 levels	[172]
5-FU, 10 μM	Quercetin, 0.1 mM	HepG2 human **hepatocellular** carcinoma cell line	↑	Increase in 5-FU-induced cell viability inhibition and apoptosis	[343]
5-FU, 125 μM	Quercetin, 50 μM	HepG2 human **hepatoma** cell line	↑	Potentiation of 5-FU-induced apoptosis (increase in caspase-3) by inhibiting Hsp27 and Hsp40 levels	[172]
5-FU, 10 μM	Quercetin, 0.1 mM	SMCC-7721 human **hepatocellular** carcinoma cell line	↑	Increase in 5-FU-induced cell viability inhibition and apoptosis	[343]
5-FU, 5 μM	Quercetin, 10-100 μM	C13* human **ovarian** cancer cell line, CDDP-resistant ov2008 cells	↓	Increase in resistance to 5-FU at 20 μM quercetin (low dose-specific protection against 5-FU cytotoxicity)	[95]
5-FU, 25 μM	Quercetin, 25, 50 μM	CYR61-AGS human **gastric** adenocarcinoma cell line, overexpressing CYR61, 5-FU-resistant	↑	Synergism in cytotoxicity (CI 0.21-0.54). Increase in apoptosis	[257]
5-FU, 500 μM	Scutellarin, 100 μM	HCT116 human **colon** cancer cell line, wild-type p53	↑	Promotion of 5-FU-evoked apoptosis through increase in p53-regulated caspase-6 activation	[351]
5-FU, 2.5 μM	Silibinin, 15 μM	KYSE270 human **esophageal** squamous cell carcinoma cell line	↑	Synergism in cell proliferation inhibition (CI 0.348)	[65]
5-FU, 10, 100, 1000 μg/ml	Silibinin, 20, 50 μM	786-O human **renal** cell carcinoma cell line	↑	Increase in 5-FU-induced cytotoxicity, 13.68-fold decrease in 5-FU LC_{50} at 50 μM silibinin	[354]
5-FU, 20 μM	Troxerutin, 5, 10, 20 μM	SGC7901 human **gastric** cancer cell line	↑	Potentiation of 5-FU suppressive effect, inhibition of colony formation. Increase in 5-FU-induced apoptosis; inhibition of migration	[328]
5-FU, 20 μM	Troxerutin, 5, 10, 20 μM	SGC7901/5-FU human **gastric** cancer cell line, 5-FU-resistant	↑	Promotion of 5-FU-induced cytotoxicity, inhibition of colony formation. Increase in apoptosis (activation of caspases-8/-9/-3, PARP cleavage, cyt c release, increase in Bax/Bcl-2 ratio, decrease in Bcl-2), inhibition of p-STAT3/NF-κB (p65 and p50). Suppression of migration	[328]

Drug	Flavonoid	Biological system	Direction of combination	Effects	Ref.
5-FU	Wogonin	SMMC-7721 human **hepatocellular** carcinoma cell line	↑	Increase in 5-FU-induced cytotoxicity and apoptosis (decrease in Bcl-2; increase in Bax, activation of caspases-3/-8/-9, PARP cleavage). Inhibition of COX-2 expression and regulation of PI3K/Akt pathway	[339]
5-FU	Wogonin	A549 human **lung** cancer cell line	~	No effect on 5-FU-induced cytotoxicity	[153]
5-FU	Wogonin	MGC-803 human **gastric** cancer cell line	↑	Increase in 5-FU-induced cytotoxicity and apoptosis (decrease in Bcl-2; increase in Bax, caspase-3, PARP cleavage). Downregulation of 5-FU catabolic enzyme DPD. Inhibition of NF-κB nuclear translocation	[330]

ABC, ATP-binding cassette; Akt, protein kinase B; AMPK, AMP-activated protein kinase; ARE, antioxidant responsive element; Bax, Bcl-2-associated X protein; Bcl-2, B-cell lymphoma 2; Bcl-xl, B-cell lymphoma-extra large; CI, combination index; COX, cyclooxygenase; cyt c, c cytochrome c; DMC, 2`,4`-dihydroxy-6`-methoxy-3`,5`-dimethylchalcone; DPD, dihydropyrimidine dehydrogenase; ER, estrogen receptor; FZD7, Frizzled homolog protein 7; GLUT, glucose transporter; GSH, glutathione; GST, glutathione S-transferase; HER2 (erbB2), human epidermal growth factor receptor 2; HIF-1α, hypoxia-inducible factor 1α; HK2, hexokinase 2; Hsp, heat shock protein; LDHA, lactate dehydrogenase A; MDR, multidrug resistance; MRP, multidrug resistance-associated protein; MSI, microsatellite instability; NF-κB, nuclear factor-κB; Nrf2, nuclear factor (erythroid-derived 2)-like 2; PARP, poly (ADP-ribose) polymerase; PDK1, pyruvate dehydrogenase kinase 1; PGE2, prostaglandin E2; P-gp, P-glycoprotein; PI3K, phosphoinositide 3-kinase; PTEN, phosphatase and tensin homolog; ROS, reactive oxygen species; STAT3, signal transducer and activator of transcription 3; TN, triple negative; TS, thymidylate synthase; ΔΨm, mitochondrial membrane potential.

Table 6.19. Effects of flavonoids on anticancer action of antimetabolites *in vivo* conditions

Drug	Flavonoid	Biological system	Direction of combination	Effects	Ref.
5-FU, 20 mg/kg, i.p.	DMC, 20, 40 mg/kg, i.p.	BEL-7402/5-FU human **hepatocellular** carcinoma cells injected s.c. into the right flanks of 4-6w old female athymic nude BALB/c mice	↑	Reversal of 5-FU resistance, increase in tumor inhibition rate, decrease in tumor weight. Increase in 5-FU concentration in tumor tissue; increase in caspase-3 activity and apoptosis	[357]
5-FU, 20 mg/kg, i.p., on alternate days for 3 weeks	Apigenin, 100 mg/kg, by gastric gavage, daily, continued for 3 weeks after 5-FU	EAC murine **mammary** adenocarcinoma cells injected i.p. into Swiss albino mice and maintained in ascitic form; ascitic fluid tumor cells injected s.c. into the right thigh of the hind limb of mice	↑	Potentiation of 5-FU cytotoxicity, decrease in tumor volume and weight. Increase in survival time of mice. Different mechanisms involving apoptosis (decrease in Mcl-1, increase in caspases-3/-9), autophagy stimulation (increase in beclin-1), increase in JNK activity and dysregulation of cellular redox status	[337]
5-FU, 20 mg/kg, i.p., for 5 consecutive days	Apigenin, 20 mg/kg, i.p., 5 days a week for 3 weeks	SK-Hep-1 human **hepatocellular** carcinoma cells injected s.c. into the left flank of 4-6w old nude male mice	↑	Promotion of growth inhibition, decrease in tumor volume and weight. Increase in apoptosis	[345]
5-FU, 60 mg/kg, i.p., every 4 days for 21 days	Genistein, 1.3 mg, i.p., every 4 days for 21 days	MIA PaCa-2 human **pancreatic** cancer cells injected s.c. into the right flank of 4-6w old female nude mice	↑	Increase in 5-FU-induced growth inhibition, apoptosis and autophagy (increase in LC3B). Decrease in tumor volume	[352]
5-FU, 30 mg/kg, i.p., thrice a week	Icariin, 40 mg/kg, i.p., thrice a week	HCT116 human **colorectal** cancer cells injected into nude mice	↑	Potentiation of 5-FU-induced growth inhibition, decrease in tumor size	[336]
5-FU, 20 mg/kg, 3-week cycle regimen	Myricetin, 25 mg/kg, 3-week cycle regimen	EC9706 human **esophageal** cancer cells injected s.c. into dorsal scapular region of 5-6w old immunodeficient female BALB/C nude mice	↑	Decrease in growth speed and tumor volume	[329]
5-FU, 20 mg/kg, every 2 days	Oroxylin A, 100 mg/kg, daily	HT-29 human **colon** cancer cells inoculated s.c. into the right axilla of 5-6w old female athymic BALB/c nude mice	↑	Decrease in tumor size and mass, retarding growth. Decrease in COX-2 expression	[347]
5-FU, 10 mg/kg, i.v., daily	Oroxylin A, 100 mg/kg, p.o., daily	H_{22} murine **hepatoma** cells inoculated s.c. at right axilla of male Kunming mice	↑	Increase in 5-FU-induced inhibitory rate, decrease in tumor volume and weight	[327]
5-FU, 12 mg/kg/day	Puerarin, 25 mg/kg/day	Eca-109 human **esophageal** cancer cells inoculated s.c. into 5-6w old male BALB/c nude mice	↑	Increase in inhibition rate, decrease in tumor volume and weight. Increase in apoptotic bodies in tumors	[353]
5-FU, 12 mg/kg, thrice a week for 3 weeks	Puerarin, 30 mg/kg, thrice a week for 3 weeks	BGC-823 human **gastric** cancer cells injected s.c. into the right dorsal area of 4-6w old male BALB/c-nu/nu mice	↑	Increase in inhibition rate, decrease in tumor volume and weight. Increase in apoptosis	[326]

Drug	Flavonoid	Biological system	Direction of combination	Effects	Ref.
5-FU, 30 mg/kg, i.p., once per 5 days	Quercetin, 40 mg/kg, i.p., daily	HepG2 human **hepatocellular** carcinoma cells injected s.c. into the left rear flank of 6w old female BALB/c nude mice	↑	Superior inhibition of tumor growth	[343]
5-FU, 20 mg/kg, i.p., twice weekly	Silibinin, 25 mg/kg, orally, daily	KYSE270 human **esophageal** cancer cells injected s.c. into the left flank of 6-8w old nude mice	↑	Synergistic decrease in tumor size (CI 0.262)	[65]
5-FU, 50 mg/kg, i.p., 2 days intervals for 4 weeks	Troxerutin, 75 mg/kg, i.p., 2 days intervals for 4 weeks	SGC7901/5-FU human **gastric** cancer cells injected s.c. into the right oxter of 5w old athymic nude male mice	↑	Increase in 5-FU-induced growth inhibition, decrease in tumor volume and weight. Decrease in p-STAT3-, p-NF-κB- and Bcl-2-positive cells in tumors; increase in cleaved caspase-3 and PARP	[328]
5-FU, 10 mg/kg, i.v., once every 2 days, 10 times in total	Wogonin, 30 mg/kg, i.v., once every 2 days, 10 times in total	SMMC-7721 human **hepatocellular** carcinoma cells inoculated s.c. into the right axilla of 5-6w old female athymic BALB/cA nude mice	↑	Increase in 5-FU-induced growth inhibition, decrease in tumor size	[339]
5-FU, 10 mg/kg, i.p., for 2 weeks	Wogonin, 15, 30 or 60 mg/kg/day, i.v., for 2 weeks	MGC-803 human **gastric** cancer cells inoculated s.c. into 5-6w old female BALB/c nude mice	↑	Increase in 5-FU-mediated tumor growth inhibitory rate	[330]
CAPE, 200 mg/kg, by gavage, daily; LDM	EGCG, 1.5 mg, i.p., daily	BGC-823 human **gastric** cancer cells injected into the right flank of BALB/c nude mice	↑	Increase in tumor reduction, decrease in tumor volume. Decrease in VEGF expression and microvessel counts	[358]
CAPE, 60 mg/kg, by gavage, twice weekly	Isorhamnetin, 1 mg/kg, i.p., thrice weekly	SNU-5 human **gastric** cancer cells implanted s.c. in the right flank of 6w old athymic nu/nu female mice	↑	Suppression of growth, reduction of tumor volume. Decrease in NF-κB activation and expression of proliferative (Ki-67) and angiogenic biomarkers (CD31). Suppression of NF-κB-regulated oncogenic gene products (p65, VEGF, COX-2, MMP-9, cyclin D1, survivin, XIAP, ICAM-1)	[359]
GEM, 125 mg/kg, i.p., twice weekly for 3 weeks	Apigenin, 50 mg/kg, i.p., 5 times a week for 3 weeks	MiaPaca-2 human **pancreatic** cancer cells inoculated s.c. into 4w old male BALB/c nude mice	↑	Potentiation of GEM-induced growth inhibition, decrease in tumor volume and weight. Decrease in BrdU incorporation staining, increase in apoptosis (TUNEL staining). Abrogation of GEM-induced activation of Akt and NF-κB pathway	[369]
GEM, 120 mg/kg, i.p., on days 1, 4, 7; 3h after EGCG 10 days	EGCG, 20 mg/kg, i.p., daily for 10 days	Mz-ChA-1 human **cholangiocarcinoma** cells injected s.c. into the right and left flanks of 8w old male athymic nu/nu mice	↑	Increase in sensitivity to GEM, decrease in tumor growth	[37]
GEM, 80 mg/kg, i.v., once every other day, 3 doses in total	Genistein, 1 mg/mouse, orally, daily for 10 days	COLO357 human **pancreatic** cancer cells injected into the parenchyma of the pancreas of female nude mice (ICR-SCID)	↑	Potentiation of GEM-induced antitumor effect, decrease in tumor weight. Downregulation of GEM-induced activation of NF-κB DNA-binding activity	[367]

Table 6.19. (Continued)

Drug	Flavonoid	Biological system	Direction of combination	Effects	Ref.
GEM, 80 mg/kg, i.v., once every other day, 3 doses in total	Genistein, 1 mg/mouse, orally, daily for 10 days	L3.6pl human **pancreatic** cancer cells injected into the parenchyma of the pancreas of female nude mice (ICR-SCID)	↑	Potentiation of GEM-induced antitumor effect, decrease in tumor weight. Downregulation of GEM-induced activation of NF-κB DNA-binding activity	[367]
GEM, 125 mg/kg, twice a week for 2 weeks	Icariin, 40 mg/kg, twice a week for 2 weeks	GBC-SD human **gallbladder** cancer cells injected s.c. into the right and left abdominal regions of 6w old female BALB/c (nu/nu) mice	↑	Potentiation of GEM-induced antitumor effect resulting in smaller tumors	[361]
GEM, 125 mg/kg, twice a week for weeks 2-6 (different days with luteolin)	Luteolin, 84 mg/kg, i.p., daily in week 1, five times a week for weeks 2-6	BxPC-3 human **pancreatic** cancer cells injected into the pancreas of 6w old male athymic nude mice	↑	Decrease in tumor mass. Reduction of PCNA. Promotion of apoptosis through inhibition of K-ras/GSK-3β/NF-κB pathway leading to reduction of bcl-2/bax ratio, cyt c release, activation of caspase-3	[370]
ARA-C, 10 mg/kg, i.p.	Genistein, 1 mg/kg, i.p.	NB4 human acute myeloid **leukemia** cells injected i.p. into recipient 4-6w old female severe combined immunodeficient mice	↑	Increase in tumor growth inhibition, improvement of mice survival	[385]
ARA-C, 10 mg/kg, i.p.	Genistein, 1 mg/kg, i.p.	HL-60 human acute myeloid **leukemia** cells injected i.p. into recipient 4-6w old female severe combined immunodeficient mice	↑	Increase in tumor growth inhibition, improvement of mice survival	[385]
AZA, 2 mg/kg, i.v., 8h infusion	Genistein, diet supplemented with 0.5% of genistein	L1210 murine **leukemia** cells injected i.v. into the lateral tail vein of male CD2F1 mice	↑	Synergism in increase in life span of mice	[387]
FLU, 35 mg/kg, i.p., 5 consecutive days for 3 cycles starting each 28 days	Deguelin, 4 mg/kg, i.g., thrice weekly for 61 days	Splenocytes from 9 months old female New Zealand Black (NZB/Ola Hsd) mice with **leukemic** hyperdiploid CD5+ B cells transferred into young 4-6w old female NZB recipients	↑	Prolongation of survival of transplanted mice	[394]

Akt, protein kinase B; Bax, Bcl-2-associated X protein; Bcl-2, B-cell lymphoma 2; BrdU, bromodeoxyuridine; CI, combination index; COX, cyclooxygenase; cyt c, cytochrome c; DMC, 2`,4`-dihydroxy-6`-methoxy-3`,5`-dimethylchalcone; EAC, Ehrlich ascites carcinoma; GSK, glycogen synthase kinase; ICAM-1, intercellular adhesion molecule 1; JNK, c-Jun N-terminal kinase; LDM, low-dose metronomic therapy; Mcl-1, myeloid cell leukemia 1; MMP, matrix metalloproteinase; NF-κB, nuclear factor-κB; NZB mice, New Zealand Black mice; PARP, poly (ADP-ribose) polymerase; PCNA, proliferating cell nuclear antigen; STAT3, signal transducer and activator of transcription 3; TUNEL, terminal deoxynucleotidyl transferase dUTP nick end labeling; VEGF, vascular endothelial growth factor; XIAP, X-linked inhibitor of apoptosis protein.

Effects of Plant Flavonoids on Chemotherapeutic Efficacy of Cancer Drugs 283

EGCG at low micromolar doses achievable after oral administration (0.1 µg/ml) markedly augmented growth inhibitory and anticlonogenic properties of 5-FU in human hypopharyngeal cancer YCU-H891 cells and to lower extent also in human nasopharyngeal cancer YCU-N861 cells. This common catechin could therefore be a potent complement for 5-FU chemotherapy in the treatment of head and neck squamous cell carcinomas [344]. Whereas EGCG enhanced 5-FU-induced cytotoxicity and reduced tumor cell viability in human colon cancer HT-29 cells [210] and colorectal cancer Caco-2 cells [334]; in another human colon cancer cell line, SW480, EGCG remained inactive in affecting antitumor activities of 5-FU [333]. No effect of EGCG on 5-FU therapeutic efficacy was observed also in human gastric cancer BGC823 cells and human bladder cancer BIU-87 cells; however, the tested concentration of EGCG was only 0.1 µg/ml that is equivalent to less than 6 cups of green tea per day in humans [333]. However, EGCG synergistically potentiated antineoplastic activities of 5-FU in human hepatocellular carcinoma Hep3B cells. The combination of EGCG and 5-FU led to activation of AMP-activated protein kinase (AMPK) followed by almost complete abrogation of drug-induced cyclooxygenase (COX)-2 overexpression and reduction of prostaglandin E2 (PGE2) secretion, besides suppression of Akt activation [332]. Cytotoxic and proapoptotic potential of 5-FU were enhanced by EGCG also in human cholangiocarcinoma Mz-ChA-1 cells, but not by another catechin, *EGC*. As the major route of metabolic excretion of EGCG is biliary, combination of EGCG and 5-FU might be of therapeutic significance in the treatment of advanced gallbladder tumors in the future [37]. The data above show that action of EGCG in combination with 5-FU depends largely on the type and molecular features of tumor cells and can reveal both positive as well as negative cooperation, requiring informed attitude by cancer patients (Table 6.18).

Current preclinical data have demonstrated only positive cooperation in antitumor action between different flavones and 5-FU. Common dietary flavone *apigenin* significantly decreased chemoresistance to 5-FU and enhanced cell growth inhibition and apoptosis in drug-resistant human breast cancer MDA-MB-453 cells overexpressing ErbB2. Such apoptosis increasing action of combined treatment was mediated via downregulation of ErbB2 level and suppression of Akt signaling [331]. Moreover, in Ehrlich ascites carcinoma (a murine mammary carcinoma with high resemblance to human tumors) bearing mice, 5-FU treatment in the presence of apigenin led to upregulation of apoptotic and autophagic markers, increase in JNK activity and dysregulation of cellular redox status, resulting in significantly smaller tumors than treatment with 5-FU alone. Moreover, lifespan of experimental animals was also prolonged by combinational therapy with apigenin and 5-FU [337]. In addition, low micromolar doses of apigenin augmented antiproliferative and cytotoxic properties of 5-FU in human head and neck squamous cell carcinoma SCC25 cells [141] and human pancreatic cancer BxPC-3 cells [140]. In human liver hepatocellular carcinoma cell lines BEL-7402 and SK-Hep-1, simultaneous exposure to apigenin and 5-FU resulted in synergistic cytotoxic responses accompanied by increase in ROS production and mitochondrial membrane depolarization, inducing mitochondrial apoptotic death. These *in vitro* results were further confirmed *in vivo* conditions using Sk-Hep-1 bearing mice, showing significantly lower tumor volumes and weights in the combined treatment versus 5-FU alone treated mice [345]. Another natural flavone, *luteolin*, also synergistically potentiated antiproliferative and proapoptotic effects of 5-FU in human hepatocellular carcinoma cell lines, Bel7402 and HepG2, associated with increase in the G1 and G2 phase cell cycle arrest. Moreover, combined treatment with luteolin and 5-FU resulted in a more significant decrease in DPD enzyme than drug alone, thereby enhancing 5-FU retention in the tumor cells and providing an additional explanation to synergistic effects [338]. Although luteolin did not sensitize human gastric cancer AGS cells to antitumor effects of 5-FU [144]; this flavone still increased 5-FU-induced cell growth inhibition in human pancreatic cancer BxPC-3 cells [140] and promoted apoptosis in MSI human colon cancer cell lines CO115 and HCT15 [341]. Flavone *baicalein* partially reversed resistance phenomenon and promoted apoptosis in 5-FU-resistant human hepatocellular carcinoma Bel7402/5-FU cells through decrease in drug efflux and increase in intracellular 5-FU concentration [314]. Also, baicalein sensitized human gastric cancer AGS cells and reversed hypoxia-induced resistance to 5-FU gradually back to the activity level observed under normoxic conditions. In fact, baicalein regulated PTEN/Akt signaling leading to attenuation of HIF-1α expression, and suppressed hypoxia-enhanced glucose uptake and lactate production through reducing the expression of several glycolysis-related enzymes, including hexokinase 2 (HK2), lactate dehydrogenase A (LDHA) and pyruvate dehydrogenase kinase 1 (PDK1) [346]. Monomethylated baicalein derivative, *oroxylin A* or 6-methoxybaicalein, enhanced 5-FU antiproliferative and proapoptotic activities in human colon cancer HT-29 cells, and reduced the sizes and weights of HT-29 tumors in nude mice compared to treatment with the drug alone. These effects were mainly related to the suppression of COX-2 expression in both HT-29 cells as well as respective xenograft tissues [347]. In addition, oroxylin A could increase the sensitivity to 5-FU-mediated growth inhibition and apoptosis also in human hepatocellular carcinoma HepG2 cells. This chemosensitization was associated with considerable downregulation of 5-FU metabolic enzymes DPD and TS, besides decrease in COX-2 level. Moreover, combined treatment with oroxylin A and 5-FU led to higher inhibitory rate in murine hepatoma H_{22} cells bearing mice as compared to counterparts receiving the drug alone [327]. Furthermore, susceptibility to 5-FU was augmented by oroxylin A also in multidrug resistant human hepatocellular carcinoma BEL7402/5-FU cells, by downregulating the expression and function of P-gp efflux pump via inhibition of NF-κB signaling cascade [348]. Thus, oroxylin A holds potential to be developed to chemoadjuvant for 5-FU therapy in the treatment of hepatocellular carcinomas. Whereas another monomethylated flavone, *wogonin*, did not affect 5-FU-mediated therapeutic efficacy in human lung cancer A549 cells [153], this natural flavone augmented cytotoxic and proapoptotic properties of 5-FU in human hepatocellular carcinoma SMMC-7721 cells through suppression of COX-2 expression and PGE2 production by inhibiting PI3K/Akt pathway. The combined treatment was effective also in nude mice implanted with SMMC-7721 cells leading to considerably smaller tumors as compared to either agent alone [339]. In addition, wogonin enhanced 5-FU-induced apoptotic death in human gastric cancer MGC-803 cells by inhibiting NF-κB translocation to the nucleus. Furthermore, wogonin was able to decrease the expression of DPD metabolic enzyme (but still not TS) and thereby increased 5-FU retention for a prolonged time inside the tumoral cells. Combination of two agents was much stronger than single drug treatment also in retarding the growth of MGC-803 xenograft tumors in mice [330]. *Hispidulin* or 6-methoxyscutellarein potentiated antitumor effects of 5-FU in human gallbladder carcinoma GBC-SD cells by downregulating P-gp expression via blocking of HIF-1α signaling [349]. The only polymethylated flavone studied so far, *nobiletin* or hexamethoxyflavone, was shown to synergistically augment the cell growth inhibitory and apoptosis-inducing properties of 5-FU in human gastric cancer SNU-16 cells. Such chemosensitizing action was achieved by modulating different intracellular pathways by nobiletin and 5-FU, both p53-dependent and -independent signaling routes [350]. Increase in 5-FU-mediated cytotoxicity by nobiletin was observed also in PTX-resistant human non-small cell lung cancer A549/T cells and human ovarian cancer A2780/T cells [276]. Sugar conjugate of flavone scutellarein, *scutellarin* or scutellarein 7-glucuronide, could augment 5-FU-evoked apoptosis in human colon cancer HCT116 cells, whereas this effect was strictly dependent on the presence of wild-type p53, regulating caspase-6 activation [351] (Table 6.18 and Table 6.19). Thus, several flavones and their methylated and glycosylated derivatives can greatly improve the therapeutic efficacy of 5-FU, mostly in tumors of human digestive system, and probably via modulation of different cellular mechanisms.

Current knowledge about the role of isoflavones on antitumor action of 5-FU is rather scarce, but so far encompasses only positive cytotoxic cooperation between these two agents. Combination of the major soy isoflavone *genistein* and 5-FU led to decreased viability of human breast cancer MCF-7 cells and human cervical cancer HeLa cells, despite the fact that 5-FU alone did not induce death in these tumor cells. Moreover, in human colon cancer HT-29 cells, genistein markedly potentiated 5-FU-induced cytotoxicity and apoptosis through stimulation of ROS generation, activation of AMPK, and abolishment of drug-induced COX-2 expression and PGE2 secretion. In addition, 5-FU-elicited increase in survival signal GLUT-1 was also diminished by combined treatment with genistein and 5-FU [335]. Genistein enhanced antitumor activities of 5-FU also in human pancreatic cancer MIA Paca-2 cells, promoting both apoptotic and autophagic cell death. This observation was further supported by the *in vivo* assays, showing that the combination of genistein and 5-FU significantly reduced xenograft tumor volume in MIA PaCa-2 bearing mice as compared to 5-FU alone treated counterparts. Similar to the *in vitro* findings, this decrease in tumor growth was accompanied by increase in apoptotic and autophagic markers in xenograft tissue [352]. In human gastric cancer MGC-803 cells, inclusion of genistein in 5-FU treatment protocols led to decrease in chemoresistance to 5-FU, being associated with downregulation of BCRP (ABCG2) expression and inhibition of ERK1/2 activity [131]. These data suggest that genistein holds potential to be clinically used as a novel adjuvant agent enhancing efficacy of 5-FU chemotherapy against a rather broad range of human tumors. Moreover, methylated isoflavone *calycosin* also potentiated 5-FU therapeutic efficacy in several human gastric cancer cell lines, i.e., BGC823, NCI-N87 and SGC7901, leading to superior antiproliferative and antimigratory activities [139]. Glycosylated isoflavone *puerarin* or daidzein 8-C-glucoside increased 5-FU-induced growth inhibition and apoptosis in human gastric cancer BGC-823 cells [326] and human esophageal cancer Eca-109 cells [353]. Moreover, combined treatment with puerarin and 5-FU exhibited significantly greater tumor growth inhibition with substantially smaller tumors also in BGC-823 bearing mice [326] and Eca-109 bearing mice as compared to either single agent [353]; suggesting that combination treatment of puerarin and 5-FU could be potential in treating upper gastrointestinal tract tumors, reducing therapeutically required drug doses and thereby mitigating toxic side effects (Table 6.18 and Table 6.19).

Furthermore, dietary flavanone *naringenin* sensitized human breast cancer HTB26 cells and human colorectal cancer SW1116 cells towards 5-FU-induced cytotoxicity [10]. Inclusion of low doses of natural flavonolignan *silibinin* in 5-FU treatment protocols led to synergistic decrease in proliferation of human esophageal cancer KYSE270 cells, and inhibited synergistically tumor growth in KYSE270 bearing mice [65]. Silibinin enhanced 5-FU-induced cytotoxicity also in human renal cell carcinoma 786-O cells [354]. Chalcone *isoliquiritigenin* potentiated antiproliferative action of 5-FU in different human breast cancer cells (MCF-7, BT-549, MDA-MB-231), particularly in triple negative BT-549 and MDA-MB-231 cells [319]. Combination of another chalcone, *licochalcone A*, and 5-FU delayed cell cycle progression and increased apoptotic death in human gastric cancer cell lines MKN-45 and SGC7901 [355]. Another chalcone, *2`,4`-dihydroxy-6`-methoxy-3`,5`-dimethylchalcone (DMC)*, reversed resistance to 5-FU in drug-resistant human hepatocellular carcinoma BEL-7402/5-FU cells, associated with inhibition of drug efflux from the cells and enhancement of intracellular 5-FU accumulation through downregulation of MRP1 and GST [299, 356]. This process was regulated by suppression of nuclear translocation and binding activity of Nrf2 to antioxidant responsive element (ARE), eventually leading to increase in apoptotic cell population [299, 356]. Moreover, combined treatment with DMC and 5-FU resulted in significantly elevated tumor inhibition rate in BEL-7402/5-FU xenografts in nude mice as compared to 5-FU alone, accompanied by promotion of drug accumulation in malignant tissues and enhanced apoptotic activities [357]. Prenylated flavonoid *icariin* augmented 5-FU-mediated growth inhibition and apoptotic death in human colorectal cancer cell lines HCT116 and HT29, through suppression of drug-induced NF-κB activation. Combination of icariin and 5-FU exhibited superior antitumor effects also in HCT116 bearing mice resulting in substantially smaller tumors as compared to mice treated with either agent alone [336] (Table 6.18 and Table 6.19).

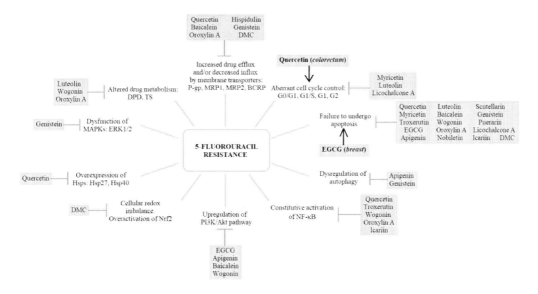

Figure 6.11. Intervention in cellular resistance mechanisms of 5-fluorouracil by plant flavonoids (Akt, protein kinase B; BCRP, breast cancer resistance protein; DMC, 2`,4`-dihydroxy-6`-methoxy-3`,5`-dimethylchalcone; DPD, dihydropyrimidine dehydrogenase; ERK, extracellular signal-regulated kinase; Hsp, heat shock protein; MAPK, mitogen-activated protein kinase; MRP, multidrug resistance-associated protein; NF-κB, nuclear factor-κB; Nrf2, nuclear factor (erythroid-derived 2)-like 2; P-gp, P-glycoprotein; PI3K, phosphoinositide 3-kinase; TS, thymidylate synthase).

Based on the current preclinical data, several flavonoids might behave as potential sensitizers for 5-FU chemotherapy against various types of human malignancies (Figure 6.11). Translation of these in vitro cell line and in vivo animal model results into the clinical settings presupposes fine-tuning of combinational treatment times, schedules and dosages in additional experimental studies and clinical trials, besides reconfirming the chemosensitizing effects. In fact, low micromolar levels of EGCG or apigenin (<5 μM), achievable in physiological conditions after oral administration of products rich in these flavonoids, can effectively sensitize different head and neck carcinoma cells to 5-FU treatment, independent on origin of the tested malignant cells, i.e., hypopharynx, nasopharynx or tongue. Cytotoxic interactions between certain flavonoids and 5-FU might be synergistic also in diverse tumoral cells derived from human digestive system neoplasms. At that, several flavonoids (luteolin, wogonin, oroxylin A) can target not only intracellular mechanisms leading to cell cycle arrest and apoptotic death, but regulate also 5-FU metabolism by modulating the respective metabolic enzymes and drug retention inside the malignant cells. However, a few specific combinations might still be contraindicated for patients with certain tumors antagonizing antineoplastic activities of

5-FU and reducing therapeutic efficacy. Until in vivo animal studies and further clinical trials will not negate the current preclinical findings, it is important for ovarian and colorectal cancer patients to avoid the exposure to quercetin and breast cancer patients to EGCG under active treatment phase with 5-FU chemotherapy.

According to the current experimental findings it is recommended for cancer patients *not to consume* dietary products or dietary supplements rich in following plant flavonoids during the active chemotherapeutic treatment phase with **5-fluorouracil**:
- **quercetin** in colorectal cancer
- **quercetin** in ovarian cancer
- **EGCG** in triple-negative breast cancer

6.2.2. Capecitabine (CAPE)

Capecitabine (CAPE) is an oral fluoropyrimidine that is quickly converted to 5-FU inside the body through which it acts [1, 358]. This cytotoxic antimetabolite is indicated for the treatment of digestive tract malignancies, including colon and gastric cancers, and locally advanced or metastatic breast tumors [1].

Only two natural flavonoids, i.e., green tea flavanol EGCG and methylated flavonol isorhamnetin, have been studied in combination with CAPE in diverse human gastric cancer cell lines or xenograft models. *Isorhamnetin* or 3`-methoxyquercetin was shown to enhance CAPE-induced cytotoxicity and apoptosis in AGS, MKN45, SNU-5 and SNU-16 cells [265, 359]. In SNU-5 bearing mice, combined treatment with isorhamnetin and CAPE led to a superior inhibition of tumor growth as compared to the drug monotherapy, accompanied by downregulation of proliferative (Ki-67) and angiogenic biomarkers (CD31). This chemosensitizing effect was related to the significant reduction of NF-κB signaling activity and its downstream gene products that are involved in tumor cell proliferation, invasion, migration and metastasis, such as survivin, VEGF, COX-2 and MMP-9 [359]. Flavanol *EGCG* was also demonstrated to increase the antitumor effects of low-dose metronomic CAPE chemotherapy in mice harboring human gastric cancer BGC-823 cells, delaying tumor growth and inhibiting angiogenesis, as observed by the lowest microvessel counts and VEGF protein levels in malignant tissue [358] (Table 6.19 and Table 6.20).

Thus, both isorhamnetin and EGCG might be important adjuvant agents for CAPE chemotherapy against gastric tumors, certainly worth of further therapeutic development.

Table 6.20. Effects of flavonoids on anticancer action of capecitabine (CAPE) *in vitro* conditions

Drug	Flavonoid	Biological system	Direction of combination	Effects	Ref.
CAPE, 10 μM	Isorhamnetin, 10 μM	AGS human **gastric** cancer cell line	↑	1.4-fold increase in CAPE-induced cytotoxicity	[265]
CAPE, 10 μM	Isorhamnetin, 10 μM	MKN45 human **gastric** cancer cell line	↑	Potentiation of CAPE-induced apoptosis. Abrogation of NF-κB activation	[359]
CAPE, 10 μM	Isorhamnetin, 10 μM	SNU-16 human **gastric** cancer cell line	↑	Potentiation of CAPE-induced apoptosis	[359]
CAPE, 10 μM	Isorhamnetin, 10 μM	SNU-5 human **gastric** cancer cell line	↑	Potentiation of CAPE-induced apoptosis	[359]

NF-κB, nuclear factor-κB.

6.2.3. Gemcitabine (GEM)

Gemcitabine (GEM) is a synthetic pyrimidine antimetabolite with antitumor activities. Since the late 1990s, GEM has been used in the treatment of several solid tumors, such as locally advanced or metastatic non-small cell lung cancer, pancreatic cancer, bladder cancer, ovarian cancer, and metastatic breast cancer [1, 360-364]. In the cells, GEM (2`,2`-difluoro-2`-deoxycytidine, dFdC) is phosphorylated by deoxycytidine kinase (DCK) to its 5`-monophosphate form (dFdCMP) and subsequently by several other enzymes to 5`-diphosphate (dFdCDP) and 5`-triphosphate derivatives (dFdCTP) [363-365]. dFdCTP is then incorporated into the DNA causing termination of chain elongation and halting DNA synthesis. Thus, GEM decreases the cellular pool of dNTP leading to a competitively higher incorporation of dFdCTP than dCTP into the DNA during the S phase (synthesis) of the cell cycle. As GEM is specific to cells in the S phase, agents that are able to regulate the cell cycle progression could potentially sensitize tumor cells to cytotoxic action of GEM [363-366]. However, the use of GEM is frequently accompanied by development of resistance resulting in relatively low response rates in the clinical settings. Resistance to GEM has been related to the upregulation of ribonucleotide reductase M2 subunit (RR-M2) that is a rate-limiting enzyme in DNA synthesis [363, 364]. Combinations of GEM with targeted therapies might improve the therapeutic efficacy and clinical outcome, especially with those agents targeting the regulatory elements of the cell cycle.

Several flavonoids have been studied in combination with GEM in different human cancer cells and xenograft tumor models (Table 6.19 and Table 6.21). The major soy isoflavone *genistein* was shown to potentiate GEM-induced growth inhibition and apoptosis in paired isogenic human pancreatic carcinoma cell line with differences in metastatic potential, i.e., COLO357 and L3.6pI. This augmentation in cell killing was

Table 6.21. Effects of flavonoids on anticancer action of gemcitabine (GEM) *in vitro* conditions

Drug	Flavonoid	Biological system	Direction of combination	Effects	Ref.
GEM, 2, 5, 10 μM	Apigenin, 25, 50 μM	AsPC-1 human **pancreatic** cancer cell line	↑	Potentiation of GEM-induced growth inhibition. Increase in apoptosis through inhibition of Akt and downregulation of NF-κB	[369]
GEM, 2, 5, 10 μM	Apigenin, 25, 50 μM	MiaPaca-2 human **pancreatic** cancer cell line	↑	Potentiation of GEM-induced growth inhibition. Increase in apoptosis through inhibition of Akt and downregulation of NF-κB	[369]
GEM, 10 μM	Apigenin, 25 μM	AsPC-1 human **pancreatic** carcinoma cell line	↑	Increase in cell proliferation inhibition. Induction of S and G2/M phase cell cycle arrest (blocking of GEM-induced upregulation of CDK2, pcdc2, cyclins A, E, B). Increase in apoptosis, abrogation of GEM-induced pAkt	[366]
GEM, 10 μM	Apigenin, 11-19 μM	BxPC-3 human **pancreatic** cancer cell line	↑	Increase in cell growth inhibition	[140]
GEM, 10 μM	Apigenin, 25 μM	CD-18 human **pancreatic** carcinoma cell line	↑	Increase in cell proliferation inhibition. Induction of S and G2/M phase cell cycle arrest (blocking of GEM-induced upregulation of CDK2, pcdc2, cyclins A, E, B). Increase in apoptosis, abrogation of GEM-induced pAkt	[366]
GEM, 0.2, 0.5, 1 μM	Baicalein, 10 μM	HPAF-II human **pancreatic** cancer cell line	↑	Synergism in cell viability reduction	[371]
GEM, 0.1, 0.2, 0.5 μM	Baicalein, 10 μM	MIA PaCa-2 human **pancreatic** cancer cell line	↑	Synergism in cell viability reduction	[371]
GEM, 2, 5, 10 μM	Baicalein, 10 μM	PANC-1 human **pancreatic** cancer cell line	↑	Synergism in cell viability reduction. Inhibition of migration	[371]
GEM, 30 μM	EGC, 1 μM	CC-LP-1 human **cholangiocarcinoma** cell line, from intrahepatic biliary tract	~	No effect on GEM-induced cytotoxicity	[37]
GEM, 30 μM	EGC, 1 μM	KMCH-1 human **cholangiocarcinoma** cell line	~	No effect on GEM-induced cytotoxicity	[37]
GEM, 30 μM	EGC, 1 μM	Mz-ChA-1 human **cholangiocarcinoma** cell line, from gallbladder cancer	~	No effect on GEM-induced cytotoxicity	[37]
GEM, 30 μM	EGCG, 1 μM	CC-LP-1 human **cholangiocarcinoma** cell line, from intrahepatic biliary tract	↑	Increase in GEM-induced apoptosis	[37]
GEM, 30 μM	EGCG, 1 μM	KMCH-1 human **cholangiocarcinoma** cell line	↑	Increase in GEM-induced apoptosis	[37]
GEM, 30 μM	EGCG, 1 μM	Mz-ChA-1 human **cholangiocarcinoma** cell line, from gallbladder cancer	↑	Increase in GEM-induced apoptosis (loss of ΔΨm, cyt c release)	[37]
GEM, 0.5 μM	EGCG, 20, 40, 60 μM	AsPC-1 human **pancreatic** cancer cell line	↑	Increase in GEM-induced cell viability inhibition and apoptosis (increase in caspase-3, PARP cleavage). Suppression of STAT3-regulated genes (VEGF, c-Myc, survivin, cyclin D1)	[375]
GEM, 0.5 μM	EGCG, 20, 40, 60 μM	PANC-1 human **pancreatic** cancer cell line	↑	Increase in GEM-induced cell viability inhibition and apoptosis (increase in caspase-3, PARP cleavage). Suppression of STAT3-regulated genes (VEGF, c-Myc, survivin, cyclin D1)	[375]
GEM, 100 nM	Fisetin, 50 μM	MiaPaca-2 human **pancreatic** carcinoma cell line	↑	Increase in GEM-induced cytotoxicity, induction of apoptosis (activation of caspases-3/-7). Inhibition of ERK-MYC signaling	[372]
GEM, 0.5 μM	Genistein, 5-60 μM	MG-63 human **osteosarcoma** cell line	↑	Synergism in growth inhibition (CI<1). Potentiation of GEM-induced apoptosis; downregulation of pAkt, decrease in Bcl-2, Bcl-xL and COX-2	[360]
GEM, 0.5 μM	Genistein, 20 μM	U2OS human **osteosarcoma** cell line, GEM-resistant	↑	Potentiation of GEM-induced growth inhibition and apoptosis. Downregulation of pAkt, abrogation of GEM-induced NF-κB activation; decrease in Bcl-xL and COX-2	[360]

Drug	Flavonoid	Biological system	Direction of combination	Effects	Ref.
GEM, 2 nM	Genistein, 10 μM	A2780 human **ovarian** cancer cell line	↑	Increase in cell viability inhibition and apoptosis (PARP cleavage, decrease in Bcl-2, Bcl-xL, survivin, c-IAP1). Decrease in NF-κB DNA binding activity	[128]
GEM, 50 nM	Genistein, 25 μM	C200 human **ovarian** cancer cell line, CDDP-resistant A2780 cells	↑	Increase in cell viability inhibition and apoptosis (PARP cleavage, decrease in Bcl-2, Bcl-xL, survivin, c-IAP1). Decrease in NF-κB DNA binding activity	[128]
GEM, 25 nM	Genistein, 25 μM	COLO357 human **pancreatic** carcinoma cell line	↑	Potentiation of GEM-induced growth inhibition and apoptosis (activation of caspase-3, PARP cleavage, cyt c release; decrease in Bcl-2, Bcl-xL). Inhibition of GEM-induced NF-κB activation and pAkt	[367]
GEM, 25 nM	Genistein, 25 μM	L3.6pl human **pancreatic** carcinoma cell line, from COLO357 cells	↑	Potentiation of GEM-induced growth inhibition and apoptosis (activation of caspase-3, PARP cleavage, cyt c release; decrease in Bcl-2, Bcl-xL). Inhibition of GEM-induced NF-κB activation and pAkt	[367]
GEM, 0.5 μM	Hispidulin, 12.5 μM	GBC-SD human **gallbladder** carcinoma cell line	↑	Increase in GEM anticancer activity. Downregulation of P-gp through repression of HIF-1α	[349]
GEM, 0.5 μM	Icariin, 40 μg/ml	GBC-SD human **gallbladder** carcinoma cell line	↑	Synergism in cell viability loss (CI 0.694). Potentiation of GEM-induced G0/G1 phase cell cycle arrest and apoptosis (increase in caspase-3; decrease in Bcl-2, Bcl-xL, survivin). Inhibition of GEM-induced NF-κB	[361]
GEM, 0.5 μM	Icariin, 40 μg/ml	SGC-996 human **gallbladder** carcinoma cell line	↑	Synergism in cell viability loss (CI 0.712). Sensitization to GEM-induced apoptosis	[361]
GEM, 5 μM	Liquiritigenin, 0.03, 0.3, 3 μM	Panc-1 human **pancreatic** adenocarcinoma cell line	↝	No effect on GEM-induced decrease in cell viability	[365]
GEM, 10 μM	Luteolin, 11-19 μM	BxPC-3 human **pancreatic** cancer cell line	↑	Increase in cell growth inhibition. Decrease in GSK-3β and NF-κB p65 expression, increase in cyt c	[140]
GEM	Luteolin	AGS human **gastric** cancer cell line	↝	No sensitization of GEM effect	[144]
GEM, 0.01-20 μg/ml	Quercetin, 50 μM	H460 human **lung** cancer cell line	↑	Augmentation of growth inhibition. Promotion of apoptosis via inhibiting HSP70 expression (increase in caspases-3/-9)	[374]
GEM, 0.01-20 μg/ml	Quercetin, 50 μM	A549 human **lung** cancer cell line	↑	Augmentation of growth inhibition. Promotion of apoptosis via inhibiting HSP70 expression (increase in caspases-3/-9)	[374]
GEM, 0.01-10 μg/ml	Quercetin, 50 μM	MiaPaCa-2 human **pancreatic** cancer cell line	↑	Increase in cell viability reduction. Increase in caspase-3 activity and LC3-II protein expression	[373]
GEM, 0.01-10 μg/ml	Quercetin, 50 μM	Panc-1 human **pancreatic** cancer cell line	↑	Increase in cell viability reduction. Increase in caspase-3 activity	[373]

Akt, protein kinase B; Bcl-2, B-cell lymphoma 2; Bcl-xl, B-cell lymphoma-extra large; CDK, cyclin-dependent kinase; CI, combination index; COX, cyclooxygenase; cyt c, cytochrome c; ERK, extracellular signal-regulated kinase; GSK, glycogen synthase kinase; HIF-1α, hypoxia-inducible factor 1α; Hsp, heat shock protein; IAP, inhibitor of apoptosis; NF-κB, nuclear factor-κB; PARP, poly (ADP-ribose) polymerase; P-gp, P-glycoprotein; STAT3, signal transducer and activator of transcription 3; VEGF, vascular endothelial growth factor; ΔΨm, mitochondrial membrane potential.

associated with suppression of constitutive and GEM-induced NF-κB DNA binding activity, and downregulation of activated Akt. Combination of genistein and GEM was more effective antitumor therapy compared to treatment with either agent alone also in mice bearing orthotopically implanted pancreatic carcinoma cells, COLO357 and L3.6pl, abrogating GEM-elicited NF-κB activation and chemosensitizing pancreatic tumors to GEM cytotoxicity [367]. Thus, genistein is able to augment GEM-based chemotherapy for pancreatic cancer, independent on metastatic behavior of pancreatic tumor cells. Moreover, a novel form of genistein with improved physicochemical properties and oral bioavailability, i.e., genistein sodium salt dihydrate or AXP107-11, was administered orally in escalating doses (400-1600 mg/day) in combination with standard GEM (1000 mg/m^2/week) to 16 treatment-naive patients with inoperable pancreatic tumors within a phase Ib clinical trial. No dose-limiting toxicities or symptoms of hematological or non-hematological toxicities related to AXP107-11 were detected over a period of 0.7-13.2 months. The median progression-free survival time of patients was 2.6 months and the median overall survival was 4.9 months. Seven patients survived longer than 6 months and three patients were alive even at the one-year follow-up. In addition, a decrease of 50% or more in cancer antigen CA 19-9 was observed in eight patients during the treatment course [368]. These limited data are attractive and encouraging providing some early signs of improved efficacy and proving the previous preclinical findings. With no doubt, further clinical trials with combined treatment of genistein and GEM against highly lethal pancreatic malignancies are greatly needed. Genistein has been demonstrated to potentiate antitumor action of GEM also in other cancer cells. In human ovarian cancer cell line A2780 and its CDDP-resistant subline C200, genistein augmented GEM-induced inhibition of cellular viability and increase in apoptotic death through suppression of NF-κB activity and downregulation of key survival factors, including survivin and cellular inhibitor of apoptosis protein 1 (cIAP1) [128]. Genistein enhanced the effect of GEM chemotherapy also in human osteosarcoma MG-63 cells and GEM-resistant osteosarcoma U2OS cells, leading to a significant reduction of growth inhibition and induction of apoptosis. Addition of genistein chemosensitized osteosarcoma cells to GEM through the same mechanism as in pancreatic and ovarian cancer cells, i.e., abrogation of GEM-induced activation of Akt/NF-κB pathway and suppression of downstream apoptosis-related proteins [360] (Table 6.19 and Table 6.21).

Similar to genistein, common dietary flavone *apigenin* strongly potentiated GEM-induced growth inhibition and apoptosis in human pancreatic cancer cell lines AsPC-1 and MiaPaca-2, mediated by downregulation of NF-κB DNA binding activity via suppression of Akt activation. Moreover, combination treatment of apigenin and GEM augmented tumor growth inhibition also in mice harboring MiaPaca-2 cells, via abrogation of GEM-induced activation of Akt and NF-κB in malignant tissues [369]. Combined treatment with apigenin and GEM regulated also the cell cycle progression in human pancreatic cancer AsPC-1 and CD-18 cells, inducing arrests at both the S and

Effects of Plant Flavonoids on Chemotherapeutic Efficacy of Cancer Drugs 293

G2/M phases, leading to increase in cell growth inhibition and apoptotic death as compared to either single agent alone [366]. Thus, apigenin might be a promising complementary agent to improve the outcome of GEM chemotherapeutic regimens for pancreatic cancer. Besides apigenin, another natural flavone *luteolin* enhanced GEM-induced growth inhibition in human pancreatic cancer BxPC-3 cells, whereas pretreatment with flavones for 24 hours was more efficient in suppressing cell proliferation than simultaneous application with the drug. This chemosensitizing effect was associated with inhibition of GSK-3β/NF-κB signaling cascade, leading to induction of apoptotic death by combined treatment with luteolin and GEM [140]. In addition, GEM in the presence of luteolin significantly reduced the proliferating cell nuclear antigen (PCNA) expression and lowered pancreatic tumor mass in BxPC-3 bearing mice. In this orthotopic model, chemosensitization by luteolin was achieved through inhibition of GSK-3β/NF-κB signaling pathway, resulting in promotion of apoptosis in tumoral tissues; suggesting that luteolin might be useful as an adjuvant agent to GEM chemotherapy against pancreatic cancer [370]. The above-described *in vitro* results recapitulated by *in vivo* findings provide a scientific rationale for therapeutic application of combined approach of flavones apigenin and luteolin with GEM for the treatment of patients suffering from pancreatic cancer. Furthermore, another flavone *baicalein* synergistically strengthened antiproliferative activities of GEM in several human pancreatic cancer cell lines, PANC-1, MIA PaCa-2 and HPAF-II [371]. On the contrary, flavone luteolin did not affect chemotherapeutic efficacy of GEM in human gastric cancer AGS cells [144]. The only methylated flavone studied so far in combination with GEM, *hispidulin* or 6-methoxyscutellarein, enhanced antitumor effects of GEM in human gallbladder carcinoma GBC-SD cells, downregulating P-gp through inhibition of HIF-1α overexpression [349] (Table 6.19 and Table 6.21).

Chemosensitization of human pancreatic cancer cells to antitumor action of GEM was achieved also in combination with a few dietary flavonols. In fact, *fisetin* promoted GEM-induced growth inhibition and apoptosis in MiaPaca-2 cells through downregulation of ERK levels [372]. Abundant natural flavonol *quercetin* enhanced GEM-elicited cell viability reduction in MiaPaCa-2 and Panc-1 cells by reducing Hsp70 expression and augmenting cell death [373]. Thus, combinations of fisetin and quercetin with GEM might be beneficial in eliminating pancreatic tumors and preventing disease recurrence. Induction of apoptosis by GEM was enhanced by quercetin also in human lung cancer A549 and H460 cells, similarly associated with inhibition of Hsp70 levels [374]. Although low micromolar doses of flavanone *liquiritigenin* were inactive in influencing GEM cytotoxicity in pancreatic cancer Panc-1 cells [365]; the major green tea flavanol *EGCG* augmented antiproliferative and proapoptotic properties of GEM in AsPC-1 and PANC-1 cells through inhibition of STAT3 signaling pathway and its several target genes, including VEGF and survivin. These data suggest that EGCG could be used as a potential chemosensitizer for GEM therapeutic efficacy in the treatment of pancreatic tumors [375]. EGCG increased GEM-induced apoptotic death also in several human cholangiocarcinoma cell lines with different origin: Mz-ChA-1 cells derived from metastatic gallbladder cancer, CC-LP-1 from intrahepatic biliary tract tumor, and KMCH-1 from combined hepatocellular and cholangiocarcinoma. EGCG in combination with GEM decreased tumor growth also in Mz-ChA-1 bearing mice as compared to the treatment with GEM alone, corroborating the *in vitro* results. As after oral administration, EGCG is excreted from the body mainly via the biliary route, intake of this common green tea flavanol can be a therapeutically important adjuvant agent for GEM chemotherapy in the treatment of biliary tract cancers. However, another flavanol *epigallocatechin (EGC)* exerted no sensitizing effects on GEM cytotoxicity in all studied cholangiocarcinoma cells [37]. Viability of human gallbladder carcinoma cell lines GBC-SD and SGC-996 was synergistically reduced also by combination of GEM and prenylated flavonoid glycoside *icariin* through augmentation of apoptotic death. In GBC-SD cells, icariin enhanced GEM-induced cell cycle arrest at the G0/G1 phase and suppressed NF-κB activity; in GBC-SD cell xenografts in nude mice, combined treatment with icariin and GEM led to significantly smaller tumors as compared to treatment with either agent alone [361]. These findings suggest that addition of icariin to GEM regimen could result in greater therapeutic effects than those observed with GEM monotherapy (Table 6.19 and Table 6.21).

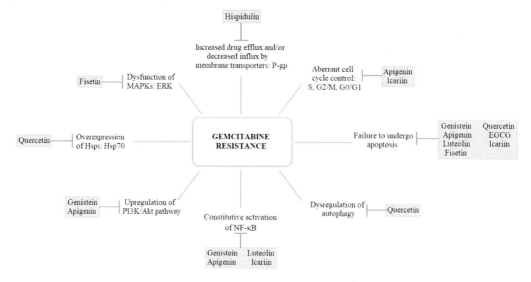

Figure 6.12. Possibilities to intervene in gemcitabine resistance with plant flavonoids (Akt, protein kinase B; ERK, extracellular signal-regulated kinase; Hsp, heat shock protein; MAPK, mitogen-activated protein kinase; NF-κB, nuclear factor-κB; P-gp, P-glycoprotein; PI3K, phosphoinositide 3-kinase).

Current promising preclinical findings about positive cooperation between different flavonoids and GEM (Figure 6.12) might open new avenues for development of novel therapeutic strategies with enhanced efficacy and improved clinical outcome. In particular, combination of genistein (but also other flavonoids like apigenin, luteolin, baicalein, fisetin, quercetin and EGCG) with GEM could provide an important therapeutic benefit for patients diagnosed with unresectable pancreatic cancer or those with resected tumors but still under high risk for disease recurrence. The results of the first clinical trial treating pancreatic cancer patients with genistein sodium salt dihydrate and GEM give promise of improving the clinical outcome and survival time of pancreatic carcinoma patients in the future; but encourage also additional clinical trials combining GEM with specific flavonoids against human pancreatic tumors. Not less important is also the further development of EGCG as an adjuvant agent for GEM chemotherapy in the clinical treatment of biliary tract cancers.

6.2.4. Cytarabine (ARA-C)

Cytarabine (ARA-C) is a pyrimidine analog that is widely employed to treat human hematological malignancies [308, 376]. This drug is a major element in the treatment of acute lymphoblastic leukemias (ALL) and acute myeloblastic leukemias (AML), including relapsed and refractory diseases, and also non-Hodgkin lymphomas [1, 377-380]. After entering the cells, this agent is rapidly converted to its active triphosphate form (Ara-CTP) that incorporates into DNA and leads to inhibition of DNA synthesis, S phase arrest of the cell cycle and eventually apoptotic death [308, 377-380]. Cytotoxic responses to ARA-C are associated also with inhibition of DNA and RNA polymerases required for DNA synthesis, and promotion of intracellular ROS generation [308, 380, 381]. Despite the positive therapeutical impact of ARA-C, its clinical use is still limited by concurrent damage to normal healthy tissues, including neurological toxicity, and acquisition of drug resistance, leading to a worse prognosis [308, 376]. Therefore, nontoxic adjuvant agents which could enhance the therapeutic efficacy and improve clinical outcome of ARA-C chemotherapy are highly needed.

Combinations of ARA-C with some natural flavonoids have been studied in different human leukemia cell lines, both *in vitro* and *in vivo* conditions (Table 6.19 and Table 6.22). These studies have shown that natural flavonols *kaempferol, myricetin* and *isorhamnetin* were able to synergistically increase antiproliferative capacity of ARA-C in murine lymphocytic leukemia L1210 cells, augmenting drug-induced apoptosis and G2/M phase arrest of the cell cycle progression [382]. Low micromolar doses of ubiquitous dietary plant flavonol *quercetin* strongly (about threefold) potentiated ARA-C-induced growth inhibition in human promyelocytic leukemia HL-60 cells and synergistically suppressed ARA-C clonogenic capacity in fresh blasts isolated from bone marrow aspirates of patients suffering from AML and ALL. However, glycosylated quercetin, *rutin* or quercetin 3-rutinoside, exerted no effects on the inhibitory action of ARA-C in HL-60 cells [383]. Despite these results obtained with human myeloid leukemia cells, rutin was shown to antagonize ARA-C cytotoxicity in murine lymphocytic leukemia L1210 cells [382]. Likewise, the sensitivity to ARA-C treatment was substantially decreased also by natural methylated flavone *5,7-dimethoxyflavone (5,7-DMF)* or dimethylchrysin in several human acute lymphoblastic leukemia cell lines, YCUB-2, YCUB-5 and YCUB-6, suggesting that combination therapy with 5,7-DMF and ARA-C is not recommended [11]. Moreover, also glycosylated citrus flavanone *naringin* was shown to strongly antagonize the cytotoxic activity of ARA-C in murine lymphocytic leukemia P388 cells, by completely blocking the ARA-C-induced DNA damage and apoptosis through inhibition of drug-elicited ROS production and increase in antioxidant enzyme effects, thereby reducing the oxidative stress [380]. On the contrary, in myeloid origin cells, i.e., in $CD34^+$ cells isolated from mononuclear cells of AML patients bone marrow, another glycosidic flavanone, *hesperidin*, enhanced ARA-C cytotoxicity [376]. The chemotherapeutic efficacy of ARA-C in these primary malignant cells was synergistically modulated also by flavonolignan *silibinin* [376]. The green tea flavanol *EGCG* strengthened cytotoxic and antiproliferative action of ARA-C in human acute promyelocytic leukemia HL-60 cells, by increasing drug-induced G1 phase cell cycle arrest and apoptotic death [381, 384]. Although EGCG exerted no effect on ARA-C cytotoxicity in human chronic myelogenous leukemia K562 cells, the peracetate-protected prodrug version of this flavanol with markedly improved bioavailability could sensitize both K562 cells as well as human T-cell leukemia Jurkat cells to ARA-C chemotherapy [308]. Soy isoflavone *genistein* worked synergistically with ARA-C in inhibiting growth of two human acute promyelocytic leukemia cell lines, HL-60 and NB4. Moreover, cotreatment with genistein and ARA-C significantly suppressed the tumor growth and prolonged survival of both NB4 and HL-60 xenograft mice [385]. In addition, rotenoid *deguelin* as low as only nanomolar doses also enhanced antileukemic and proapoptotic action of ARA-C in human acute myeloid leukemia U937 cells and primary blasts isolated from AML patients, by dephosphorylating Akt in these cells possessing an active PI3K/Akt pathway. However, in parental HL60PT cells with no active PI3K/Akt signaling network, deguelin remained ineffective in modulating ARA-C-induced cytotoxicity [211] (Table 6.19 and Table 6.22). Possibilities to intervene in ARA-C resistance by plant-derived flavonoids are summarized in Figure 6.13.

Current preclinical studies have demonstrated that several dietary flavonoids can behave antagonistically in combination with ARA-C therapy suggesting that leukemia patients, particularly those suffering from lymphocytic leukemias, who are receiving ARA-C chemotherapy should be especially cautious in consuming food products and supplements rich in certain flavonoids, such as naringin, rutin and 5,7-dimethoxyflavone. Further in vivo investigations are urgently required to prove or disprove the current in vitro findings. To date, no such contraindicated combinations between flavonoids and ARA-C are found in acute myeloid leukemia cells, where combined treatment reveals rather positive cooperation.

Table 6.22. Effects of flavonoids on anticancer action of cytarabine (ARA-C) *in vitro* conditions

Drug	Flavonoid	Biological system	Direction of combination	Effects	Ref.
ARA-C	5,7-DMF	YCUB-2 human acute lymphoblastic **leukemia** cell line	↓	Antagonism with ARA-C	[11]
ARA-C	5,7-DMF	YCUB-5 human acute lymphoblastic **leukemia** cell line	↓	Antagonism with ARA-C	[11]
ARA-C	5,7-DMF	YCUB-6 human acute lymphoblastic **leukemia** cell line	↓	Antagonism with ARA-C	[11]
ARA-C, 0.1 µM	Deguelin, 10 nM	Acute myeloid **leukemia** blasts isolated from AML patients	↑	Increase in ARA-C-induced apoptosis. Decrease in pAkt level	[211]
ARA-C, 0.3 µM	Deguelin, 10, 100 nM	HL60PT human **leukemia** cell line	~	No effect on ARA-C-induced apoptosis	[211]
ARA-C, 0.3 µM	Deguelin, 10, 100 nM	U937 human acute myeloid **leukemia** cell line	↑	Increase in ARA-C-induced apoptosis. Downregulation of Akt phosphorylation	[211]
ARA-C, 5, 10, 20 nM	EGCG, 20, 25 µM	HL-60 human promyelocytic **leukemia** cell line	↑	Additive cytostatic activity	[381]
ARA-C, 0.1-0.8 µM	EGCG, 20 µM	HL-60 human acute promyelocytic **leukemia** cell line	↑	Increase in ARA-C-induced cytotoxicity, G1 phase cell cycle arrest and apoptosis. Nullifying the rescue effect of dCdR, downregulation of bcl-2, increase in intracellular Ca^{2+}	[384]
ARA-C, 300 nM	EGCG with peracetate protecting groups (Pro-EGCG), 20 µM	Jurkat human T-cell **leukemia** cell line	↑	Sensitization of cells to ARA-C, increase in cell death	[308]
ARA-C, 200 nM	EGCG	K562 human chronic myelogenous **leukemia** cell line	~	No effect on ARA-C cytotoxicity	[308]
ARA-C, 200 nM	EGCG with peracetate protecting groups (Pro-EGCG), 20 µM	K562 human chronic myelogenous **leukemia** cell line	↑	Sensitization of cells to ARA-C, increase in cell death	[308]
ARA-C, 10-1000 nM	Genistein, 20 µM	HL-60 human acute promyelocytic **leukemia** cell line	↑	Synergism in growth inhibition (CI 0.51) when treated concurrently. Increase in ARA-C-induced morphological cytotoxic effect	[385]
ARA-C, 10-1000 nM	Genistein, 20 µM	NB4 human acute promyelocytic **leukemia** cell line	↑	Synergism in growth inhibition (CI 0.68) when treated concurrently. Increase in ARA-C-induced morphological cytotoxic effect	[385]
ARA-C, 100 nM-1 µM	Hesperidin, 25 µM	CD34+ cells isolated from MNCs of acute myelogenous **leukemia** patient`s bone marrow	↑	Synergism in cytotoxicity, about 5.9-fold decrease in ARA-C IC_{50}	[376]
ARA-C, 0.05, 0.1, 0.25 µM	Isorhamnetin, 10, 20 µM	L1210 murine **leukemia** cell line	↑	Synergism in antiproliferative activity (CI<1). Potentiation of ARA-C-induced apoptosis, increase in G2/M phase cell cycle arrest	[382]
ARA-C, 0.05, 0.1, 0.25 µM	Kaempferol, 10, 20 µM	L1210 murine **leukemia** cell line	↑	Synergism in antiproliferative activity (CI<1). Potentiation of ARA-C-induced apoptosis, increase in G2/M phase cell cycle arrest	[382]
ARA-C, 0.05, 0.1, 0.25 µM	Myricetin, 10, 20 µM	L1210 murine **leukemia** cell line	↑	Synergism in antiproliferative activity (CI<1). Potentiation of ARA-C-induced apoptosis, increase in G2/M phase cell cycle arrest	[382]

Table 6.22. (Continued)

Drug	Flavonoid	Biological system	Direction of combination	Effects	Ref.
ARA-C, 1 µM	Naringin, 0.1-1 mM	P388 murine **leukemia** cell line	↓	Complete prevention of ARA-C-induced cytotoxicity. Decrease in ARA-C-induced ROS production and oxidative stress. Attenuation of ARA-C-induced apoptosis and DNA damage	[380]
ARA-C, 1-100 nM	Quercetin, 1 µM	HL-60 human promyelocytic **leukemia** cell line	↑	Potentiation of ARA-c-induced inhibitory activity	[383]
ARA-C, 1-100 nM	Quercetin, 0.1 µM	Blasts isolated from bone marrow aspirates of **leukemia** patients (AML, ALL)	↑	Synergistic inhibitory activity on CFU-L	[383]
ARA-C, 1-100 nM	Rutin, 1 µM	HL-60 human promyelocytic **leukemia** cell line	~	No effect on ARA-C inhibitory capacity	[383]
ARA-C, 0.05, 0.1, 0.25 µM	Rutin, 10, 20 µM	L1210 murine **leukemia** cell line	↓	Antagonism in antiproliferative activity (CI>1)	[382]
ARA-C, 100 nM-1 µM	Silibinin, 10 µM	CD34+ cells isolated from MNCs of acute myelogenous **leukemia** patient`s bone marrow	↑	Synergism in cytotoxicity, about 4.5-fold decrease in ARA-C IC_{50}	[376]

Akt, protein kinase B; Bcl-2, B-cell lymphoma 2; CFU-L, colony forming unit-leukemic; CI, combination index; dCdR, deoxycytidine; DMF, dimethoxyflavone; MNC, mononuclear cells; ROS, reactive oxygen species.

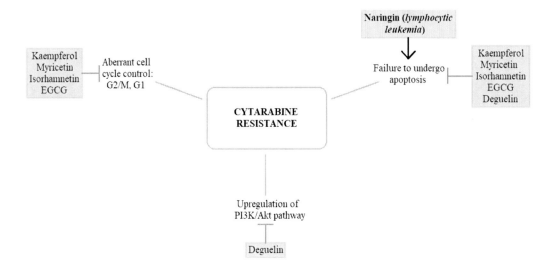

Figure 6.13. Modulation of cytarabine resistance by plant-derived natural flavonoids (Akt, protein kinase B; PI3K, phosphoinositide 3-kinase).

According to the current experimental findings it is recommended for cancer patients *not to consume* dietary products or dietary supplements rich in following plant flavonoids during the active chemotherapeutic treatment phase with **cytarabine**:
- **5,7-dimethoxyflavone** in acute lymphoblastic leukemia
- **rutin** in lymphocytic leukemia
- **naringin** in lymphocytic leukemia

6.2.5. Decitabine (AZA)

Decitabine (AZA) is a pyrimidine antagonist that works as a hypomethylating agent as well. This drug is clinically indicated for the treatment of older patients with acute myeloid leukemia (AML); however, it has shown some limited efficacy also against breast tumors [1, 386, 387]. Pharmacological action of AZA is mediated by its phosphorylation and incorporation into DNA, leading to formation of cytotoxic DNA adducts [386, 387]. At lower doses, AZA acts also as a demethylating agent, by inhibiting the activity of DNA methyltransferase enzymes (DNMTs) or degrading DNMT1 via proteasomal pathway, thereby contributing to reduced proliferation and apoptosis [386, 387]. However, higher pharmacological doses of AZA cause significant toxicity to normal healthy tissues and are often involved in the development of drug-resistant clones [386, 387]. Therefore, development of combination chemotherapy applying non-toxic adjuvant agents in therapeutic protocols of AZA might overcome these limitations and bring about improvement of clinical outcome.

Current preclinical findings have shown that inclusion of soy isoflavone *genistein* in AZA chemotherapy could synergistically decrease the clonogenicity in human myeloid leukemia HL-60 cells, human lymphoid leukemia MOLT-3 cells, but also in murine lymphoid leukemia cell line L1210 and its drug-resistant subline L1210/ARA-C. Although the exact mechanism responsible for this cooperation remains to be clarified, it may be clinically useful for eradicating the clonogenic potential of leukemic cells, especially due to submicromolar doses of genistein used in these assays. Moreover, combined treatment with genistein and AZA led to a synergistic prolongation of lifespan of mice with L1210 leukemia [387]. Besides these antileukemic experiments, combination of flavonoids and AZA has been studied also in some solid tumor cell lines. As a result, it was demonstrated that green tea flavanol *EGCG* augmented AZA-induced growth inhibition in both estrogen receptor-positive as well as -negative breast cancer cell lines, MCF-7 and MDA-MB-231 respectively, at least partially through epigenetic mechanisms by causing alterations in DNA methylation pattern. These effects were associated with increase in pre-G1 cell population and decrease in tumorigenic potential of MCF-7 cells [386]. Combination of natural flavonolignan *silibinin* and AZA restored the levels of E-cadherin in human non-small cell lung cancer H1299 cells which harbor epigenetically silenced E-cadherin expression, modulating thus epithelial-mesenchymal transition (EMT) events and leading to a substantial inhibition of invasive and migratory potential of these malignant pulmonary cells. As E-cadherin has been reported to be epigenetically silenced through methylation in about 18% of non-small cell lung cancer tumor specimens, inclusion of silibinin in AZA hypomethylating therapy might be an effective clinical regimen for the treatment of lung tumors in the future [388] (Table 6.19 and Table 6.23)

300   *Katrin Sak*

Table 6.23. Effects of flavonoids on anticancer action of decitabine (AZA)
***in vitro* conditions**

Drug	Flavonoid	Biological system	Direction of combination	Effects	Ref.
AZA, 5 µM	EGCG, 50 µM	MCF-7 human **breast** cancer cell line, ER-positive	↑	Potentiation of growth inhibition. Increase in percentage of pre-G1 cell population, decrease in number and size of colonies. Synergistic targeting of epigenetic regulatory genes, greater effects on DNA methylation and histone modification	[386]
AZA, 5 µM	EGCG, 50 µM	MDA-MB-231 human **breast** cancer cell line, ER-negative	↑	Potentiation of growth inhibition. Increase in percentage of pre-G1 cell population	[386]
AZA, 44 nM	Genistein, 0.1, 1 µM	HL-60 human myeloid **leukemia** cell line	↑	Synergistic loss of clonogenicity	[387]
AZA, 4.4 nM	Genistein, 0.1, 1 µM	L1210 murine lymphoid **leukemia** cell line	↑	Synergistic loss of clonogenicity	[387]
AZA, 4.4 nM	Genistein, 0.1, 1 µM	L1210/ARA-C murine lymphoid **leukemia** cell line, ARA-C- and AZA-resistant	↑	Increase in loss of clonogenicity	[387]
AZA, 44 nM	Genistein, 0.1, 1 µM	MOLT-3 human lymphoid **leukemia** cell line	↑	Synergistic loss of clonogenicity	[387]
AZA, 5 µM	Silibinin, 3.75-12.5 µM	H1299 human non-small cell **lung** cancer cell line	↑	Upregulation of E-cadherin levels. Inhibition of migration and invasion	[388]

ER, estrogen receptor.

Based on the currently available preclinical findings, addition of certain flavonoids, such as genistein, EGCG or silibinin, to AZA treatment protocols might confer improvement of antineoplastic action by reducing disease progression and metastasis, at least in part through restoration of expression of methylation-silenced proteins important in controlling proliferation, migration and death of malignant cells.

6.2.6. Methotrexate (MTX)

Methotrexate (MTX) is an antifolate drug that is commonly used in the treatment of most malignancies, including acute lymphocytic leukemia, lymphomas and certain solid tumors. Moreover, this drug is indicated also for some non-neoplastic disorders, such as psoriasis or rheumatoid arthritis [1, 325, 389, 390]. After entering the cells, MTX targets the enzyme dihydrofolate reductase, thereby reducing nucleotide synthesis, inducing cell cycle arrest and inhibiting cell growth via apoptotic death [325, 334, 390, 391]. Prolonged treatment with this antifolate has been related to acquisition of resistance, attenuation of therapeutic efficacy and progression of disease [389, 390]; highlighting the necessity to identify novel adjuvant agents that could modulate the cellular pathways involved in MTX resistance and prevent the development of resistance phenomenon.

Several flavonoids have been tested in combination with MTX in some *in vitro* cancer cell lines. These studies have revealed diverse results, showing both positive,

Effects of Plant Flavonoids on Chemotherapeutic Efficacy of Cancer Drugs 301

negative as well as no cooperation between certain natural flavonoids and MTX (Table 6.24). Addition of dietary flavonol *fisetin* in MTX treatment protocols did not show any effect on the drug-induced cytotoxicity in human non-small cell lung cancer A549 cells [323]. Glycosylated flavonol *rutin* or quercetin 3-O-rutinoside was also inactive in modulating therapeutic efficacy of MTX in human hormone receptor-positive breast cancer MCF-7 cells, but significantly enhanced drug cytotoxicity in triple negative human breast cancer MDA-MB-231 cells by inhibiting P-gp and BCRP efflux pumps. Inactivity of rutin in MCF-7 cells was explained by only poor expression of these transporter proteins at cellular surface, being overexpressed in MDA-MB-231 cells [8].

Table 6.24. Effects of flavonoids on anticancer action of methotrexate (MTX) *in vitro* conditions

Drug	Flavonoid	Biological system	Direction of combination	Effects	Ref.
MTX	Alopecurone B, 10 μM	MG-63/DOX human **osteosarcoma** cell line, MDR, DOX-resistant	↑	Increase in sensitivity to MTX, 2.78-fold decrease in MTX IC_{50}	[235]
MTX, 3.125, 6.25, 12.5 nM	Baicalein, 50 μM	CCRF-CEM human childhood acute lymphoblastic **leukemia** cell line	~	No effect on MTX-induced cytotoxicity	[391]
MTX, 1, 5, 10 μM	EGCG, 30, 60 μM	JAR human placenta **choriocarcinoma** cell line	↑	Increase in cytotoxicity. Decrease in metastatic HER2 protein synthesis. Increase in caspase-3 activation and Bax gene (not protein)	[325]
MTX	Fisetin, 10-50 μM	A549 human non-small cell **lung** cancer cell line, wild-type p53	~	No increase in cell viability reduction	[323]
MTX, 0.01 μM	Genistein, 50 μM	L1210 murine **leukemia** cell line	↓	Protection of cells from MTX cytotoxicity. Decrease in phosphorylation of 66 kDa membrane protein, decrease in MTX uptake and influx rate	[389]
MTX, 2 μM	Rutin, 20 μM	MCF-7 human **breast** cancer cell line, HER2-negative, ER- and PR-positive	~	No effect on MTX efficacy	[8]
MTX, 2 μM	Rutin, 20 μM	MDA-MB-231 human TN **breast** cancer cell line	↑	Increase in MTX-induced cytotoxicity. Inhibition of P-gp and BCRP pumps	[8]
MTX, 800 μM	Silibinin (SDH), 25-200 μM	hRD, MTX-R human **rhabdomyosarcoma** cell line, MTX-resistant	↑	Reversal of MTX resistance. 1.12-fold decrease in MTX IC_{50} at 25 μM, 2.24-fold at 50 μM, 7.94-fold at 100 μM, 17.8-fold at 200 μM SDH	[390]

Bax, Bcl-2-associated X protein; BCRP, breast cancer resistance protein; ER, estrogen receptor; HER2 (erbB2) human epidermal growth factor receptor 2; MDR, multidrug resistance; P-gp, P-glycoprotein; PR, progesterone receptor; SDH, silibinin di-hemisuccinate; TN, triple negative.

Also, green tea flavanol *EGCG* acted as a potential chemosensitizer to MTX cytotoxicity, resulting in a greater decrease in proliferation and inhibition of metastatic HER2 protein synthesis in human placenta choriocarcinoma JAR cells as compared to MTX alone. In addition, this combination induced apoptotic death in JAR cells, but not via mitochondrial pathway [325]. Furthermore, flavonolignan *silibinin* (in the form of silibinin di-hemisuccinate, SDH) reversed resistance to MTX in drug-resistant human rhabdomyosarcoma MTX-R hRD cells [390] and flavonostilbene *alopecurone B* increased sensitivity to MTX in multidrug-resistant human osteosarcoma MG-63/DOX cells [235]. Nevertheless, whereas flavone *baicalein* did not affect MTX cytotoxicity in human childhood acute lymphoblastic leukemia CCRF-CEM cells [391]; soy isoflavone *genistein* significantly decreased antileukemic activities of MTX in murine lymphocytic leukemia L1210 cells suppressing drug influx into the cells. Such protective effect of genistein from MTX cytotoxicity made the cells chemoresistant to drug therapeutic efficacy and certainly needs further studies in human lymphocytic leukemia cell lines [389] (Table 6.24).

Despite its rather extensive use in clinical oncology, our current knowledge about the possible role of flavonoids on MTX cytotoxicity is still rather poor revealing both positive, negative and also no cooperation depending on malignant cells; highlighting the necessity of cancer patients to be cautious in consuming products rich in flavonoids during the active treatment phase with MTX.

According to the current experimental findings it is recommended for cancer patients *not to consume* dietary products or dietary supplements rich in following plant flavonoids during the active chemotherapeutic treatment phase with **methotrexate**:
- **genistein** in lymphocytic leukemia

6.2.7. Fludarabine (FLU)

Fludarabine (FLU) is a purine nucleoside analog that is widely used for the treatment of chronic lymphocytic leukemia (CLL) [1, 392].

Only a few flavonoids have been studied in combination with FLU in B-cell CLL preclinical models (Table 6.19 and Table 6.25). Based on these assays, abundant dietary flavonol *quercetin* was shown to be able to ameliorate the resistance to FLU in mononuclear cells (MNCs) isolated from peripheral blood of B-CLL patients, by enhancing cell growth inhibitory and proapoptotic properties of FLU [392]. Soy isoflavone *genistein* also augmented FLU-induced cytotoxicity and apoptosis in MNCs derived from patients with B-cell CLL, whereas ZAP-70 could represent as a target for this therapy. In addition, expression of interleukin-10 (IL-10) in malignant cells was negatively correlated with the ability of apoptosis induction by combined treatment with genistein and FLU [393]. Natural rotenoid *deguelin* augmented FLU-induced DNA damage and apoptotic death in both peripheral blood mononuclear cells (PBMCs) isolated from CLL patients as well as in CLL-like splenic MNCs derived from New Zealand Black (NZB) mice. Moreover, inclusion of deguelin in FLU treatment schemes significantly increased survival time of young NZB mice transplanted with leukemic splenocytes from aged NZB mice as compared to the treatment with either agent alone [394] (Table 6.19 and Table 6.25).

Effects of Plant Flavonoids on Chemotherapeutic Efficacy of Cancer Drugs 303

Table 6.25. Effects of flavonoids on anticancer action of fludarabine (FLU)
***in vitro* conditions**

Drug	Flavonoid	Biological system	Direction of combination	Effects	Ref.
FLU, 0-50 μM	Deguelin, 0-100 μM	B-cell chronic lymphocytic **leukemia**-like splenic MNCs from NZB mice	↑	Mild synergism on apoptosis induction	[394]
FLU, 0-50 μM	Deguelin, 0-100 μM	PBMCs from chronic lymphocytic **leukemia** patients	↑	Mild synergism on apoptosis induction. Increase in FLU-induced DNA damage	[394]
FLU, 3 μM	Genistein, 15-60 μM	MNCs from patients with B-cell chronic lymphocytic **leukemia**	↑	Potentiation of FLU-induced cytotoxicity. Increase in apoptosis (more apoptosis in cells with high ZAP-70 expression; negative correlation with basal IL-10 expression)	[393]
FLU, 14 μM	Quercetin, 25 μM	MNCs from peripheral blood of patients with B-cell chronic lymphocytic **leukemia**	↑	6-fold increase in cell viability reduction. Increase in apoptosis (activation of caspase-3)	[392]

IL, interleukin; MNC, mononuclear cell; NZB mice, New Zealand Black mice; PBMC, peripheral blood mononuclear cell.

As only very few preclinical data are available so far on the positive cooperation between natural flavonoids and FLU, further studies are certainly needed before giving any dietary advice to patients suffering from CLL undergoing treatment with FLU chemotherapy.

6.2.8. Tiazofurin (TCAR)

Tiazofurin (TCAR) is a synthetic purine nucleoside that is still under investigation for its potential clinical use in the fight against different cancers. TCAR is an inhibitor of inosine 5`-monophosphate (IMP) dehydrogenase, reducing nucleotide biosynthesis, and leading to S phase arrest of the cell cycle progression and apoptotic cell death [395-397].

It is well known that TCAR reduces biosynthesis and depletes intracellular pool of guanosine 5`-triphosphate (GTP). As GTP is required for functioning of enzymes in phosphoinositide pathway, TCAR suppresses also the signal transduction activity and level of inositol 1,4,5-triphosphate (IP_3) in cells [395-397]. When combined with dietary flavonol *quercetin*, reduction of IP_3 induced by TCAR was significantly enhanced, probably explaining also the synergistic inhibition of cell growth and colony formation in human ovarian carcinoma cell line OVCAR-5, treated sequentially with TCAR and quercetin [397]. Likewise, pretreatment of OVCAR-5 cells with TCAR for 12 hours before addition of soy isoflavone *genistein* led to a synergistic inhibition of cell growth and clonogenicity [396]. Genistein potentiated TCAR-induced cytotoxicity also in human leukemia K562 cells by synergistically inhibiting the growth and elevating differentiation induction of these multipotent cells [395]. Thus, lower doses of TCAR might be employed in the presence of quercetin or genistein to achieve therapeutic efficacy of the drug, thereby decreasing also the potential side effects (Table 6.26).

Table 6.26. Effects of flavonoids on anticancer action of tiazofurin (TCAR)
***in vitro* conditions**

Drug	Flavonoid	Biological system	Direction of combination	Effects	Ref.
TCAR, 5-15 µM	Genistein, 10-30 µM	K562 human **leukemia** cell line	↑	Synergism in growth inhibition and differentiation when pretreated with TCAR for 12h	[395]
TCAR, 10, 20, 40 µM	Genistein, 10, 20, 40 µM	OVCAR-5 human **ovarian** carcinoma cell line	↑	Synergism in growth inhibition and cytotoxicity when pretreated with TCAR for 12h	[396]
TCAR, 2-10 µM	Quercetin, 10-30 µM	OVCAR-5 human **ovarian** carcinoma cell line	↑	Synergistic inhibition of cell growth and clonogenicity when pretreated with TCAR for 12h. Reduction of IP$_3$ concentration in cells	[397]

IP$_3$, inositol 1, 4, 5-trisphosphate.

The role of several flavonoids on cytotoxic action of antimetabolites has been studied in numerous preclinical works with some promising results definitely worth of further therapeutic development. In fact, if further in vivo research and additional clinical trials will corroborate the positive cooperation between genistein and gemcitabine against pancreatic tumors, this combination might have substantial therapeutic benefit for pancreatic cancer patients improving clinical outcome and prolonging survival time. It is equally important to develop novel strategies for clinical management of biliary tract tumors using EGCG as a natural adjuvant for gemcitabine chemotherapy and for head and neck carcinomas combining EGCG or apigenin with 5-fluorouracil, among other attractive combinational approaches. However, as current preclinical studies have revealed also several antagonistic activities in addition of certain flavonoids to chemotherapeutic regimens with antimetabolites, patients should be well-informed and aware of possible risks before deciding to consume food products rich in flavonoids or flavonoids-containing dietary supplements during the active treatment phase with different antimetabolites. Such antagonistic combinations might attenuate the therapeutic efficacy of conventional drugs promoting development of resistance and further progression of neoplasms. Based on the current preclinical findings, a special precaution is definitely needed by patients with acute lymphocytic leukemia under cytarabine chemotherapy.

6.3. DRUGS WHICH TARGET MICROTUBULES

Microtubules are essential components of cellular life, intervening in proliferation, signaling, transport and trafficking of eukaryotic cells. These highly dynamic hollow cylindrical polymers are composed of two proteins, α- and β-tubulins [1, 398-400]. When cell cycle progresses from interphase into mitosis, the cytoskeleton microtubules form well-organized and functional bipolar mitotic spindles that attach to chromosomes at the kinetochore, facilitating the chromosomal separation at anaphase. Balanced microtubule dynamics is crucial for spindle assembly, mitotic checkpoint, proper chromosomal segregation and cell division [398, 399]. Therefore, microtubules represent attractive targets for cancer therapy. In general, antineoplastic agents which act on microtubules can be subdivided into two groups: periwinkle alkaloids or vinca alkaloids (vinblastine, vincristine) that inhibit microtubule polymerization and destabilize microtubules, and taxanes (paclitaxel, docetaxel, cabazitaxel) that inhibit microtubule depolymerization and stabilize microtubules [1, 161, 398, 399, 401, 402]. Although both drug classes interfere with microtubule dynamics in different ways, they have a roughly similar final action on the functioning of the mitotic spindle, becoming disrupted during the transition from metaphase to anaphase, resulting in arrested mitosis (cell cycle arrest) and apoptotic cell death [1, 398]. Despite microtubules-targeting agents are widely used in cancer therapy against various types of tumors, resistance to these compounds is frequently encountered in the clinical settings and therefore, new strategies to overcome resistance phenomenon and improve therapeutic efficacy are continually investigated [398, 399, 402, 403]. Clinical use of microtubules-interfering agents is limited also by serious side effects on normal non-tumoral tissues [399, 402]; altogether demonstrating that novel adjuvant agents, preferably from natural sources, are highly needed to enhance the therapeutic efficacy and clinical outcome of treatment regimens with vinca alkaloids and taxanes.

6.3.1. Vinblastine (VBL)

Vinblastine (VBL) is a natural vinca alkaloid isolated from the Madagascar periwinkle (*Catharanthus roseus* (L.) G.Don) first in 1958 and is used in the clinical settings already for decades. VBL is indicated for the treatment of Hodgkin and non-Hodgkin lymphoma, but may be used also in the management of several solid tumors, including breast, ovarian, renal, bladder and testicle cancers as well as sarcomas [1, 398]. The main cytotoxic action of VBL comes from its ability to bind to tubulin and inhibit polymerization of tubulin to form microtubules. This process causes M phase cell cycle arrest and disruption of proper formation of mitotic spindle, blocking cell division and inducing apoptotic death [1, 398]. However, administration of VBL is frequently associated with adverse side effects, such as changes in sensation, neutropenia, weakness, depression and headaches. In addition, clinical use of VBL is limited also by development of resistance.

The role of natural flavonoids on therapeutic efficacy of VBL has been studied in several human cancer cell lines *in vitro* conditions (Table 6.27). Green tea flavanol *EGCG* potentiated VBL cytotoxicity in human breast cancer MCF-7 cells. This chemosensitizing action was associated with activation of proapoptotic arms of the endoplasmic reticulum stress (ERS) response via abrogation of GRP78 by EGCG, leading to enhancement of VBL-induced JNK and caspase-7 activation [398]. EGCG potentiated VBL cytotoxicity also in human metastatic renal cell carcinoma Caki-1 cells, by inducing upregulation of a tumor suppressor gene, connexin (Cx) 32, further leading to reduction of P-gp level and function. This process occurred via inactivation of Src oncoprotein and subsequent activation of JNK signaling. Connexins are the constituent proteins of gap junctions mediating communication, controlling growth and keeping cellular homeostasis; but they exert also tumor suppressive effect in a gap junctions-independent manner potentiating cytotoxicity of antineoplastic agents [404]. Susceptibility to VBL cytotoxicity was increased also by monomethylated flavone *oroxylin A* in NCI/ADR-RES cells, reducing P-gp-mediated drug efflux [405]. However, another methylated flavone, *wogonin*, did not affect antitumor action of VBL in human lung cancer A549 cells [153]. Several flavonoids, such as flavonols *quercetin* and *kaempferol* and isoflavones *genistein* and *daidzein*, markedly enhanced VBL-induced cytotoxicity in P-gp-overexpressing multidrug resistant human cervical carcinoma KB-V1 cells, reducing efflux and increasing intracellular accumulation of the drug. At that, flavonols were more potent than isoflavones in decreasing P-gp function and differently from isoflavones, flavonols suppressed also P-gp expression, suggesting that structural peculiarities at flavonoid skeleton can take part in regulating the transcriptional activity of MDR1 gene. Moreover, glycosylated form of genistein, *genistin* or genistein 7-glucoside, modulated neither drug transport nor cytotoxicity of VBL. None of the tested flavonoids exerted any chemosensitizing effects to VBL in the parental drug-sensitive KB-3-1 cells with no P-gp expression [406]. Likewise, several flavonoids, such as *flavone, 4`,7-dimethoxyflavone (4`,7-DMF)* and *biochanin A* (but still not *chrysin, baptigenin Ψ* and *4`,7-dimethoxyisoflavone*), reversed resistance to VBL in P-gp-overexpressing human acute lymphoblastic leukemia CEM/VBL100 cells, whereas both flavone and 4`,7-DMF significantly inhibited VBL-stimulated P-gp ATPase activity. Moreover, flavone and 4`,7-DMF remained inactive in affecting VBL cytotoxicity in parental sensitive CCRF-CEM cells [312] (Table 6.27).

The in vitro findings reported so far demonstrate either positive or no cooperation between dietary flavonoids and VBL in diverse human malignant cell lines, improving the therapeutic potential of VBL mostly in drug-resistant cancer cells (Figure 6.14). Although the chemosensitizing action of certain flavonoids towards VBL cytotoxicity is

Effects of Plant Flavonoids on Chemotherapeutic Efficacy of Cancer Drugs 307

often associated with suppression of P-gp efflux pump, other cellular mechanisms might be involved as well.

Table 6.27. Effects of flavonoids on anticancer action of vinblastine (VBL) *in vitro* conditions

Drug	Flavonoid	Biological system	Direction of combination	Effects	Ref.
VBL, 0.05-1.25 μM	4`,7-DMF, 10, 20 μM	CCRF-CEM human acute lymphoblastic **leukemia** cell line	~	No effect on VBL cytotoxicity	[312]
VBL, 0.05-1.25 μM	4`,7-DMF, 10, 20 μM	CEM/VBL100 human acute lymphoblastic **leukemia** cell line, VBL-resistant, overexpressing P-gp	↑	Decrease in VBL IC_{50}. Inhibition of VBL-stimulated P-gp ATPase activity, increase in VBL cellular accumulation	[312]
VBL, 0.05-1.25 μM	4`,7-dimethoxyisoflavone, 10, 20 μM	CEM/VBL100 human acute lymphoblastic **leukemia** cell line, VBL-resistant, overexpressing P-gp	~	No significant decrease in VBL IC_{50}. Increase in VBL cellular accumulation	[312]
VBL, 0.05-1.25 μM	Baptigenin Ψ, 10, 20 μM	CEM/VBL100 human acute lymphoblastic **leukemia** cell line, VBL-resistant, overexpressing P-gp	~	No significant decrease in VBL IC_{50}	[312]
VBL, 0.05-1.25 μM	Biochanin A, 10, 20 μM	CEM/VBL100 human acute lymphoblastic **leukemia** cell line, VBL-resistant, overexpressing P-gp	↑	Decrease in VBL IC_{50}. Increase in VBL cellular accumulation	[312]
VBL, 0.05-1.25 μM	Chrysin, 10, 20 μM	CEM/VBL100 human acute lymphoblastic **leukemia** cell line, VBL-resistant, overexpressing P-gp	~	No significant decrease in VBL IC_{50}. Increase in VBL cellular accumulation	[312]
VBL	Daidzein, 10, 30 μM	KB 3-1 human **cervical** carcinoma cell line, no P-gp expression	~	No effect on VBL cytotoxicity	[406]
VBL	Daidzein, 10, 30 μM	KB-V1 human **cervical** carcinoma cell line, MDR KB 3-1 cells, VBL-resistant, overexpressing P-gp/MDR1	↑	Sensitization to VBL, decrease in VBL IC_{50}. Decrease in VBL efflux, increase in VBL cellular accumulation	[406]
VBL, 0.25 μM	EGCG, 10 μM	MCF-7 human **breast** cancer cell line	↑	Promotion of VBL-induced cytotoxicity. Potentiation of proapoptotic signals (JNK phosphorylation, cleavage of caspase-7 and PARP), increase in apoptosis	[398]
VBL, 5, 10, 20 μM	EGCG, 2.5 μM	Caki-1 human metastatic **renal** cell carcinoma cell line	↑	Potentiation of VBL-induced cytotoxicity. Restoration of Cx32 leading to suppression of P-gp due to inactivation of Src and activation of JNK	[404]
VBL, 0.05-1.25 μM	Flavone, 10, 20 μM	CCRF-CEM human acute lymphoblastic **leukemia** cell line	~	No effect on VBL cytotoxicity	[312]
VBL, 0.05-1.25 μM	Flavone, 10, 20 μM	CEM/VBL100 human acute lymphoblastic **leukemia** cell line, VBL-resistant, overexpressing P-gp	↑	Decrease in VBL IC_{50}. Inhibition of VBL-stimulated P-gp ATPase activity, increase in VBL cellular accumulation	[312]
VBL	Genistein, 10, 30 μM	KB 3-1 human **cervical** carcinoma cell line, no P-gp expression	~	No effect on VBL cytotoxicity	[406]

Table 6.27. (Continued)

Drug	Flavonoid	Biological system	Direction of combination	Effects	Ref.
VBL	Genistein, 10, 30 μM	KB-V1 human **cervical** carcinoma cell line, MDR KB 3-1 cells, VBL-resistant, overexpressing P-gp/MDR1	↑	Sensitization to VBL. Decrease in VBL efflux, increase in VBL cellular accumulation	[406]
VBL	Genistin, 10, 30 μM	KB 3-1 human **cervical** carcinoma cell line, no P-gp expression	~	No effect on VBL cytotoxicity	[406]
VBL	Genistin 10, 30 μM	KB-V1 human **cervical** carcinoma cell line, MDR KB 3-1 cells, VBL-resistant, overexpressing P-gp/MDR1	~	No effect on VBL-induced cell growth inhibition	[406]
VBL	Kaempferol, 10, 30 μM	KB 3-1 human **cervical** carcinoma cell line, no P-gp expression	~	No effect on VBL cytotoxicity	[406]
VBL	Kaempferol, 10, 30 μM	KB-V1 human **cervical** carcinoma cell line, MDR KB 3-1 cells, VBL-resistant, overexpressing P-gp/MDR1	↑	Sensitization to VBL, decrease in VBL IC_{50}. Decrease in P-gp level, decrease in VBL efflux, increase in VBL cellular accumulation	[406]
VBL, 0.001-10 μM	Oroxylin A, 10 μM	NCI/ADR-RES expressing P-gp, no MRP1	↑	Overcoming P-gp-mediated MDR. About 5-fold decrease in VBL IC_{50}	[405]
VBL	Quercetin, 10, 30 μM	KB 3-1 human **cervical** carcinoma cell line, no P-gp expression	~	No effect on VBL cytotoxicity	[406]
VBL	Quercetin, 10, 30 μM	KB-V1 human **cervical** carcinoma cell line, MDR KB 3-1 cells, VBL-resistant, overexpressing P-gp/MDR1	↑	Sensitization to VBL. Decrease in P-gp level, decrease in VBL efflux, increase in VBL cellular accumulation	[406]
VBL, 10, 100 μM	Wogonin, 25 μM	A549 human **lung** cancer cell line	~	No effect on VBL cytotoxicity	[153]

Cx, connexin; DMF, dimethoxyflavone; JNK, c-Jun N-terminal kinase; MDR, multidrug resistance; MRP, multidrug resistance-associated protein; PARP, poly (ADP-ribose) polymerase; P-gp, P-glycoprotein.

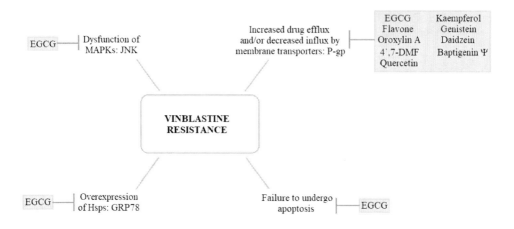

Figure 6.14. Modulation of vinblastine resistance by plant flavonoids (DMF, dimethoxyflavone; GRP, glucose-regulated protein; Hsp, heat shock protein; JNK, c-Jun N-terminal kinase; MAPK, mitogen-activated protein kinase; P-gp, P-glycoprotein).

Effects of Plant Flavonoids on Chemotherapeutic Efficacy of Cancer Drugs 309

6.3.2. Vincristine (VCR)

Vincristine (VCR) is another natural vinca alkaloid isolated from the leaves of Madagascar periwinkle (*Catharanthus roseus* (L.) G.Don) first in 1961 [407, 408]. VCR was approved by the FDA already in 1963 and is nowadays indicated for the treatment of acute lymphoblastic leukemia, Hodgkin and non-Hodgkin lymphomas, as well as different solid tumors, including lung, breast and cervical cancers, sarcomas, and pediatric tumors like neuroblastoma and nephroblastoma [1, 409]. This antimitotic cytotoxic agent binds to the tubulin and inhibits the polymerization process of the tubulin to form microtubules in the mitotic spindle, leading to an arrest of the dividing cells at metaphase and rushing the cells towards apoptotic death [1, 407, 408]. However, VCR binds also to neuronal tubulin, disrupting axonal microtubules and thereby resulting in neurotoxicity, manifesting as sensory loss, numbness, tingling and hearing changes. Such toxic side effects limit the use of maximum clinical doses of VCR [391, 409], highlighting the necessity to include non-toxic adjuvant agents in the treatment protocols of VCR chemotherapy against different human cancers.

A variety of flavonoids has been studied in combination with VCR in different preclinical cancer models, both *in vitro* cancer cell lines as well as *in vivo* xenograft models (Table 6.28 and Table 6.29). Dietary flavonol *quercetin* at only 0.7 µM physiologically achievable concentration enhanced antitumor activity of VCR in human breast cancer MCF-7 cells and eliminated breast cancer stem cells (BCSCs). Moreover, combined treatment with quercetin and VCR significantly reversed resistance to VCR in multidrug resistant (MDR) MCF-7/DOX cells by downregulating P-gp and eliminating BCSCs, mediated by inhibition of Y-box binding protein 1 (YB-1) nuclear translocation [250]. Also, quercetin augmented synergistically VCR-induced growth inhibition in human estrogen receptor (ER)-negative breast cancer MDA-MB-231 cells, revealing the highest synergism at molar ratio of quercetin and VCR of 1:2. Coencapsulation of both agents into liposomes enabled to maintain the synergistic ratio of quercetin and VCR throughout the study, suggesting that the same therapeutic effects could be attained at substantially lower drug doses when combined with quercetin as compared to VCR monotherapy [408]. Strong synergism in growth inhibition was observed also when ER-negative, progesterone receptor (PR)-negative and HER2-overexpressing human breast cancer JIMT-1 cells were treated with combination of quercetin and VCR, at the molar ratio of 1:2. Moreover, liposomal coencapsulation prolonged plasma circulation time of both agents and maintained the optimal synergistic ratio to be delivered to the malignant site *in vivo* conditions, leading to the most efficient tumor growth inhibition and increased survival of JIMT-1 bearing mice [410]. As hormone receptor-negative and HER2-overexpressing breast tumors currently lack effective treatment options, combination of quercetin and VCR might provide a therapeutically important strategy to improve the clinical outcome of breast cancer patients in the future. Quercetin coloaded with VCR into lipid-polymeric nanocarriers (LPNs) exerted superior antitumor activities also in human Burkitt`s lymphoma cell line Raji and bypassed resistance in VCR-resistant subline Raji/VCR. Moreover, these dual-loaded nanoparticles led to almost complete growth inhibition of tumor xenografts in Raji/VCR bearing mice as compared to single drugs containing LPNs. As quercetin and VCR delivered by nanoparticles were accumulated in the tumor tissue, free drugs administered as solutions were mainly biodistributed in heart and kidneys, leading to higher systemic toxicity. Therefore, the use of nanocarriers in co-delivering quercetin and VCR might contribute to decrease in side effects, besides augmenting therapeutic efficacy [409]. Quercetin enhanced sensitivity to VCR also in VCR-resistant human oral cancer KB/VCR cells which overexpress P-gp efflux pump, by reducing proliferation, promoting apoptosis and decreasing migratory and invasive abilities of malignant cells through downregulation of P-gp expression [407] (Table 6.28 and Table 6.29).

Table 6.28. Effects of flavonoids on anticancer action of vincristine (VCR)
***in vitro* conditions**

Drug	Flavonoid	Biological system	Direction of combination	Effects	Ref.
VCR, 0.75, 1.5 nM	(-)-Hydnocarpin, 10 μM	697 human pre-B acute lymphoblastic **leukemia** cell line	↑	Potentiation of VCR-induced cytotoxicity	[414]
VCR, 3 nM	(-)-Hydnocarpin, 5, 10 μM	697-R human pre-B acute lymphoblastic **leukemia** cell line, MDR, expressing P-gp	↑	Re-sensitization to VCR, increase in growth inhibition	[414]
VCR	5,7-DMF	YCUB-2 human acute lymphoblastic **leukemia** cell line	↑	Additive effect on cell proliferation reduction	[11]
VCR	5,7-DMF	YCUB-5 human acute lymphoblastic **leukemia** cell line	↑↓	Antagonistic effect on cell proliferation reduction (at ratio 40:1 DMF:VCR), additive effect (at ratios 80:1, 160:1, 320:1)	[11]
VCR	5,7-DMF	YCUB-6 human acute lymphoblastic **leukemia** cell line	↓	Antagonistic effect on cell proliferation reduction	[11]
VCR	Alopecurone B, 10 μM	MG-63/DOX human **osteosarcoma** cell line, MDR, DOX-resistant	↑	Sensitization to VCR, 6.36-fold decrease in VCR IC$_{50}$	[235]
VCR, 2 μM	Apigenin, 100 μM	TF1 human **erythroleukemia** cell line	↓	Decrease in VCR-induced cytotoxicity and apoptosis when pretreated with apigenin for 24h	[411]
VCR, 1.25, 2.5, 5 nM	Baicalein, 50 μM	CCRF-CEM human childhood acute lymphoblastic **leukemia** cell line	↑	Increase in antileukemic effect, increase in apoptosis	[391]
VCR, 25 μg/ml	EGCG, 1, 10, 50 μg/ml	ALL-1 human B-lineage acute lymphoblastic **leukemia** cell line, chemotherapy-resistant	↑	Chemosensitization, additive antileukemic potency	[415]

Effects of Plant Flavonoids on Chemotherapeutic Efficacy of Cancer Drugs 311

Drug	Flavonoid	Biological system	Direction of combination	Effects	Ref.
VCR, 25 µg/ml	EGCG, 1, 10, 50 µg/ml	NALM-6 human B-lineage acute lymphoblastic **leukemia** cell line, chemotherapy-resistant	↑	Chemosensitization, additive antileukemic potency	[415]
VCR, 25 µg/ml	EGCG, 1, 10, 50 µg/ml	REH human B-lineage acute lymphoblastic **leukemia** cell line, chemotherapy-resistant	↑	Chemosensitization, additive antileukemic potency	[415]
VCR, 0-1000 ng/ml	Genistein, 3, 10 µM	K562 human **leukemia** cell line, no expression of BCRP, P-gp or MRP1	~	No effect on VCR-induced growth inhibition	[197]
VCR, 0-1000 ng/ml	Genistein, 3, 10 µM	K562/MDR human **leukemia** cell line, expressing P-gp, no BCRP or MRP1, VCR-resistant	~	No reversal of (P-gp-mediated) VCR resistance	[197]
VCR, 0.01 µM	Genistein, 6 µM	CRL-8805 human **medulloblastoma** cell line	↑	Mild-to-moderate improvement of VCR antiproliferative effect. 1.06-fold increase in growth inhibition, 1.4-fold increase in clonogenic survival inhibition	[135]
VCR, 0.05, 0.1 µM	Genistein, 6 µM	HTB-186 human **medulloblastoma** cell line	↑	Mild-to-moderate improvement of VCR antiproliferative effect. 1.4-fold increase in growth inhibition at 0.1 µM VCR, 1.4-fold increase in clonogenic survival inhibition (0.05 µM VCR)	[135]
VCR, 0.01 µM	Genistein, 6 µM	MED-1 human **medulloblastoma** cell line	↑~	Mild (or no) improvement of VCR antiproliferative effect. 1.09-fold increase in growth inhibition, 1.13-fold increase in clonogenic survival inhibition	[135]
VCR, 0.01-100 µM	Heptamethoxy-flavone, 2, 20 µM	K562/ADM human chronic myelogenous **leukemia** cell line, DOX-resistant	↑	Increase in VCR-induced growth inhibition. Increase in VCR cellular uptake	[412]
VCR, 0-1000 ng/ml	Naringenin, 3, 10 µM	K562 human **leukemia** cell line, no expression of BCRP, P-gp or MRP1	~	No effect on VCR-induced growth inhibition	[197]
VCR, 0-1000 ng/ml	Naringenin, 3, 10 µM	K562/MDR human **leukemia** cell line, expressing P-gp, no BCRP or MRP1, VCR-resistant	~	No reversal of (P-gp-mediated) VCR resistance	[197]
VCR, 0.01-100 µM	Nobiletin, 2, 20 µM	K562/ADM human chronic myelogenous **leukemia** cell line, DOX-resistant	↑	Increase in VCR-induced growth inhibition. Increase in VCR cellular uptake	[412]
VCR, 0-20 µg/ml, co-loaded into LPNs	Quercetin, 0-20 µg/ml, co-loaded into LPNs	Raji human Burkitt`s **lymphoma** cell line	↑	Increase in antitumor activity	[409]
VCR, 0-20 µg/ml, co-loaded into LPNs	Quercetin, 0-20 µg/ml, co-loaded into LPNs	Raji/VCR human Burkitt`s **lymphoma** cell line, VCR-resistant	↑	Increase in antitumor activity, synergism in cytotoxicity at VCR:quercetin weight ratios 2:1, 1:1, 1:2	[409]
VCR	Quercetin	JIMT-1 human **breast** cancer cell line, ER-, PR-, trastuzumab-insensitive	↑	Synergism in growth inhibition (CI<1; most synergistic effect at molar ratio 2:1, VCR:quercetin)	[410]
VCR, co-encapsulated into liposomes	Quercetin, co-encapsulated into liposomes	JIMT-1 human **breast** cancer cell line, ER-, PR-, trastuzumab-insensitive	↑	Synergistic increase in cell killing (CI<1; at VCR:quercetin molar ratio 2:1)	[410]

Table 6.28 (Continued)

Drug	Flavonoid	Biological system	Direction of combination	Effects	Ref.
VCR, 0.005-10 µg/ml	Quercetin, 0.7 µM	MCF-7 human **breast** cancer cell line	↑	1.21-fold increase in VCR antitumor activity. Elimination of BCSCs (CD44+/CD24-/low)	[250]
VCR, 0.005-10 µg/ml	Quercetin, 0.7 µM	MCF-7/Dox human **breast** cancer cell line, DOX-resistant	↑	Reversal of MDR, 3.15-fold increase in VCR antitumor activity. Downregulation of P-gp. Elimination of BCSCs (CD44+/CD24-/low). Inhibition of YB-1 nuclear translocation	[250]
VCR	Quercetin	MDA-MB-231 human **breast** cancer cell line, ER-negative	↑	Synergism in cytotoxicity (CI<1; the most optimal ratio 2:1, VCR:quercetin)	[408]
VCR, co-encapsulated into liposomes	Quercetin, co-encapsulated into liposomes	MDA-MB-231 human **breast** cancer cell line, ER-negative	↑	Synergistic increase in cell killing (CI<0.113, at VCR:quercetin molar ratio 2:1)	[408]
VCR, 0.375 µM	Quercetin, 25-100 µM	KB/VCR human **oral** cancer cell line, VCR-resistant, overexpressing P-gp	↑	Sensitization to VCR. Downregulation of P-gp. Increase in apoptosis, decrease in migration and invasion rates	[407]
VCR, 0.01-200 µM	Sinensetin	AML-2/D100 human acute myelogenous **leukemia** cell line, DNR-resistant, overexpressing P-gp	↑	Reversal of resistance, 72.28-fold chemosensitization. Decrease in P-gp, increase in VCR cellular accumulation	[413]
VCR	Sinensetin	AML-2/DX100 human acute myelogenous **leukemia** cell line, DOX-resistant, overexpressing MRP1	~	No chemosensitizing activity	[413]
VCR, 0.01-100 µM	Tangeretin, 2, 20 µM	K562/ADM human chronic myelogenous **leukemia** cell line, DOX-resistant	↑	Increase in VCR-induced growth inhibition. Increase in VCR cellular uptake	[412]
VCR, 1 nM	Taxifolin, 80, 100 µM	HeLaS3 human **cervical** carcinoma cell line	~	No effect on VCR-induced cell viability inhibition	[304]
VCR, 100, 1000 nM	Taxifolin, 80, 100 µM	KB-vin human **cervical** cancer cell line, MDR	↑	Additive to synergistic reduction of cell viability (CI 0.56-1.00). Increase in VCR-induced apoptosis. Decrease in ABCB1 expression and P-gp efflux function	[304]

ABC, ATP-binding cassette; BCRP, breast cancer resistance protein; BCSC, breast cancer stem cell; CI, combination index; DMF, dimethoxyflavone; ER, estrogen receptor; LPN, lipid-polymeric nanocarrier; MDR, multidrug resistance; MRP, multidrug resistance-associated protein; P-gp, P-glycoprotein; PR, progesterone receptor; YB-1, Y-box binding protein 1.

Soy isoflavone *genistein* at typical dietary plasma levels (6 µM) improved antiproliferative and anticlonogenic properties of VCR to some small extent in human medulloblastoma cell lines CRL-8805, HTB-186 and MED-1. Such chemosensitization might confer reduction of VCR therapeutic dosage recommendations for treatment of medulloblastomas of early childhood, with subsequent decrease in the risk of potentially devastating treatment sequelae [135]. However, neither genistein nor citrus flavanone *naringenin* modulated VCR induced growth inhibition in human leukemia cell line K562 or its VCR-resistant P-gp-overexpressing subline K562/MDR [197]. Whereas natural flavone *baicalein* synergistically enhanced antileukemic and proapoptotic effects of VCR in human childhood acute lymphoblastic leukemia (ALL) CCRF-CEM cells [391]; pretreatment of human erythroleukemia TF1 cells with the common dietary flavone *apigenin* markedly decreased VCR-induced chemotherapeutic sensitivity, cytotoxicity and apoptosis. This antagonistic action was associated with the ability of malignant cells to escape the antimitotic effects of VCR after being blocked in the G0/G1 phase of the cell cycle by apigenin. Moreover, such negative interference with chemotherapeutic efficacy suggests that erythroleukemia patients should certainly take cation in dietary intake of apigenin-containing products during the treatment with VCR [411]. Another flavone *5,7-dimethoxyflavone (5,7-DMF)* also protected human ALL YCUB-5 and YCUB-6 cells against cytotoxicity induced by VCR, whereas this antagonistic action was dependent on the ratio of two agents. Therefore, combination therapy of VCR with 5,7-DMF is not recommended for ALL patients [11]. On the contrary, polymethylated flavones *tangeretin, nobiletin* and *heptamethoxyflavone*, even at low 2 µM concentration, all enhanced VCR-induced growth inhibition in a DOX-resistant variant of human chronic myelogenous leukemia K562 cells, i.e., K562/ADM. This chemosensitizing action was at least in part associated with increased cellular uptake of VCR through P-gp inhibition [412]. Likewise, another natural polymethylated flavone, *sinensetin*, reversed resistance to VCR in P-gp-overexpressing DNR-resistant human acute myelogenous leukemia AML-2/D100 cells, by downregulating P-gp levels and enhancing intracellular drug accumulation. However, sinensetin remained inactive in modulating VCR cytotoxicity in MRP1-overexpressing DOX-resistant AML-2/DX100 cells [413]. Thus, polymethylated flavones might be potential candidates for clinical application as reversal agents for VCR resistance in different myelogenous leukemia cells. Susceptibility of human pre-B ALL cell line 697 and its MDR subline 697-R to VCR-induced cytotoxicity was enhanced by a natural flavonolignan *hydnocarpin* [414]. Moreover, the major green tea flavanol *EGCG* also sensitized several chemotherapy-resistant human B-lineage ALL cell lines, such as ALL-1, NALM-6 and REH, towards antileukemic action of VCR; probably via inhibiting antiapoptotic functions of GRP78 protein. Induction of GRP78 in malignant cells has been associated with adaption to chronic metabolic and hypoxic stress of the tumor microenvironment and resistance to chemotherapy. Also, upregulated expression of this protein has been considered as a potential biomarker for cancer aggressiveness. Therefore, suppression of GRP78 by EGCG in ALL cells might lead to augmentation of VCR cytotoxic efficacy [415]. Besides the effects of flavonoids on antileukemic action of VCR, flavanonol *taxifolin* increased VCR-induced cell viability and apoptosis in human MDR cervical cancer KB-vin cell through inhibition of expression and function of P-gp (ABCB1) efflux pump. However, taxifolin did not affect VCR cytotoxicity in drug sensitive human cervical cancer HeLaS3 cells [304]. Last but not least, flavonostilbene *alopecurone B* sensitized human MDR osteosarcoma MG-

63/DOX cells to antitumor action of VCR, allowing to reduce the therapeutically effective drug dosage for the clinical application [235] (Table 6.28).

Table 6.29. Effects of flavonoids on anticancer action of vincristine (VCR) *in vivo* conditions

Drug	Flavonoid	Biological system	Direction of combination	Effects	Ref.
VCR, 20 mg/kg, i.v. every 7 days, co-loaded into LPNs	Quercetin, 20 mg/kg, i.v., every 7 days, co-loaded into LPNs	Raji/VCR human **lymphoma** cells injected s.c. into the right flank of 6-8w old male BALB/c mice	↑	Almost complete suppression of tumor growth	[409]
VCR, 1.33 mg/kg, co-encapsulated into liposomes (molar ratio VCR:quercetin 2:1)	Quercetin, 0.24 mg/kg, co-encapsulated into liposomes (molar ratio VCR:quercetin 2:1)	JIMT-1 human **breast** cancer cells injected s.c. into the upper back area of SCID mice	↑	Potentiation of tumor growth inhibition, slowing of tumor growth. Increase in mice survival	[410]

LPN, lipid-polymeric nanocarrier.

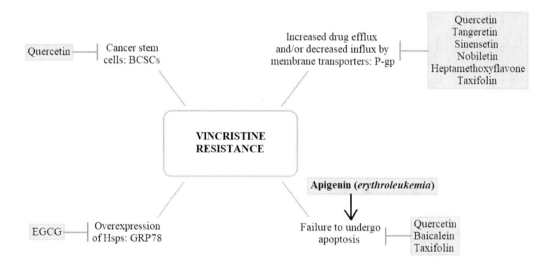

Figure 6.15. Modulation of vincristine resistance by dietary plant flavonoids (BCSC, breast cancer stem cell; GRP, glucose-regulated protein; Hsp, heat shock protein; P-gp, P-glycoprotein).

Possibilities to intervene in chemoresistance to VCR by different plant flavonoids are summarized in Figure 6.15. Based on the current preclinical data, several combinations of these natural dietary polyphenols and VCR are worth of further therapeutic development, especially combination of quercetin and VCR in the management of both hormone-positive as well as hormone-negative breast tumors. Such combined treatment might allow to use substantially lower doses of VCR to attain the same therapeutic effects as using monotherapy, with substantially fewer side effects, including neurotoxicity. Moreover, coencapsulation of both quercetin and VCR into liposomes might provide prolonged plasma circulation and coordinated drug release in tumoral tissue, making the clinical applications more realistic in the future. However, some antagonistic antileukemic activities described in combining VCR with certain natural flavones clearly show that cancer patients should be extremely cautious when taking the initiative to consume products rich in flavonoids during the active treatment phase with VCR therapy; especially erythroleukemia patients towards apigenin- and acute lymphoblastic leukemia patients towards 5,7-dimethoxyflavone-containing food items or dietary supplements. Consumption of such products might lead to undesired decrease in therapeutic efficacy and impairment of clinical success.

> According to the current experimental findings it is recommended for cancer patients *not to consume* dietary products or dietary supplements rich in following plant flavonoids during the active chemotherapeutic treatment phase with **vincristine**:
> - **apigenin** in erythroleukemia
> - **5,7-dimethoxyflavone** in acute lymphoblastic leukemia

6.3.3. Paclitaxel (PTX)

Paclitaxel (PTX) is a microtubule-targeted agent that was first isolated from the bark of the Pacific Yew tree (*Taxus brevifolia* Nutt.) already in the 1960s [1, 323, 416-418]. PTX is indicated for the treatment of breast, ovarian and non-small cell lung cancer, and Kaposi`s sarcoma; but has shown efficacy also against various other solid tumors, including head and neck, bladder, prostate, pancreatic and esophageal cancer and melanoma [1, 187, 323, 417-428]. PTX binds to the β-subunit of tubulin, promotes tubulin assembly, stabilizes microtubules and disrupts the formation of normal spindle at metaphase, thereby blocking mitosis and inducing cell cycle arrest at the G2/M phase. PTX can also induce formation of ROS, affect mitochondria, diminish mitochondrial functionality and result in apoptosis, in all conferring drug cytotoxicity on malignant cells [130, 161, 187, 400, 403, 416-418, 421, 423, 425-427, 429-433]. Although this mitotic inhibitor has been widely used both as monotherapy as well as in combination with other cytotoxic antineoplastic agents, tumors often are, or rapidly become, resistant, leading to relapse and progression of the disease. Chemoresistance to PTX is mediated by multiple mechanisms, being often associated with upregulation of P-gp membrane transporter and drug efflux out of the cells, but could also result from the changes in tubulin expression [187, 398, 418, 419, 426-428, 434]. In addition, clinical application of PTX at optimum doses and for a prolonged time has been impeded also by several adverse side effects, including hypersensitivity reactions, myelosuppression, neurotoxicity, cardiac rhythm disorder, hair loss, pain in the joints and muscles, fatigue, diarrhea, nausea and vomiting. The severity of side effects depends on administered drug doses and can seriously worsen the quality of life of cancer patients, resulting in dosage reduction and discontinuation of the treatment [161, 323, 419, 425, 433, 435-437]. Therefore, development of new strategies to manage these obstacles and improve therapeutic efficacy of PTX by using proper natural adjuvant agents is highly needed.

A number of flavonoids have been studied in combination with PTX in diverse preclinical cancer models, revealing different types of interactions. Pretreatment of human hepatoma HA22T/VGH cells with abundant natural flavonol *quercetin* for 24 hours before addition of PTX induced enhancement of cytotoxic and proapoptotic properties of PTX [432]. However, quercetin revealed bimodal effects on PTX-induced antitumor action in human colorectal cancer HCT116 cells. While prolonged exposure to quercetin suppressed colony formation and clonogenicity in combination with PTX, quercetin still protected malignant cells from PTX effects in short-term assays. Quercetin completely inhibited the PTX activity to induce G2/M phase cell cycle arrest and restored drug-induced loss in viability. Quercetin-treated cells did not respond to the cell cycle effects of PTX, accompanied by inhibition of cyclin B1 accumulation at the microtubule organizing center to initiate mitosis. Although this antagonism of chemotherapeutic action of PTX by quercetin was not long-lasting, further studies are urgently needed to examine *in vivo* effects followed by coadministration of quercetin and PTX in colorectal cancer preclinical models [438]. Quercetin markedly abrogated therapeutic effects of PTX also in human breast cancer MCF-7 cells and human cervical cancer HeLa cells. In fact, cotreatment of these cells with 15 μM quercetin and PTX led to protection of malignant cells from drug-mediated death. Quercetin completely abolished PTX-elicited Bcl-2 and p38 phosphorylation and prevented PTX-induced change in relative mobility of the apoptosis signal-regulating kinase 1 (Ask1), a stress response kinase [400]. However, submicromolar doses of quercetin (0.7 μM) still enhanced PTX-induced antitumor activities in human breast cancer MCF-7 cells, by eliminating breast cancer stem cells (BCSCs). In DOX-resistant subline of these cells, i.e., MCF-7/Dox, quercetin reversed multidrug resistance by downregulating P-gp and eliminating BCSCs through inhibition of YB-1 nuclear translocation [250]. Chemosensitivity to PTX was markedly enhanced by quercetin also in P-gp-overexpressing multidrug resistant (MDR) human cervical carcinoma KB-V1 cells [406] and PTX-resistant KB CH^{R}8-5 cells [439], but not in parental drug sensitive KB-3-1 cells with no P-gp expression [406]; suggesting that quercetin could reverse PTX resistance by inhibition of P-gp expression and transport function [406, 439]. Likewise, low micromolar doses of quercetin (1 μM and 5 μM, achievable after oral administration) increased chemosensitivity to PTX in several human ovarian cancer cell lines, i.e., A2780P, OVCAR-3, EFO27 and SKOV-3 cells [94]. However, somewhat higher doses of quercetin (10-100 μM) have still been shown to promote the survival of PTX-treated human ovarian cancer C13* cells, attenuating therapeutic efficacy and increasing chemoresistance to PTX, probably via suppressing ROS-induced injury. This antagonistic effect on PTX cytotoxicity suggests that ovarian cancer patients should be especially cautious towards quercetin supplements during PTX chemotherapy [95]. Another common dietary flavonol, *fisetin*, strongly antagonized PTX cytotoxicity in human breast cancer MCF-7 cells; but led to a synergistic loss of cell viability in several other human malignant cells, such as colon cancer LoVo cells and non-small cell lung cancer A549 and H1299 cells. In A549 cells, synergistic action of fisetin and PTX was at least partially associated with enhancement of PTX-induced mitotic catastrophe through promotion of multipolar spindle formation and the switch from cytoprotective autophagy to autophagic cell death. Thus, combinational effect of fisetin and PTX was strictly dependent on the type of cancer cells, but specific factors determining this interaction are still remained unknown [323]. In addition, fisetin was shown to significantly enhance antimigratory and antiinvasive properties of PTX in A549 cells through substantial disorganization of actin and vimentin cytoskeleton and modulation of metastasis-related genes, including downregulation of matrix metallo-proteinase (MMP)-2 and upregulation of E-cadherin. These antimetastatic effects could be, at least partially, mediated through the inhibition of PI3K/AKT/mTOR signaling pathway [422]. Therefore, fisetin could be an important adjuvant agent for PTX chemotherapy in the treatment of non-small cell lung tumors in the future. Considering emerging evidence highlighting the drawback of PTX therapy, namely, its metastasis-promoting effects in several *in vitro* and *in vivo* cancer models, including lung cancer [422], increase in antimetastatic properties of PTX in the presence of fisetin might be of great clinical significance. Natural flavonol *myricetin* increased PTX-induced cytotoxicity in human ovarian cancer A2780 and OVCAR3 cells by downregulating MDR1 expression [431]. Flavonol *morin* sensitized human prostate cancer DU145 and PC-3 cells towards cell viability repressing and proapoptotic effects of PTX through inhibition of microRNA (miR)-155 and elevation of downstream GATA binding protein 3 (GATA3) expression. Differently from prostate cancer cell lines, GATA3 has been shown to be highly expressed in normal human and mouse prostate tissues, being involved in regulation of prostate-specific antigen (PSA) levels. Moreover, morin promoted chemosensitivity to PTX also in DU145 bearing mice, leading to significantly smaller tumors as compared to treatments with either agent alone [426]. Combined treatment of P-gp-overexpressing human MDR cervical cancer KB-V1 cells with flavonol *kaempferol* and PTX led to enhancement of PTX cytotoxicity, but did not affect antitumor potential of the drug in parental KB-3-1 cells with no P-gp expression [406]. Likewise, glycosylated flavonol *rutin* or quercetin 3-rutinoside reversed resistance to PTX in P-gp-overexpressing human PTX-resistant cervical cancer KB CH^{R}8-5 cells by downregulating P-gp expression and inhibiting drug efflux out of the cells [439]. The only methylated flavonol studied so far in combination with PTX, *rhamnetin* or 7-methoxyquercetin, improved susceptibility of human hepatocellular carcinoma HepG2 cells and also MDR HepG2/ADR cells to chemotherapeutic efficacy of PTX. In HepG2 cells, rhamnetin enhanced miR-34a level and in turn reduced endogenous Notch-1 expression, besides potentiation of PTX-induced G2/M phase cell cycle arrest [207] (Table 6.30 and Table 6.31).

Table 6.30. Effects of flavonoids on anticancer action of paclitaxel (PTX) *in vitro* conditions

Drug	Flavonoid	Biological system	Direction of combination	Effects	Ref.
PTX, 4 nM	Apigenin, 15 µM	Hep3B human negroid **hepatocyte** carcinoma cell line	↑	Sensitization to PTX, increase in PTX cytotoxicity	[435]
PTX, 4 nM	Apigenin, 15 µM	A549 human **lung** epithelial carcinoma cell line	↑	Sensitization to PTX, increase in PTX cytotoxicity	[435]
PTX, 4 nM	Apigenin, 15 µM	HeLa human **cervical** epithelial carcinoma cell line	↑	Synergism in cell viability reduction (CI 0.3918). Increase in PTX-induced apoptosis (cleavage of caspase-3 and PARP). Suppression of SOD activity leading to ROS accumulation and cleavage of caspase-2	[435]
PTX, 0.05, 0.1 µM	Baicalein, 1, 10 µM	C3L5 murine **breast** cancer cell line	↑	Increase in cell growth inhibition and apoptosis	[447]
PTX	Baicalein	MCF-7 human **breast** cancer cell line	~	No effect on PTX cytotoxicity	[420]
PTX, co-encapsulated in NE	Baicalein, co-encapsulated in NE	MCF-7 human **breast** cancer cell line	~	No effect on PTX cytotoxicity (at weight ratio 1:1)	[420]
PTX	Baicalein	MCF-7/Tax human **breast** cancer cell line, PTX-resistant	↑	Synergism in cytotoxicity (CI<1), strongest effect at weight ratio 1:1. Increase in PTX cellular uptake. Increase in ROS, induction of apoptosis (activation of caspase-3)	[420]
PTX, co-encapsulated in NE	Baicalein, co-encapsulated in NE	MCF-7/Tax human **breast** cancer cell line, PTX-resistant	↑	Increase in PTX cytotoxicity (at weight ratio 1:1). Increase in PTX cellular uptake. Increase in ROS, induction of apoptosis (activation of caspase-3)	[420]
PTX, 10-200 µM, co-loaded in NPs	Baicalein, co-loaded in NPs	A549 human **lung** cancer cell line	↑	Increase in PTX cytotoxicity, synergism at weight ratio 1:5 (PTX:baicalein, CI 0.707)	[417]
PTX, 10-200 µM, co-loaded in NPs	Baicalein, co-loaded in NPs	A549/PTX human **lung** cancer cell line, PTX-resistant	↑	Overcoming MDR. Increase in PTX cytotoxicity, synergism at weight ratio 1:5 (PTX:baicalein, CI 0.513)	[417]
PTX, 1-1000 nM	Baicalein, 10 µM	A2780 human **ovarian** cancer cell line	↑~	Increase in growth inhibition up to 50 nM PTX, no effect with 100-1000 nM PTX. Induction of mitochondrial apoptosis, inhibition of Akt/β-catenin signaling	[419]
PTX, 1-1000 nM	Baicalein, 10 µM	OVCAR human **ovarian** cancer cell line	↑~	Increase in growth inhibition up to 500 nM PTX, no effect with 1000 nM PTX	[419]
PTX, 10 nM	Baicalein, 10 µM	SKOV3 human **ovarian** cancer cell line	↑	Promotion of apoptosis (increase in caspase-3 activity, PARP cleavage) and necrosis	[419]
PTX	Daidzein, 10, 30 µM	KB-3-1 human **cervical** carcinoma cell line, no expression of P-gp	~	No effect on PTX cytotoxicity	[406]
PTX	Daidzein, 10, 30 µM	KB-V1 human **cervical** carcinoma cell line, MDR KB-3-1 cells, VBL-resistant, overexpressing P-gp/MDR1	~	No effect on PTX-induced cell growth inhibition	[406]
PTX, 0.01, 0.1, 1 µM	Dihydromyricetin, 50 µM	A2780/PTX human **ovarian** cancer cell line, PTX-resistant, wild-type p53	↑	Sensitization to PTX. Increase in PTX-induced apoptosis (PARP cleavage), p53-mediated downregulation of survivin	[303]
PTX, 1 µM	EGCG, 20 µM	4T1 murine **breast** cancer cell line	↑	Increase in cell viability reduction and apoptosis. Potentiation of JNK activation, suppression of PTX-induced GRP78 expression	[418]
PTX, 0.7-50 ng/ml	EGCG, 1 µg/ml	BT-474 human **breast** cancer cell line, overexpressing HER2	↑	Enhancement of growth inhibitory effects of PTX	[441]

Drug	Flavonoid	Biological system	Direction of combination	Effects	Ref.
PTX, 0.5 µM	EGCG, 10 µM	MCF-7 human **breast** cancer cell line	↑	Promotion of PTX-induced cytotoxicity. Potentiation of proapoptotic signals (JNK phosphorylation, caspase-7 and PARP cleavage), increase in apoptosis	[398]
PTX, 0.14-4.6 µM	EGCG, 5.6-180 µM	MDA-MB231 human **breast** cancer cell line	↑↓	Biphasic behavior: anti-sensitization of PTX effect at 5.6-45 µM EGCG (CI 2.55 at 45 µM EGCG, 1.1 µM PTX); pro-sensitization at 90, 180 µM EGCG	[444]
PTX, 1 µM	EGCG, 20 µM	MDA-MB-231 human **breast** cancer cell line	↑	Increase in cell viability reduction	[418]
PTX, 10 µM	EGCG, 50 µM	MDA-MB-231 human **breast** cancer cell line	↑	Increase in PTX cytotoxicity	[421]
PTX, 10 µM, co-loaded into liposomes	EGCG, 50 µM, co-loaded into liposomes	MDA-MB-231 human **breast** cancer cell line	↑	Increase in PTX cytotoxicity and apoptosis (activation of caspase-3). Suppression of MMP-2/-9 and invasion	[421]
PTX, 10 nM, co-encapsulated into PLGA-Casein NPs	EGCG, 40-120 µM, co-encapsulated into PLGA-Casein NPs	MDA-MB-231 human **breast** cancer cell line, PTX-resistant	↑	Synergism in cytotoxicity (CI 0.81). Increase in apoptosis and p21 level; inhibition of PTX-induced NF-κB activation, regulation of downstream genes (MMP9, VEGFA, BIRC5). Decrease in PTX-induced P-gp	[443]
PTX, 0.7-50 ng/ml	EGCG, 0.1 µg/ml	YCU-H891 human **head and neck** squamous cell carcinoma cell line, overexpressing HER2	↑	Increase in PTX-induced cell growth inhibition	[441]
PTX, 1-7.5 nM	EGCG, 75-150 µM	NCI-H460 human non-small cell **lung** cancer cell line	↑↓	Sequence-dependent effect: Synergism in growth inhibition when pretreated with PTX doses >5 nM (CI<1); promotion of apoptosis (decrease in Bcl2, cleavage of caspase-3 and PARP). Antagonism with concurrent and pre-treatment with EGCG (CI>1)	[429]
PTX, 0.1 µM	EGCG, 1, 10, 100 µM	PC-3 human **prostate** cancer cell line, hormone-refractory, AR-negative	↑	Synergism in cytotoxicity (CI 0.642). Induction of apoptosis (increase in caspase-9, decrease in Bcl-2, loss of ΔΨm). Suppression of Akt/NF-κB pathway	[403]
PTX, 6.25 nM	EGCG, 30, 50 µM	PC-3ML human **prostate** cancer cell line, single clone derived from bone marrow metastases	↑	Synergism in growth inhibition. Increase in p53, p73, p21 and caspase-3 expression; increase in apoptosis	[442]
PTX, 0.1-0.5 µM	Fisetin, 10-50 µM	MCF-7 human **breast** adenocarcinoma cell line	↓	Antagonistic effect on cell viability reduction	[323]
PTX, 0.1-0.5 µM	Fisetin, 10-50 µM	LoVo human **colon** adenocarcinoma cell line	↑	Synergistic decrease in cell viability	[323]
PTX, 0.1 µM	Fisetin, 10 µM	A549 human non-small cell **lung** cancer cell line	↑	Decrease in migration and invasion, rearrangement of actin and vimentin cytoskeleton, modulation of metastasis-related genes (decrease in N-cadherin, fibronectin, MMP-2, uPA, SLUG, TWIST; increase in E-cadherin, occludin, ZO-1). Suppression of PI3K and mTOR expression	[422]
PTX, 0.1-0.5 µM	Fisetin, 10-50 µM	A549 human non-small cell **lung** cancer cell line, wild-type p53	↑	Synergistic decrease in cell viability. Induction of mitotic catastrophe and autophagic cell death	[323]

Table 6.30. (Continued)

Drug	Flavonoid	Biological system	Direction of combination	Effects	Ref.
PTX, 0.1-0.5 μM	Fisetin, 10-50 μM	H1299 human non-small cell **lung** cancer cell line, p53-deficient	↑	Synergistic decrease in cell viability	[323]
PTX, 10 nM	Genistein, 1 μM	MCF-7 human **breast** cancer cell line, high ERα/ERβ ratio	↓	Decrease in sensitivity to PTX, increase in cell viability	[130]
PTX, 10 nM	Genistein, 1 μM	T47D human **breast** cancer cell line, low ERα/ERβ ratio	~	No effect on PTX cytotoxicity	[130]
PTX, 1-1000 nM	Genistein, 74 μM	OV2008 human **ovarian** tumor cell line	↓	About 3-fold increase in colony survival. Inhibition of PTX-induced apoptosis (blocking of PTX-induced bcl-2α suppression)	[424]
PTX, 0.1 μM	Genistein, 1, 10, 100 μM	PC-3 human **prostate** cancer cell line, hormone-refractory, AR-negative	↑	Synergism in cytotoxicity (CI<1). Induction of apoptosis (increase in caspase-9, decrease in Bcl-2, loss of ΔΨm). Suppression of Akt/NF-κB pathway	[403]
PTX	Genistein, 10, 30 μM	KB-3-1 human **cervical** carcinoma cell line, no expression of P-gp	~	No effect on PTX cytotoxicity	[406]
PTX	Genistein, 10, 30 μM	KB-V1 human **cervical** carcinoma cell line, MDR KB-3-1 cells, VBL-resistant, overexpressing P-gp/MDR1	↑	Increase in PTX cytotoxicity at 30 μM genistein	[406]
PTX	Genistin, 10, 30 μM	KB-3-1 human **cervical** carcinoma cell line, no expression of P-gp	~	No effect on PTX cytotoxicity	[406]
PTX	Genistin, 10, 30 μM	KB-V1 human **cervical** carcinoma cell line, MDR KB-3-1 cells, VBL-resistant, overexpressing P-gp/MDR1	~	No effect on PTX-induced cell growth inhibition	[406]
PTX, 10 nM	Icariside II, 10 μM	U87 human **glioma** cell line	↑	Augmentation of cell viability reduction	[430]
PTX, 10, 100 nM	Icariside II, 10 μM	A375 human **melanoma** cell line	↑	Augmentation of cell viability reduction. Promotion of PTX-induced apoptosis (caspase-3 cleavage). Decrease in IL-8 and VEGF production; inhibition of PTX-induced activation of TLR4-MyD88-ERK signaling and NF-κB nuclear translocation	[430]
PTX, 10 nM	Icariside II, 10 μM	B16 murine **melanoma** cell line	↑	Augmentation of cell viability reduction. Inhibition of PTX-induced increase in TLR4 and p-ERK levels	[430]
PTX, 0.125 μg/ml	Isoliquiritigenin, 25 μM	BT-549 human TN **breast** cancer cell line	↑	Synergism in cell proliferation inhibition	[319]
PTX, 0.125 μg/ml	Isoliquiritigenin, 25 μM	MCF-7 human **breast** cancer cell line, ER-positive	↑	Synergism in cell proliferation inhibition	[319]
PTX, 0.125 μg/ml	Isoliquiritigenin, 25 μM	MDA-MB-231 human TN **breast** cancer cell line	↑	Synergism in cell proliferation inhibition	[319]
PTX, 3.125-25 nM	Isoxanthohumol, 5.75-23 μM	A375 human **melanoma** cell line	↑	Synergistic sensitization of cells to PTX treatment	[171]
PTX, 3.125-25 nM	Isoxanthohumol, 5.75-23 μM	B16 murine **melanoma** cell line	↑	Synergistic sensitization of cells to PTX treatment	[171]
PTX, 3.125-25 nM	Isoxanthohumol, 5.75-23 μM	B16F10 murine metastatic **melanoma** cell line, highly invasive B16 cells	↑	Synergistic sensitization of cells to PTX treatment	[171]

Drug	Flavonoid	Biological system	Direction of combination	Effects	Ref.
PTX	Kaempferol, 10, 30 µM	KB-3-1 human **cervical** carcinoma cell line, no expressing P-gp	~	No effect on PTX cytotoxicity	[406]
PTX	Kaempferol, 10, 30 µM	KB-V1 human **cervical** carcinoma cell line, MDR KB-3-1 cells, VBL-resistant, overexpressing P-gp/MDR1	↑	Increase in PTX cytotoxicity at 30 µM kaempferol	[406]
PTX, 40 nM	Luteolin, 5, 10, 15 µM	MDA-MB-231 human metastatic E2-independent **breast** cancer cell line, ER-, HER/neu-negative	↑	Increase in PTX cytotoxicity and apoptosis (activation of caspases-8/-3, PARP cleavage), increase in Fas expression due to blocking of STAT3	[425]
PTX, 40 nM	Luteolin, 5, 10, 15 µM	MDA-MB-453 human metastatic E2-independent **breast** cancer cell line, ER-negative, HER/neu-positive	↑	Increase in PTX-induced cytotoxicity and apoptosis	[425]
PTX, 0.3 nM	Luteolin, 5, 10 µM	SCC-4 human **tongue** squamous cell carcinoma cell line	↑	Increase in PTX cytotoxicity	[445]
PTX, 6.25-100 µM	Luteolin, 15.625 µM	A2780IAP-X10 human **ovarian** cancer cell line, PTX-resistant	↑	59-fold reduction of PTX IC$_{50}$. Reversal of EMT (increase in E-cadherin; decrease in N-cadherin, vimentin, Slug, Snail, Twist1) through reduction of p-FAK/p-ERK/p65 signaling	[446]
PTX, 6.25-100 µM	Luteolin, 15.625 µM	A2780IAP-X22 human **ovarian** cancer cell line, PTX-resistant	↑	2.4-fold reduction of PTX IC$_{50}$. Reversal of EMT (decrease in N-cadherin, vimentin, Twist1) through reduction of p-FAK/p-ERK/p65 signaling	[446]
PTX	Luteolin	AGS human **gastric** cancer cell line	~	No sensitization of cells to PTX treatment	[144]
PTX, 0-100 nM	Morin, 50 µM	DU145 human **prostate** cancer cell line	↑	Increase in cell viability reduction and apoptosis. Suppression of miR-155, elevation of GATA3 level	[426]
PTX, 0-100 nM	Morin, 50 µM	PC-3 human **prostate** cancer cell line	↑	Promotion of cell viability reduction and apoptosis. Suppression of miR-155, elevation of GATA3 level	[426]
PTX, 100 nM	Myricetin, 5 µM	A2780 human **ovarian** cancer cell line	↑	Increase in PTX cytotoxicity. Downregulation of MDR1	[431]
PTX, 100 nM	Myricetin, 5 µM	OVCAR3 human **ovarian** cancer cell line	↑	Increase in PTX cytotoxicity. Downregulation of MDR1	[431]
PTX	Nobiletin	A549 human non-small cell **lung** carcinoma cell line	↑	Synergism in cell proliferation inhibition (CI<1)	[175]
PTX	Nobiletin, 0.5-9 µM	A549 human non-small cell **lung** cancer cell line	~	No effect on sensitivity to PTX	[276]
PTX	Nobiletin, 0.5-9 µM	A549/T human non-small cell **lung** cancer cell line, PTX-resistant, overexpressing ABCB1	↑	Sensitization to PTX, decrease in PTX IC$_{50}$	[276]
PTX	Nobiletin	H460 human non-small cell **lung** carcinoma cell line	↑	Synergism in cell proliferation inhibition (CI<1)	[175]
PTX	Nobiletin, 0.5-9 µM	A2780 human **ovarian** cancer cell line	~	No effect on sensitivity to PTX	[276]
PTX	Nobiletin, 0.5-9 µM	A2780/T human **ovarian** cancer cell line, PTX-resistant, overexpressing ABCB1	↑	Synergism in cytotoxicity (CI<1). Inhibition of colony formation, potentiation of apoptosis, increase in G2/M phase cell cycle arrest. Accumulation of p53. Intracellular accumulation of PTX and nobiletin. Inhibition of AKT/ERK and Nrf2 pathways	[276]

Table 6.30. (Continued)

Drug	Flavonoid	Biological system	Direction of combination	Effects	Ref.
PTX	Orobol, 0.1 mM	2008 human **ovarian** cancer cell line	↑~	18.9-fold increase in chemosensitivity when treated with PTX for 2h, promotion of apoptosis; no effect at 24h treatment	[427]
PTX	Orobol, 0.1 mM	2008/C13*5.25 human **ovarian** cancer cell line, CDDP-resistant	↑	2.5-fold increase in chemosensitivity when treated with PTX for 2h	[427]
PTX, 0.001-10 μM	Oroxylin A, 10 μM	NCI/ADR-RES expressing P-gp, no MRP1	↑	Overcoming of P-gp-mediated MDR, 5-fold decrease in PTX IC_{50}. Increase in PTX cellular accumulation	[405]
PTX, 10 nM	Phloretin, 50, 100 μM	Hep G2 human **hepatocellular** carcinoma cell line, wild-type p53	↑	Increase in PTX-induced apoptosis (activation of caspase-3/-8/-9, PARP cleavage, increase in t-Bid, Bax, p53, cyt c release; decrease in Bcl-2)	[436]
PTX, 5, 10 nM	Prenylated chalcone 2 (PC2), 4.16 μM	MCF-7 human **breast** adenocarcinoma cell line	↑	Increase in PTX cytotoxicity, almost complete abolishment of colony formation	[399]
PTX, 5, 10 nM	Prenylated chalcone 2 (PC2), 1.07 μM	NCI-H460 human non-small cell **lung** cancer cell line	↑	Increase in PTX cytotoxicity, almost complete abolishment of colony formation	[399]
PTX, 10 nM	Quercetin, 15 μM	MCF-7 human **breast** cancer cell line	↓	Protection from PTX-induced cell death. Blocking of PTX-induced p38 and Bcl-2 phosphorylation, affecting PTX-induced Ask1 modification	[400]
PTX, 0.005-10 μg/ml	Quercetin, 0.7 μM	MCF-7 human **breast** cancer cell line	↑	1.68-fold increase in PTX antitumor activity. Elimination of BCSCs (CD44$^+$/CD24$^{-/low}$)	[250]
PTX, 0.005-10 μg/ml	Quercetin, 0.7 μM	MCF-7/Dox human **breast** cancer cell line (DOX-resistant)	↑	Reversal of MDR, 2.45-fold increase in PTX antitumor activity. Downregulation of P-gp. Elimination of BCSCs (CD44$^+$/CD24$^{-/low}$). Inhibition of YB-1 nuclear translocation	[250]
PTX, 0.6-5 nM	Quercetin, 25 μM	HCT116 human **colorectal** cancer cell line, wild-type p53	↑↓	Bimodal effect: Inhibition of clonogenicity (long term effect). Cytoprotective activity; abolishment of PTX-induced G2/M phase cell cycle arrest, decrease in cyclin B1 level (short term effect)	[438]
PTX, 0.1 μM	Quercetin, 40, 60, 80 μM	HA22T/VGH human **hepatoma** cell line	↑	Increase in PTX-induced cytotoxicity and apoptosis	[432]
PTX, 2.9 μM	Quercetin, 1, 5 μM	A2780P human **ovarian** cancer cell line	↑	Increase in sensitivity of cells to PTX	[94]
PTX, 3 μM	Quercetin, 10-100 μM	C13* human **ovarian** cancer cell line, CDDP-resistant ov2008 cells	↓	Promotion of cell survival	[95]
PTX, 2.9 μM	Quercetin, 1, 5 μM	EFO27 human **ovarian** cancer cell line, PTX-resistant	↑	Increase in sensitivity of cells to PTX	[94]
PTX, 2.9 μM	Quercetin, 1, 5 μM	OVCAR-3 human **ovarian** cancer cell line	↑	Increase in sensitivity of cells to PTX	[94]
PTX, 2.9 μM	Quercetin, 1, 5 μM	SKOV-3 human **ovarian** cancer cell line, PTX-resistant	↑	Increase in sensitivity of cells to PTX	[94]
PTX, 10 nM	Quercetin, 15 μM	HeLa human **cervical** cancer cell line	↓	Protection from PTX-induced cell death. Blocking of PTX-induced p38 and Bcl-2 phosphorylation, affecting PTX-induced Ask1 modification	[400]
PTX	Quercetin, 10, 30 μM	KB-3-1 human **cervical** carcinoma cell line, no expression of P-gp	~	No effect on PTX cytotoxicity	[406]

Drug	Flavonoid	Biological system	Direction of combination	Effects	Ref.
PTX	Quercetin, 10, 30 µM	KB-V1 human **cervical** carcinoma cell line, MDR KB-3-1 cells, VBL-resistant, overexpressing of P-gp/MDR1	↑	Increase in PTX cytotoxicity at 30 µM quercetin	[406]
PTX	Quercetin, 1, 5, 10 µM	KB CHf8-5 human **cervical** carcinoma cell line, PTX-resistant KB 3-1 cells, overexpressing ABCB1	↑	1.59-fold increase in sensitivity to PTX at 1 µM, 2.27-fold at 5 µM, 5.41-fold at 10 µM quercetin. Inhibition of P-gp efflux activity, downregulation of ABCB1 (P-gp) expression	[439]
PTX, 0.001-1 µM	Rhamnetin, 3 µM	HepG2 human **hepatocellular** carcinoma cell line	↑	Increase in anchorage-independent cell growth inhibition and G2/M phase cell cycle arrest. miR-34a-mediated Notch1 suppression	[207]
PTX, 0.001-1 µM	Rhamnetin, 3 µM	HepG2/ADR human **hepatocellular** carcinoma cell line, MDR, DOX-resistant	↑	Sensitization of cells to PTX, decrease in PTX IC$_{50}$	[207]
PTX, 0-4 µM	Rubone, 5 µM	DU145 human advanced **prostate** cancer cell line, androgen-refractory	~	No effect on PTX cytotoxicity	[434]
PTX, 0-4 µM	Rubone, 5 µM	DU145-TXR human advanced **prostate** cancer cell line, androgen-refractory, PTX-resistant	↑	Reversal of PTX resistance, sensitization of cells to PTX. Upregulation of miR-34a via p53-independent pathway. Inhibition of invasion and migration. Downregulation of aldehyde activity (as CSC marker)	[434]
PTX, 0-4 µM	Rubone, 5 µM	PC3 human advanced **prostate** cancer cell line, androgen-refractory	~	No effect on PTX cytotoxicity	[434]
PTX, 0-4 µM	Rubone, 5 µM	PC3-TXR human advanced **prostate** cancer cell line, androgen-refractory, PTX-resistant, p53-null	↑	Reversal of PTX resistance, 27.68-fold decrease in PTX IC$_{50}$. Upregulation of miR-34a via p53-independent pathway. Inhibition of invasion and migration. Downregulation of aldehyde activity (as CSC marker)	[434]
PTX	Rutin, 1, 5, 10 µM	KB CHf8-5 human **cervical** carcinoma cell line, PTX-resistant KB 3-1 cells, overexpressing ABCB1	↑	1.02-fold increase in sensitivity to PTX at 1 µM, 2.94-fold at 5 µM, 4.26-fold at 10 µM rutin. Downregulation of ABCB1 (P-gp), inhibition of P-gp efflux activity	[439]
PTX, 20-150 nM	Silibinin, 50-350 µM	4T1 murine metastatic TN **breast** cancer cell line, ER-negative	↑	Synergism in growth inhibition (CI 0.43-0.96). Increase in G2/M phase cell cycle arrest. Inhibition of migration, elevation of relative E-cadherin/N-cadherin ratio. Decrease in serpin PN-1 level	[437]
PTX, 10-40 nM	Silibinin, 150 µM	MCF-7 human **breast** cancer cell line	↑	Synergism in antiproliferative activity (CI<1). Increase in apoptosis (decrease in Bcl-2; increase in Bax, p53, BRCA1, ATM)	[161]
PTX	Silibinin	MCF-7 human **breast** adenocarcinoma cell line	↑	Synergism in anticancer effect (CI 0.8)	[163]
PTX, 250 nM	Silibinin, 400 µM	MCF-7/PAC human **breast** adenocarcinoma cell line, PTX-resistant	↑	Moderate synergism in cell viability reduction (CI 0.81). Increase in Bax; decrease in Bcl-2 and survivin expression	[163]
PTX, 50-200 nM	Silibinin, 20, 50 µM	786-O human **renal** cell carcinoma cell line	↑	Sensitization to PTX, 2.25-fold increase in PTX cytotoxicity at 50 µM silibinin	[354]
PTX, 1-10000 nM	Silibinin, 25-200 µM	A2780 human **ovarian** carcinoma cell line, no expression P-gp	↑	1.77-fold decrease in PTX IC$_{50}$ at 200 µM silibinin	[448]
PTX, 0.02 µM	Silibinin, 50 µM	SKOV-3 human **ovarian** cancer cell line	↑	Increase in growth inhibition. Upregulation of p53 and p21 genes	[433]

Table 6.30. (Continued)

Drug	Flavonoid	Biological system	Direction of combination	Effects	Ref.
PTX, 1-10000 nM	Silibinin, 25-200 µM	A2780/taxol human **ovarian** carcinoma cell line, PTX-resistant, expressing P-gp	↑	Reversal of PTX resistance; 5.96-fold decrease in PTX IC$_{50}$ at 200 µM silibinin. Increase in PTX-induced apoptosis and G2/M phase cell cycle arrest. Downregulation of survivin and P-gp. Reduction of invasive potential (suppression of MMP-2/-9)	[448]
PTX, 0.001-10 nM	Silibinin, 25, 50 µM	AGS human **gastric** cancer cell line	↑	Synergism in growth inhibition (CI<1)	[449]
PTX, 0.001-10 nM	Silibinin, 25, 50 µM	BGC-823 human **gastric** cancer cell line	↑	Synergism in growth inhibition (CI<1)	[449]
PTX, 0.001-10 nM	Silibinin, 25, 50 µM	SGC-7901 human **gastric** cancer cell line	↑	Synergism in growth inhibition (CI<1). Increase in PTX-induced G2/M phase cell cycle arrest (decrease in Cdc2, Cdc25C) and apoptosis via death receptor-mediated pathway (increase in Fas/FasL, Bax; decrease in Bcl-2, activation of caspases-3/-8, PARP cleavage)	[449]
PTX, 10 nM	Taxifolin, 80, 100 µM	HeLaS3 human **cervical** carcinoma cell line	~	No effect on PTX-induced cell viability reduction	[304]
PTX, 100, 1000 nM	Taxifolin, 80, 100 µM	KB-vin human **cervical** cancer cell line, MDR	↑	Additivity to synergism in cell viability reduction (CI 0.66-0.95). Decrease in ABCB1 expression and P-gp efflux function	[304]
PTX, 0.5-500 nM	Tectorigenin, 25, 100 µM	A2780 human **ovarian** cancer cell line, no expressing of ER	↑	Synergistic increase in PTX anticancer potency	[428]
PTX, 0.5-500 nM	Tectorigenin, 25, 100 µM	A2780^{TR} human **ovarian** cancer cell line, no expressing ER, PTX-resistant	↑	Synergistic increase in cell growth inhibition and apoptosis (activation of caspases-3/-9/-8). Inactivation of Akt/IKK/IκB/NF-κB signaling	[428]
PTX, 0.5-500 nM	Tectorigenin, 25, 100 µM	MPSC1 human **ovarian** cancer cell line, no expressing ER	↑	Synergistic increase in PTX anticancer potency	[428]
PTX, 0.5-500 nM	Tectorigenin, 25, 100 µM	MPSC1^{TR} human **ovarian** cancer cell line, no expressing ER, PTX-resistant	↑	Synergistic increase in cell growth inhibition and apoptosis (activation of caspases-3/-9/-8). Inactivation of Akt/IKK/IκB/NF-κB signaling	[428]
PTX, 0.5-500 nM	Tectorigenin, 25, 100 µM	SKOV3 human **ovarian** cancer cell line	↑	Synergistic increase in PTX anticancer potency	[428]
PTX, 0.5-500 nM	Tectorigenin, 25, 100 µM	SKOV3^{TR} human **ovarian** cancer cell line, PTX-resistant	↑	Synergistic increase in PTX anticancer potency	[428]
PTX	Wogonin	BGC-823 human **gastric** cancer cell line	↑	Synergism in cell growth inhibition, increase in apoptosis	[155]
PTX	Wogonin	HGC-27 human **gastric** cancer cell line	↑	Synergism in cell growth inhibition, increase in apoptosis	[155]
PTX	Wogonin	MGC-803 human **gastric** cancer cell line	↑	Synergism in cell growth inhibition, increase in apoptosis	[155]
PTX	Wogonin	MKN-45 human **gastric** cancer cell line	↑	Synergism in cell growth inhibition, increase in apoptosis	[155]

ABC, ATP-binding cassette; Akt, protein kinase B; AR, androgen receptor; Ask1, apoptosis signal-regulating kinase 1; ATM, ataxia telangiectasia mutated; Bax, Bcl-2-associated X protein; Bcl-2, B-cell lymphoma 2; BCSC, breast cancer stem cell; BIRC5, Baculovirus inhibitor of apoptosis repeat-containing 5; BRCA, breast cancer gene; Cdc, cell division cycle; CI, combination index; CSC, cancer stem cell; cyt c, cytochrome c; E2, estradiol; EMT, epithelial-mesenchymal transition; ER, estrogen receptor; ERK, extracellular signal-regulated kinase; FAK, focal adhesion kinase; FasL, Fas ligand; GATA3, GATA binding protein 3; GRP, glucose-regulated protein; HER2 (erbB2), human epidermal growth factor receptor 2; IKK, IκB kinase; IL-8, interleukin; IκB, nuclear factor of kappa light polypeptide gene enhancer in B-cells inhibitor; JNK, c-Jun N-terminal kinase; MDR, multidrug resistance; miR, microRNA; MMP, matrix metalloproteinase; MRP, multidrug resistance-associated protein; mTOR, mammalian target of rapamycin; NE, nanoemulsion; NF-κB, nuclear factor-κB; NP, nanoparticle; Nrf2, nuclear factor (erythroid-derived 2)-like 2; PARP, poly (ADP-ribose) polymerase; P-gp, P-glycoprotein; PI3K, phosphoinositide 3-kinase; PLGA, poly(lactic-co-glycolic acid); PN-1, protease nexin-1; ROS, reactive oxygen species; SOD, superoxide dismutase; STAT3, signal transducer and activator of transcription 3; TLR4, Toll-like receptor 4; TN, triple negative; uPA, urokinase-type plasminogen activator; VEGF, vascular endothelial growth factor; YB-1, Y-box binding protein 1; ΔΨm, mitochondrial membrane potential.

Table 6.31. Effects of flavonoids on anticancer action of paclitaxel (PTX) *in vivo* conditions

Drug	Flavonoid	Biological system	Direction of combination	Effects	Ref.
PTX, via tail vein on days 0, 4, 8, 12, co-encapsulated in NE	Baicalein, via tail vein on days 0, 4, 8, 12, co-encapsulated in NE	MCF-7/Tax human **breast** cancer cells injected into 6-8w old female Balb/C nude mice	↑	Increase in PTX antitumor activity and tumor inhibition rate, decrease in tumor volumes	[420]
PTX, 10 mg/kg, via tail vein, once every 4 days, co-loaded in NPs	Baicalein, 50 mg/kg, via tail vein, once every 4 days, co-loaded in NPs	A549/PTX human **lung** cancer cells injected into the right armpits of 4-6w old Kunming mice	↑	Increase in tumor growth inhibition	[417]
PTX, 10 mg/kg, i.p., every two days	EGCG, 30 mg/kg, i.p., daily	4T1 murine **breast** cancer cells injected s.c. to 6-7w old female Balb/c mice	↑	Increase in tumor growth inhibition. Promotion of apoptosis, decrease in metastatic foci in lung. Overcoming PTX-induced GRP78 expression, potentiation of JNK phosphorylation	[418]
PTX, 20 mg/kg, i.p., weekly	EGCG, 228 mg/kg, i.p., at day 1 on weekly basis	PC-3ML human **prostate** cancer cells injected i.p. in 5-6w old CD17 SCID mice	↑	Decrease in tumor volume, increase in mice survival rates. Increase in p53, p73, p21; promotion of apoptosis. Blocking of bone metastases (when PC-3ML cells were injected via tail vein)	[442]
PTX, i.p., for 7 consecutive days, co-loaded into NPs	Genistein, i.p., for 7 consecutive days, co-loaded into NPs	EAC murine **mammary** adenocarcinoma cells injected i.p. into 6-8w old Swiss male mice; EAC maintained in ascitic form in Swiss mice	↑	Increase in tumor growth inhibition. Antiangiogenic effect (decrease in VEGF levels)	[440]
PTX, 3 mg/kg, 5 times every second day	Isoxanthohumol, 20 mg/kg, for 10 consecutive days	B16 murine **melanoma** cells inoculated s.c. in the dorsal right lumbosacral region of syngeneic C57BL/6 mice	↑	Synergistic reduction of tumor volume	[171]
PTX, 1 mg/kg, i.p., thrice per week	Luteolin, 3 mg/kg, i.p., thrice per week	MDA-MB-231 human **breast** cancer cells injected s.c. into the mammary fat pad of 6w old female athymic nude mice (BALB/cAnN.Cg-Fox-nlnu/CrlNarf)	↑	Increase in reduction of tumor size and weight	[425]
PTX, 1 mg/kg, i.p., every 2 days	Luteolin, 3 mg/kg, i.p., every 2 days	SCC-4 human **oral** cancer cells injected s.c. into the right front axilla of 5-6w old immunodeficient nude male BALB/c nu/nu mice	↑	Synergism in tumor growth inhibition	[445]
PTX, 50 µg/kg, via tail vein, daily for 15 days	Morin, 50 mg/kg, via tail vein, daily for 15 days	DU145 human **prostate** cancer cells injected into both sides of posterior flanks in nude mice	↑	Increase in reduction of tumor size and weight	[426]
PTX, 1 mg/kg, i.p., thrice weekly for 6 weeks	Phloretin, 10 mg/kg, i.p., thrice weekly for 6 weeks	Hep G2 human **hepatocellular** carcinoma cells injected s.c. between the scapulae of 6-7w old NOD-SCID mice	↑	Potentiation of PTX-induced reduction of tumor volume and weight (more than 5-fold decrease in tumor volume)	[436]
PTX, i.v., every other day for 5 doses, co-loaded into PEG-PCD micelles	Rubone, i.v., every other day for 5 doses, co-loaded into PEG-PCD micelles	PC3-TXR human **prostate** cancer cells (expressing GFP and Luc) injected into the lower abdomen (dorsal prostate lobe) of 8w old male nude mice	↑	Increase in tumor growth inhibition, decrease in tumor size. Upregulation of miR-34a via p53-independent pathway; reversal of E-cadherin, cyclin D1 and SIRT1 expression	[434]
PTX, 2 mg/kg, i.p., every other day	Silibinin, 200 mg/kg, by oral gavage, every other day	4T1 murine **breast** cancer cells (carrying COX-2 promoter-driven Luc) injected via tail vein into 6w old female BALB/cByJNar1 mice	↑	Sensitization of tumors to PTX treatment. Increase in PTX-induced inhibition of VEGF and PCNA level	[437]
PTX, 10 or 20 mg/kg, i.p., once a week for 2 weeks	Wogonin, 60 mg/kg, i.p., once a day for 2 weeks	BGC-823 human **gastric** cancer cells injected s.c. into the right oxter of 6w old female BALB/c athymic nu/nu mice	↑	Increase in PTX efficacy, inhibition of tumor volume and weight	[155]

COX, cyclooxygenase; EAC, Ehrlich ascites carcinoma; GRP, glucose-regulated protein; JNK, c-Jun N-terminal kinase; Luc, luciferase; miR, microRNA; NE, nanoemulsion; NP, nanoparticle; PCNA, proliferating cell nuclear antigen; PEG-PCD, poly(ethylene glycol)-block-poly(2-methyl-2-carboxyl-propylene carbonate-graft-dodecanol); SIRT1, sirtuin 1; VEGF, vascular endothelial growth factor.

Soy isoflavone *genistein* promoted colony survival and suppressed PTX-induced apoptosis in human ovarian cancer OV2008 cells, rendering malignant cells more resistant to cytotoxic action of this antimitotic drug and requiring precaution by ovarian cancer patients [424]. Among several other cellular action mechanisms, genistein can exert its functions through interaction with estrogen receptors (ERs), ERα and ERβ, whereas the ratio of ERα/ERβ is a critical factor determining the action of genistein in breast cancer cells. In fact, genistein decreased the sensitivity to PTX-induced cytotoxicity and increased viability of human breast cancer MCF-7 cells with a high ERα/ERβ ratio, but still remained inactive in modulating antitumor potential of PTX in T47D cells with a low ERα/ERβ ratio. Therefore, consumption of genistein containing food products or supplements may be contraindicated for women receiving PTX chemotherapy whose breast tumor has a high ERα/ERβ ratio [130]. Coencapsulation of genistein and PTX into nanoparticles increased tumor growth inhibition in Ehrlich ascites carcinoma (murine mammary adenocarcinoma) bearing mice, through potentiation of cytotoxic and antiangiogenic properties [440]. Genistein synergistically enhanced PTX-induced cytotoxicity and apoptosis also in human androgen receptor (AR)-negative prostate cancer PC-3 cells through suppression of Akt activity and NF-κB nuclear translocation. Combined treatment with genistein and PTX could thus allow to reduce the therapeutic dose of PTX and thereby decrease its toxic side effects on normal tissues [403]. Genistein, but not another isoflavone *daidzein* and glycosylated isoflavone *genistin* or genistein 7-glucoside, increased PTX-induced cytotoxicity in P-gp-overexpressing MDR human cervical cancer KB-V1 cells; whereas none of these isoflavones affected antitumor action of PTX in parental drug sensitive KB-3-1 cells [406]. Pretreatment with isoflavone *orobol* for 1.5 hours before addition of PTX for another 2 hours enhanced chemosensitivity in human ovarian cancer cell line 2008 as well as its CDDP-resistant subline 2008/C13*5.25. This chemosensitization was at least partially associated with promotion of apoptotic signaling pathway [427]. Monomethylated isoflavone *tectorigenin* synergistically increased anticancer activities of PTX in several human ovarian cancer cell lines A2780, MPSC1 and SKOV3 as well as their PTX-resistant sublines A2780[TR], MPSC1[TR] and SKOV3[TR]. Combined treatment of PTX-resistant A2780[TR] and MPSC1[TR] cells with tectorigenin and PTX led to potentiation of drug-induced apoptotic death through inactivation of Akt, inhibition of nuclear translocation of NF-κB and expression of its chemoresistance-related downstream genes, including XIAP, Bcl-2 and COX-2. As these ovarian cancer cell lines did not expressed estrogen receptors (ERs), estrogen-ER system could not be involved in sensitizing effects of PTX cytotoxicity by tectorigenin [428]. Based on the above-described preclinical data, certain isoflavones tend to augment antitumor action of PTX in malignant cells with no expression of estrogen-androgen receptors, whereas in ER-expressing models the interaction can be antagonistic (Table 6.30 and Table 6.31).

The major green tea flavanol *EGCG*, even in the range of submicromolar doses (0.2 µM) that can be readily obtained in the human plasma after administration of a single oral dose of green tea extract, increased growth inhibitory properties of PTX in HER2-overexpressing human head and neck squamous cell carcinoma YCU-H891 cells. As overexpression of HER2 is associated with aggressive phenotypes of several tumor types, being involved in increased metastatic ability and resistance to different conventional chemotherapeutic drugs, including taxanes, inclusion of EGCG in PTX treatment protocols might be of clinical significance in the treatment of head and neck carcinomas in the future [441]. EGCG synergistically augmented PTX-induced cytotoxicity and apoptosis also in hormone-refractory human prostate cancer PC-3 cells through inactivation of Akt and suppression of NF-κB translocation into the nucleus [403]. PC-3 cells possess a strong capability to metastasize to bone marrow. In single clone of PC-3 cells derived from bone marrow metastases, PC-3ML, EGCG synergistically enhanced growth inhibitory and proapoptotic properties of PTX by increasing expression of apoptosis-related p53, p73 and p21 genes. Moreover, the percent of apoptotic cells in xenograft tumor tissue was significantly increased by combined treatment of PC-3ML bearing mice with EGCG and PTX, accompanied by decrease in tumor volume, increase in overall survival rates of experimental animals and blocking of bone metastases. Therefore, combination of EGCG and PTX might provide a novel attractive therapeutic strategy for the treatment of patients with advanced and metastatic prostate tumors [442]. Cytotoxic and proapoptotic activities of PTX were significantly potentiated by EGCG also in human breast cancer MCF-7 cells, mediated via downregulation of drug-induced GRP78 expression resulting in increase in JNK and caspase-7 activation [398]. Likewise, PTX-induced GRP78 expression was suppressed in the presence of EGCG in murine breast cancer 4T1 cells, followed by potentiation of JNK phosphorylation, leading to increased reduction of cell viability and apoptotic death. Combined treatment of 4T1 bearing mice with EGCG and PTX resulted in substantially greater tumor growth inhibition than treatment with either agent alone, associated with promotion of apoptosis, decrease in tumor burden and reduction of pulmonary metastases. At that, EGCG suppressed PTX-increased GRP78 expression in xenograft tumor tissues enhancing sensitivity of breast cancer cells to therapeutic efficacy of this microtubules-interfering drug [418]. In addition, low micromolar doses of EGCG (2.2 µM) augmented growth inhibitory properties of PTX in HER2-overexpressing human breast cancer BT-474 cells [441]. EGCG enhanced antitumor properties of PTX also in estrogen-independent human breast cancer MDA-MB-231 cells, potentiating drug-induced cell viability reduction and cytotoxic responses [418, 421]. Moreover, co-loading of EGCG and PTX into liposomes resulted in further increase in cytotoxic and proapoptotic activities of PTX, with suppression of cellular invasion through inhibition of MMP-2 and MMP-9 enzymes; being in turn more effective than individual agents-loaded liposomes [421]. Coencapsulation of EGCG and PTX into poly(lactic-co-glycolic acid) (PLGA)-casein nanoparticles led to synergistic cytotoxic and apoptotic responses in MDA-MB-231 cells, inhibiting drug-induced NF-κB activation and its downstream key genes involved in survival, angiogenesis and metastasis processes. Also, PTX-induced P-gp levels were downregulated by treating breast cancer cells with dual-loaded nanoparticles [443]. As poor bioavailability of EGCG is still a limiting factor for its clinical use, novel nanocarrier-based drug delivery systems can make an important progress in application of combinational therapies of EGCG and conventional antineoplastic drugs in the treatment of human cancers. However, this issue might be more complicated as EGCG was demonstrated to exert biphasic impact on PTX cytotoxicity in MDA-MB-231 cells, depending on the doses of agents. In fact, lower doses of EGCG revealed antagonistic effects in combinations with PTX in MDA-MB-231 cells, while higher concentrations of EGCG were able to sensitize these breast cancer cells to PTX cytotoxicity [444]. As the available preclinical findings about the combined effects of EGCG and PTX in MDA-MB-231 cells are somewhat inconsistent, it is possible that different subclones of this estrogen-independent human breast cancer cell line are in circulation, in turn pointing to heterogeneity of the disease. Therefore, as long as further confirmative data will be available, it would be reasonable of patients with estrogen-independent breast tumors to avoid the exposure to EGCG while receiving PTX chemotherapy, with the aim not to impair the therapeutic outcome. Furthermore, in human non-small cell lung cancer NCI-H460 cells, EGCG revealed schedule-dependent effects on antitumor action of PTX. Synergistic growth inhibition with apoptotic death were observed when cells were pretreated with the drug for 24 hours before addition of EGCG; however, pretreatment of the cells with EGCG for 24 hours followed by PTX treatment and also concurrent treatment with both agents antagonized the cytotoxicity of antineoplastic drug, rendering lung cancer cells more resistant to PTX chemotherapy [429]. Thus, as EGCG can diminish the therapeutic efficacy of PTX against lung tumors, patients should be extremely cautious when consuming green tea or taking green tea supplements during the active treatment phase with PTX (Table 6.30 and Table 6.31).

Common dietary flavone *apigenin* enhanced chemosensitivity to PTX in human lung cancer A549 cells, human hepatocellular carcinoma Hep3B cells and human cervical cancer HeLa cells. In HeLa cells, apigenin synergistically potentiated PTX-induced cell viability reduction and apoptosis by promoting ROS accumulation and caspase-2 activation through inhibition of enzymatic activity of superoxide dismutase (SOD). Thus, combined use of apigenin and PTX might be an effective way to reduce the dose of PTX in the treatment of different types of human cancers, thereby decreasing also the severity of adverse reactions on the patients [435]. Although another natural flavone *luteolin* did not affect antitumor activity of PTX in human gastric cancer AGS cells [144], addition of luteolin to PTX treatment protocols led to increased cytotoxicity of this antimitotic drug in human oral squamous cell carcinoma SCC-4 cells. Moreover, combined treatment with luteolin and PTX resulted in synergistic inhibition of xenograft tumor growth also in

SCC-4 bearing mice [445]. In addition, luteolin significantly augmented PTX-induced cytotoxicity in PTX-resistant human ovarian cancer A2780IAP-X10 and A2780IAP-X22 cells. This chemosensitization was associated with reversal of epithelial-mesenchymal transition (EMT) by downregulating mesenchymal phenotype and upregulating epithelial characteristics, through reduction of focal adhesion kinase (FAK) and ERK activities leading to suppression of p65 translocation into the nucleus. At that, the morphology of resistant cells was also changed by addition of luteolin, as elongated, spindle-shaped, pseudopodia forming cells were turned into more cobblestone-like cells with less intercellular space. Therefore, luteolin could be applied as a potential adjuvant agent for PTX chemotherapy against recurrent and chemoresistant ovarian tumors [446]. Luteolin potentiated PTX-induced cytotoxicity also in estrogen-independent human breast cancer cell lines MDA-MB-231 and MDA-MB-453. Coadministration of luteolin and PTX in MDA-MB-231 cells inactivated signal transducer and activator of transcription 3 (STAT3) leading to enhanced apoptotic death as compared to the treatment with PTX alone. Moreover, combined treatment with luteolin and PTX substantially reduced tumor size and weight also in an orthotopic tumor model of MDA-MB-231 cells in nude mice; suggesting that luteolin-PTX combination is worth of further therapeutic development for the treatment of estrogen-independent breast tumors, reducing side effects while maintaining or even enhancing PTX clinical efficacy [425]. Despite the fact that flavone *baicalein* did not modulate PTX cytotoxicity in drug sensitive parental human breast cancer MCF-7 cells, baicalein synergistically enhanced antitumor activities of PTX in PTX-resistant MCF-7 cells, i.e., MCF-7/Tax, increasing ROS level and inducing apoptosis, besides enhancing intracellular drug accumulation. Coencapsulation of baicalein and PTX into nanoemulsions at a synergistic weight ratio of 1:1 led to further improvement of PTX cytotoxicity in drug-resistant breast cancer cells. This nanoformulation increased PTX antitumor activity also in MCF-7/Tax bearing mice, inhibiting tumor growth and leading to significantly smaller tumors as compared to PTX monotherapy [420]. Inclusion of baicalein, only at 1 μM concentration, in PTX treatment schemes increased growth inhibitory and proapoptotic activities of PTX also in murine breast cancer C3L5 cells [447]. In addition, combined treatment with baicalein and lower doses of PTX (less than 1 μM) revealed superior antitumor effects in several human ovarian cancer cell lines (A2780, OVCAR, SKOV3) as compared to treatment with the drug alone. In A2780 cells, baicalein augmented PTX-mediated mitochondrial apoptosis by inhibiting Akt/β-catenin signaling pathway. In SKOV3 cells, combined treatment with baicalein and PTX led to increased rate of cellular apoptosis and necrosis [419]. Furthermore, cotreatment of human lung cancer A549 cells and PTX-resistant A549/PTX cells with baicalein and PTX dual-loaded nanoparticles (at optimal weight ratio of 5:1) led to synergistic antitumor effects, with circumvention of multidrug resistance (MDR) phenotype in drug resistant cells. *In vivo* results further confirmed the *in vitro* findings, showing that treatment of A549/PTX drug-resistant human lung cancer xenografts bearing mice with dual agents-loaded nanoparticles significantly increased tumor growth inhibition [417]. Thus, baicalein might be an important adjunct for PTX therapy exerting its effects as a chemoresistance reversal agent. Monomethylated baicalein, *oroxylin A* or 6-methoxybaicalein, enhanced susceptibility of NCI/ADR-RES cells to PTX cytotoxicity by increasing P-gp-mediated cellular accumulation of the drug [405]. Another monomethylated flavone *wogonin* synergistically augmented growth inhibitory and proapoptotic activities of PTX in several human gastric cancer cell lines, i.e., BGC-823, HGC-27, MGC-803 and MKN-45; and increased chemotherapeutic efficacy of this microtubules-interfering drug also in BGC-823 bearing mice, leading to substantially smaller xenograft tumors than in mice treated with PTX alone [155]. Polymethylated citrus flavone *nobiletin* or hexamethoxyflavone synergistically increased inhibitory effects of PTX in human non-small cell lung cancer cell lines A549 and H460 [175]. However, later studies still specified that achievable plasma concentrations of nobiletin (0.5-9 µM) significantly sensitized P-gp (ABCB1)-overexpressing drug-resistant human lung cancer A549/T cells and human ovarian cancer A2780/T cells to PTX, but did not modulate antitumor action of PTX in parental sensitive A549 and A2780 cells. In A2780/T cells, addition of 9 µM nobiletin reduced half-maximal inhibitory concentration (IC_{50}) of PTX by 432.9-fold and this chemosensitization was related to inhibition of PI3K/AKT and MAPK/ERK pathways and downregulation of Nrf2 expression, leading to enhanced inhibition of cell growth and colony formation, and promotion of apoptotic death. In addition, combined treatment of A2780/T cells with nobiletin and PTX resulted in markedly increased proportion of G2/M phase-arrested cells; besides resulting in intracellular drug accumulation through affecting ATPase activity of P-gp (ABCB1) efflux pump [276]. Therefore, nobiletin has the potential to be used in combination therapies with PTX for the treatment of PTX-resistant tumors, particularly those overexpressing P-gp transporter protein (Table 6.30 and Table 6.31).

The role of natural flavonolignan *silibinin* on the chemotherapeutic efficacy of PTX has also been studied in different preclinical cancer models. In human breast cancer MCF-7 cells, the interaction between silibinin and PTX was synergistic via inhibition of proliferation and induction of apoptotic death [161, 163]. Silibinin potentiated PTX cytotoxicity also in PTX-resistant MCF-7 cells, i.e., MCF-7/PAC, by suppressing growth and regulating the expression of proapoptotic and antiapoptotic proteins, including decrease in oncogenic survivin [163]. Combined treatment of highly metastatic triple-negative (TN) murine breast cancer 4T1 cells with silibinin and PTX led to synergistic growth inhibition and enhanced G2/M phase cell cycle arrest. Silibinin also potentiated PTX-induced suppression of cellular migration and motility through downregulation of serpin protease nexin-1 (PN-1) and N-cadherin, upregulation of E-cadherin and inhibition of MMP-9 activity. *In vivo* studies with mice bearing 4T1 breast cancer cells (with a COX-2 promoter-driven luciferase reporter gene for monitoring of cellular migration and location) revealed increased chemotherapeutic efficacy of PTX in the presence of silibinin, reducing the percentage of cells positive for angiogenic (VEGF) and proliferative biomarkers (PCNA) [437]. Silibinin enhanced PTX-induced cytotoxicity also in human ovarian carcinoma A2780 cells. In P-gp-expressing PTX-resistant subclone, A2780/taxol, addition of silibinin to PTX treatment reversed drug resistance, increased PTX-induced G2/M phase cell cycle arrest and apoptosis through downregulation of P-gp and survivin overexpression; besides reduction of cellular invasion via suppression of MMP-2 and MMP-9 protein levels [448]. In human ovarian cancer SKOV-3 cells, cotreatment with silibinin and PTX led to increase in cell growth inhibition by upregulation of tumor suppressor genes p53 and p21, as compared to the treatment of either agent alone [433]. Silibinin synergistically enhanced PTX-induced growth inhibition also in several human gastric cancer cell lines, such as AGS, BGC-823 and SGC-7901. In the latest cell line, combined treatment with silibinin and PTX resulted in superior increase in G2/M phase cell cycle arrest and apoptosis through the death receptor-mediated extrinsic signaling pathway [449]. In addition, silibinin was able to chemosensitize to PTX cytotoxicity also in human renal cell carcinoma 786-O cells [354]. Thus, silibinin could be a beneficial adjuvant agent to enhance the therapeutic potential of PTX chemotherapy, especially for the treatment of tumors refractory to PTX alone, allowing to reduce the required drug dosages (Table 6.30 and Table 6.31).

Flavanonol *ampelopsin* or dihydromyricetin reversed drug resistance and augmented PTX-induced apoptotic death in PTX-resistant human ovarian cancer A2780/PTX cells, by inhibiting survivin expression via p53 activation. Thus, p53 status in ovarian tumor cells might be an important factor determining the sensitivity to ampelopsin supplementation [303]. As another flavanonol *taxifolin* did not modulate PTX cytotoxicity in drug sensitive human cervical cancer HeLaS3 cells; addition of taxifolin to PTX treatment protocols markedly enhanced cell viability reduction in MDR human cervical cancer KB-vin cells through suppression of expression and efflux function of P-gp (ABCB1) transport protein [304]. Natural chalcone *isoliquiritigenin* augmented synergistically antiproliferative properties of PTX in different human breast cancer cell lines, both in triple negative (TN) BT-549 and MDA-MB-231 cells as well as estrogen receptor (ER)-positive MCF-7 cells [319]. Chalcone *rubone* strongly reversed PTX resistance in drug-resistant human advanced prostate cancer cell lines DU145-TXR and PC3-TXR, but did not modulate PTX cytotoxicity in the respective parental lines DU145 and PC3. In DU145-TXR and PC3-TXR cells, coadministration of low micromolar doses of rubone (5 μM) and PTX led to upregulation of the tumor suppressor gene miR-34a via a p53-independent pathway, followed by restoration of the expression of miR-34a targeted genes; resulting in inhibition of cellular growth, invasion and migration. Moreover, combined treatment with rubone and PTX killed both cancer stem-like cells as well as bulk tumor cells. In addition, administration of micelles loaded with both rubone and PTX suppressed prostate tumor growth in orthotopic model obtained via injection of p53-null PC3-TXR cells to dorsal prostate lobe of nude mice. This *in vivo* chemosensitization was accompanied by reversing of the expression of miR-34a, cyclin D1, sirtuin 1 and E-cadherin. As clinical management of prostate tumors with PTX often fails due to the development of chemoresistance phenomenon caused by significant downregulation of miR-34a, addition of rubone as a specific non-toxic natural miR-34a modulator to PTX treatment regimens might lead to chemosensitization and improvement of PTX therapeutic efficacy for treatment of androgen refractory metastatic prostate cancers [434]. Chalcone *phloretin* interacted with PTX chemotherapy in human hepatocellular carcinoma preclinical models, augmenting PTX-induced apoptotic death in HepG2 cells, and leading to more than fourfold decrease in tumor weight in HepG2 bearing mice cotreated with phloretin and PTX as compared to treatment with PTX alone [436]. *Prenylated chalcone 2 (PC2)* increased PTX cytotoxicity in human breast cancer MCF-7 cells and human lung cancer NCI-H460 cells, by enhancing the effect of PTX on microtubule assembly and abrogating the colony formation ability of malignant cells [399]. Prenylated flavonoid *isoxanthohumol* synergistically sensitized aggressive human melanoma A375 cells, nonmetastatic murine melanoma B16 cells and its highly invasive subclone, B16F10, to antitumor action of PTX. Such synergistic interaction was further confirmed *in vivo* conditions in a subcutaneous model of mice injected with B16 melanoma cells, leading to significantly smaller tumors by combined treatment as compared to treatment with either single agents. Thus, isoxanthohumol might be a promising candidate for combinational chemotherapy with PTX against aggressive advanced melanomas [171]. Likewise, glycosylated prenylated flavonoid *icariside II* potentiated PTX cytotoxicity in A375 and B16 melanoma cells. In A375 cells, icariside II promoted PTX-induced apoptosis, and reduced production of interleukin (IL)-8 and VEGF; mediated at least in part through suppression of drug-induced increase in Toll-like receptor 4 (TLR4) cell survival pathway, including inhibition of downstream ERK signaling and NF-κB nuclear translocation. Moreover, combined treatment with icariside II and PTX augmented cell viability reduction also in human glioma U87 cells [430] (Table 6.30 and Table 6.31).

There are many possibilities for interactions to occur between plant-derived dietary flavonoids and PTX (Figure 6.16). Without doubt, certain synergistic combinations of these dietary polyphenols and PTX need further in vitro and in vivo studies before starting clinical trials, such as fisetin-PTX against non-small cell lung tumors, EGCG-PTX against head and neck carcinomas or advanced prostate tumors, luteolin-PTX against drug-resistant ovarian tumors or breast carcinomas, baicalein-PTX and nobiletin-PTX against different PTX-resistant tumors, rubone-PTX against metastatic taxane-resistant prostate tumors, and isoxanthohumol-PTX against advanced melanomas. Such combined approaches might lead to reduction of therapeutically efficient doses of PTX, thereby decreasing toxic side effects on normal healthy tissues and improving quality of life of patients. However, due to several antagonistic combinations reported in preclinical studies, cancer patients should take an extreme caution avoiding dietary exposure to certain contraindicated flavonoids during the active treatment phase with PTX. Antagonistic action of different flavonoids, such as quercetin, fisetin, genistein and EGCG, on antitumor effects of PTX in certain cancer models is probably mediated through modulation of multiple intracellular signaling cascades and acting on diverse molecular targets, depending on dosage of agents, time schedule and molecular characteristics of specific malignant cells, including expression of sex hormone receptors. As these antagonistic combinations have shown to result in almost complete abolishment of therapeutic efficacy of PTX, cancer patients must be counselled in the future concerning these contraindicated plant-derived dietary components when undergoing PTX chemotherapy.

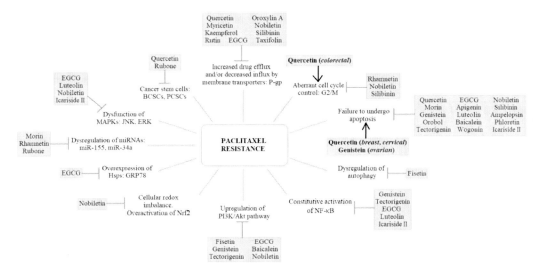

Figure 6.16. Intervention in cellular resistance mechanisms of paclitaxel by plant flavonoids (Akt, protein kinase B; BCSC, breast cancer stem cell; ERK, extracellular signal-regulated kinase; GRP, glucose-regulated protein; Hsp, heat shock protein; JNK, c-Jun N-terminal kinase; MAPK, mitogen-activated protein kinase; miR, microRNA; NF-κB, nuclear factor-κB; Nrf2, nuclear factor (erythroid-derived 2)-like 2; PCSC, prostate cancer stem cell; P-gp, P-glycoprotein; PI3K, phosphoinositide 3-kinase).

According to the current experimental findings it is recommended for cancer patients *not to consume* dietary products or dietary supplements rich in following plant flavonoids during the active chemotherapeutic treatment phase with **paclitaxel**:
- **quercetin** in estrogen receptor-positive breast cancer
- **fisetin** in estrogen receptor-positive breast cancer
- **genistein** in estrogen receptor-positive breast cancer
- **EGCG** in estrogen receptor-negative breast cancer
- **quercetin** in ovarian cancer
- **genistein** in ovarian cancer
- **quercetin** in cervical cancer
- **quercetin** in colorectal cancer
- **EGCG** in non-small cell lung cancer (*concurrent treatment or pretreatment with flavonoid*)

6.3.4. Docetaxel (DOC)

Docetaxel (DOC), a semisynthetic derivative of PTX, is a member of the family of taxanes. DOC has been routinely used as a first- and second-line treatment for different types of cancers, including tumors in the prostate, breast, stomach, lung and the upper aerodigestive tract; alone or in combination with other chemotherapeutic agents [1, 62, 450-453]. DOC is a microtubule stabilizer agent, exerting its cytotoxicity by binding to the β-subunit of tubulin and promoting the assembly of tubulin into stable microtubule bundles, while concurrently inhibiting their disassembly; thereby leading to mitotic arrest, abrogating tumor progression and inducing apoptosis [451-457]. However, prolonged use of DOC can lead to the development of drug resistance and cause serious side effects, including hair loss, neurosensory and neuromotor symptoms, low blood cell counts, edema, muscle pain and vomiting [450-452]. Therefore, novel approaches have been searched to interfere with DOC chemotherapy and potentiate its therapeutic efficacy at lower drug doses using non-toxic natural compounds.

Table 6.32. Effects of flavonoids on anticancer action of docetaxel (DOC) *in vitro* conditions

Drug	Flavonoid	Biological system	Direction of combination	Effects	Ref.
DOC	Alopecurone B, 10 μM	MG-63/DOX human **osteosarcoma** cell line, MDR, DOX-resistant	↑	Sensitization to DOC, 2.99-fold decrease in DOC IC$_{50}$	[235]
DOC, 5, 10, 20 nM	Baicalein, 10 μM	HPAF-II human **pancreatic** cancer cell line	↑	Synergistic decrease in cell viability	[371]
DOC, 5, 10, 20 nM	Baicalein, 10 μM	MIA PaCa-2 human **pancreatic** cancer cell line	↑	Synergistic decrease in cell viability	[371]
DOC, 2, 5, 10 nM	Baicalein, 10 μM	PANC-1 human **pancreatic** cancer cell line	↑	Synergistic decrease in cell viability. Increase in S phase cell cycle arrest and apoptosis. Inhibition migration	[371]
DOC, 2 nM	Baicalein, 50, 100 μM	8505c human anaplastic **thyroid** cancer cell line, mutant p53	↑	Increase in DOC-induced antiproliferative activity and apoptosis (increase in Bax, caspase-3; decrease in Bcl-2). Decrease in angiogenic (VEGF, TGF-β) and invasive proteins (E-cadherin, N-cadherin) through inhibition of ERK and Akt/mTOR pathways	[450]
DOC, 0-10 μM, co-loaded into Tf-decorated SLNs	Baicalin, 0-10 μM, co-loaded into Tf-decorated SLNs	A549/DTX human non-small cell **lung** cancer cell line, DOC-resistant	↑	Synergism in cytotoxicity	[451]
DOC, 0.625-10 ng/ml	Chrysin, 10-100 μM	A549 human non-small cell **lung** cancer cell line	↑↓	Synergism in cytotoxicity when pretreated with DOC for 24h. Upregulation of apoptosis-related proteins (p53, p21, p27, IGFBP-4/-6, TRAILR-1/-3/-4). Antagonistic effect when pretreated with chrysin for 24h	[452]
DOC, 5 nM	EGCG, 40 μM	LAPC-4-AI human **prostate** cancer cell line, androgen-independent	↑	Increase in DOC-induced antiproliferative effect	[457]
DOC, 3.12 nM	EGCG, 30, 50 μM	PC-3ML human **prostate** cancer cell line, single clone derived from bone marrow metastases	↑	Synergism in growth inhibition. Increase in p53, p73, p21 and caspase-3 expression; increase in apoptosis	[442]
DOC, 1 nM	Genistein, 30 μM	MDA-MB-231 human **breast** cancer cell line	↑	Synergism in cell growth inhibition (CI 0.577). Increase in apoptosis	[62]

Effects of Plant Flavonoids on Chemotherapeutic Efficacy of Cancer Drugs 335

Drug	Flavonoid	Biological system	Direction of combination	Effects	Ref.
DOC, 2 nM	Genistein, 15 μM	H460 human **lung** cancer cell line	↑	Synergism in cell growth inhibition (CI 0.788). Increase in apoptosis	[62]
DOC, 1 nM	Genistein, 10 μM	A2780 human **ovarian** cancer cell line	↑	Increase in cell viability reduction and apoptosis (PARP cleavage; decrease in Bcl-2, Bcl-xL, survivin, cIAP1). Inactivation of NF-κB DNA binding activity	[128]
DOC, 2 nM	Genistein, 25 μM	C200 human **ovarian** cancer cell line, CDDP-resistant A2780 cells	↑	Increase in cell viability reduction and apoptosis (PARP cleavage; decrease in Bcl-2, Bcl-xL, survivin, cIAP1). Inactivation of NF-κB DNA binding activity	[128]
DOC, 1 nM	Genistein, 30 μM	BxPC-3 human **pancreatic** cancer cell line	↑	Synergism in cell growth inhibition (CI 0.651). Increase in apoptosis, blocking of DOC-induced NF-κB activation	[62]
DOC, 1 nM	Genistein, 30 μM	BxPC-3 human **pancreatic** cancer cell line	↑	Potentiation of DOC-induced growth inhibition and apoptosis. Abrogation of DOC-induced NF-κB activation	[132]
DOC, 1 nM	Genistein, 30 μM	PC-3 human **prostate** cancer cell line	↑	Potentiation of DOC-induced growth inhibition. Regulation of OPG/RANK/RANKL/MMP-9 signaling	[455]
DOC, 1 nM	Genistein, 30 μM	PC-3 human **prostate** cancer cell line	↑	Synergism in cell growth inhibition (CI 0.773). Increase in apoptosis (upregulation of $p21^{WAF1}$; downregulation of survivin, Bcl-2, Bcl-xL), blocking of DOC-induced NF-κB activation	[62]
DOC	Nobiletin, 0.5-9 μM	A549/T human non-small cell **lung** cancer cell line, PTX-resistant, overexpressing ABCB1	↑	Sensitization to DOC, decrease in DOC IC_{50}	[276]
DOC	Nobiletin, 0.5-9 μM	A2780/T human **ovarian** cancer cell line, PTX-resistant, overexpressing ABCB1	↑	Sensitization to DOC, decrease in DOC IC_{50}	[276]
DOC, 5 nM	Quercetin, 5 μM	LAPC-4-AI human **prostate** cancer cell line, androgen-independent	↑	Increase in DOC-induced antiproliferative effect	[457]
DOC, 5-200 μg/ml, co-loaded into HA-modified PLGA-PEI NPs	Quercetin, co-loaded into HA-modified PLGA-PEI NPs	4T1 murine highly metastatic **breast** cancer cell line	↑	Improvement of DOC cytotoxicity, decrease in colony formation, promotion of apoptosis. Downregulation of p-Akt and MMP-9; inhibition of migration and invasion	[456]
DOC, 2.5-5 nM	Silibinin, 10-40 μM	DU145 human **prostate** cancer cell line, mutant p53	~↓	Little if any increase in DOC efficacy, neutral or antagonistic pattern (CI 0.898-2.54)	[321]
DOC, 2.5-5 nM	Silibinin, 10-40 μM	LNCaP human **prostate** cancer cell line, wild-type p53	~↓	Little if any increase in DOC efficacy, neutral or antagonistic pattern (CI 921-2.32)	[321]
DOC, 2.5-5 nM	Silibinin, 10-40 μM	PC-3 human **prostate** cancer cell line, mutant p53	~↓	Little if any increase in DOC efficacy, neutral or antagonistic pattern (CI 0.895-4.47)	[321]
DOC	Tricin	PC-3 human metastatic **prostate** cancer cell line, hormone-resistant	↑	Synergism in antiproliferative effect (CI<1)	[458]
DOC, 5, 10 nM	Vicenin-2, 5, 10 μM	LNCaP human **prostate** carcinoma cell line, androgen-dependent, AR-positive	↑	Synergism in cell growth inhibition and decrease in clonogenic potential (CI<1). Potentiation of DOC-induced decrease in AR levels	[459]
DOC, 5, 10 nM	Vicenin-2, 5, 10 μM	PC-3 human **prostate** carcinoma cell line, androgen-independent, AR-negative	↑	Synergism in cell growth inhibition and decrease in clonogenic potential (CI<1)	[459]

ABC, ATP-binding cassette; Akt, protein kinase B; AR, androgen receptor; Bax, Bcl-2-associated X protein; Bcl-2, B-cell lymphoma 2; Bcl-xl, B-cell lymphoma-extra large; CI, combination index; cIAP1, cellular inhibitor of apoptosis protein 1; ERK, extracellular signal-regulated kinase; HA, hyaluronic acid; IGFBP, insulin-like growth factor binding protein; MMP, matrix metalloproteinase; mTOR, mammalian target of rapamycin; NF-κB, nuclear factor-κB; NP, nanoparticle; OPG, osteoprotegerin; PARP, poly (ADP-ribose) polymerase; PEI, polyethyleneimine; PLGA, poly(lactic-co-glycolic acid); RANK, receptor activator of nuclear factor-κB; RANKL, RANK ligand; SLN, solid lipid nanoparticle; Tf, transferrin; TGF-β, transforming growth factor β; TRAILR, TNF-related apoptosis-inducing ligand receptor; VEGF, vascular endothelial growth factor.

Interactions with several flavonoids and DOC have been studied in different preclinical cancer systems, both *in vitro* cancer cell lines as well as *in vivo* animal models (Table 6.32 and Table 6.33). Dietary flavone *chrysin* was shown to increase DOC-induced cytotoxicity in human non-small cell lung cancer A549 cells, when the cells were pretreated with the antimitotic drug for 24 hours prior to the addition of flavone. Posttreatment with chrysin augmented DOC-induced tumor growth delay also in A549-derived xenograft mice model, leading to apoptotic death and decrease in tumor weight. However, in reverse order, i.e., pretreatment of the cells with chrysin for 24 hours before addition of DOC, antagonistic interaction was observed with decrease in DOC therapeutic efficacy. Therefore, based on these findings, it would be reasonable for lung cancer patients to avoid the exposure to chrysin containing products during the active treatment phase with DOC [452]. Another natural flavone *baicalein* synergistically enhanced DOC-induced decrease in cell viability of different human pancreatic cancer cell lines HPAF-II, MIA PaCa-2 and PANC-1. In fact, cotreatment of PANC-1 cells with baicalein and DOC led to increase in S phase cell cycle arrest and apoptosis, besides suppression of cellular migration, as compared to DOC monotherapy. These data suggest that baicalein might be a potential adjuvant agent to strengthen the therapeutic effects and improve the outcome of DOC regimen in the clinical treatment of pancreatic tumors [371]. In addition, baicalein augmented antiproliferative, proapoptotic, antiangiogenic and antiinvasive activities of DOC in human anaplastic thyroid cancer 8505c cells, through inhibition of ERK and Akt/mTOR signaling pathways. Combined treatment with both agents led to enhanced suppression of angiogenic markers, such as VEGF and transforming growth factor β (TGF-β), and invasive proteins, including N-cadherin, more than treatment with DOC alone [450]. Citrus flavone *nobiletin* or hexamethoxyflavone sensitized P-gp-overexpressing PTX-resistant human non-small cell lung cancer A549/T cells and human ovarian cancer A2780/T cells to therapeutic efficacy of DOC, probably via modulation of multiple proteins and signaling pathways, including suppression of P-gp (ABCB1) transporter activity [276]. Dimethylated flavone *tricin* synergistically enhanced antiproliferative properties of DOC in human metastatic hormone refractory prostate cancer PC-3 cells [458]. Furthermore, diglycosylated flavone *vicenin-2* increased growth inhibitory and anticlonogenic properties of DOC in both androgen receptor (AR)-negative PC-3 cells as well as androgen-dependent human prostate cancer LNCaP cells, by downregulating AR levels in LNCaP cells. Combined treatment of PC3 bearing mice with vicenin-2 and DOC led to synergistic tumor regression, accompanied by enhanced decrease in proliferative (Ki67) and angiogenic markers (CD31) and increase in apoptotic markers, among effects on other signaling proteins [459]. Another sugar-conjugated flavone, *baicalin* or baicalein 7-glucuronide, synergistically augmented DOC cytotoxicity in DOC-resistant human non-small cell lung cancer A549/DTX cells, when both agents were co-loaded into transferrin-decorated solid lipid nanoparticles. Moreover, treatment

Effects of Plant Flavonoids on Chemotherapeutic Efficacy of Cancer Drugs 337

of A549/DTX bearing mice with this dual nanoformulation led to almost complete suppression of xenograft tumor growth [451] (Table 6.32 and Table 6.33).

Table 6.33. Effects of flavonoids on anticancer action of docetaxel (DOC) *in vivo* conditions

Drug	Flavonoid	Biological system	Direction of combination	Effects	Ref.
DOC, 10 mg in dual Tf-decorated SLNs, i.v., via tail vein, every 3 days	Baicalin, 10 mg in dual Tf-decorated SLNs, i.v., via tail vein, every 3 days	A549/DTX human **lung** cancer cells injected s.c. into the right flank of BALB/c nude mice	↑	Almost complete suppression of tumor growth, the best tumor inhibition rate	[452]
DOC, 10 mg/kg, i.v., once on day 1	Chrysin, 50 mg/kg, orally, 5 days a week	A549 human **lung** cancer cells implanted s.c. in the right leg of 4w old female ICR mice	↑	Increase in DOC-induced tumor growth delay, decrease in tumor weight. Potentiation of apoptosis	[452]
DOC, 5 or 12.5 mg/kg, i.p., weekly	EGCG, 228 mg/kg, i.p., weekly	PC-3ML human **prostate** cancer cells injected i.p. in 5-6w old CD17 SCID mice	↑	Decrease in tumor volume, increase in mice survival rates. Increase in p53, p73, p21; promotion of apoptosis. Blocking of bone metastases (when PC-3ML cells were injected via tail vein)	[442]
DOC, 0.5 mg/kg, i.p., thrice a week	EGCG, 1.5 mg, i.p., daily	BGC-823 human **gastric** cancer cells injected into the right flank of BALB/c nude mice	↑	Potentiation of LDM DOC antitumor activities, increase in tumor growth delay, decrease in tumor volume. Decrease in MVD, improvement of DOC-induced antiangiogenic effects (decrease in CD31 and VEGF)	[453]
DOC, 30 mg/kg, topically to skin over the tumors, loaded into EGCG-nanoethosomes	EGCG, topically to skin over the tumors, as DOC-loaded EGCG-nanoethosomes	A375 human **melanoma** cells injected subcutaneously in the armpit of the left forelimb of 4w old male hairless mice (HRS/J)	↑	Increase in tumor growth inhibition, decrease in tumor volume. Improvement of DOC transdermal delivery, prolongation of its MRT	[460]
DOC, 5 mg/kg, i.v., a total of 3 doses in 6 days	Genistein, 1 g/kg diet, stopped with completion of DOC treatment	PC-3 human **prostate** cancer cells injected intraosseously directly into the marrow of surface of previously implanted bone of 4w old male homozygous CB-17 SCID/SCID mice	↑	Increase in DOC-induced tumor growth inhibition. Inhibition of osteolysis	[455]
DOC, 5 mg/kg, i.v., 3 doses every 48h, after 4 days of genistein	Genistein, 1 g/kg diet, for a total of 10 days	PC-3 human **prostate** cancer cells injected s.c. to 4w old male homozygous CB-17 scid/scid mice	↑	Sensitization of cells to DOC, increase in apoptosis (PARP cleavage). Blocking of DOC-induced NF-κB activation	[62]
DOC, 0.01 mg/kg, by oral gavage, alternate day with vicenin-2	Vicenin-2, 1 mg/kg, by oral gavage, alternate day with DOC	PC3 human **prostate** cancer cells injected s.c. into one flank of each 11w old athymic nude nu/nu mice	↑	Synergism in growth inhibition, decrease in tumor weight. Decrease in proliferation (Ki67) and angiogenesis marker (CD31); increase in E-cadherin level and apoptosis marker (PARP cleavage). Decrease in pAkt, pRb, PCNA, cyclin D1, fibronectin, IGF-1R	[459]

Akt, protein kinase B; IGF-1R, insulin like growth factor 1 receptor; LDM, low-dose metronomic therapy; MRT, mean residence time; MVD, microvessel density; NF-κB, nuclear factor-κB; PARP, poly (ADP-ribose) polymerase; PCNA, proliferating cell nuclear antigen; Rb, retinoblastoma; SLN, solid lipid nanoparticle; Tf, transferrin; VEGF, vascular endothelial growth factor.

Soy isoflavone *genistein* enhanced DOC-induced cell viability reduction and apoptosis in human ovarian cancer cell line A2780 and its CDDP-resistant subclone C200, when the cells were pretreated with genistein before addition of DOC. This chemosensitization effect was associated with inactivation of NF-κB signaling and suppression of downstream key survival factors, including survivin and cIAP1 [128]. Pretreatment with genistein synergistically augmented cell growth inhibitory and proapoptotic activities of DOC also in human breast cancer MDA-MB-231 cells, human lung cancer H460 cells and human prostate cancer PC-3 cells. In PC-3 cells, genistein completely abrogated DOC-stimulated NF-κB DNA binding activity, being at least partially responsible for sensitization of tumor cells to DOC. Moreover, genistein increased chemosensitivity to DOC therapy also in PC-3 bearing mice, blocking drug-induced NF-κB activation and resulting in better cancer cell killing effect [62]. In addition, genistein potentiated antiinvasive and antimetastatic activities of DOC in human prostate cancer PC-3 cells, by upregulating DOC-suppressed osteoprotegerin (OPG) expression and downregulating DOC-elevated MMP-9 levels. Although DOC is a cytotoxic drug, DOC-triggered decrease in OPG and increase in MMP-9 might promote metastatic cancer cell growth in the bone environment. Opposite effects of genistein on these bone remodeling- and tumor bone metastasis-related genes could contribute to the antimetastatic activity by preventing bone matrix degradation. Indeed, addition of genistein in DOC treatment regimen resulted in increased tumor growth inhibition in mice model intraosseously inoculated with PC-3 cells, indicating that dietary genistein significantly suppressed osteolysis and growth of prostate cancer bone metastasis [455]. These findings indicate that inclusion of genistein in DOC therapeutic regimen might improve the clinical outcome of the treatment of metastatic prostate tumors. Genistein enhanced DOC-induced growth inhibition and apoptosis also in human pancreatic cancer BxPC-3 cells through complete abrogation of DOC-induced NF-κB activation; showing that efficient therapeutic effects should be achievable with lower doses of DOC in the presence of genistein, allowing to mitigate toxic side effects on normal tissues [62, 132] (Table 6.32 and Table 6.33).

The major green tea flavanol, *EGCG*, augmented DOC-induced antiproliferative effects in androgen-independent human prostate cancer LAPC-4-A1 cells [457]. In human prostate cancer PC-3ML cells derived from bone marrow metastases, combined treatment with EGCG and DOC resulted in synergistic enhancement of therapeutic efficacy through increase in apoptosis-related genes p53, p73 and p21, and promotion of apoptotic death. EGCG potentiated antitumor action of DOC also in mice model implanted intraperitoneally with PC-3ML cells, reducing the tumor burden and markedly prolonging overall survival rates of experimental animals. In addition, bone metastases were significantly suppressed by combined treatment of mice that were intravenously inoculated with PC-3ML cells via tail vein. Therefore, EGCG in combination with relatively low doses of DOC might provide a novel therapeutic approach for the treatment of patients with highly aggressive and metastatic prostate tumors [442]. EGCG potentiated antitumor activities of DOC also in human gastric cancer BGC-823 mouse xenograft model. When DOC was administered as low-dose metronomic therapy (LDM), addition of EGCG led to significant increase in tumor growth delay, associated with smaller tumors with lower microvessel density and improved antiangiogenic effects on newly formed blood vessels [453]. Furthermore, co-loading of both EGCG and DOC into nanoethosomes resulted in augmentation of tumor growth inhibition in human melanoma A375 cells bearing mice as compared to DOC monotherapy. This chemosensitization was related to significantly shrunken tumors, suggesting that EGCG-nanoethosomes possess a great potential as drug carriers through the skin and prolonged exposure of tumors to the antineoplastic agent under the skin. Moreover, transdermal drug delivery can avoid gastrointestinal toxicities and thereby improve patient compliance [460] (Table 6.32 and Table 6.33).

Coencapsulation of abundant dietary flavonol *quercetin* and DOC into hyaluronic acid (HA)-modified PLGA-polyethyleneimine (PEI) nanoparticles resulted in synergistic cytotoxic, proapoptotic, antiinvasive and antimigratory effects in murine breast cancer 4T1 cells. This antitumor synergism was accompanied by downregulation of phosphorylated Akt and MMP-9 levels [456]. Therapeutic effects of DOC were augmented by quercetin also in human castration-resistant prostate cancer LAPC-4-A1 cells [457]. However, natural flavonolignan *silibinin*, at doses that are achievable in human plasma after oral administration, exhibited preferably antagonistic cytotoxic interactions when combined with DOC in different human prostate cancer cell lines, i.e., LNCaP, DU145 and PC-3 [321]. These findings suggest that men with prostate tumors should avoid the exposure to silibinin containing products during the active treatment phase with DOC, with the aim not to impair the therapeutic efficacy of this microtubules-interfering antineoplastic drug. Last but not least, addition of flavonostilbene *alopecurone B* in DOC treatment regimens led to sensitization of multidrug resistant (MDR) human osteosarcoma MG-63/DOX cells to DOC chemotherapy [235] (Table 6.32).

Based on the current preclinical findings, structurally different flavonoids affect DOC cytotoxicity in various ways, depending on the concentrations of agents, time schedule and specific characteristics of malignant cells (Figure 6.17). Alongside with promising synergistic combinations, such as baicalein-DOC against pancreatic tumors and genistein-DOC or EGCG-DOC against metastatic prostate cancers, antagonistic interactions have also been described in combining certain flavonoids (chrysin, silibinin) and DOC chemotherapy. Therefore, cancer patients should be extremely cautious in consuming plant-derived products rich in these bioactive compounds in the period of chemotherapeutic treatment with DOC. In particular, patients suffering from prostate tumors and receiving DOC chemotherapy should abstain from consuming dietary supplements containing milk thistle flavonolignan silibinin.

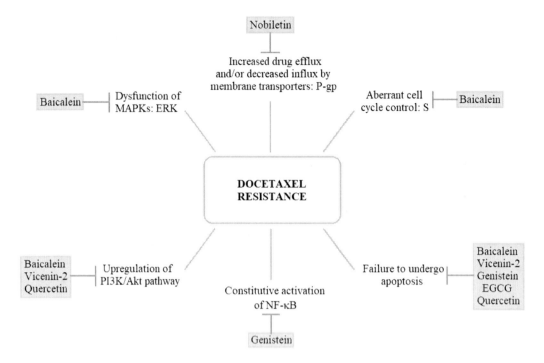

Figure 6.17. Modulation of docetaxel resistance by plant-derived natural flavonoids (Akt, protein kinase B; ERK, extracellular signal-regulated kinase; MAPK, mitogen-activated protein kinase; NF-κB, nuclear factor-κB; P-gp, P-glycoprotein; PI3K, phosphoinositide 3-kinase).

> According to the current experimental findings it is recommended for cancer patients *not to consume* dietary products or dietary supplements rich in following plant flavonoids during the active chemotherapeutic treatment phase with **docetaxel**:
> - **chrysin** in non-small cell lung cancer (*pretreatment with flavonoid*)
> - **silibinin** in prostate cancer

6.3.5. Cabazitaxel (CBZ)

Cabazitaxel (CBZ) is a semisynthetic taxane approved for the treatment of patients with hormone-resistant metastatic prostate tumors, after failure of DOC-based chemotherapy [1].

Only a couple of studies have been performed exploring the role of flavonoids fisetin and genistein on the therapeutic efficacy of CBZ in different preclinical prostate cancer models, both *in vitro* and *in vivo* conditions (Table 6.34 and Table 6.35). Natural flavonol *fisetin* was shown to synergistically increase antiproliferative and anticlonogenic activities of CBZ in human prostate cancer cell lines 22Rv1, C4-2 and PC-3M-luc-6. In 22Rv1 cells, fisetin promoted CBZ-induced apoptotic death; whereas in 22Rv1 bearing mice, combined treatment with fisetin and CBZ strengthened tumor growth inhibition and enhanced median survival rate of experimental animals as compared to the treatment with

Effects of Plant Flavonoids on Chemotherapeutic Efficacy of Cancer Drugs 341

either agent alone. This synergism was achieved by reducing proliferative markers (Ki67, PCNA) and enhancing apoptotic proteins. In PC-3M-luc-6 mouse xenograft model, enhanced therapeutic efficacy and tumor growth inhibition observed by combined treatment with fisetin and CBZ was associated with decrease in proliferative (Ki67, PCNA), angiogenic (VEGF, CD31, MVD) and metastatic markers (MMP-2, MMP-9, uPA), leading to reduction of metastatic foci in the excised liver tissue of combined treated mice. Thus, fisetin might enhance the antitumor efficacy of CBZ against prostate tumors through affecting multiple targets and regulating several cellular signaling mechanisms involved in antiproliferative, proapoptotic, antiinvasive and antimetastatic effects [402]. Soy isoflavone *genistein* synergistically augmented CBZ cytotoxicity in several human metastatic castration-resistant prostate cancer cell lines, i.e., ARCaP$_M$, C4-2 and PC3. Moreover, genistein significantly enhanced CBZ-induced growth retardation also in PC3-luciferase tumors in athymic nude mice, suppressing proliferation and promoting apoptotic death of malignant cells [461] (Table 6.34 and Table 6.35).

Table 6.34. Effects of flavonoids on anticancer action of cabazitaxel (CBZ)
***in vitro* conditions**

Drug	Flavonoid	Biological system	Direction of combination	Effects	Ref.
CBZ, 5 nM	Fisetin, 20 µM	22Rv1 human **prostate** cancer cell line	↑	Synergism in cell viability reduction, suppression of colony formation. Increase in apoptosis (decrease in Mcl-1; increase in Bax, PARP cleavage). Decrease in PCNA	[402]
CBZ, 5 nM	Fisetin, 20 µM	C4-2 human **prostate** cancer cell line	↑	Synergism in cell viability reduction, suppression of colony formation	[402]
CBZ, 5 nM	Fisetin, 20 µM	NCI/ADR-RES	↑	Decrease in colony formation, increase in apoptosis. Downregulation of P-gp	[402]
CBZ, 5 nM	Fisetin, 20 µM	PC-3M-luc-6 human **prostate** cancer cell line, androgen-independent	↑	Synergism in cell viability reduction, suppression of colony formation	[402]
CBZ, 0-100 nM	Genistein, 5, 10 µg/ml	ARCaP$_M$ human metastatic castration-resistant **prostate** cancer cell line	↑	Sensitization to CBZ. Synergism in cell viability reduction at 100 nM CBZ and 5 µg/ml genistein (CI 0.612)	[461]
CBZ, 0-100 nM	Genistein, 5, 10 µg/ml	C4-2 human metastatic castration-resistant **prostate** cancer cell line	↑	Sensitization to CBZ. Synergism in cell viability reduction at 100 nM CBZ and 5 µg/ml genistein (CI 0.589)	[461]
CBZ, 0-100 nM	Genistein, 5, 10 µg/ml	PC3 human metastatic castration-resistant **prostate** cancer cell line	↑	Sensitization to CBZ. Synergism in cell viability reduction at 20 nM CBZ and 5 µg/ml genistein (CI 0.693)	[461]

Bax, Bcl-2-associated X protein; CI, combination index; Luc, luciferase; Mcl-1, myeloid cell leukemia 1; PARP, poly (ADP-ribose) polymerase; PCNA, proliferating cell nuclear antigen; P-gp, P-glycoprotein.

Although the current knowledge about the combinational activities of flavonoids and CBZ in preclinical prostate cancer models is still very scarce, reports with fisetin and genistein have shown synergistic interactions and chemosensitizing effects to this microtubules-interfering antineoplastic drug. As CBZ is used for the treatment of metastatic androgen refractory prostate tumors after failure of DOC-based chemotherapy, increase in therapeutic efficacy by inclusion of natural non-toxic

342   *Katrin Sak*

flavonoids in CBZ regimen might be of great clinical significance in the management of advanced and resistant prostate cancers in the future.

Numerous combinations of structurally diverse natural flavonoids and different microtubules targeting chemotherapeutic drugs have been studied in preclinical assays with both cancer cell lines and xenograft models, revealing additive to synergistic but also antagonistic interactions. Several combinations are worth of further in vivo studies and clinical trials, particularly quercetin and vincristine against molecularly different breast tumor subtypes, fisetin and paclitaxel against non-small cell lung cancer, baicalein and docetaxel against pancreatic tumor, EGCG and taxanes (paclitaxel, docetaxel) against advanced prostate tumor, or genistein and taxanes (docetaxel, cabazitaxel) against metastatic prostate tumor. However, due to specific antagonistic interactions observed in preclinical assays, cancer patients should be advised about the possible adverse effects of certain plant-derived compounds on the therapeutic efficacy of antimitotic drugs (vincristine, paclitaxel, docetaxel) before they are undergoing active chemotherapeutic treatment phase. This would allow patients to make well-informed and more proper choices concerning their diets during the treatment period; with the aim not to contravene therapeutic efficacy, but rather enhance clinical outcome, improve quality of life and prolong overall survival time.

Table 6.35. Effects of flavonoids on anticancer action of cabazitaxel (CBZ) *in vivo* conditions

Drug	Flavonoid	Biological system	Direction of combination	Effects	Ref.
CBZ, 5 mg/kg, i.p., once a week	Fisetin, 20 mg/kg, i.p., thrice a week	22Rv1 human **prostate** cancer cells injected s.c. into 6-8w old athymic nude male mice	↑	Increase in tumor growth inhibition, increase in median survival of mice. Decrease in proliferative markers (PCNA, Ki67), induction of apoptosis (increase in Bax, decrease in Bcl-2)	[402]
CBZ, 5 mg/kg, i.p., once a week	Fisetin, 20 mg/kg, i.p., thrice a week	PC-3M-luc-6 human **prostate** cancer cells injected s.c. into 6-8w old athymic nude male mice	↑	Increase in tumor growth inhibition, decrease in tumor volume. Decrease in proliferative markers (PCNA, Ki67), MVD and angiogenesis (decrease in VEGF, CD31). Decrease in metastasis incidence in excised liver, decrease in metastatic markers (MMP-2/-9, uPA)	[402]
CBZ, 5 mg/kg, i.p., once a week	Genistein, 100 mg/kg, i.p., thrice a week	PC3-luc human **prostate** cancer cells injected s.c. into 6w old athymic nude BALB/c mice	↑	Increase in tumor growth suppression, decrease in tumor sizes. Increase in apoptosis (increase in Bax), decrease in proliferative marker Ki67	[461]

Bax, Bcl-2-associated X protein; Bcl-2, B-cell lymphoma 2; Luc, luciferase; MMP, matrix metalloproteinase; MVD, microvessel density; PCNA, proliferating cell nuclear antigen; uPA, urokinase-type plasminogen activator; VEGF, vascular endothelial growth factor.

6.4. Unclassified Drugs

There is a certain number of cytotoxic chemotherapeutic drugs which do not fit any of the above-mentioned categories of traditional anticancer agents. As interactions with flavonoids have been reported for these drugs in different preclinical cancer models, they are concerned in this subsection.

6.4.1. Bleomycin (BLM)

Bleomycin (BLM) is indicated for the treatment of Hodgkin and non-Hodgkin lymphomas, but also of testicular tumors and overall of epidermoid carcinomas [1]. BLM was isolated from the bacterium *Streptomyces verticillus* and is actually a mixture of glycopeptides. This drug attacks on deoxyribose moieties of DNA, producing free radicals and inducing DNA strand breaks, eventually leading to apoptotic death [1, 462]. However, toxicity of BLM to normal cells has remained a major problem in its clinical use, especially impaired lung function that may evolve in its terminal phase to lethal pulmonary fibrosis [1, 462].

**Table 6.36. Effects of flavonoids on anticancer action of unclassified drugs
in vitro conditions**

Drug	Flavonoid	Biological system	Direction of combination	Effects	Ref.
BLM	Alopecurone B, 10 μM	MG-63/DOX human **osteosarcoma** cell line, MDR, DOX-resistant	↑	Sensitization to BLM, 2.29-fold decrease in BLM IC_{50}	[235]
BLM, 1, 3 μg/ml	Genistein, 3, 5 μg/ml	HL-60 human **leukemia** cell line	↑	Increase in BLM-induced cytotoxicity. Increase in frequency of BLM-induced MN frequency and DNA damage	[462]
BLM, 0-100 μM	Luteolin, 5 μM	A549 human non-small cell **lung** cancer cell line	↑	Synergism in sensitization to BLM (CI<1), decrease in BLM IC_{50}. Inhibition of Nrf2	[181]
DHE, 25 μg/ml	EGCG, 50 μM	BA murine **mammary** carcinoma cell line	↑	Increase in DHE cytotoxicity, improvement of PDT efficacy. Increase in apoptosis (increased activation of JNK, caspases-3/-7, PARP cleavage), decrease in GRP78 and survivin expression. Attenuation of PDT-induced PGE2 expression	[464]
DHE, 0.1-50 μg/ml	Genistein, 25 μM	SNU 80 human anaplastic **thyroid** cancer cell line,	↑	Increase in cell growth inhibition and apoptosis (elevation of ROS; increase in Bax, caspases-3/-8/-9/-12, cyt c, PARP, AIF, CHOP)	[465]
ASP	5,7-DMF	YCUB-2 human acute lymphoblastic **leukemia** cell line	↓	Antagonism in cytotoxicity	[11]
ASP	5,7-DMF	YCUB-5 human acute lymphoblastic **leukemia** cell line	↓	Antagonism in cytotoxicity	[11]
ASP	5,7-DMF	YCUB-6 human acute lymphoblastic **leukemia** cell line	↓	Antagonism in cytotoxicity	[11]

AIF, apoptosis-inducing factor; Bax, Bcl-2-associated X protein; CHOP, CCAAT/enhancer binding protein homologues protein; CI, combination index; cyt c, cytochrome c; DMF, dimethoxyflavone; GRP, glucose-regulated protein; JNK, c-Jun N-terminal kinase; MDR, multidrug resistance; MN, micronuclei; Nrf2, nuclear factor (erythroid-derived 2)-like 2; PARP, poly (ADP-ribose) polymerase; PDT, photodynamic therapy; PGE2, prostaglandin E2; ROS, reactive oxygen species.

A few dietary flavonoids have been shown to augment BLM-induced cytotoxic activities in different human cancer cells. At low micromolar physiological doses (5 μM), natural flavone *luteolin* synergistically enhanced antitumor effects of BLM in human non-small cell lung cancer A549 cells by downregulating Nrf2 expression [181]. Pretreatment of human leukemia HL-60 cells with soy isoflavone *genistein* sensitized them to BLM chemotherapy, increasing drug-induced micronuclei frequency and DNA damage [462]. Flavonostilbene *alopecurone B* strengthened BLM cytotoxicity in multidrug resistant (MDR) human osteosarcoma MG-63/DOX cells [235] (Table 6.36).

Considering severe pulmonary toxicity related to administration of BLM, new strategies to reduce therapeutically efficient drug doses by inclusion of natural non-toxic flavonoids (luteolin, genistein) in BLM-based chemotherapeutic regimens might be of great clinical significance. However, further combinational studies are needed, investigating the role of more varied flavonoids on BLM cytotoxicity in diverse malignant models.

6.4.2. Photofrin (DHE)

Photofrin (DHE) or porfimer sodium is a photosensitizing chemotherapeutic agent used in photodynamic therapy (PDT) [1]. DHE is activated by light and is used for the local treatment of non-small cell lung cancer and esophageal cancer [1]. After intravenous administration of the prodrug DHE, a laser beam is applied to the tumor, producing cytotoxic free radicals and extensive oxidative stress, thereby stimulating death of malignant cells [1, 463-465]. Such cell killing process is associated with inflammatory reactions, vascular damage and hypoxia within photoexcited tumoral tissue [464]. However, although the main aim of PDT is to destroy tumoral cells without causing any adverse effects on normal healthy tissues, the major constraint of this therapy involves the need for the patient to prevent exposure to intense light, including the sun, for a period of at least a month [1, 465].

The effect of couple dietary flavonoids, i.e., EGCG and genistein, has been explored in combination with DHE-based PDT in preclinical cancer models. The major green tea flavanol *EGCG* significantly augmented cytotoxicity in murine mammary carcinoma BA cells exposed to DHE-mediated PDT, by significantly promoting apoptotic death. This sensitization effect was achieved via suppression of PDT-induced prosurvival proteins GRP78 and survivin, besides reducing prostaglandin E2 (PGE2) levels. Moreover, combined treatment of BA tumors in mice with EGCG and DHE led to enhanced PDT responsiveness and improved tumor cure rate; accompanied by production of proapoptotic reaction and decrease in expression of PDT-induced inflammatory and angiogenic molecules within the tumor microenvironment (PGE2, MMP-2, MMP-9, VEGF) [464]. Soy isoflavone *genistein* improved DHE-mediated PDT tumoricidal

Effects of Plant Flavonoids on Chemotherapeutic Efficacy of Cancer Drugs 345

activity in human thyroid cancer SNU 80 cells as compared to the PDT treatment alone. This potentiation of antitumor effects was associated with elevation of ROS generation, increase in growth inhibition and promotion of apoptotic death in combined treated cells, via regulation of expression of different apoptosis-related proteins [465] (Table 6.36).

Thus, specific flavonoids (EGCG, genistein) could improve the DHE-mediated PDT efficacy through multiple mechanisms, suggesting that consuming products rich in these plant-derived dietary compounds during the administration of DHE might be beneficial for PDT responsiveness leading to improved clinical outcome.

6.4.3. Asparaginase (ASP)

Asparaginase (ASP) is an important component of the treatment protocols for acute lymphoblastic leukemia (ALL), but has also been used for some non-Hodgkin lymphomas. On the one hand, ASP is extracted from the cultures of *Escherichia coli* and can be considered as anticancer antibiotic; on the other hand, ASP is the only antineoplastic drug with an enzymatic nature, thus revealing its double particularity. As differently from normal cells, malignant lymphoid cells are unable to synthesize amino acid asparagine and rely on extracellular asparagine, destroying circulating asparagine by ASP leads to inhibition of protein synthesis and apoptotic death [1].

The only combinational study of flavonoids and ASP was focused on the natural flavone *5,7-dimethoxyflavone (5,7-DMF)*. As a result, antagonistic interaction of 5,7-DMF and ASP was described in several human ALL cell lines, i.e., YCUB-2, YCUB-5 and YCUB-6, leading to decrease in ASP therapeutic efficacy [11] (Table 6.36).

Combination therapy with 5,7-DMF and ASP is not recommended and therefore, it would be reasonable of patients with acute lymphoblastic leukemia to avoid the intake of products containing 5,7-DMF when undergoing chemotherapy with ASP, with the aim not to reduce the drug therapeutic efficacy.

According to the current experimental findings it is recommended for cancer patients *not to consume* dietary products or dietary supplements rich in following plant flavonoids during the active chemotherapeutic treatment phase with **asparaginase**:
- **5,7-dimethoxyflavone** in acute lymphoblastic leukemia

REFERENCES

[1] Tredaniel J. *Cancer Drugs. A practical approach to drugs available to us.* ESKA Publishing, 2015. 352 pp.

[2]   Raina K, Agarwal R. Combinatorial strategies for cancer eradication by silibinin and cytotoxic agents: efficacy and mechanisms. *Acta Pharmacol Sin* 2007; 28: 1466-75.

[3]   Zhao H, Yuan X, Li D, Chen H, Jiang J, Wang Z, Sun X, Zheng Q. Isoliquiritigen enhances the antitumour activity and decreases the genotoxic effect of cyclophosphamide. *Molecules* 2013; 18: 8786-98.

[4]   Hosseinimehr SJ, Jalayer Z, Naghshvar F, Mahmoudzadeh A, Hesperidin inhibits cyclophosphamide-induced tumor growth delay in mice. *Integr Cancer Ther* 2012; 11: 251-6.

[5]   Smith ML, Murphy K, Doucette CD, Greenshields AL, Hoskin DW. The dietary flavonoid fisetin causes cell cycle arrest, caspase-dependent apoptosis, and enhanced cytotoxicity of chemotherapeutic drugs in triple-negative breast cancer cells. *J Cell Biochem* 2016; 117: 1913-25.

[6]   Touil YS, Seguin J, Scherman D, Chabot GG. Improved antiangiogenic and antitumour activity of the combination of the natural flavonoid fisetin and cyclophosphamide in Lewis lung carcinoma-bearing mice. *Cancer Chemother Pharmacol* 2011; 68: 445-55.

[7]   Seguin J, Brulle L, Boyer R, Lu YM, Ramos Romano M, Touil YS, Scherman D, Bessodes M, Mignet N, Chabot GG. Liposomal encapsulation of the natural flavonoid fisetin improves bioavailability and antitumor efficacy. *Int J Pharm* 2013; 444: 146-54.

[8]   Iriti M, Kubina R, Cochis A, Sorrentino R, Varoni EM, Kabala-Dzik A, Azzimonti B, Dziedzic A, Rimondini L, Wojtyczka RD. Rutin, a quercetin glycoside, restores chemosensitivity in human breast cancer cells. *Phytother Res* 2017; 31: 1529-38.

[9]   Di Lorenzo G, Pagliuca M, Perillo T, Zarrella A, Verde A, De Placido S, Buonerba C. Complete response and fatigue improvement with the combined use of cyclophosphamide and quercetin in a patient with metastatic bladder cancer: A case report. *Medicine (Baltimore)* 2016; 95: e2598.

[10]   Abaza MS, Orabi KY, Al-Quattan E, Al-Attiyah RJ. Growth inhibitory and chemo-sensitization effects of naringenin, a natural flavanone purified from Thymus vulgaris, on human breast and colorectal cancer. *Cancer Cell Int* 2015; 15: 46.

[11]   Goto H, Yanagimachi M, Goto S, Takeuchi M, Kato H, Yokosuka T, Kajiwara R, Yokota S. Methylated chrysin reduced cell proliferation, but antagonized cytotoxicity of other anticancer drugs in acute lymphoblastic leukemia. *Anticancer Drugs* 2012; 23: 417-25.

[12]   Wietrzyk J, Mazurkiewicz M, Madej J, Dzimira S, Grynkiewicz G, Radzikowski C, Opolski A. Genistein alone or combined with cyclophosphamide may stimulate 16/C transplantable mouse mammary cancer growth. *Med Sci Monit* 2004; 10: BR414-9.

[13] Wietrzyk J, Boratynski J, Grynkiewicz G, Ryczynski A, Radzikowski C, Opolski A. Antiangiogenic and antitumour effects in vivo of genistein applied alone or combined with cyclophosphamide. *Anticancer Res* 2001; 21: 3893-6.

[14] Wietrzyk J, Opolski A, Madej J, Radzikowski C. The antitumor effect of postoperative treatment with genistein alone or combined with cyclophosphamide in mice bearing transplantable tumors. *Acta Pol Pharm* 2000; 57 Suppl: 5-8.

[15] Wietrzyk J, Opolski A, Madej J, Radzikowski C. Antitumour and antimetastatic effect of genistein alone or combined with cyclophosphamide in mice transplanted with various tumours depends on the route of tumour transplantation. *In Vivo* 2000; 14: 357-62.

[16] Chen TC, Wang W, Golden EB, Thomas S, Sivakumar W, Hofman FM, Louie SG, Schönthal AH. Green tea epigallocatechin gallate enhances therapeutic efficacy of temozolomide in orthotopic mouse glioblastoma models. *Cancer Lett* 2011; 302: 100-8.

[17] Sang DP, Li RJ, Lan Q. Quercetin sensitizes human glioblastoma cells to temozolomide in vitro via inhibition of Hsp27. *Acta Pharmacol Sin* 2014; 35: 832-8.

[18] Zhang P, Sun S, Li N, Ho ASW, Kiang KMY, Zhang X, Cheng YS, Poon MW, Lee D, Pu JKS, Leung GKK. Rutin increases the cytotoxicity of temozolomide in glioblastoma via autophagy inhibition. *J Neurooncol* 2017; 132: 393-400.

[19] Pyrko P, Schönthal AH, Hofman FM, Chen TC, Lee AS. The unfolded protein response regulator GRP78/BiP as a novel target for increasing chemosensitivity in malignant gliomas. *Cancer Res* 2007; 67: 9809-16.

[20] Thangasamy T, Sittadjody S, Mitchell GC, Mendoza EE, Radhakrishnan VM, Limesand KH, Burd R. Quercetin abrogates chemoresistance in melanoma cells by modulating deltaNp73. *BMC Cancer* 2010; 10: 282.

[21] Jakubowicz-Gil J, Langner E, Rzeski W. Kinetic studies of the effects of Temodal and quercetin on astrocytoma cells. *Pharmacol Rep* 2011; 63: 403-16.

[22] Jakubowicz-Gil J, Langner E, Wertel I, Piersiak T, Rzeski W. Temozolomide, quercetin and cell death in the MOGGCCM astrocytoma cell line. *Chem Biol Interact* 2010; 188: 190-203.

[23] Yang L, Wang Y, Guo H, Guo M. Synergistic anti-cancer effects of icariin and temozolomide in glioblastoma. *Cell Biochem Biophys* 2015; 71: 1379-85.

[24] Jakubowicz-Gil J, Langner E, Badziul D, Wertel I, Rzeski W. Apoptosis induction in human glioblastoma multiforme T98G cells upon temozolomide and quercetin treatment. *Tumour Biol* 2013; 34: 2367-78.

[25] Hu J, Wang J, Wang G, Yao Z, Dang X. Pharmacokinetics and antitumor efficacy of DSPE-PEG2000 polymeric liposomes loaded with quercetin and temozolomide: Analysis of their effectiveness in enhancing the chemosensitization of drug-resistant glioma cells. *Int J Mol Med* 2016; 37: 690-702.

[26] Zhang Y, Wang SX, Ma JW, Li HY, Ye JC, Xie SM, Du B, Zhong XY. EGCG inhibits properties of glioma stem-like cells and synergizes with temozolomide through downregulation of P-glycoprotein inhibition. *J Neurooncol* 2015; 121: 41-52.

[27] Wang Y, Liu W, He X, Fei Z. Hispidulin enhances the anti-tumor effects of temozolomide in glioblastoma by activating AMPK. *Cell Biochem Biophys* 2015; 71: 701-6.

[28] Elhag R, Mazzio EA, Soliman KF. The effect of silibinin in enhancing toxicity of temozolomide and etoposide in p53 and PTEN-mutated resistant glioma cell lines. *Anticancer Res* 2015; 35: 1263-9.

[29] Thangasamy T, Sittadjody S, Limesand KH, Burd R. Tyrosinase overexpression promotes ATM-dependent p53 phosphorylation by quercetin and sensitizes melanoma cells to dacarbazine. *Cell Oncol* 2008; 30: 371-87.

[30] Liu JD, Chen SH, Lin CL, Tsai SH, Liang YC. Inhibition of melanoma growth and metastasis by combination with (-)-epigallocatechin-3-gallate and dacarbazine in mice. *J Cell Biochem* 2001; 83: 631-42.

[31] Zhang K, Wong KP. Glutathione conjugation of chlorambucil: measurement and modulation by plant polyphenols. *Biochem J* 1997; 325: 417-22.

[32] Zhang K, Wong KP, Chow P. Conjugation of chlorambucil with GSH by GST purified from human colon adenocarcinoma cells and its inhibition by plant polyphenols. *Life Sci* 2003; 72: 2629-40.

[33] Khoshyomn S, Nathan D, Manske GC, Osler TM, Penar PL. Synergistic effect of genistein and BCNU on growth inhibition and cytotoxicity of glioblastoma cells. *J Neurooncol* 2002; 57: 193-200.

[34] Hoffman R, Graham L, Newlands ES. Enhanced anti-proliferative action of busulphan by quercetin on the human leukaemia cell line K562. *Br J Cancer* 1989; 59: 347-8.

[35] Jiang YY, Wang HJ, Wang J, Tashiro S, Onodera S, Ikejima T. The protective effect of silibinin against mitomycin C-induced intrinsic apoptosis in human melanoma A375-S2 cells. *J Pharmacol Sci* 2009; 111: 137-46.

[36] Parkins CS, Denekamp J, Chaplin DJ. Enhancement of mitomycin-C cytotoxicity by combination with flavone acetic acid in a murine tumour. *Anticancer Res* 1993; 13: 1437-42.

[37] Lang M, Henson R, Braconi C, Patel T. Epigallocatechin-gallate modulates chemotherapy-induced apoptosis in human cholangiocarcinoma cells. *Liver Int* 2009; 29: 670-7.

[38] Chen Z, Huang C, Ma T, Jiang L, Tang L, Shi T, Zhang S, Zhang L, Zhu P, Li J, Shen A. Reversal effect of quercetin on multidrug resistance via FZD7/β-catenin pathway in hepatocellular carcinoma cells. *Phytomedicine* 2018; 43: 37-45.

[39] Jiang YY, Yang R, Wang HJ, Huang H, Wu D, Tashiro S, Onodera S, Ikejima T. Mechanism of autophagy induction and role of autophagy in antagonizing mitomycin C-induced cell apoptosis in silibinin treated human melanoma A375-S2 cells. *Eur J Pharmacol* 2011; 659: 7-14.

[40] Xu Z, Mei J, Tan Y. Baicalin attenuates DDP (cisplatin) resistance in lung cancer by downregulating MARK2 and p-Akt. *Int J Oncol* 2017; 50: 93-100.

[41] Su YK, Huang WC, Lee WH, Bamodu OA, Zucha MA, Astuti I, Suwito H, Yeh CT, Lin CM. Methoxyphenyl chalcone sensitizes aggressive epithelial cancer to cisplatin through apoptosis induction and cancer stem cell eradication. *Tumour Biol* 2017; 39: 1010428317691689.

[42] Singh VK, Arora D, Satija NK, Khare P, Roy SK, Sharma PK. Intricatinol synergistically enhances the anticancerous activity of cisplatin in human A549 cells via p38 MAPK/p53 signalling. *Apoptosis* 2017; 22: 1273-86.

[43] Nessa MU, Beale P, Chan C, Yu JQ, Huq F. Synergism from combinations of cisplatin and oxaliplatin with quercetin and thymoquinone in human ovarian tumour models. *Anticancer Res* 2011; 31: 3789-97.

[44] Yang Z, Liu Y, Liao J, Gong C, Sun C, Zhou X, Wei X, Zhang T, Gao Q, Ma D, Chen G. Quercetin induces endoplasmic reticulum stress to enhance cDDP cytotoxicity in ovarian cancer: involvement of STAT3 signaling. *FEBS J* 2015; 282: 1111-25.

[45] Jiang L, Zhang Q, Ren H, Ma S, Lu C, Liu B, Liu J, Liang J, Li M, Zhu R. Dihydromyricetin enhances the chemo-sensitivity of nedaplatin via regulation of the p53/Bcl-2 pathway in hepatocellular carcinoma cells. *PLoS One* 2015; 10: e0124994.

[46] Hagen RM, Chedea VS, Mintoff CP, Bowler E, Morse HR, Ladomery MR. Epigallocatechin-3-gallate promotes apoptosis and expression of the caspase 9a splice variant in PC3 prostate cancer cells. *Int J Oncol* 2013; 43: 194-200.

[47] Vittorio O, Brandl M, Cirillo G, Spizzirri UG, Picci N, Kavallaris M, Iemma F, Hampel S. Novel functional cisplatin carrier based on carbon nanotubes-quercetin nanohybrid induces synergistic anticancer activity against neuroblastoma in vitro. *RSC Adv* 2014; 4: 31378.

[48] Kiartivich S, Wei Y, Liu J, Soiampornkul R, Li M, Zhang H, Dong J. Regulation of cytotoxicity and apoptosis-associated pathways contributes to the enhancement of efficacy of cisplatin by baicalein adjuvant in human A549 lung cancer cells. *Oncol Lett* 2017; 13: 2799-804.

[49] Wang Y, Wang Q, Zhang S, Zhang Y, Tao L. Baicalein increases the cytotoxicity of cisplatin by enhancing gap junction intercellular communication. *Mol Med Rep* 2014; 10: 515-21.

[50] Kim EH, Jang H, Roh JL. A novel polyphenol conjugate sensitizes cisplatin-resistant head and neck cancer cells to cisplatin via Nrf2 inhibition. *Mol Cancer Ther* 2016; 15: 2620-9.

[51] Patricia Moreno-Londono A, Bello-Alvarez C, Pedraza-Chaverri J. Isoliquiritigenin pretreatment attenuates cisplatin induced proximal tubular cells (LLC-PK1) death and enhances the toxicity induced by this drug in bladder cancer T24 cell line. *Food Chem Toxicol* 2017; 109: 143-54.

[52] Tang B, Du J, Wang J, Tan G, Gao Z, Wang Z, Wang L. Alpinetin suppresses proliferation of human hepatoma cells by the activation of MKK7 and elevates sensitization to cis-diammined dichloridoplatium. *Oncol Rep* 2012; 27: 1090-6.

[53] Liu R, Ji P, Liu B, Qiao H, Wang X, Zhou L, Deng T, Ba Y. Apigenin enhances the cisplatin cytotoxic effect through p53-modulated apoptosis. *Oncol Lett* 2017; 13: 1024-30.

[54] Erdogan S, Turkekul K, Serttas R, Erdogan Z. The natural flavonoid apigenin sensitizes human CD44+ prostate cancer stem cells to cisplatin therapy. *Biomed Pharmacother* 2017; 88: 210-7.

[55] Xu YY, Wu TT, Zhou SH, Bao YY, Wang QY, Fan J, Huang YP. Apigenin suppresses GLUT-1 and p-AKT expression to enhance the chemosensitivity to cisplatin of laryngeal carcinoma Hep-2 cells: an in vitro study. *Int J Clin Exp Pathol* 2014; 7: 3938-47.

[56] Guo XF, Liu JP, Ma SQ, Zhang P, Sun WD. Avicularin reversed multidrug-resistance in human gastric cancer through enhancing Bax and BOK expressions. *Biomed Pharmacother* 2018; 103: 67-74.

[57] Li X, Huang JM, Wang JN, Xiong XK, Yang XF, Zou F. Combination of chrysin and cisplatin promotes the apoptosis of Hep G2 cells by up-regulating p53. *Chem Biol Interact* 2015; 232: 12-20.

[58] Yunos NM, Beale P, Yu JQ, Huq F. Synergism from sequenced combinations of curcumin and epigallocatechin-3-gallate with cisplatin in the killing of human ovarian cancer cells. *Anticancer Res* 2011; 31: 1131-40.

[59] Zhuo W, Zhang L, Zhu Y, Zhu B, Chen Z. Fisetin, a dietary bioflavonoid, reverses acquired Cisplatin-resistance of lung adenocarcinoma cells through MAPK/Survivin/Caspase pathway. *Am J Transl Res* 2015; 7: 2045-52.

[60] Lee H, Lee D, Kang KS, Song JH, Choi YK. Inhibition of intracellular ROS accumulation by formononetin attenuates cisplatin-mediated apoptosis in LLC-PK1 cells. *Int J Mol Sci* 2018; 19: E813.

[61] Yu S, Gong LS, Li NF, Pan YF, Zhang L. Galangin (GG) combined with cisplatin (DDP) to suppress human lung cancer by inhibition of STAT3-regulated NF-κB and Bcl-2/Bax signaling pathways. *Biomed Pharmacother* 2018; 97: 213-24.

[62] Li Y, Ahmed F, Ali S, Philip PA, Kucuk O, Sarkar FH. Inactivation of nuclear factor kappaB by soy isoflavone genistein contributes to increased apoptosis

induced by chemotherapeutic agents in human cancer cells. *Cancer Res* 2005; 65: 6934-42.

[63] Lee CK, Son SH, Park KK, Park JH, Lim SS, Kim SH, Chung WY. Licochalcone A inhibits the growth of colon carcinoma and attenuates cisplatin-induced toxicity without a loss of chemotherapeutic efficacy in mice. *Basic Clin Pharmacol Toxicol* 2008; 103: 48-54.

[64] Li QC, Liang Y, Hu GR, Tian Y. Enhanced therapeutic efficacy and amelioration of cisplatin-induced nephrotoxicity by quercetin in 1,2-dimethyl hydrazine-induced colon cancer in rats. *Indian J Pharmacol* 2016; 48: 168-71.

[65] Li J, Li B, Xu WW, Chan KW, Guan XY, Qin YR, Lee NP, Chan KT, Law S, Tsao SW, Cheung AL. Role of AMPK signaling in mediating the anticancer effects of silibinin in esophageal squamous cell carcinoma. *Expert Opin Ther Targets* 2016; 20: 7-18.

[66] Dhima IT, Peschos D, Simos YV, Gkiouli MI, Palatianou ME, Ragos VN, Kalfakakou V, Evangelou AM, Karkabounas SC. Modulation of cisplatin cytotoxic activity against leiomyosarcoma cells by epigallocatechin-3-gallate. *Nat Prod Res* 2018; 32: 1337-42.

[67] Yi JL, Shi S, Shen YL, Wang L, Chen HY, Zhu J, Ding Y. Myricetin and methyl eugenol combination enhances the anticancer activity, cell cycle arrest and apoptosis induction of cis-platin against HeLa cervical cancer cell lines. *Int J Clin Exp Pathol* 2015; 8: 1116-27.

[68] Kim EH, Jang H, Shin D, Baek SH, Roh JL. Targeting Nrf2 with wogonin overcomes cisplatin resistance in head and neck cancer. *Apoptosis* 2016; 21: 1265-78.

[69] Varela-Castillo O, Cordero P, Gutierrez-Iglesias G, Palma I, Rubio-Gayosso I, Meaney E, Ramirez-Sanchez I, Villarreal F, Ceballos G, Najera N. Characterization of the cytotoxic effects of the combination of cisplatin and flavanol (-)-epicatechin on human lung cancer cell line A549. An isobolographic approach. *Exp Oncol* 2018; 40: 19-23.

[70] Wang X, Jiang P, Wang P, Yang CS, Wang X, Feng Q. EGCG enhances cisplatin sensitivity by regulating expression of the copper and cisplatin influx transporter CTR1 in ovary cancer. *PLoS One* 2015; 10: e0125402.

[71] Bieg D, Sypniewski D, Nowak E, Bednarek I. Morin decreases galectin-3 expression and sensitizes ovarian cancer cells to cisplatin. *Arch Gynecol Obstet* 2018; 298: 1181-94.

[72] He F, Wang Q, Zheng XL, Yan JQ, Yang L, Sun H, Hu LN, Lin Y, Wang X. Wogonin potentiates cisplatin-induced cancer cell apoptosis through accumulation of intracellular reactive oxygen species. *Oncol Rep* 2012; 28: 601-5.

[73] Yellepeddi VK, Vangara KK, Kumar A, Palakurthi S. Comparative evaluation of small-molecule chemosensitizers in reversal of cisplatin resistance in ovarian cancer cells. *Anticancer Res* 2012; 32: 3651-8.

[74] Chen SF, Nieh S, Jao SW, Liu CL, Wu CH, Chang YC, Yang CY, Lin YS. Quercetin suppresses drug-resistant spheres via the p38 MAPK-Hsp27 apoptotic pathway in oral cancer cells. *PLoS One* 2012; 7: e49275.

[75] Zhou DH, Wang X, Feng Q. EGCG enhances the efficacy of cisplatin by downregulating hsa-miR-98-5p in NSCLC A549 cells. *Nutr Cancer* 2014; 66: 636-44.

[76] Zhao JL, Zhao J, Jiao HJ. Synergistic growth-suppressive effects of quercetin and cisplatin on HepG2 human hepatocellular carcinoma cells. *Appl Biochem Biotechnol* 2014; 172: 784-91.

[77] Gao C, Zhou Y, Jiang Z, Zhao Y, Zhang D, Cong X, Cao R, Li H, Tian W. Cytotoxic and chemosensitization effects of Scutellarin from traditional Chinese herb Scutellaria altissima L. in human prostate cancer cells. *Oncol Rep* 2017; 38: 1491-9.

[78] Chan MM, Soprano KJ, Weinstein K, Fong D. Epigallocatechin-3-gallate delivers hydrogen peroxide to induce death of ovarian cancer cells and enhances their cisplatin susceptibility. *J Cell Physiol* 2006; 207: 389-96.

[79] Jiang P, Wu X, Wang X, Huang W, Feng Q. NEAT1 upregulates EGCG-induced CTR1 to enhance cisplatin sensitivity in lung cancer cells. *Oncotarget* 2016; 7: 43337-51.

[80] Wang H, Luo Y, Qiao T, Wu Z, Huang Z. Luteolin sensitizes the antitumor effect of cisplatin in drug-resistant ovarian cancer via induction of apoptosis and inhibition of cell migration and invasion. *J Ovarian Res* 2018; 11: 93.

[81] Arafa el-SA, Zhu Q, Barakat BM, Wani G, Zhao Q, El-Mahdy MA, Wani AA. Tangeretin sensitizes cisplatin-resistant human ovarian cancer cells through downregulation of phosphoinositide 3-kinase/Akt signaling pathway. *Cancer Res* 2009; 69: 8910-7.

[82] Daker M, Ahmad M, Khoo AS. Quercetin-induced inhibition and synergistic activity with cisplatin – a chemotherapeutic strategy for nasopharyngeal carcinoma cells. *Cancer Cell Int* 2012; 12: 34.

[83] Lim J, Lee SH, Cho S, Lee IS, Kang BY, Choi HJ. 4-methoxychalcone enhances cisplatin-induced oxidative stress and cytotoxicity by inhibiting the Nrf2/ARE-mediated defense mechanism in A549 lung cancer cells. *Mol Cells* 2013; 36: 340-6.

[84] Cipak L, Novotny L, Cipakova I, Rauko P. Differential modulation of cisplatin and doxorubicin efficacies in leukemia cells by flavonoids. *Nutr Res* 2003; 23: 1045-57.

[85] Cipak L, Berczeliova E, Paulikova H. Effects of flavonoids on glutathione and glutathione-related enzymes in cisplatin-treated L1210 leukemia cells. *Neoplasma* 2003; 50: 443-6.

[86] Cipak L, Rauko P, Miadokova E, Cipakova I, Novotny L. Effects of flavonoids on cisplatin-induced apoptosis of HL-60 and L1210 leukemia cells. *Leuk Res* 2003; 27: 65-72.

[87] Kuo CY, Zupko I, Chang FR, Hunyadi A, Wu CC, Weng TS, Wang HC. Dietary flavonoid derivatives enhance chemotherapeutic effect by inhibiting the DNA damage response pathway. *Toxicol Appl Pharmacol* 2016; 311: 99-105.

[88] Sharma R, Gatchie L, Williams IS, Jain SK, Vishwakarma RA, Chaudhuri B, Bharate SB. Glycyrrhiza glabra extract and quercetin reverses cisplatin resistance in triple-negative MDA-MB-468 breast cancer cells via inhibition of cytochrome P450 1B1 enzyme. *Bioorg Med Chem Lett* 2017; 27: 5400-3.

[89] Hofmann J, Doppler W, Jakob A, Maly K, Posch L, Uberall F, Grunicke HH. Enhancement of the antiproliferative effect of cis-diamminedichloroplatinum(II) and nitrogen mustard by inhibitors of protein kinase C. *Int J Cancer* 1988; 42: 382-8.

[90] Scambia G, Ranelletti FO, Benedetti Panici P, Paintelli M, Bonanno G, De Vincenzo R, Ferrandina G, Maggiano N, Capelli A, Mancuso S. Inhibitory effect of quercetin on primary ovarian and endometrial cancers and synergistic activity with cis-diamminedichloroplatinum (II). *Gynecol Oncol* 1992; 45: 13-9.

[91] Scambia G, Ranelletti FO, Benedetti Panici P, Bonanno G, De Vincenzo R, Piantelli M, Mancuso S. Synergistic antiproliferative activity of quercetin and cisplatin on ovarian cancer cell growth. *Anticancer Drugs* 1990; 1: 45-8.

[92] Chan MM, Fong D, Soprano KJ, Holmes WF, Heverling H. Inhibition of growth and sensitization to cisplatin-mediated killing of ovarian cancer cells by polyphenolic chemopreventive agents. *J Cell Physiol* 2003; 194: 63-70.

[93] Wang Y, Han A, Chen E, Singh RK, Chichester CO, Moore RG, Singh AP, Vorsa N. The cranberry flavonoids PAC DP-9 and quercetin aglycone induce cytotoxicity and cell cycle arrest and increase cisplatin sensitivity in ovarian cancer cells. *Int J Oncol* 2015; 46: 1924-34.

[94] Maciejczyk A, Surowiak P. Quercetin inhibits proliferation and increases sensitivity of ovarian cancer cells to cisplatin and paclitaxel. *Ginekol Pol* 2013; 84: 590-5.

[95] Li N, Sun C, Zhou B, Xing H, Ma D, Chen G, Weng D. Low concentration of quercetin antagonizes the cytotoxic effects of anti-neoplastic drugs in ovarian cancer. *PLoS One* 2014; 9: e100314.

[96] Jakubowicz-Gil J, Paduch R, Piersiak T, Glowniak K, Gawron A, Kandefer-Szerszen M. The effect of quercetin on pro-apoptotic activity of cisplatin in HeLa cells. *Biochem Pharmacol* 2005; 69: 1343-50.

[97] Sharma H, Sen S, Singh N. Molecular pathways in the chemosensitization of cisplatin by quercetin in human head and neck cancer. *Cancer Biol Ther* 2005; 4: 949-55.

[98] Kuhar M, Imran S, Singh N. Curcumin and quercetin combined with cisplatin to induce apoptosis in human laryngeal carcinoma Hep-2 cells through the mitochondrial pathway. *J Cancer Mol* 2007; 3: 121-8.

[99] Borska S, Gebarowska E, Wysocka T, Drag-Zalesinska M, Zabel M. The effects of quercetin vs cisplatin on proliferation and the apoptotic process in A549 and SW1271 cell lines in in vitro conditions. *Folia Morphol (Warsz)* 2004; 63: 103-5.

[100] Kuhar M, Sen S, Singh N. Role of mitochondria in quercetin-enhanced chemotherapeutic response in human non-small cell lung carcinoma H-520 cells. *Anticancer Res* 2006; 26: 1297-303.

[101] Demiroglu-Zergeroglu A, Basara-Cigerim B, Kilic E, Yanikkaya-Demirel G. The investigation of effects of quercetin and its combination with Cisplatin on malignant mesothelioma cells in vitro. *J Biomed Biotechnol* 2010; 2010: 851589.

[102] Zhang X, Guo Q, Chen J, Chen Z. Quercetin enhances cisplatin sensitivity of human osteosarcoma cells by modulating microRNA-217-KRAS axis. *Mol Cells* 2015; 38: 638-42.

[103] Hofmann J, Fiebig HH, Winterhalter BR, Berger DP, Grunicke H. Enhancement of the antiproliferative activity of cis-diamminedichloroplatinum(II) by quercetin. *Int J Cancer* 1990; 45: 536-9.

[104] Caltagirone S, Rossi C, Poggi A, Ranelletti FO, Natali PG, Brunetti M, Aiello FB, Piantelli M. Flavonoids apigenin and quercetin inhibit melanoma growth and metastatic potential. *Int J Cancer* 2000; 87: 595-600.

[105] Sung B, Pandey MK, Aggarwal BB. Fisetin, an inhibitor of cyclin-dependent kinase 6, down-regulates nuclear factor-kappaB-regulated cell proliferation, antiapoptotic and metastatic gene products through the suppression of TAK-1 and receptor-interacting protein-regulated IkappaBalpha kinase activation. *Mol Pharmacol* 2007; 71: 1703-14.

[106] Tripathi R, Samadder T, Gupta S, Surolia A, Shaha C. Anticancer activity of a combination of cisplatin and fisetin in embryonal carcinoma cells and xenograft tumors. *Mol Cancer Ther* 2011; 10: 255-68.

[107] Zhang BY, Wang YM, Gong H, Zhao H, Lv XY, Yuan GH, Han SR. Isorhamnetin flavonoid synergistically enhances the anticancer activity and apoptosis induction by cis-platin and carboplatin in non-small cell lung carcinoma (NSCLC). *Int J Clin Exp Pathol* 2015; 8: 25-37.

[108] Yuan CH, Filippova M, Krstenansky JL, Duerksen-Hughes PJ. Flavonol and imidazole derivatives block HPV16 E6 activities and reactivate apoptotic pathways in HPV+ cells. *Cell Death Dis* 2016; 7: 2060.

[109] Nakatsuma A, Fukami T, Suzuki T, Furuishi T, Tomono K, Hidaka S. Effects of kaempferol on the mechanisms of drug resistance in the human glioblastoma cell line T98G. *Pharmazie* 2010; 65: 379-83.

[110] Luo H, Daddysman MK, Rankin GO, Jiang BH, Chen YC. Kaempferol enhances cisplatin`s effect on ovarian cancer cells through promoting apoptosis caused by down regulation of cMyc. *Cancer Cell Int* 2010; 10: 16.

[111] Zhu X, Ji M, Han Y, Guo Y, Zhu W, Gao F, Yang X, Zhang C. PGRMC1-dependent autophagy by hyperoside induces apoptosis and sensitizes ovarian cancer cells to cisplatin treatment. *Int J Oncol* 2017; 50: 835-46.

[112] Li J, Wang Y, Lei JC, Hao Y, Yang Y, Yang CX, Yu JQ. Sensitisation of ovarian cancer cells to cisplatin by flavonoids from Scutellaria barbata. *Nat Prod Res* 2014; 28: 683-9.

[113] Flores-Perez A, Marchat LA, Sanchez LL, Romero-Zamora D, Arechaga-Ocampo E, Ramirez-Torres N, Chavez JD, Carlos-Reyes A, Astudillo-de la Vega H, Ruiz-Garcia E, Gonzales-Perez A, Lopez-Camarillo C. Differential proteomic analysis reveals that EGCG inhibits HDGF and activates apoptosis to increase the sensitivity of non-small cells lung cancer to chemotherapy. *Proteomics Clin Appl* 2016; 10: 172-82.

[114] Zhang Y, Wang X, Han L, Zhou Y, Sun S. Green tea polyphenol EGCG reverse cisplatin resistance of A549/DDP cell line through candidate genes demethylation. *Biomed Pharmacother* 2015; 69: 285-90.

[115] Deng PB, Hu CP, Xiong Z, Yang HP, Li YY. Treatment with EGCG in NSCLC leads to decreasing interstitial fluid pressure and hypoxia to improve chemotherapy efficacy through rebalance of Ang-1 and Ang-2. *Chin J Nat Med* 2013; 11: 245-53.

[116] Singh M, Bhatnagar P, Mishra S, Kumar P, Shukla Y, Gupta KC. PLGA-encapsulated tea polyphenols enhance the chemotherapeutic efficacy of cisplatin against human cancer cells and mice bearing Ehrlich ascites carcinoma. *Int J Nanomedicine* 2015; 10: 6789-809.

[117] Singh M, Bhatnagar P, Srivastava AK, Kumar P, Shukla Y, Gupta KC. Enhancement of cancer chemosensitization potential of cisplatin by tea polyphenols poly(lactide-co-glycolide) nanoparticles. *J Biomed Nanotechnol* 2011; 7: 202.

[118] Mazumder ME, Beale P, Chan C, Yu JQ, Huq F. Epigallocatechin gallate acts synergistically in combination with cisplatin and designed trans-palladiums in ovarian cancer cells. *Anticancer Res* 2012; 32: 4851-60.

[119] Singh M, Bhui K, Singh R, Shukla Y. Tea polyphenols enhance cisplatin chemosensitivity in cervical cancer cells via induction of apoptosis. *Life Sci* 2013; 93: 7-16.

[120] Foygel K, Sekar TV, Paulmurugan R. Monitoring the antioxidant mediated chemosensitization and ARE-signaling in triple negative breast cancer therapy. *PLoS One* 2015; 10: e0141913.

[121] Hu F, Wei F, Wang Y, Wu B, Fang Y, Xiong B. EGCG synergizes the therapeutic effect of cisplatin and oxaliplatin through autophagic pathway in human colorectal cancer cells. *J Pharmacol Sci* 2015; 128: 27-34.

[122] Mayr C, Wagner A, Neureiter D, Pichler M, Jakab M, Illig R, Berr F, Kiesslich T. The green tea catechin epigallocatechin gallate induces cell cycle arrest and shows potential synergism with cisplatin in biliary tract cancer cells. *BMC Complement Altern Med* 2015; 15: 194.

[123] Lee SH, Nam HJ, Kang HJ, Kwon HW, Lim YC. Epigallocatechin-3-gallate attenuates head and neck cancer stem cell traits through suppression of Notch pathway. *Eur J Cancer* 2013; 49: 3210-8.

[124] Shervington A, Pawar V, Menon S, Thakkar D, Patel R. The sensitization of glioma cells to cisplatin and tamoxifen by the use of catechin. *Mol Biol Rep* 2009; 36: 1181-6.

[125] Liu D, Yan L, Wang L, Tai W, Wang W, Yang C. Genistein enhances the effect of cisplatin on the inhibition of non-small cell lung cancer A549 cell growth *in vitro* and *in vivo*. *Oncol Lett* 2014; 8: 2806-10.

[126] Lei W, Mayotte JE, Levitt ML. Enhancement of chemosensitivity and programmed cell death by tyrosine kinase inhibitors correlates with EGFR expression in non-small cell lung cancer cells. *Anticancer Res* 1999; 19: 221-8.

[127] Marverti G, Andrews PA. Stimulation of cis-diamminedichloroplatinum(II) accumulation by modulation of passive permeability with genistein: an altered response in accumulation-defective resistant cells. *Clin Cancer Res* 1996; 2: 991-9.

[128] Solomon LA, Ali S, Banerjee S, Munkarah AR, Morris RT, Sarkar FH. Sensitization of ovarian cancer cells to cisplatin by genistein: the role of NF-kappaB. *J Ovarian Res* 2008; 1: 9.

[129] Hu XJ, Xie MY, Kluxen FM, Diel P. Genistein modulates the anti-tumor activity of cisplatin in MCF-7 breast and HT-29 colon cancer cells. *Arch Toxicol* 2014; 88: 625-35.

[130] Pons DG, Nadal-Serrano M, Torrens-Mas M, Oliver J, Roca P. The phytoestrogen genistein affects breast cancer cells treatment depending on the ERα/ERβ ratio. *J Cell Biochem* 2016; 117: 218-29.

[131] Huang W, Wan C, Luo Q, Huang Z, Luo Q. Genistein-inhibited cancer stem cell-like properties and reduced chemoresistance of gastric cancer. *Int J Mol Sci* 2014; 15: 3432-43.

[132] Li Y, Ellis KL, Ali S, El-Rayes BF, Nedeljkovic-Kurepa A, Kucuk O, Philip PA, Sarkar FH. Apoptosis-inducing effect of chemotherapeutic agents is potentiated by

soy isoflavone genistein, a natural inhibitor of NF-kappaB in BxPC-3 pancreatic cancer cell line. *Pancreas* 2004; 28: e90-5.

[133] Chen P, Hu MD, Deng XF, Li B. Genistein reinforces the inhibitory effect of Cisplatin on liver cancer recurrence and metastasis after curative hepatectomy. *Asian Pac J Cancer Prev* 2013; 14: 759-64.

[134] Belcher SM, Burton CC, Cookman CJ, Kirby M, Miranda GL, Saeed FO, Wray KE. Estrogen and soy isoflavonoids decrease sensitivity of medulloblastoma and central nervous system primitive neuroectodermal tumor cells to chemotherapeutic cytotoxicity. *BMC Pharmacol Toxicol* 2017; 18: 63.

[135] Khoshyomn S, Manske GC, Lew SM, Wald SL, Penar PL. Synergistic action of genistein and cisplatin on growth inhibition and cytotoxicity of human medulloblastoma cells. *Pediatr Neurosurg* 2000; 33: 123-31.

[136] Tamura S, Bito T, Ichihashi M, Ueda M. Genistein enhances the cisplatin-induced inhibition of cell growth and apoptosis in human malignant melanoma cells. *Pigment Cell Res* 2003; 16: 470-6.

[137] Isonishi S, Saitou M, Yasuda M, Ochiai K, Tanaka T. Enhancement of sensitivity to cisplatin by orobol is associated with increased mitochondrial cytochrome c release in human ovarian carcinoma cells. *Gynecol Oncol* 2003; 90: 413-20.

[138] Shiotsuka S, Isonishi S. Differential sensitization by orobol in proliferating and quiescent human ovarian carcinoma cells. *Int J Oncol* 2001; 18: 337-42.

[139] Zhou L, Wu Y, Guo Y, Li Y, Li N, Yang Y, Qin X. Calycosin enhances some chemotherapeutic drugs inhibition of Akt signaling pathway in gastric cells. *Cancer Invest* 2017; 35: 289-300.

[140] Johnson JL, Gonzalez de Mejia E. Interactions between dietary flavonoids apigenin or luteolin and chemotherapeutic drugs to potentiate anti-proliferative effect on human pancreatic cancer cells, in vitro. *Food Chem Toxicol* 2013; 60: 83-91.

[141] Chan LP, Chou TH, Ding HY, Chen PR, Chiang FY, Kuo PL, Liang CH. Apigenin induces apoptosis via tumor necrosis factor receptor- and Bcl-2-mediated pathway and enhances susceptibility of head and neck squamous cell carcinoma to 5-fluorouracil and cisplatin. *Biochim Biophys Acta* 2012; 1820: 1081-91.

[142] Shi R, Huang Q, Zhu X, Ong YB, Zhao B, Lu J, Ong CN, Shen HM. Luteolin sensitizes the anticancer effect of cisplatin via c-Jun NH2-terminal kinase-mediated p53 phosphorylation and stabilization. *Mol Cancer Ther* 2007; 6: 1338-47.

[143] Chian S, Li YY, Wang XJ, Tang XW. Luteolin sensitizes two oxaliplatin-resistant colorectal cancer cell lines to chemotherapeutic drugs via inhibition of the Nrf2 pathway. *Asian Pac J Cancer Prev* 2014; 15: 2911-6.

[144] Wu B, Zhang Q, Shen W, Zhu J. Anti-proliferative and chemosensitizing effects of luteolin on human gastric cancer AGS cell line. *Mol Cell Biochem* 2008; 313: 125-32.

[145] Ryu S, Park S, Lim W, Song G. Effects of luteolin on canine osteosarcoma: Suppression of cell proliferation and synergy with cisplatin. *J Cell Physiol* 2019; 234: 9504-14.

[146] Jia WZ, Zhao JC, Sun XL, Yao ZG, Wu HL, Xi ZQ. Additive anticancer effects of chrysin and low dose cisplatin in human malignant glioma cell (U87) proliferation and evaluation of the mechanistic pathway. *J BUON* 2015; 20: 1327-36.

[147] Kachadourian R, Leitner HM, Day BJ. Selected flavonoids potentiate the toxicity of cisplatin in human lung adenocarcinoma cells: a role for glutathione depletion. *Int J Oncol* 2007; 31: 161-8.

[148] Mehnath S, Arjama M, Rajan M, Annamalai G, Jeyaraj M. Co-encapsulation of dual drug loaded in MLNPs: Implication on sustained drug release and effectively inducing apoptosis in oral carcinoma cells. *Biomed Pharmacother* 2018; 104: 661-71.

[149] Lu C, Wang H, Chen S, Yang R, Li H, Zhang G. Baicalein inhibits cell growth and increases cisplatin sensitivity of A549 and H460 cells via miR-424-3p and targeting PTEN/PI3K/Akt pathway. *J Cell Mol Med* 2018; 22: 2478-87.

[150] Yu M, Qi B, Xiaoxiang W, Xu J, Liu X. Baicalein increases cisplatin sensitivity of A549 lung adenocarcinoma cells via PI3K/Akt/NF-κB pathway. *Biomed Pharmacother* 2017; 90: 677-85.

[151] Lee SW, Song GS, Kwon CH, Kim YK. Beneficial effect of flavonoid baicalein in cisplatin-induced cell death of human glioma cells. *Neurosci Lett* 2005; 382: 71-5.

[152] Qian C, Wang Y, Zhong Y, Tang J, Zhang J, Li Z, Wang Q, Hu R. Wogonin-enhanced reactive oxygen species-induced apoptosis and potentiated cytotoxic effects of chemotherapeutic agents by suppression Nrf2-mediated signaling in HepG2 cells. *Free Radic Res* 2014; 48: 607-21.

[153] Enomoto R, Koshiba C, Suzuki C, Lee E. Wogonin potentiates the antitumor action of etoposide and ameliorates its adverse effects. *Cancer Chemother Pharmacol* 2011; 67: 1063-72.

[154] Lee E, Enomoto R, Suzuki C, Ohno M, Ohashi T, Miyauchi A, Tanimoto E, Maeda K, Hirano H, Yokoi T, Sugahara C. Wogonin, a plant flavone, potentiates etoposide-induced apoptosis in cancer cells. *Ann N Y Acad Sci* 2007; 1095: 521-6.

[155] Wang T, Gao J, Yu J, Shen L. Synergistic inhibitory effect of wogonin and low-dose paclitaxel on gastric cancer cells and tumor xenografts. *Chin J Cancer Res* 2013; 25: 505-13.

[156] Hou X, Bai X, Gou X, Zeng H, Xia C, Zhuang W, Chen X, Zhao Z, Huang M, Jin J. 3`,4`,5`,5,7-pentamethoxyflavone sensitizes Cisplatin-resistant A549 cells to Cisplatin by inhibition of Nrf2 pathway. *Mol Cells* 2015; 38: 396-401.

[157] Yoshimizu N, Otani Y, Saikawa Y, Kubota T, Yoshida M, Furukawa T, Kumai K, Kameyama K, Fujii M, Yano M, Sato T, Ito A, Kitajima M. Anti-tumour effects of nobiletin, a citrus flavonoid, on gastric cancer include: antiproliferative effects,

induction of apoptosis and cell cycle deregulation. *Aliment Pharmacol Ther* 2004; 20 Suppl1: 95-101.

[158] Wang HC, Lee AY, Chou WC, Wu CC, Tseng CN, Liu KY, Lin WL, Chang FR, Chuang DW, Hunyadi A, Wu YC. Inhibition of ATR-dependent signaling by protoapigenone and its derivative sensitizes cancer cells to interstrand cross-link-generating agents in vitro and in vivo. *Mol Cancer Ther* 2012; 11: 1443-53.

[159] Shi H, Wu Y, Wang Y, Zhou M, Yan S, Chen Z, Gu D, Cai Y. Liquiritigenin potentiates the inhibitory effects of cisplatin on invasion and metastasis via downregulation of MMP-2/9 and PI3K/AKT signaling pathway in B16F10 melanoma cells and mice model. *Nutr Cancer* 2015; 67: 761-70.

[160] Wu L, Yang W, Zhang SN, Lu JB. Alpinetin inhibits lung cancer progression and elevates sensitization drug-resistant lung cancer cells to cis-diammined dichloridoplatium. *Drug Des Devel Ther* 2015; 9: 6119-27.

[161] Chavoshi H, Vahedian V, Saghaei S, Pirouzpanah MB, Raeisi M, Samadi N. Adjuvant therapy with silibinin improves the efficacy of paclitaxel and cisplatin in MCF-7 breast cancer cells. *Asian Pac J Cancer Prev* 2017; 18: 2243-7.

[162] Tyagi AK, Agarwal C, Chan DC, Agarwal R. Synergistic anti-cancer effects of silibinin with conventional cytotoxic agents doxorubicin, cisplatin and carboplatin against human breast carcinoma MCF-7 and MDA-MB468 cells. *Oncol Rep* 2004; 11: 493-9.

[163] Molavi O, Narimani F, Asiaee F, Sharifi S, Tarhriz V, Shayanfar A, Hejazi M, Lai R. Silibinin sensitizes chemo-resistant breast cancer cells to chemotherapy. *Pharm Biol* 2017; 55: 729-39.

[164] Scambia G, De Vincenzo R, Ranelletti FO, Panici PB, Ferrandina G, D`Agostino G, Fattorossi A, Bombardelli E, Mancuso S. Antiproliferative effect of silybin on gynaecological malignancies: synergism with cisplatin and doxorubicin. *Eur J Cancer* 1996; 32A: 877-82.

[165] Giacomelli S, Gallo D, Apollonio P, Ferlini C, Distefano M, Morazzoni P, Riva A, Bombardelli E, Mancuso S, Scambia G. Silybin and its bioavailable phospholipid complex (IdB 1016) potentiate in vitro and in vivo the activity of cisplatin. *Life Sci* 2002; 70: 1447-59.

[166] Dhanalakshmi S, Agarwal P, Glode LM, Agarwal R. Silibinin sensitizes human prostate carcinoma DU145 cells to cisplatin- and carboplatin-induced growth inhibition and apoptotic death. *Int J Cancer* 2003; 106: 699-705.

[167] Sadava D, Kane SE. Silibinin reverses drug resistance in human small-cell lung carcinoma cells. *Cancer Lett* 2013; 339: 102-6.

[168] Zhang L, Yang X, Li X, Li C, Zhao L, Zhou Y, Hou H. Butein sensitizes HeLa cells to cisplatin through the AKT and ERK/p38 MAPK pathways by targeting FoxO3a. *Int J Mol Med* 2015; 36: 957-66.

[169] Hu FW, Yu CC, Hsieh PL, Liao YW, Lu MY, Chu PM. Targeting oral cancer stemness and chemoresistance by isoliquiritigenin-mediated GRP78 regulation. *Oncotarget* 2017; 8: 93912-23.

[170] Ma L, Wang R, Nan Y, Li W, Wang Q, Jin F. Phloretin exhibits an anticancer effect and enhances the anticancer ability of cisplatin on non-small cell lung cancer cell lines by regulating expression of apoptotic pathways and matrix metalloproteinases. *Int J Oncol* 2016; 48: 843-53.

[171] Krajnovic T, Kaluderovic GN, Wessjohann LA, Mijatovic S, Maksimovic-Ivanic D. Versatile antitumor potential of isoxanthohumol: Enhancement of paclitaxel activity in vivo. *Pharmacol Res* 2016; 105: 62-73.

[172] Sharma A, Upadhyay AK, Bhat MK. Inhibition of Hsp27 and Hsp40 potentiates 5-fluorouracil and carboplatin mediated cell killing in hepatoma cells. *Cancer Biol Ther* 2009; 8: 2106-13.

[173] Kluger HM, McCarthy MM, Alvero AB, Sznol M, Ariyan S, Camp RL, Rimm DL, Mor G. The X-linked inhibitor of apoptosis protein (XIAP) is up-regulated in metastatic melanoma, and XIAP cleavage by Phenoxodiol is associated with Carboplatin sensitization. *J Transl Med* 2007; 5: 6.

[174] Lu L, Yang LN, Wang XX, Song CL, Qin H, Wu YJ. Synergistic cytotoxicity of ampelopsin sodium and carboplatin in human non-small cell lung cancer cell line SPC-A1 by G1 cell cycle arrested. *Chin J Integr Med* 2017; 23: 125-31.

[175] Uesato S, Yamashita H, Maeda R, Hirata Y, Yamamoto M, Matsue S, Nagaoka Y, Shibano M, Taniguchi M, Baba K, Ju-ichi M. Synergistic antitumor effect of a combination of paclitaxel and carboplatin with nobiletin from Citrus depressa on non-small-cell lung cancer cell lines. *Planta Med* 2014; 80: 452-7.

[176] Yunos NM, Beale P, Yu JQ, Huq F. Synergism from the combination of oxaliplatin with selected phytochemicals in human ovarian cancer cell lines. *Anticancer Res* 2011; 31: 4283-9.

[177] Wang Z, Sun X, Feng Y, Liu X, Zhou L, Sui H, Ji Q, E Q, Chen J, Wu L, Li Q. Dihydromyricetin reverses MRP2-mediated MDR and enhances anticancer activity induced by oxaliplatin in colorectal cancer cells. *Anticancer Drugs* 2017; 28: 281-8.

[178] Qu Q, Qu J, Guo Y, Zhou BT, Zhou HH. Luteolin potentiates the sensitivity of colorectal cancer cell lines to oxaliplatin through the PPARγ/OCTN2 pathway. *Anticancer Drugs* 2014; 25: 1016-27.

[179] Li N, Zhang Z, Jiang G, Sun H, Yu D. Nobiletin sensitizes colorectal cancer cells to oxaliplatin by PI3K/Akt/MTOR pathway. *Front Biosci (Landmark Ed)* 2019; 24: 303-12.

[180] Hong ZP, Wang LG, Wang HJ, Ye WF, Wang XZ. Wogonin exacerbates the cytotoxic effect of oxaliplatin by inducing nitrosative stress and autophagy in human gastric cancer cells. *Phytomedicine* 2018; 39: 168-75.

[181] Tang X, Wang H, Fan L, Wu X, Xin A, Ren H, Wang XJ. Luteolin inhibits Nrf2 leading to negative regulation of the Nrf2/ARE pathway and sensitization of human lung carcinoma A549 cells to therapeutic drugs. *Free Radic Biol Med* 2011; 50: 1599-609.

[182] Dhivya S, Khandelwal N, Abraham SK, Premkumar K. Impact of anthocyanidins on mitoxantrone-induced cytotoxicity and genotoxicity: An in vitro and in vivo analysis. *Integr Cancer Ther* 2016; 15: 525-34.

[183] Papazisis KT, Kalemi TG, Zambouli D, Geromichalos GD, Lambropoulos AF, Kotsis A, Boutis LL, Kortsaris AH. Synergistic effects of protein tyrosine kinase inhibitor genistein with camptothecins against three cell lines in vitro. *Cancer Lett* 2006; 233: 255-64.

[184] Liang G, Tang A, Lin X, Li L, Zhang S, Huang Z, Tang H, Li QQ. Green tea catechins augment the antitumor activity of doxorubicin in an in vivo mouse model for chemoresistant liver cancer. *Int J Oncol* 2010; 37: 111-23.

[185] Staedler D, Idrizi E, Kenzaoui BH, Juillerat-Jeanneret L. Drug combinations with quercetin: doxorubicin plus quercetin in human breast cancer cells. *Cancer Chemother Pharmacol* 2011; 68: 1161-72.

[186] Yoshikawa M, Ikegami Y, Sano K, Yoshida H, Mitomo H, Sawada S, Ishikawa T. Transport of SN-38 by the wild type of human ABC transporter ABCG2 and its inhibition by quercetin, a natural flavonoid. *J Exp Ther Oncol* 2004; 4: 25-35.

[187] Reinicke KE, Kuffel MJ, Goetz MP, Ames MM. Synergistic interactions between aminoflavone, paclitaxel and camptothecin in human breast cancer cells. *Cancer Chemother Pharmacol* 2010; 66: 575-83.

[188] Hörmann V, Kumi-Diaka J, Durity M, Rathinavelu A. Anticancer activities of genistein-topotecan combination in prostate cancer cells. *J Cell Mol Med* 2012; 16: 2631-6.

[189] Tang Q, Ji F, Sun W, Wang J, Guo J, Guo L, Li Y, Bao Y. Combination of baicalein and 10-hydroxy camptothecin exerts remarkable synergetic anti-cancer effects. *Phytomedicine* 2016; 23: 1778-86.

[190] Wang Y, Wang H, Zhang W, Shao C, Xu P, Shi CH, Shi JG, Li YM, Fu Q, Xue W, Lei YH, Gao JY, Wang JY, Gao XP, Li JQ, Yuan JL, Zhang YT. Genistein sensitizes bladder cancer cells to HCPT treatment in vitro and in vivo via ATM/NF-κB/IKK pathway-induced apoptosis. *PLoS One* 2013; 8: e50175.

[191] Yu Y, Kong R, Cao H, Yin Z, Liu J, Nan X, Phan AT, Ding T, Zhao H, Wong STC. Two birds, one stone: hesperetin alleviates chemotherapy-induced diarrhea and potentiates tumor inhibition. *Oncotarget* 2018; 9: 27958-73.

[192] Lei CS, Hou YC, Pai MH, Lin MT, Yeh SL. Effects of quercetin combined with anticancer drugs on metastasis-associated factors of gastric cancer cells: in vitro and in vivo studies. *J Nutr Biochem* 2018; 51: 105-13.

[193] Ambrosini G, Seelman SL, Qin LX, Schwartz GK. The cyclin-dependent kinase inhibitor flavopiridol potentiates the effects of topoisomerase I poisons by suppressing Rad51 expression in a p53-dependent manner. *Cancer Res* 2008; 68: 2312-20.

[194] Motwani M, Jung C, Sirotnak FM, She Y, Shah MA, Gonen M, Schwartz GK. Augmentation of apoptosis and tumor regression by flavopiridol in the presence of CPT-11 in Hct116 colon cancer monolayers and xenografts. *Clin Cancer Res* 2001; 7: 4209-19.

[195] Fekrazad HK, Verschraegen CF, Royce M, Smith HO, Chyi Lee F, Rabinowitz I. A phase I study of flavopiridol in combination with gemcitabine and irinotecan in patients with metastatic cancer. *Am J Clin Oncol* 2010; 33: 393-7.

[196] Knezevic AH, Dikic D, Lisicic D, Kopjar N, Orsolic N, Karabeg S, Benkovic V. Synergistic effects of irinotecan and flavonoids on Ehrlich ascites tumour-bearing mice. *Basic Clin Pharmacol Toxicol* 2011; 109: 343-9.

[197] Imai Y, Tsukahara S, Asada S, Sugimoto Y. Phytoestrogens/flavonoids reverse breast cancer resistance protein/ABCG2-mediated multidrug resistance. *Cancer Res* 2004; 64: 4346-52.

[198] Akbas SH, Timur M, Ozben T. The effect of quercetin on topotecan cytotoxicity in MCF-7 and MDA-MB 231 human breast cancer cells. *J Surg Res* 2005; 125: 49-55.

[199] Alvero AB, Brown D, Montagna M, Matthews M, Mor G. Phenoxodiol-Topotecan co-administration exhibit significant anti-tumor activity without major adverse side effects. *Cancer Biol Ther* 2007; 6: 612-7.

[200] Schumacher M, Hautzinger A, Rossmann A, Holzhauser S, Popovic D, Hertrampf A, Kuntz S, Boll M, Wenzel U. Chrysin blocks topotecan-induced apoptosis in Caco-2 cells in spite of inhibition of ABC-transporters. *Biochem Pharmacol* 2010; 80: 471-9.

[201] Fatma S, Talegaonkar S, Igbal Z, Panda AK, Negi LM, Goswami DG, Tariq M. Novel flavonoid-based biodegradable nanoparticles for effective oral delivery of etoposide by P-glycoprotein modulation: an in vitro, ex vivo and in vivo investigations. *Drug Deliv* 2016; 23: 500-11.

[202] Papiez MA, Bukowska-Strakova K, Krzysciak W, Baran J. (-)-Epicatechin enhances etoposide-induced antileukaemic effect in rats with acute myeloid leukaemia. *Anticancer Res* 2012; 32: 2905-13.

[203] Coutinho L, Oliveira H, Pacheco AR, Almeida L, Pimentel F, Santos C, Ferreira de Oliveira JM. Hesperetin-etoposide combinations induce cytotoxicity in U2OS cells: Implications on therapeutic developments for osteosarcoma. *DNA Repair (Amst)* 2017; 50: 36-42.

[204] Lee E, Enomoto R, Koshiba C, Hirano H. Inhibition of P-glycoprotein by wogonin is involved with the potentiation of etoposide-induced apoptosis in cancer cells. *Ann N Y Acad Sci* 2009; 1171: 132-6.

[205] Ferreira de Oliveira JMP, Pacheco AR, Coutinho L, Oliveira H, Pinho S, Almeida L, Fernandes E, Santos C. Combination of etoposide and fisetin results in anti-cancer efficiency against osteosarcoma cell models. *Arch Toxicol* 2018; 92: 1205-14.

[206] Mahbub AA, Le Maitre CL, Haywood-Small SL, Cross NA, Jordan-Mahy N. Polyphenols act synergistically with doxorubicin and etoposide in leukaemia cell lines. *Cell Death Discov* 2015; 1: 15043.

[207] Jia H, Yang Q, Wang T, Cao Y, Jiang QY, Ma HD, Sun HW, Hou MX, Yang YP, Feng F. Rhamnetin induces sensitization of hepatocellular carcinoma cells to a small molecular kinase inhibitor or chemotherapeutic agents. *Biochim Biophys Acta* 2016; 1860: 1417-30.

[208] Cai X, Liu X. Inhibition of Thr-55 phosphorylation restores p53 nuclear localization and sensitizes cancer cells to DNA damage. *Proc Natl Acad Sci USA* 2008; 105: 16958-63.

[209] Ermakova SP, Kang BS, Choi BY, Choi HS, Schuster TF, Ma WY, Bode AM, Dong Z. (-)-Epigallocatechin gallate overcomes resistance to etoposide-induced cell death by targeting the molecular chaperone glucose-regulated protein 78. *Cancer Res* 2006; 66: 9260-9.

[210] Hwang JT, Ha J, Park IJ, Lee SK, Baik HW, Kim YM, Park OJ. Apoptotic effect of EGCG in HT-29 colon cancer cells via AMPK signal pathway. *Cancer Lett* 2007; 247: 115-21.

[211] Bortul R, Tazzari PL, Billi AM, Tabellini G, Mantovani I, Cappellini A, Grafone T, Martinelli G, Conte R, Martelli AM. Deguelin, a PI3K/AKT inhibitor, enhances chemosensitivity of leukaemia cells with an active PI3K/AKT pathway. *Br J Haematol* 2005; 129: 677-86.

[212] Punia R, Raina K, Agarwal R, Singh RP. Acacetin enhances the therapeutic efficacy of doxorubicin in non-small-cell lung carcinoma cells. *PLoS One* 2017; 12: e0182870.

[213] Liu Q, Li J, Pu G, Zhang F, Liu H, Zhang Y. Co-delivery of baicalein and doxorubicin by hyaluronic acid decorated nanostructured lipid carriers for breast cancer therapy. *Drug Deliv* 2016; 23: 1364-8.

[214] Cheng T, Liu J, Ren J, Huang F, Ou H, Ding Y, Zhang Y, Ma R, An Y, Liu J, Shi L. Green tea catechin-based complex micelles combined with doxorubicin to overcome cardiotoxicity and multidrug resistance. *Theranostics* 2016; 6: 1277-92.

[215] Zhu H, Luo P, Fu Y, Wang J, Dai J, Shao J, Yang X, Chang L, Weng Q, Yang B, He Q. Dihydromyricetin prevents cardiotoxicity and enhances anticancer activity induced by adriamycin. *Oncotarget* 2015; 6: 3254-67.

[216] Rudolfova P, Hanusova V, Skalova L, Bartikova H, Matouskova P, Bousova I. Effect of selected catechins on doxorubicin antiproliferative efficacy and hepatotoxicity in vitro. *Acta Pharm* 2014; 64: 199-209.

[217] Zhang FY, Du GJ, Zhang L, Zhang CL, Lu WL, Liang W. Naringenin enhances the anti-tumor effect of doxorubicin through selectively inhibiting the activity of multidrug resistance-associated proteins but not P-glycoprotein. *Pharm Res* 2009; 26: 914-25.

[218] Heeba GH, Mahmoud ME. Dual effects of quercetin in doxorubicin-induced nephrotoxicity in rats and its modulation of the cytotoxic activity of doxorubicin on human carcinoma cells. *Environ Toxicol* 2016; 31: 624-36.

[219] Czepas J, Gwozdzinski K. The flavonoid quercetin: possible solution for anthracycline-induced cardiotoxicity and multidrug resistance. *Biomed Pharmacother* 2014; 68: 1149-59.

[220] Tsai LC, Hsieh HY, Lu KY, Wang SY, Mi FL. EGCG/gelatin-doxorubicin gold nanoparticles enhance therapeutic efficacy of doxorubicin for prostate cancer treatment. *Nanomedicine (Lond)* 2016; 11: 9-30.

[221] Chen L, Ye HL, Zhang G, Yao WM, Chen XZ, Zhang FC, Liang G. Autophagy inhibition contributes to the synergistic interaction between EGCG and doxorubicin to kill the hepatoma Hep3B cells. *PLoS One* 2014; 9: e85771.

[222] Budak-Alpdogan T, Chen B, Warrier A, Medina DJ, Moore D, Bertino JR. Retinoblastoma tumor suppressor gene expression determines the response to sequential flavopiridol and doxorubicin treatment in small-cell lung carcinoma. *Clin Cancer Res* 2009; 15: 1232-40.

[223] Xue JP, Wang G, Zhao ZB, Wang Q, Shi Y. Synergistic cytotoxic effect of genistein and doxorubicin on drug-resistant human breast cancer MCF-7/Adr cells. *Oncol Rep* 2014; 32: 1647-53.

[224] Wang G, Zhang D, Yang S, Wang Y, Tang Z, Fu X. Co-administration of genistein with doxorubicin-loaded polypeptide nanoparticles weakens the metastasis of malignant prostate cancer by amplifying oxidative damage. *Biomater Sci* 2018; 6: 827-35.

[225] Donia TIK, Gerges MN, Mohamed TM. Amelioration effect of Egyptian sweet orange hesperidin on Ehrlich ascites carcinoma (EAC) bearing mice. *Chem Biol Interact* 2018; 285: 76-84.

[226] Sun L, Chen W, Qu L, Wu J, Si J. Icaritin reverses multidrug resistance of HepG2/ADR human hepatoma cells via downregulation of MDR1 and P-glycoprotein expression. *Mol Med Rep* 2013; 8: 1883-7.

[227] Li S, Yuan S, Zhao Q, Wang B, Wang X, Li K. Quercetin enhances chemo-therapeutic effect of doxorubicin against human breast cancer cells while reducing toxic side effects of it. *Biomed Pharmacother* 2018; 100: 441-7.

[228] Mihaila M, Bostan M, Hotnog D, Ferdes M, Brasoveanu LL. Real-time analysis of quercetin, resveratrol and/or doxorubicin effects in MCF-7 cells. *Rom Biotechnol Lett* 2013; 18: 8106-14.

[229] Brito AF, Ribeiro M, Abrantes AM, Pires AS, Teixo RJ, Tralhao JG, Botelho MF. Quercetin in cancer treatment, alone or in combination with conventional therapeutics? *Curr Med Chem* 2015; 22: 3025-39.

[230] Du G, Lin H, Yang Y, Zhang S, Wu X, Wang M, Ji L, Lu L, Yu L, Han G. Dietary quercetin combining intratumoral doxorubicin injection synergistically induces rejection of established breast cancer in mice. *Int Immunopharmacol* 2010; 10: 819-26.

[231] Fang J, Zhang S, Xue X, Zhu X, Song S, Wang B, Jiang L, Qin M, Liang H, Gao L. Quercetin and doxorubicin co-delivery using mesoporous silica nanoparticles enhance the efficacy of gastric carcinoma chemotherapy. *Int J Nanomedicine* 2018; 13: 5113-26.

[232] Cote B, Carlson LJ, Rao DA, Alani AWG. Combinatorial resveratrol and quercetin polymeric micelles mitigate doxorubicin induced cardiotoxicity in vitro and in vivo. *J Control Release* 2015; 213: 128-33.

[233] Singh RP, Mallikarjuna GU, Sharma G, Dhanalakshmi S, Tyagi AK, Chan DC, Agarwal C, Agarwal R. Oral silibinin inhibits lung tumor growth in athymic nude mice and forms a novel chemocombination with doxorubicin targeting nuclear factor kappaB-mediated inducible chemoresistance. *Clin Cancer Res* 2004; 10: 8641-7.

[234] Rastegar H, Ahmadi Ashtiani H, Anjarani S, Bokaee S, Khaki A, Javadi L. The role of milk thistle extract in breast carcinoma cell line (MCF-7) apoptosis with doxorubicin. *Acta Med Iran* 2013; 51; 591-8.

[235] Xia YZ, Ni K, Guo C, Zhang C, Geng YD, Wang ZD, Yang L, Kong LY. Alopecurone B reverses doxorubicin-resistant human osteosarcoma cell line by inhibiting P-glycoprotein and NF-kappa B signaling. *Phytomedicine* 2015; 22: 344-51.

[236] Stammler G, Volm M. Green tea catechins (EGCG and EGC) have modulating effects on the activity of doxorubicin in drug-resistant cell lines. *Anticancer Drugs* 1997; 8: 265-8.

[237] Kwak MS, Yu SJ, Yoon JH, Lee SH, Lee SM, Lee JH, Kim YJ, Lee HS, Kim CY. Synergistic anti-tumor efficacy of doxorubicin and flavopiridol in an in vivo hepatocellular carcinoma model. *J Cancer Res Clin Oncol* 2015; 141: 2037-45.

[238] Sato Y, Sasaki N, Saito M, Endo N, Kugawa F, Ueno A. Luteolin attenuates doxorubicin-induced cytotoxicity to MCF-7 human breast cancer cells. *Biol Pharm Bull* 2015; 38: 703-9.

[239] Yurtcu E, Iseri Ö, Sahin F. Genotoxic and cytotoxic effects of doxorubicin and silymarin on human hepatocellular carcinoma cells. *Hum Exp Toxicol* 2014; 33: 1269-76.

[240] Zhang Q, Wei D, Liu J. In vivo reversal of doxorubicin resistance by (-)-epigallocatechin gallate in a solid human carcinoma xenograft. *Cancer Lett* 2004; 208: 179-86.

[241] Yurtcu E, Darcansov Iseri O, Iffet Sahin F. Effects of silymarin and silymarin-doxorubicin applications on telomerase activity of human hepatocellular carcinoma cell line HepG2. *J BUON* 2015; 20: 555-61.

[242] Brechbuhl HM, Kachadourian R, Min E, Chan D, Day BJ. Chrysin enhances doxorubicin-induced cytotoxicity in human lung epithelial cancer cell lines: the role of glutathione. *Toxicol Appl Pharmacol* 2012; 258: 1-9.

[243] Mei Y, Wei D, Liu J. Reversal of cancer multidrug resistance by tea polyphenol in KB cells. *J Chemother* 2003; 15: 260-5.

[244] Wei D, Mei Y, Liu J. Quantification of doxorubicin and validation of reversal effect of tea polyphenols on multidrug resistance in human carcinoma cells. *Biotechnol Lett* 2003; 25: 291-4.

[245] Namazi Sarvestani N, Sepehri H, Delphi L, Moridi Farimani M. Eupatorin and salvigenin potentiate doxorubicin-induced apoptosis and cell cycle arrest in HT-29 and SW948 human colon cancer cells. *Asian Pac J Cancer Prev* 2018; 19: 131-9.

[246] Du G, Lin H, Wang M, Zhang S, Wu X, Lu L, Ji L, Yu L. Quercetin greatly improved therapeutic index of doxorubicin against 4T1 breast cancer by its opposing effects on HIF-1α in tumor and normal cells. *Cancer Chemother Pharmacol* 2010; 65: 277-87.

[247] Zhang B, Yu X, Xia H. The flavonoid luteolin enhances doxorubicin-induced autophagy in human osteosarcoma U2OS cells. *Int J Clin Exp Med* 2015; 8: 15190-7.

[248] Li SZ, Li K, Zhang JH, Dong Z. The effect of quercetin on doxorubicin cytotoxicity in human breast cancer cells. *Anticancer Agents Med Chem* 2013; 13: 352-5.

[249] Li SZ, Qiao SF, Zhang JH, Li K. Quercetin increase the chemosensitivity of breast cancer cells to doxorubicin via PTEN/Akt pathway. *Anticancer Agents Med Chem* 2015; 15: 1185-9.

[250] Li S, Zhao Q, Wang B, Yuan S, Wang X, Li K. Quercetin reversed MDR in breast cancer cells through down-regulating P-gp expression and eliminating cancer stem cells mediated by YB-1 nuclear translocation. *Phytother Res* 2018; 32: 1530-6.

[251] Minaei A, Sabzichi M, Ramezani F, Hamishehkar H, Samadi N. Co-delivery with nano-quercetin enhances doxorubicin-mediated cytotoxicity against MCF-7 cells. *Mol Biol Rep* 2016; 43: 99-105.

[252] Scambia G, Ranelletti FO, Panici PB, De Vincenzo R, Bonanno G, Ferrandina G, Piantelli M, Bussa S, Rumi C, Cianfriglia M, Mancuso S. Quercetin potentiates the effect of adriamycin in a multidrug-resistant MCF-7 human breast-cancer cell line: P-glycoprotein as a possible target. *Cancer Chemother Pharmacol* 1994; 34: 459-64.

[253] Zhang J, Luo Y, Zhao X, Li X, Li K, Chen D, Qiao M, Hu H, Zhao X. Co-delivery of doxorubicin and the traditional Chinese medicine quercetin using biotin-PEG2000-DSPE modified liposomes for the treatment of multidrug resistant breast cancer. *RSC Adv* 2016; 6: 113173.

[254] Lv L, Liu C, Chen C, Yu X, Chen G, Shi Y, Qin F, Qu J, Qiu K, Li G. Quercetin and doxorubicin co-encapsulated biotin receptor-targeting nanoparticles for minimizing drug resistance in breast cancer. *Oncotarget* 2016; 7: 32184-99.

[255] Mohana S, Ganesan M, Rajendra Prasad N, Ananthakrishnan D, Velmurugan D. Flavonoids modulate multidrug resistance through wnt signaling in P-glycoprotein overexpressing cell lines. *BMC Cancer* 2018; 18: 1168.

[256] Liu Z, Balasubramanian V, Bhat C, Vahermo M, Mäkilä E, Kemell M, Fontana F, Janoniene A, Petrikaite V, Salonen J, Yli-Kauhaluoma J, Hirvonen J, Zhang H, Santos HA. Quercetin-based modified porous silicon nanoparticles for enhanced inhibition of doxorubicin-resistant cancer cells. *Adv Healthc Mater* 2017; 6: 1601009.

[257] Hyun HB, Moon JY, Cho SK. Quercetin suppresses CYR61-mediated multidrug resistance in human gastric adenocarcinoma AGS cells. *Molecules* 2018; 23: E209.

[258] Wang G, Zhang J, Liu L, Sharma S, Dong Q. Quercetin potentiates doxorubicin mediated antitumor effects against liver cancer through p53/Bcl-xl. *PLoS One* 2012; 7: e51764.

[259] Daglioglu C. Enhancing tumor cell response to multidrug resistance with pH-sensitive quercetin and doxorubicin conjugated multifunctional nanoparticles. *Colloids Surf B Biointerfaces* 2017; 156: 175-85.

[260] Zanini C, Giribaldi G, Madili G, Carta F, Crescenzio N, Bisaro B, Doria A, Foglia L, di Montezemolo LC, Timeus F, Turrini F. Inhibition of heat shock proteins (HSP) expression by quercetin and differential doxorubicin sensitization in neuroblastoma and Ewing`s sarcoma cell lines. *J Neurochem* 2007; 103: 1344-54.

[261] Critchfield JW, Welsh CJ, Phang JM, Yeh GC. Modulation of adriamycin accumulation and efflux by flavonoids in HCT-15 colon cells. Activation of P-glycoprotein as a putative mechanism. *Biochem Pharmacol* 1994; 48: 1437-45.

[262] Chen FY, Cao LF, Wan HX, Zhang MY, Cai JY, Shen LJ, Zhong JH, Zhong H. Quercetin enhances adriamycin cytotoxicity through induction of apoptosis and regulation of mitogen-activated protein kinase/extracellular signal-regulated kinase/c-Jun N-terminal kinase signaling in multidrug-resistant leukemia K562 cells. *Mol Med Rep* 2015; 11: 341-8.

[263] Angelini A, Di Ilio C, Castellani ML, Conti P, Cuccurullo F. Modulation of multidrug resistance p-glycoprotein activity by flavonoids and honokiol in human doxorubicin- resistant sarcoma cells (MES-SA/DX-5): implications for natural sedatives as chemosensitizing agents in cancer therapy. *J Biol Regul Homeost Agents* 2010; 24: 197-205.

[264] Zhang S, Morris ME. Effects of the flavonoids biochanin A, morin, phloretin, and silymarin on P-glycoprotein-mediated transport. *J Pharmacol Exp Ther* 2003; 304: 1258-67.

[265] Ramachandran L, Manu KA, Shanmugam MK, Li F, Siveen KS, Vali S, Kapoor S, Abbasi T, Surana R, Smoot DT, Ashktorab H, Tan P, Ahn KS, Yap CW, Kumar AP, Sethi G. Isorhamnetin inhibits proliferation and invasion and induces apoptosis through the modulation of peroxisome proliferator-activated receptor γ activation pathway in gastric cancer. *J Biol Chem* 2012; 287: 38028-40.

[266] Brantley E, Amis L, Davis W. Apigenin augments the growth inhibitory effects of doxorubicin in breast cancer cells derived from African American patients. *Cancer Epidemiol Biomarkers Prev* 2007; 16: B81.

[267] Gao AM, Ke ZP, Wang JN, Yang JY, Chen SY, Chen H. Apigenin sensitizes doxorubicin-resistant hepatocellular carcinoma BEL-7402/ADM cells to doxorubicin via inhibiting PI3K/Akt/Nrf2 pathway. *Carcinogenesis* 2013; 34: 1806-14.

[268] Gao AM, Zhang XY, Hu JN, Ke ZP. Apigenin sensitizes hepatocellular carcinoma cells to doxorubic through regulating miR-520b/ATG7 axis. *Chem Biol Interact* 2018; 280: 45-50.

[269] Sabzichi M, Hamishehkar H, Ramezani F, Sharifi S, Tabasinezhad M, Pirouzpanah M, Ghanbari P, Samadi N. Luteolin-loaded phytosomes sensitize human breast carcinoma MDA-MB 231 cells to doxorubicin by suppressing Nrf2 mediated signalling. *Asian Pac J Cancer Prev* 2014; 15: 5311-6.

[270] Wang HW, Lin CP, Chiu JH, Chow KC, Kuo KT, Lin CS, Wang LS. Reversal of inflammation-associated dihydrodiol dehydrogenases (AKR1C1 and AKR1C2) overexpression and drug resistance in nonsmall cell lung cancer cells by wogonin and chrysin. *Int J Cancer* 2007; 120: 2019-27.

[271] Gao AM, Ke ZP, Shi F, Sun GC, Chen H. Chrysin enhances sensitivity of BEL-7402/ADM cells to doxorubic by suppressing PI3K/Akt/Nrf2 and ERK/Nrf2 pathway. *Chem Biol Interact* 2013; 206: 100-8.

[272] Xu X, Zhang X, Zhang Y, Yang L, Liu Y, Huang S, Lu L, Kong L, Li Z, Guo Q, Zhao L. Wogonin reversed resistant human myelogenous leukemia cells via inhibiting Nrf2 signaling by Stat3/NF-κB inactivation. *Sci Rep* 2017; 7: 39950.

[273] Zhong Y, Zhang F, Sun Z, Zhou W, Li ZY, You QD, Guo QL, Hu R. Drug resistance associates with activation of Nrf2 in MCF-7/DOX cells, and wogonin

reverses it by down-regulating Nrf2-mediated cellular defense response. *Mol Carcinog* 2013; 52: 824-34.

[274] Fu P, Du F, Liu Y, Hong Y, Yao M, Zheng S. Wogonin increases doxorubicin sensitivity by down-regulation of IGF-1R/AKT signaling pathway in human breast cancer. *Cell Mol Biol (Noisy-le-grand)* 2015; 61: 123-7.

[275] Wang Y, Miao H, Li W, Yao J, Sun Y, Li Z, Zhao L, Guo Q. CXCL12/CXCR4 axis confers adriamycin resistance to human chronic myelogenous leukemia and oroxylin A improves the sensitivity of K562/ADM cells. *Biochem Pharmacol* 2014; 90: 212-25.

[276] Ma W, Feng S, Yao X, Yuan Z, Liu L, Xie Y. Nobiletin enhances the efficacy of chemotherapeutic agents in ABCB1 overexpression cancer cells. *Sci Rep* 2015; 5: 18789.

[277] Meiyanto E, Hermawan A, Junedi S, Fitriasari A, Susidarti RA. Nobiletin increased cytotoxic activity of doxorubicin on Mcf-7 cells but not on T47d cells. *Int J Phytomed* 2011; 3: 129-37.

[278] Zheng J, Asakawa T, Chen Y, Zheng Z, Chen B, Lin M, Liu T, Hu J. Synergistic effect of baicalin and adriamycin in resistant HL-60/ADM leukaemia cells. *Cell Physiol Biochem* 2017; 43: 419-30.

[279] Mei Y, Qian F, Wei D, Liu J. Reversal of cancer multidrug resistance by green tea polyphenols. *J Pharm Pharmacol* 2004; 56: 1307-14.

[280] Mei Y, Wei D, Liu J. Reversal of multidrug resistance in KB cells with tea polyphenol antioxidant capacity. *Cancer Biol Ther* 2005; 4: 468-73.

[281] Qian F, Wei D, Zhang Q, Yang S. Modulation of P-glycoprotein function and reversal of multidrug resistance by (-)-epigallocatechin gallate in human cancer cells. *Biomed Pharmacother* 2005; 59: 64-9.

[282] Liu L, Ju Y, Wang J, Zhou R. Epigallocatechin-3-gallate promotes apoptosis and reversal of multidrug resistance in esophageal cancer cells. *Pathol Res Pract* 2017; 213: 1242-50.

[283] Stearns ME, Amatangelo MD, Varma D, Sell C, Goodyear SM. Combination therapy with epigallocatechin-3-gallate and doxorubicin in human prostate tumor modeling studies: inhibition of metastatic tumor growth in severe combined immunodeficiency mice. *Am J Pathol* 2010; 177: 3169-79.

[284] Wen Y, Zhao RQ, Zhang YK, Gupta P, Fu LX, Tang AZ, Liu BM, Chen ZS, Yang DH, Liang G. Effect of Y6, an epigallocatechin gallate derivative, on reversing doxorubicin drug resistance in human hepatocellular carcinoma cells. *Oncotarget* 2017; 8: 29760-70.

[285] Vittorio O, Le Grand M, Makharza SA, Curcio M, Tucci P, Iemma F, Nicoletta FP, Hampel S, Cirillo G. Doxorubicin synergism and resistance reversal in human neuroblastoma BE(2)C cell lines: An in vitro study with dextran-catechin nanohybrids. *Eur J Pharm Biopharm* 2018; 122: 176-85.

[286] Nazari M, Ghorbani A, Hekmat-Doost A, Jeddi-Tehrani M, Zand H. Inactivation of nuclear factor-κB by citrus flavanone hesperidin contributes to apoptosis and chemo-sensitizing effect in Ramos cells. *Eur J Pharmacol* 2011; 650: 526-33.

[287] Lim HA, Kim JH, Kim JH, Sung MK, Kim MK, Park JH, Kim JS. Genistein induces glucose-regulated protein 78 in mammary tumor cells. *J Med Food* 2006; 9: 28-32.

[288] Monti E, Sinha BK. Antiproliferative effect of genistein and adriamycin against estrogen-dependent and -independent human breast carcinoma cell lines. *Anticancer Res* 1994; 14: 1221-6.

[289] Satoh H, Nishikawa K, Suzuki K, Asano R, Virgona N, Ichikawa T, Hagiwara K, Yano T. Genistein, a soy isoflavone, enhances necrotic-like cell death in a breast cancer cell treated with a chemotherapeutic agent. *Res Commun Mol Pathol Pharmacol* 2003; 113-114: 149-58.

[290] Dash TK, Konkimalla VB. Formulation and optimization of doxorubicin and biochanin A combinational liposomes for reversal of chemoresistance. *AAPS PharmSciTech* 2017; 18: 1116-24.

[291] Liu Q, Sun Y, Zheng JM, Yan XL, Chen HM, Chen JK, Huang HQ. Formononetin sensitizes glioma cells to doxorubicin through preventing EMT via inhibition of histone deacetylase 5. *Int J Clin Exp Pathol* 2015; 8: 6434-41.

[292] Ji BS, He L. CJY, an isoflavone, reverses P-glycoprotein-mediated multidrug-resistance in doxorubicin-resistant human myelogenous leukaemia (K562/DOX) cells. *J Pharm Pharmacol* 2007; 59: 1011-5.

[293] Li X, Wan L, Wang F, Pei H, Zheng L, Wu W, Ye H, Wang Y, Chen L. Barbigerone reverses multidrug resistance in breast MCF-7/ADR cells. *Phytother Res* 2018; 32: 733-40.

[294] Tyagi AK, Singh RP, Agarwal C, Chan DC, Agarwal R. Silibinin strongly synergizes human prostate carcinoma DU145 cells to doxorubicin-induced growth inhibition, G2-M arrest, and apoptosis. *Clin Cancer Res* 2002; 8: 3512-9.

[295] Catanzaro D, Gabbia D, Cocetta V, Biagi M, Ragazzi E, Montopoli M, Carrara M. Silybin counteracts doxorubicin resistance by inhibiting GLUT1 expression. *Fitoterapia* 2018; 124: 42-8.

[296] Li WG, Wang HQ. Inhibitory effects of Silibinin combined with doxorubicin in hepatocellular carcinoma; an in vivo study. *J BUON* 2016; 21: 917-24.

[297] Molavi O, Samadi N, Wu C, Lavasanifar A, Lai R. Silibinin suppresses NPM-ALK, potently induces apoptosis and enhances chemosensitivity in ALK-positive anaplastic large cell lymphoma. *Leuk Lymphoma* 2016; 57: 1154-62.

[298] Qian F, Ye CL, Wei DZ, Lu YH, Yang SL. In vitro and in vivo reversal of cancer cell multidrug resistance by 2`,4`-dihydroxy-6`-methoxy-3`,5`-dimethylchalcone. *J Chemother* 2005; 17: 309-14.

[299] Huang HY, Niu JL, Zhao LM, Lu YH. Reversal effect of 2`,4`-dihydroxy-6`-methoxy-3`,5`-dimethylchalcone on multi-drug resistance in resistant human hepatocellular carcinoma cell line BEL-7402/5-FU. *Phytomedicine* 2011; 18: 1086-92.

[300] Chen X, Wu Y, Jiang Y, Zhou Y, Wang Y, Yao Y, Yi C, Gou L, Yang J. Isoliquiritigenin inhibits the growth of multiple myeloma via blocking IL-6 signaling. *J Mol Med (Berl)* 2012; 90: 1311-9.

[301] Wang ZD, Wang RZ, Xia YZ, Kong LY, Yang L. Reversal of multidrug resistance by icaritin in doxorubicin-resistant human osteosarcoma cells. *Chin J Nat Med* 2018; 16: 20-8.

[302] Wang Z, Yang L, Xia Y, Guo C, Kong L. Icariin enhances cytotoxicity of doxorubicin in human multidrug-resistant osteosarcoma cells by inhibition of ABCB1 and down-regulation of the PI3K/Akt pathway. *Biol Pharm Bull* 2015; 38: 277-84.

[303] Xu Y, Wang S, Chan HF, Lu H, Lin Z, He C, Chen M. Dihydromyricetin induces apoptosis and reverses drug resistance in ovarian cancer cells by p53-mediated downregulation of survivin. *Sci Rep* 2017; 7: 46060.

[304] Chen HJ, Chung YL, Li CY, Chang YT, Wang CCN, Lee HY, Lin HY, Hung CC. Taxifolin resensitizes multidrug resistance cancer cells via uncompetitive inhibition of P-glycoprotein function. *Molecules* 2018; 23: E3055.

[305] Wang A, Wang W, Chen Y, Ma F, Wei X, Bi Y. Deguelin induces PUMA-mediated apoptosis and promotes sensitivity of lung cancer cells (LCCs) to doxorubicin (Dox). *Mol Cell Biochem* 2018; 442: 177-86.

[306] Xu XD, Zhao Y, Zhang M, He RZ, Shi XH, Guo XJ, Shi CJ, Peng F, Wang M, Shen M, Wang X, Li X, Qin RY. Inhibition of autophagy by deguelin sensitizes pancreatic cancer cells to doxorubicin. *Int J Mol Sci* 2017; 18: E370.

[307] Lee JJ, Koh KN, Park CJ, Jang S, Im HJ, Kim N. The combination of flavokawain B and daunorubicin induces apoptosis in human myeloid leukemic cells by modifying NF-κB. *Anticancer Res* 2018; 38: 2771-8.

[308] Davenport A, Frezza M, Shen M, Ge Y, Huo C, Chan TH, Dou QP. Celastrol and an EGCG pro-drug exhibit potent chemosensitizing activity in human leukemia cells. *Int J Mol Med* 2010; 25: 465-70.

[309] Borska S, Chmielewska M, Wysocka T, Drag-Zalesinska M, Zabel M, Dziegiel P. In vitro effect of quercetin on human gastric carcinoma: targeting cancer cells death and MDR. *Food Chem Toxicol* 2012; 50: 3375-83.

[310] Borska S, Sopel M, Chmielewska M, Zabel M, Dziegiel P. Quercetin as a potential modulator of P-glycoprotein expression and function in cells of human pancreatic carcinoma line resistant to daunorubicin. *Molecules* 2010; 15: 857-70.

[311] Huang W, Ding L, Huang Q, Hu H, Liu S, Yang X, Hu X, Dang Y, Shen S, Li J, Ji X, Jiang S, Liu JO, Yu L. Carbonyl reductase 1 as a novel target of (-)-

epigallocatechin gallate against hepatocellular carcinoma. *Hepatology* 2010; 52: 703-14.

[312] Tran VH, Marks D, Duke RK, Bebawy M, Duke CC, Roufogalis BD. Modulation of P-glycoprotein-mediated anticancer drug accumulation, cytotoxicity, and ATPase activity by flavonoid interactions. *Nutr Cancer* 2011; 63: 435-43.

[313] den Boer ML, Pieters R, Kazemier KM, Janka-Schaub GE, Henze G, Veerman AJ. The modulating effect of PSC 833, cyclosporin A, verapamil and genistein on in vitro cytotoxicity and intracellular content of daunorubicin in childhood acute lymphoblastic leukemia. *Leukemia* 1998; 12: 912-20.

[314] Li J, Duan B, Guo Y, Zhou R, Sun J, Bie B, Yang S, Huang C, Yang J, Li Z. Baicalein sensitizes hepatocellular carcinoma cells to 5-FU and Epirubicin by activating apoptosis and ameliorating P-glycoprotein activity. *Biomed Pharmacother* 2018; 98: 806-12.

[315] Lo YL. A potential daidzein derivative enhances cytotoxicity of epirubicin on human colon adenocarcinoma Caco-2 cells. *Int J Mol Sci* 2012; 14: 158-76.

[316] Lo YL, Wang W. Formononetin potentiates epirubicin-induced apoptosis via ROS production in HeLa cells in vitro. *Chem Biol Interact* 2013; 205: 188-97.

[317] Gyemant N, Tanaka M, Antus S, Hohmann J, Csuka O, Mandoky L, Molnar J. In vitro search for synergy between flavonoids and epirubicin on multidrug-resistant cancer cells. *In Vivo* 2005; 19: 367-74.

[318] Wang Z, Wang N, Liu P, Chen Q, Situ H, Xie T, Zhang J, Peng C, Lin Y, Chen J. MicroRNA-25 regulates chemoresistance-associated autophagy in breast cancer cells, a process modulated by the natural autophagy inducer isoliquiritigenin. *Oncotarget* 2014; 5: 7013-26.

[319] Wang N, Wang Z, Peng C, You J, Shen J, Han S, Chen J. Dietary compound isoliquiritigenin targets GRP78 to chemosensitize breast cancer stem cells via β-catenin/ABCG2 signaling. *Carcinogenesis* 2014; 35: 2544-54.

[320] Pan XW, Li L, Huang Y, Huang H, Xu DF, Gao Y, Chen L, Ren JZ, Cao JW, Hong Y, Cui XG. Icaritin acts synergistically with epirubicin to suppress bladder cancer growth through inhibition of autophagy. *Oncol Rep* 2016; 35: 334-42.

[321] Flaig TW, Su LJ, Harrison G, Agarwal R, Glode LM. Silibinin synergizes with mitoxantrone to inhibit cell growth and induce apoptosis in human prostate cancer cells. *Int J Cancer* 2007; 120: 2028-33.

[322] An G, Morris ME. Effects of single and multiple flavonoids on BCRP-mediated accumulation, cytotoxicity and transport of mitoxantrone in vitro. *Pharm Res* 2010; 27: 1296-308.

[323] Klimaszewska-Wisniewska A, Halas-Wisniewska M, Tadrowski T, Gagat M, Grzanka D, Grzanka A. Paclitaxel and the dietary flavonoid fisetin: a synergistic combination that induces mitotic catastrophe and autophagic cell death in A549 non-small cell lung cancer cells. *Cancer Cell Int* 2016; 16: 10.

[324] Zhang S, Yang X, Morris ME. Flavonoids are inhibitors of breast cancer resistance protein (ABCG2)-mediated transport. *Mol Pharmacol* 2004; 65: 1208-16.

[325] Telli E, Genc H, Tasa BA, Sinan Özalp S, Tansu Koparal A. In vitro evaluation of combination of EGCG and Erlotinib with classical chemotherapeutics on JAR cells. *In Vitro Cell Dev Biol Anim* 2017; 53: 651-8.

[326] Guo XF, Yang ZR, Wang J, Lei XF, Lv XG, Dong WG. Synergistic antitumor effect of puerarin combined with 5-fluorouracil on gastric carcinoma. *Mol Med Rep* 2015; 11: 2562-8.

[327] Zhao L, Chen Z, Wang J, Yang L, Zhao Q, Wang J, Qi Q, Mu R, You QD, Guo QL. Synergistic effect of 5-fluorouracil and the flavanoid oroxylin A on HepG2 human hepatocellular carcinoma and on H22 transplanted mice. *Cancer Chemother Pharmacol* 2010; 65: 481-9.

[328] Xu GY, Tang XJ. Troxerutin (TXN) potentiated 5-Fluorouracil (5-Fu) treatment of human gastric cancer through suppressing STAT3/NF-κB and Bcl-2 signaling pathways. *Biomed Pharmacother* 2017; 92: 95-107.

[329] Wang L, Feng J, Chen X, Guo W, Du Y, Wang Y, Zang W, Zhang S, Zhao G. Myricetin enhance chemosensitivity of 5-fluorouracil on esophageal carcinoma in vitro and in vivo. *Cancer Cell Int* 2014; 14: 71.

[330] Zhao Q, Wang J, Zou MJ, Hu R, Zhao L, Qiang L, Rong JJ, You QD, Guo QL. Wogonin potentiates the antitumor effects of low dose 5-fluorouracil against gastric cancer through induction of apoptosis by down-regulation of NF-kappaB and regulation of its metabolism. *Toxicol Lett* 2010; 197: 201-10.

[331] Choi EJ, Kim GH. 5-Fluorouracil combined with apigenin enhances anticancer activity through induction of apoptosis in human breast cancer MDA-MB-453 cells. *Oncol Rep* 2009; 22: 1533-7.

[332] Yang XW, Wang XL, Cao LQ, Jiang XF, Peng HP, Lin SM, Xue P, Chen D. Green tea polyphenol epigallocatehin-3-gallate enhances 5-fluorouracil-induced cell growth inhibition of hepatocellular carcinoma cells. *Hepatol Res* 2012; 42: 494-501.

[333] Qiao J, Gu C, Shang W, Du J, Yin W, Zhu M, Wang W, Han M, Lu W. Effect of green tea on pharmacokinetics of 5-fluorouracil in rats and pharmacodynamics in human cell lines in vitro. *Food Chem Toxicol* 2011; 49: 1410-5.

[334] Navarro-Peran E, Cabezas-Herrera J, Campo LS, Rodriguez-Lopez JN. Effects of folate cycle disruption by the green tea polyphenol epigallocatechin-3-gallate. *Int J Biochem Cell Biol* 2007; 39: 2215-25.

[335] Hwang JT, Ha J, Park OJ. Combination of 5-fluorouracil and genistein induces apoptosis synergistically in chemo-resistant cancer cells through the modulation of AMPK and COX-2 signaling pathways. *Biochem Biophys Res Commun* 2005; 332: 433-40.

[336] Shi DB, Li XX, Zheng HT, Li DW, Cai GX, Peng JJ, Gu WL, Guan ZQ, Xu Y, Cai SJ. Icariin-mediated inhibition of NF-κB activity enhances the in vitro and in vivo antitumour effect of 5-fluorouracil in colorectal cancer. *Cell Biochem Biophys* 2014; 69: 523-30.

[337] Gaballah HH, Gaber RA, Mohamed DA. Apigenin potentiates the antitumor activity of 5-FU on solid Ehrlich carcinoma: Crosstalk between apoptotic and JNK-mediated autophagic cell death platforms. *Toxicol Appl Pharmacol* 2017; 316: 27-35.

[338] Xu H, Yang T, Liu X, Tian Y, Chen X, Yuan R, Su S, Lin X, Du G. Luteolin synergizes the antitumor effects of 5-fluorouracil against human hepatocellular carcinoma cells through apoptosis induction and metabolism. *Life Sci* 2016; 144: 138-47.

[339] Zhao L, Sha YY, Zhao Q, Yao J, Zhu BB, Lu ZJ, You QD, Guo QL. Enhanced 5-fluorouracil cytotoxicity in high COX-2 expressing hepatocellular carcinoma cells by wogonin via the PI3K/Akt pathway. *Biochem Cell Biol* 2013; 91: 221-9.

[340] Chuang-Xin L, Wen-Yu W, Yao C, Xiao-Yan L, Yun Z. Quercetin enhances the effects of 5-fluorouracil-mediated growth inhibition and apoptosis of esophageal cancer cells by inhibiting NF-κB. *Oncol Lett* 2012; 4: 775-8.

[341] Xavier CP, Lima CF, Rohde M, Pereira-Wilson C. Quercetin enhances 5-fluorouracil-induced apoptosis in MSI colorectal cancer cells through p53 modulation. *Cancer Chemother Pharmacol* 2011; 68: 1449-57.

[342] Samuel T, Fadlalla K, Mosley L, Katkoori V, Turner T, Manne U. Dual-mode interaction between quercetin and DNA-damaging drugs in cancer cells. *Anticancer Res* 2012; 32: 61-71.

[343] Dai W, Gao Q, Qiu J, Yuan J, Wu G, Shen G. Quercetin induces apoptosis and enhances 5-FU therapeutic efficacy in hepatocellular carcinoma. *Tumour Biol* 2016; 37: 6307-13.

[344] Masuda M, Suzui M, Weinstein IB. Effects of epigallocatechin-3-gallate on growth, epidermal growth factor receptor signaling pathways, gene expression, and chemosensitivity in human head and neck squamous cell carcinoma cell lines. *Clin Cancer Res* 2001; 7: 4220-9.

[345] Hu XY, Liang JY, Guo XJ, Liu L, Guo YB. 5-Fluorouracil combined with apigenin enhances anticancer activity through mitochondrial membrane potential ($\Delta\Psi$m)-mediated apoptosis in hepatocellular carcinoma. *Clin Exp Pharmacol Physiol* 2015; 42: 146-53.

[346] Chen F, Zhuang M, Zhong C, Peng J, Wang X, Li J, Chen Z, Huang Y. Baicalein reverses hypoxia-induced 5-FU resistance in gastric cancer AGS cells through suppression of glycolysis and the PTEN/Akt/HIF-1α signaling pathway. *Oncol Rep* 2015; 33: 457-63.

[347] Ha J, Zhao L, Zhao Q, Yao J, Zhu BB, Lu N, Ke X, Yang HY, Li Z, You QD, Guo QL. Oroxylin A improves the sensitivity of HT-29 human colon cancer cells to 5-FU through modulation of the COX-2 signaling pathway. *Biochem Cell Biol* 2012; 90: 521-31.

[348] Yang HY, Zhao L, Yang Z, Zhao Q, Qiang L, Ha J, Li ZY, You QD, Guo QL. Oroxylin A reverses multi-drug resistance of human hepatoma BEL7402/5-FU cells via downregulation of P-glycoprotein expression by inhibiting NF-κB signaling pathway. *Mol Carcinog* 2012; 51: 185-95.

[349] Gao H, Xie J, Peng J, Han Y, Jiang Q, Han M, Wang C. Hispidulin inhibits proliferation and enhances chemosensitivity of gallbladder cancer cells by targeting HIF-1α. *Exp Cell Res* 2015; 332: 236-46.

[350] Moon JY, Cho M, Ahn KS, Cho SK. Nobiletin induces apoptosis and potentiates the effects of the anticancer drug 5-fluorouracil in p53-mutated SNU-16 human gastric cancer cells. *Nutr Cancer* 2013; 65: 286-95.

[351] Chan JY, Tan BK, Lee SC. Scutellarin sensitizes drug-evoked colon cancer cell apoptosis through enhanced caspase-6 activation. *Anticancer Res* 2009; 29: 3043-7.

[352] Suzuki R, Kang Y, Li X, Roife D, Zhang R, Fleming JB, Genistein potentiates the antitumor effect of 5-Fluorouracil by inducing apoptosis and autophagy in human pancreatic cancer cells. *Anticancer Res* 2014; 34: 4685-92.

[353] Wang J, Yang ZR, Guo XF, Song J, Zhang JX, Wang J, Dong WG. Synergistic effects of puerarin combined with 5-fluorouracil on esophageal cancer. *Mol Med Rep* 2014; 10: 2535-41.

[354] Chang HR, Chen PN, Yang SF, Sun YS, Wu SW, Hung TW, Lian JD, Chu SC, Hsieh YS. Silibinin inhibits the invasion and migration of renal carcinoma 786-O cells in vitro, inhibits the growth of xenografts in vivo and enhances chemosensitivity to 5-fluorouracil and paclitaxel. *Mol Carcinog* 2011; 50: 811-23.

[355] Lin X, Tian L, Wang L, Li W, Xu Q, Xiao X. Antitumor effects and the underlying mechanism of licochalcone A combined with 5-fluorouracil in gastric cancer cells. *Oncol Lett* 2017; 13: 1695-701.

[356] Wei X, Mo X, An F, Ji X, Lu Y. 2`,4`-Dihydroxy-6`-methoxy-3`,5`-dimethylchalcone, a potent Nrf2/ARE pathway inhibitor, reverses drug resistance by decreasing glutathione synthesis and drug efflux in BEL-7402/5-FU cells. *Food Chem Toxicol* 2018; 119: 252-9.

[357] Huang HY, Niu JL, Lu YH. Multidrug resistance reversal effect of DMC derived from buds of Cleistocalyx operculatus in human hepatocellular tumor xenograft model. *J Sci Food Agric* 2012; 92: 135-40.

[358] Wu H, Xin Y, Xu C, Xiao Y. Capecitabine combined with (-)-epigallocatechin-3-gallate inhibits angiogenesis and tumor growth in nude mice with gastric cancer xenografts. *Exp Ther Med* 2012; 3: 650-4.

[359] Manu KA, Shanmugam MK, Ramachandran L, Li F, Siveen KS, Chinnathambi A, Zayed ME, Alharbi SA, Arfuso F, Kumar AP, Ahn KS, Sethi G. Isorhamnetin augments the anti-tumor effect of capeciatbine through the negative regulation of NF-κB signaling cascade in gastric cancer. *Cancer Lett* 2015; 363: 28-36.

[360] Zhang B, Shi ZL, Liu B, Yan XB, Feng J, Tao HM. Enhanced anticancer effect of gemcitabine by genistein in osteosarcoma: the role of Akt and nuclear factor-kappaB. *Anticancer Drugs* 2010; 21: 288-96.

[361] Zhang DC, Liu JL, Ding YB, Xia JG, Chen GY. Icariin potentiates the antitumor activity of gemcitabine in gallbladder cancer by suppressing NF-κB. *Acta Pharmacol Sin* 2013; 34: 301-8.

[362] Li Y, Huang X, Huang Z, Feng J. Phenoxodiol enhances the antitumor activity of gemcitabine in gallbladder cancer through suppressing Akt/mTOR pathway. *Cell Biochem Biophys* 2014; 70: 1337-42.

[363] Jung CP, Motwani MV, Schwartz GK. Flavopiridol increases sensitization to gemcitabine in human gastrointestinal cancer cell lines and correlates with down-regulation of ribonucleotide reductase M2 subunit. *Clin Cancer Res* 2001; 7: 2527-36.

[364] Ali S, El-Rayes BF, Aranha O, Sarkar FH, Philip PA. Sequence dependent potentiation of gemcitabine by flavopiridol in human breast cancer cells. *Breast Cancer Res Treat* 2005; 90: 25-31.

[365] Wu W, Xia Q, Luo RJ, Lin ZQ, Xue P. In vitro study of the antagonistic effect of low-dose liquiritigenin on gemcitabine-induced capillary leak syndrome in pancreatic adenocarcinoma via inhibiting ROS-mediated signalling pathways. *Asian Pac J Cancer Prev* 2015; 16: 4369-76.

[366] Strouch MJ, Milam BM, Melstrom LG, McGull JJ, Salabat MR, Ujiki MB, Ding XZ, Bentrem DJ. The flavonoid apigenin potentiates the growth inhibitory effects of gemcitabine and abrogates gemcitabine resistance in human pancreatic cancer cells. *Pancreas* 2009; 38: 409-15.

[367] Banerjee S, Zhang Y, Ali S, Bhuiyan M, Wang Z, Chiao PJ, Philip PA, Abbruzzese J, Sarkar FH. Molecular evidence for increased antitumor activity of gemcitabine by genistein in vitro and in vivo using an orthotopic model of pancreatic cancer. *Cancer Res* 2005; 65: 9064-72.

[368] Löhr JM, Karimi M, Omazic B, Kartalis N, Verbeke CS, Berkenstam A, Frödin JE. A phase I dose escalation trial of AXP107-11, a novel multi-component crystalline form of genistein, in combination with gemcitabine in chemotherapy-naive patients with unresectable pancreatic cancer. *Pancreatology* 2016; 16: 640-5.

[369] Lee SH, Ryu JK, Lee KY, Woo SM, Park JK, Yoo JW, Kim YT, Yoon YB. Enhanced anti-tumor effect of combination therapy with gemcitabine and apigenin in pancreatic cancer. *Cancer Lett* 2008; 259: 39-49.

[370] Johnson JL, Dia VP, Wallig M, Gonzalez de Mejia E. Luteolin and gemcitabine protect against pancreatic cancer in an orthotopic mouse model. *Pancreas* 2015; 44: 144-51.

[371] Liu P, Feng J, Sun M, Yuan W, Xiao R, Xiong J, Huang X, Xiong M, Chen W, Yu X, Sun Q, Zhao X, Zhang Q, Shao L. Synergistic effects of baicalein with gemcitabine or docetaxel on the proliferation, migration and apoptosis of pancreatic cancer cells. *Int J Oncol* 2017; 51: 1878-86.

[372] Kim N, Kang MJ, Lee SH, Son JH, Lee JE, Paik WH, Ryu JK, Kim YT. Fisetin enhances the cytotoxicity of gemcitabine by down-regulating ERK-MYC in MiaPaca-2 human pancreatic cancer cells. *Anticancer Res* 2018; 38: 3527-33.

[373] Hyun JJ, Lee HS, Keum B, Seo YS, Jeen YT, Chun HJ, Um SH, Kim CD. Expression of heat shock protein 70 modulates the chemoresponsiveness of pancreatic cancer. *Gut Liver* 2013; 7: 739-46.

[374] Lee SH, Lee EJ, Min KH, Hur GY, Lee SH, Lee SY, Kim JH, Shin C, Shim JJ, In KH, Kang KH, Lee SY. Quercetin enhances chemosensitivity to gemcitabine in lung cancer cells by inhibiting heat shock protein 70 expression. *Clin Lung Cancer* 2015; 16: e235-43.

[375] Tang SN, Fu J, Shankar S, Srivastava RK. EGCG enhances the therapeutic potential of gemcitabine and CP690550 by inhibiting STAT3 signaling pathway in human pancreatic cancer. *PLoS One* 2012; 7: e31067.

[376] Desai UN, Shah KP, Mirza SH, Panchal DK, Parikh SK, Rawal RM. Enhancement of the cytotoxic effects of cytarabine in synergism with hesperidine and silibinin in acute myeloid leukemia: An in-vitro approach. *J Cancer Res Ther* 2015; 11: 352-7.

[377] Karp JE, Ross DD, Yang W, Tidwell ML, Wei Y, Greer J, Mann DL, Nakanishi T, Wright JJ, Colevas AD. Timed sequential therapy of acute leukemia with flavopiridol: in vitro model for a phase I clinical trial. *Clin Cancer Res* 2003; 9: 307-15.

[378] Karp JE, Passaniti A, Gojo I, Kaufmann S, Bible K, Garimella TS, Greer J, Briel J, Smith BD, Gore SD, Tidwell ML, Ross DD, Wright JJ, Colevas AS, Bauer KS. Phase I and pharmacokinetic study of flavopiridol followed by 1-beta-D-arabinofuranosylcytosine and mitoxantrone in relapsed and refractory adult acute leukemias. *Clin Cancer Res* 2005; 11: 8403-12.

[379] Karp JE, Smith BD, Levis MJ, Gore SD, Greer J, Hattenburg C, Briel J, Jones RJ, Wright JJ, Colevas AD. Sequential flavopiridol, cytosine arabinoside, and mitoxantrone: a phase II trial in adults with poor-risk acute myelogenous leukemia. *Clin Cancer Res* 2007; 13: 4467-73.

[380] Kanno S, Shouji A, Hirata R, Asou K, Ishikawa M. Effects of naringin on cytosine arabinoside (Ara-C)-induced cytotoxicity and apoptosis in P388 cells. *Life Sci* 2004; 75: 353-65.

[381] Saiko P, Steinmann MT, Schuster H, Graser G, Bressler S, Giessrigl B, Lackner A, Grusch M, Krupitza G, Bago-Horvath Z, Jaeger W, Fritzer-Szekeres M, Szekeres T. Epigallocatechin gallate, ellagic acid, and rosmarinic acid perturb dNTP pools and inhibit de novo DNA synthesis and proliferation of human HL-60 promyelocytic leukemia cells: Synergism with arabinofuranosylcytosine. *Phytomedicine* 2015; 22: 213-22.

[382] Nadova S, Miadokova E, Cipak L. Flavonoids potentiate the efficacy of cytarabine through modulation of drug-induced apoptosis. *Neoplasma* 2007; 54: 202-6.

[383] Teofili L, Pierelli L, Iovino MS, Leone G, Scambia G, De Vincenzo R, Benedetti-Panici P, Menichella G, Macri E, Piantelli M, Ranelletti FO, Larocca LM. The combination of quercetin and cytosine arabinoside synergistically inhibits leukemic cell growth. *Leuk Res* 1992; 16: 497-503.

[384] Xu F, Zhen YS. (-)-Epigallocatechin-3-gallate enhances anti-tumor effect of cytosine arabinoside on HL-60 cells. *Acta Pharmacol Sin* 2003; 24: 163-8.

[385] Shen J, Tai YC, Zhou J, Stephen Wong CH, Cheang PT, Fred Wong WS, Xie Z, Khan M, Han JH, Chen CS. Synergistic antileukemia effect of genistein and chemotherapy in mouse xenograft model and potential mechanism through MAPK signaling. *Exp Hematol* 2007; 35: 75-83.

[386] Tyagi T, Treas JN, Mahalingaiah PK, Singh KP. Potentiation of growth inhibition and epigenetic modulation by combination of green tea polyphenol and 5-aza-2`-deoxycytidine in human breast cancer cells. *Breast Cancer Res Treat* 2015; 149: 655-68.

[387] Raynal NJ, Charbonneau M, Momparler LF, Momparler RL. Synergistic effect of 5-Aza-2`-deoxycytidine and genistein in combination against leukemia. *Oncol Res* 2008; 17: 223-30.

[388] Mateen S, Raina K, Agarwal C, Chan D, Agarwal R. Silibinin synergizes with histone deacetylase and DNA methyltransferase inhibitors in upregulating E-cadherin expression together with inhibition of migration and invasion of human non-small cell lung cancer cells. *J Pharmacol Exp Ther* 2013; 345: 206-14.

[389] Xuan Y, Hacker MP, Tritton TR, Bhushan A. Modulation of methotrexate resistance by genistein in murine leukemia L1210 cells. *Oncol Rep* 1998; 5: 419-21.

[390] Hussain SA, Marouf BH. Silibinin improves the cytotoxicity of methotrexate in chemo resistant human rhabdomyosarcoma cell lines. *Saudi Med J* 2013; 34: 1145-50.

[391] Chen YJ, Wu CS, Shieh JJ, Wu JH, Chen HY, Chung TW, Chen YK, Lin CC. Baicalein triggers mitochondria-mediated apoptosis and enhances the antileukemic effect of vincristine in childhood acute lymphoblastic leukemia CCRF-CEM cells. *Evid Based Complement Alternat Med* 2013: 2013: 124747.

[392] Russo M, Spagnuolo C, Volpe S, Mupo A, Tedesco I, Russo GL. Quercetin induced apoptosis in association with death receptors and fludarabine in cells isolated from chronic lymphocytic leukaemia patients. *Br J Cancer* 2010; 103: 642-8.

[393] Mansour A, Chang VT, Srinivas S, Harrison J, Raveche E. Correlation of ZAP-70 expression in B cell leukemias to the ex vivo response to a combination of fludarabine/genistein. *Cancer Immunol Immunother* 2007; 56: 501-14.

[394] Rebolleda N, Losada-Fernandez I, Perez-Chacon G, Castejon R, Rosado S, Morado M, Vallejo-Cremades MT, Martinez A, Vargas-Nunez JA, Perez-Aciego P. Synergistic activity of deguelin and fludarabine in cells from chronic lymphocytic leukemia patients and in the New Zealand Black murine model. *PLoS One* 2016; 11: e0154159.

[395] Li W, Weber G. Synergistic action of tiazofurin and genistein on growth inhibition and differentiation of K-562 human leukemic cells. *Life Sci* 1998; 63: 1975-81.

[396] Li W, Weber G. Synergistic action of tiazofurin and genistein in human ovarian carcinoma cells. *Oncol Res* 1998; 10: 117-22.

[397] Shen F, Herenyiova M, Weber G. Synergistic down-regulation of signal transduction and cytotoxicity by tiazofurin and quercetin in human ovarian carcinoma cells. *Life Sci* 1999; 64: 1869-76.

[398] Wang J, Yin Y, Hua H, Li M, Luo T, Xu L, Wang R, Liu D, Zhang Y, Jiang Y. Blockade of GRP78 sensitizes breast cancer cells to microtubules-interfering agents that induce the unfolded protein response. *J Cell Mol Med* 2009; 13: 3888-97.

[399] Fonseca J, Marques S, Silva PM, Brandao P, Cidade H, Pinto MM, Bousbaa H. Prenylated chalcone 2 acts as an antimitotic agent and enhances the chemosensitivity of tumor cells to paclitaxel. *Molecules* 2016; 21: E982.

[400] Marone M, D`Andrilli G, Das N, Ferlini C, Chatterjee S, Scambia G. Quercetin abrogates taxol-mediated signaling by inhibiting multiple kinases. *Exp Cell Res* 2001; 270: 1-12.

[401] Motwani M, Rizzo C, Sirotnak F, She Y, Schwartz GK. Flavopiridol enhances the effect of docetaxel in vitro and in vivo in human gastric cancer cells. *Mol Cancer Ther* 2003; 2: 549-55.

[402] Mukhtar E, Adhami VM, Siddiqui IA, Verma AK, Mukhtar H. Fisetin enhances chemotherapeutic effect of cabazitaxel against human prostate cancer cells. *Mol Cancer Ther* 2016; 15: 2863-74.

[403] Ping SY, Hour TC, Lin SR, Yu DS. Taxol synergizes with antioxidants in inhibiting hormal refractory prostate cancer cell growth. *Urol Oncol* 2010; 28: 170-9.

[404] Sato A, Sekine M, Kobayashi M, Virgona N, Ota M, Yano T. Induction of the connexin 32 gene by epigallocatechin-3-gallate potentiates vinblastine-induced cytotoxicity in human renal carcinoma cells. *Chemotherapy* 2013; 59: 192-9.

[405] Go WJ, Ryu JH, Qiang F, Han HK. Evaluation of the flavonoid oroxylin A as an inhibitor of P-glycoprotein-mediated cellular efflux. *J Nat Prod* 2009; 72: 1616-9.

[406] Limtrakul P, Khantamat O, Pintha K. Inhibition of P-glycoprotein function and expression by kaempferol and quercetin. *J Chemother* 2005; 17: 86-95.

[407] Yuan Z, Wang H, Hu Z, Huang Y, Yao F, Sun S, Wu B. Quercetin inhibits proliferation and drug resistance in KB/VCR oral cancer cells and enhances its sensitivity to vincristine. *Nutr Cancer* 2015; 67: 126-36.

[408] Wong MY, Chiu GN. Simultaneous liposomal delivery of quercetin and vincristine for enhanced estrogen-receptor-negative breast cancer treatment. *Anticancer Drugs* 2010; 21: 401-10.

[409] Zhu B, Yu L, Yue Q. Co-delivery of vincristine and quercetin by nanocarriers for lymphoma combination chemotherapy. *Biomed Pharmacother* 2017; 91: 287-94.

[410] Wong MY, Chiu GN. Liposome formulation of co-encapsulated vincristine and quercetin enhanced antitumor activity in a trastuzumab-insensitive breast tumor xenograft model. *Nanomedicine* 2011; 7: 834-40.

[411] Ruela-de-Sousa RR, Fuhler GM, Blom N, Ferreira CV, Aoyama H, Peppelenbosch MP. Cytotoxicity of apigenin on leukemia cell lines: implications for prevention and therapy. *Cell Death Dis* 2010; 1: e19.

[412] Ohtani H, Ikegawa T, Honda Y, Kohyama N, Morimoto S, Shoyama Y, Juichi M, Naito M, Tsuruo T, Sawada Y. Effects of various methoxyflavones on vincristine uptake and multidrug resistance to vincristine in P-gp-overexpressing K562/ADM cells. *Pharm Res* 2007; 24: 1936-43.

[413] Choi CH, Sun KH, An CS, Yoo JC, Hahm KS, Lee IH, Sohng JK, Kim YC. Reversal of P-glycoprotein-mediated multidrug resistance by 5,6,7,3`,4`-pentamethoxyflavone (Sinensetin). *Biochem Biophys Res Commun* 2002; 295: 832-40.

[414] Bueno Perez L, Pan L, Sass E, Gupta SV, Lehman A, Kinghorn AD, Lucas DM. Potentiating effect of the flavonolignan (-)-hydnocarpin in combination with vincristine in a sensitive and P-gp-expressing acute lymphoblastic leukemia cell line. *Phytother Res* 2013; 27: 1735-8.

[415] Uckun FM, Qazi S, Ozer Z, Garner AL, Pitt J, Ma H, Janda KD. Inducing apoptosis in chemotherapy-resistant B-lineage acute lymphoblastic leukaemia cells by targeting HSPA5, a master regulator of the anti-apoptotic unfolded protein response signalling network. *Br J Haematol* 2011; 153: 741-52.

[416] Hemalswarya S, Doble M. Potential synergism of natural products in the treatment of cancer. *Phytother Res* 2006; 20: 239-49.

[417] Wang W, Xi M, Duan X, Wang Y, Kong F. Delivery of baicalein and paclitaxel using self-assembled nanoparticles: synergistic antitumor effect in vitro and in vivo. *Int J Nanomedicine* 2015; 10: 3737-50.

[418] Luo T, Wang J, Yin Y, Hua H, Jing J, Sun X, Li M, Zhang Y, Jiang Y. (-)-Epigallocatechin gallate sensitizes breast cancer cells to paclitaxel in a murine model of breast carcinoma. *Breast Cancer Res* 2010; 12: R8.

[419] Pan Q, Xue M, Xiao SS, Wan YJ, Xu DB. A combination therapy with baicalein and taxol promotes mitochondria-mediated cell apoptosis: Involving in Akt/β-catenin signaling pathway. *DNA Cell Biol* 2016; 35: 646-56.

[420] Meng L, Xia X, Yang Y, Ye J, Dong W, Ma P, Jin Y, Liu Y. Co-encapsulation of paclitaxel and baicalein in nanoemulsions to overcome multidrug resistance via oxidative stress augmentation and P-glycoprotein inhibition. *Int J Pharm* 2016; 513: 8-16.

[421] Ramadass SK, Anantharaman NV, Subramanian S, Sivasubramanian S, Madhan B. Paclitaxel/epigallocatechin gallate coloaded liposome: a synergistic delivery to control the invasiveness of MDA-MB-231 breast cancer cells. *Colloids Surf B Biointerfaces* 2015; 125: 65-72.

[422] Klimaszewska-Wisniewska A, Halas-Wisniewska M, Grzanka A, Grzanka D. Evaluation of anti-metastatic potential of the combination of fisetin with paclitaxel on A549 non-small cell lung cancer cells. *Int J Mol Sci* 2018; 19: E661.

[423] Motwani M, Delohery TM, Schwartz GK. Sequential dependent enhancement of caspase activation and apoptosis by flavopiridol on paclitaxel-treated human gastric and breast cancer cells. *Clin Cancer Res* 1999; 5: 1876-83.

[424] Liu Y, Bhalla K, Hill C, Priest DG. Evidence for involvement of tyrosine phosphorylation in taxol-induced apoptosis in a human ovarian tumor cell line. *Biochem Pharmacol* 1994; 48: 1265-72.

[425] Yang MY, Wang CJ, Chen NF, Ho WH, Lu FJ, Tseng TH. Luteolin enhances paclitaxel-induced apoptosis in human breast cancer MDA-MB-231 cells by blocking STAT3. *Chem Biol Interact* 2014; 213: 60-8.

[426] Li B, Jin X, Meng H, Hu B, Zhang T, Yu J, Chen S, Guo X, Wang W, Jiang W, Wang J. Morin promotes prostate cancer cells chemosensitivity to paclitaxel through miR-155/GATA3 axis. *Oncotarget* 2017; 8: 47849-60.

[427] Isonishi S, Saitou M, Saitou M, Yasuda M, Tanaka T. Differential regulation of the cytotoxicity activity of paclitaxel by orobol and platelet derived growth factor in human ovarian carcinoma cells. *Oncol Rep* 2007; 18: 195-201.

[428] Yang YI, Lee KT, Park HJ, Kim TJ, Choi YS, Shih IeM, Choi JH. Tectorigenin sensitizes paclitaxel-resistant human ovarian cancer cells through downregulation of the Akt and NFκB pathway. *Carcinogenesis* 2012; 33: 2488-98.

[429] Park S, Kim JH, Hwang YI, Jung KS, Jang YS, Jang SH. Schedule-dependent effect of epigallocatechin-3-gallate (EGCG) with paclitaxel on H460 cells. *Tuberc Respir Dis (Seoul)* 2014; 76: 114-9.

[430] Wu J, Guan M, Wong PF, Yu H, Dong J, Xu J. Icariside II potentiates paclitaxel-induced apoptosis in human melanoma A375 cells by inhibiting TLR4 signaling pathway. *Food Chem Toxicol* 2012; 50: 3019-24.

[431] Zheng AW, Chen YQ, Zhao LQ, Feng JG. Myricetin induces apoptosis and enhances chemosensitivity in ovarian cancer cells. *Oncol Lett* 2017; 13: 4974-8.

[432] Chang YF, Chi CW, Wang JJ. Reactive oxygen species production is involved in quercetin-induced apoptosis in human hepatoma cells. *Nutr Cancer* 2006; 55: 201-9.

[433] Pashaei-Asl F, Pashaei-Asl R, Khodadadi K, Akbarzadeh A, Ebrahimie E, Pashaiasl M. Enhancement of anticancer activity by silibinin and paclitaxel combination on the ovarian cancer. *Artif Cells Nanomed Biotechnol* 2018; 46: 1483-7.

[434] Wen D, Peng Y, Lin F, Singh RK, Mahato RI. Micellar delivery of miR-34a modulator rubone and paclitaxel in resistant prostate cancer. *Cancer Res* 2017; 77: 3244-54.

[435] Xu Y, Xin Y, Diao Y, Lu C, Fu J, Luo L, Yin Z. Synergistic effects of apigenin and paclitaxel on apoptosis of cancer cells. *PLoS One* 2011; 6: e29169.

[436] Yang KC, Tsai CY, Wang YJ, Wei PL, Lee CH, Chen JH, Wu CH, Ho YS. Apple polyphenol phloretin potentiates the anticancer actions of paclitaxel through induction of apoptosis in human hep G2 cells. *Mol Carcinog* 2009; 48: 420-31.

[437] Ho BY, Lin CH, Apaya MK, Chao WW, Shyur LF. Silibinin and paclitaxel cotreatment significantly suppress the activity and lung metastasis of triple negative 4T1 mammary tumor cell in mice. *J Tradit Complement Med* 2011; 2: 301-11.

[438] Samuel T, Fadlalla K, Turner T, Yehualaeshet TE. The flavonoid quercetin transiently inhibits the activity of taxol and nocodazole through interference with the cell cycle. *Nutr Cancer* 2010; 62: 1025-35.

[439] Mohana S, Ganesan M, Agilan B, Karthikeyan R, Srithar G, Beaulah Mary R, Ananthakrishnan D, Velmurugan D, Rajendra Prasad N, Ambudkar SV. Screening dietary flavonoids for the reversal of P-glycoprotein-mediated multidrug resistance in cancer. *Mol Biosyst* 2016; 12: 2458-70.

[440] Mendes LP, Gaeti MP, de Avila PH, de Sousa Vieira M, Dos Santos Rodrigues B, de Avila Marcelino RI, Dos Santos LC, Valadares MC, Lima EM. Multicompartimental nanoparticles for co-encapsulation and multimodal drug delivery to tumor cells and neovasculature. *Pharm Res* 2014; 31: 1106-19.

[441] Masuda M, Suzui M, Lim JT, Weinstein IB. Epigallocatechin-3-gallate inhibits activation of HER-2/neu and downstream signaling pathways in human head and neck and breast carcinoma cells. *Clin Cancer Res* 2003; 9: 3486-91.

[442] Stearns ME, Wang M. Synergistic effects of the green tea extract epigallocatechin-3-gallate and taxane in eradication of malignant human prostate tumors. *Transl Oncol* 2011; 4: 147-56.

[443] Narayanan S, Mony U, Vijaykumar DK, Koyakutty M, Paul-Prasanth B, Menon D. Sequential release of epigallocatechin gallate and paclitaxel from PLGA-casein core/shell nanoparticles sensitizes drug-resistant breast cancer cells. *Nanomedicine* 2015; 11: 1399-406.

[444] Garcia-Vilas JA, Quesada AR, Medina MA. Screening of synergistic interactions of epigallocatechin-3-gallate with antiangiogenic and antitumor compounds. *Synergy* 2016; 3: 5-13.

[445] Yang SF, Yang WE, Chang HR, Chu SC, Hsieh YS. Luteolin induces apoptosis in oral squamous cancer cells. *J Dent Res* 2008; 87: 401-6.

[446] Dia VP, Pangloli P. Epithelial-to-mesenchymal transition in paclitaxel-resistant ovarian cancer cells is downregulated by luteolin. *J Cell Physiol* 2017; 232: 391-401.

[447] Akmal Y, Senthil M, Yan J, Xing Q, Wang Y, Somlo G, Yim J. Combination of a natural compound (baicalein) and paclitaxel results in synergistic apoptosis in mouse breast cancer cells. *J Surg Res* 2011; 165: 218-9.

[448] Zhou L, Liu P, Chen B, Wang Y, Wang X, Chiriva Internati M, Wachtel MS, Frezza EE. Silibinin restores paclitaxel sensitivity to paclitaxel-resistant human ovarian carcinoma cells. *Anticancer Res* 2008; 28: 1119-27.

[449] Zhang Y, Ge Y, Ping X, Yu M, Lou D, Shi W. Synergistic apoptotic effects of silibinin in enhancing paclitaxel toxicity in human gastric cancer cell lines. *Mol Med Rep* 2018; 18: 1835-41.

[450] Park CH, Han SE, Nam-Goong IS, Kim YI, Kim ES. Combined effects of baicalein and docetaxel on apoptosis in 8505c anaplastic thyroid cancer cells via downregulation of the ERK and Akt/mTOR pathways. *Endocrinol Metab (Seoul)* 2018; 33: 121-32.

[451] Li S, Wang L, Li N, Liu Y, Su H. Combination lung cancer chemotherapy: Design of a pH-sensitive transferrin-PEG-Hz-lipid conjugate for the co-delivery of docetaxel and baicalin. *Biomed Pharmacother* 2017; 95: 548-55.

[452] Lim HK, Kim KM, Jeong SY, Choi EK, Jung J. Chrysin increases the therapeutic efficacy of docetaxel and mitigates docetaxel-induced edema. *Integr Cancer Ther* 2017; 16: 496-504.

[453] Wu H, Xin Y, Xiao Y, Zhao J. Low-dose docetaxel combined with (-)-epigallocatechin-3-gallate inhibits angiogenesis and tumor growth in nude mice with gastric cancer xenografts. *Cancer Biother Radiopharm* 2012; 27: 204-9.

[454] Guo J, Zhou AW, Fu YC, Verma UN, Tripathy D, Frenkel EP, Becerra CR. Efficacy of sequential treatment of HCT116 colon cancer monolayers and xenografts with docetaxel, flavopiridol, and 5-fluorouracil. *Acta Pharmacol Sin* 2006; 27: 1375-81.

[455] Li Y, Kucuk O, Hussain M, Abrams J, Cher ML, Sarkar FH. Antitumor and antimetastatic activities of docetaxel are enhanced by genistein through regulation of osteoprotegerin/receptor activator of nuclear factor-kappaB (RANK)/RANK ligand/MMP-9 signaling in prostate cancer. *Cancer Res* 2006; 66: 4816-25.

[456] Li J, Zhang J, Wang Y, Liang X, Wusiman Z, Yin Y, Shen Q. Synergistic inhibition of migration and invasion of breast cancer cells by dual docetaxel/quercetin-loaded nanoparticles via Akt/MMP-9 pathway. *Int J Pharm* 2017; 523: 300-9.

[457] Wang P, Henning SM, Heber D, Vadgama JV. Sensitization of docetaxel in prostate cancer cells by green tea and quercetin. *J Nutr Biochem* 2015; 26: 408-15.

[458] Ghasemi S, Lorigooini Z, Wibowo J, Amini-Khoei H. Tricin isolated from Allium atroviolaceum potentiated the effect of docetaxel on PC3 cell proliferation: role of miR-21. *Nat Prod Res* 2019; 33: 1828-31.

[459] Nagaprashantha LD. Vatsyayan R, Singhal J, Fast S, Roby R, Awasthi S, Singhal SS. Anti-cancer effects of novel flavonoid vicenin-2 as a single agent and in synergistic combination with docetaxel in prostate cancer. *Biochem Pharmacol* 2011; 82: 1100-9.

[460] Liao B, Ying H, Yu C, Fan Z, Zhang W, Shi J, Ying H, Ravichandran N, Xu Y, Yin J, Jiang Y, Du Q. (-)-Epigallocatechin gallate (EGCG)-nanoethosomes as a transdermal delivery system for docetaxel to treat implanted human melanoma cell tumors in mice. *Int J Pharm* 2016; 512: 22-31.

[461] Zhang S, Wang Y, Chen Z, Kim S, Iqbal S, Chi A, Ritenour C, Wang YA, Kucuk O, Wu D. Genistein enhances the efficacy of cabazitaxel chemotherapy in metastatic castration-resistant prostate cancer cells. *Prostate* 2013; 73: 1681-9.

[462] Lee R, Kim YJ, Lee YJ, Chung HW. The selective effect of genistein on the toxicity of bleomycin in normal lymphocytes and HL-60 cells. *Toxicology* 2004; 195: 87-95.

[463] Mohan A, Narayanan S, Sethuraman S, Krishnan UM. Combinations of plant polyphenols & anti-cancer molecules: a novel treatment strategy for cancer chemotherapy. *Anticancer Agents Med Chem* 2013; 13: 281-95.

[464] Ferrario A, Luna M, Rucker N, Wong S, Gomer CJ. Pro-apoptotic and anti-inflammatory properties of the green tea constituent epigallocatechin gallate increase photodynamic therapy responsiveness. *Lasers Surg Med* 2011; 43: 644-50.

[465] Ahn JC, Biswas R, Chung PS. Combination with genistein enhances the efficacy of photodynamic therapy against human anaplastic thyroid cancer cells. *Lasers Surg Med* 2012; 44: 840-9.

Chapter 7

CONCLUSION AND FURTHER PERSPECTIVES TO IMPROVE CANCER THERAPEUTIC OUTCOME

Numerous preclinical *in vitro* and *in vivo* findings presented in the Chapter 6 of this book about the combinational treatment of cancer cells with traditional cytotoxic agents and plant-derived dietary flavonoids introduce a compelling rationale for the development of novel strategies for clinical management of human malignancies in the future. Several structurally different plant secondary metabolites have the ability to sensitize certain types of cancer cells towards conventional chemotherapeutics, providing evidence for rational design of new combinational treatment approaches using these non-toxic compounds derived from natural resources.

Chemotherapy with cytotoxic agents remains one of the major treatment modalities and cornerstones in cancer therapy. Unfortunately, occurrence or acquisition of drug resistance and appearance of severe adverse side effects during the treatment of many tumors with cytotoxic antineoplastic agents constitute impediments limiting their clinical application and leading to failure of the treatment. These obstacles offer important challenges for the global cancer research. However, up to now, none of the compounds have been approved for the clinical use to efficiently modulate and reverse multidrug resistance phenomenon or overcome systemic toxicity [1]. Therefore, in recent years, attempts to augment therapeutic efficacy by using a combinational approach and inclusion of natural flavonoids in the chemotherapeutic protocols are gaining continuously increasing interest and attention as a novel promising strategy to sensitize malignant cells to anticancer action [2-4]. A number of findings presented in this book highlight the importance of this combinational approach for suppression of cancer growth and combating malignant disorders. Limitless potential and power of plant natural products to provide lead compounds for discovery of anticancer drugs and potential adjuvant agents are illustrated also by the fact that more than 60% of all clinically approved chemotherapeutic drugs have been isolated from natural sources, such as camptothecin, etoposide, vinca alkaloids vinblastine and vincristine, and paclitaxel [5, 6]. Combined application of flavonoids and cytotoxic drugs might result in enhanced anticancer responses in different types of tumoral cells, allowing to reduce current standard chemotherapeutic dosage recommendations and subsequently decrease the risk of potentially devastating treatment sequelae, i.e., mitigating serious adverse side effects [7-9]. As a result, the quality of life of patients will probably be improved, accompanied by fewer interruptions or discontinuations of treatment processes. In addition, inclusion of flavonoids in the chemotherapeutic treatment regimens confers reversal of drug resistance phenomenon, altogether leading to better clinical outcome and prolonged overall survival of patients. Potential benefits of addition of flavonoids in the chemotherapeutic treatment regimens are summarized in Figure 7.1. Therefore, certain flavonoids might be used as promising adjuvant agents for chemotherapeutic treatment regimens against diverse malignant disorders and would guide further development and optimization of therapeutic protocols to benefit cancer patients.

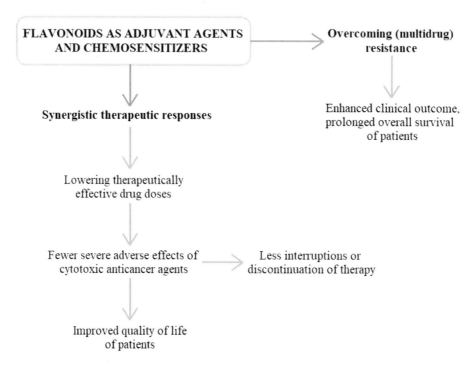

Figure 7.1. New therapeutic avenues opened up by addition of properly chosen flavonoids in the chemotherapeutic treatment regimens against different malignancies.

However, not only positive cooperation and chemosensitizing action have been attributed to natural flavonoids in the combined treatment of cancer cells with antineoplastic agents. In certain cases, flavonoids can exert also undesired opposite effects, antagonizing therapeutic activities of cytotoxic drugs, leading to decrease or even abolishment of treatment efficacy and promoting development of drug resistance. Such negative combinations are described in detail in the Chapter 6 at subsections devoted to specific chemotherapeutic drugs with special warnings to patients suffering from different tumors. There are diverse molecular mechanisms possibly underlying these antagonistic interactions, including antioxidant action of flavonoids, modulation of pharmacokinetic properties of drugs or promotion of drug efflux from the cancer cells through regulation of transporter proteins, among others. As there is no ethical basis to initiate clinical trials with these antagonistic combinations that are probably harmful for patients, the only possibility here is to trust the findings obtained from preclinical studies with *in vitro* cancer cell lines and *in vivo* xenograft tumors in animals. Therefore, due to counteractive action of certain flavonoids concerning therapeutic effects of conventional drugs, cancer patients should be well-informed and conscious about these combinations, to be able to avoid the exposure to specific plant-derived food products and dietary supplements during the active treatment phase with certain cytotoxic antineoplastic agents. As self-initiative consumption of plant-based supplements is rather frequent among cancer patients, the information compiled in this book concerning recommendable (synergistic) and unrecommendable (antagonistic) combinations of flavonoids and chemotherapeutic drugs could assist patients to make safer and more conscious choices. Abstinence from contraindicated dietary products by patients going under chemotherapeutic treatment with certain drugs is required, with the aim not to detrimentally affect the clinical success.

Apart from structural peculiarities of flavonoids and standard antineoplastic drugs, several aspects are decisive in determining their combinational effects in preclinical malignant systems, i.e., synergistic, additive or antagonistic interactions. These key factors include concentrations of both agents, sequence of their addition (pre- or posttreatment or simultaneous administration) and timing schedule; besides certain molecular characteristics of cancer cells, such as expression and function of different transporter proteins or hormonal receptors, among others. The properly chosen dosage of flavonoids and fine-tuned treatment schedule in combination with chemotherapeutic drugs are very important to achieve the desired therapeutic benefits. Therefore, further chemotherapeutic protocols comprising flavonoids as adjuvant agents must be strictly optimized to attain maximized therapeutic effects.

In general, flavonoids alone exert their anticancer activities at micromolar doses, mainly at higher than 10 μM, which are hardly achievable via oral consumption of food products rich in these plant secondary metabolites. However, when used in combinational treatment regimens, essentially lower non-toxic concentrations of flavonoids have been shown to affect the therapeutic efficacy of conventional chemotherapeutics, indicating that flavonoids at typical physiological dietary plasma levels might be able to modulate antineoplastic action of traditional drugs. Therefore, the actual application of dietary polyphenolic constituents in anticancer therapy may lie more in combinational therapy with cytotoxic drugs than in monotherapy. This evidence-based opinion makes the addition of flavonoids as adjuvant agents during the administration of chemotherapeutic drugs an especially attractive and promising approach in the development of further modern anticancer treatment protocols. At that, flavonoids act on multiple molecular targets in malignant systems and modulate several signal transduction pathways involved in survival of cancer cells. Since tumorigenesis is a complex process associated with hundreds of gene mutations and multiple dysfunctions, it is probably impossible to control cancer growth and progression by affecting single or few signaling cascades [10]. Resistance to chemotherapy also represents a complex and complicated phenomenon implicating alterations in a variety of cellular mechanisms, including modulation of expression and function of drug efflux pumps on cellular membrane [11]. Therefore, simultaneous targeting of the multifaceted machinery of cancer and exerting the diversity of anticancer activities by natural flavonoids are essential advantages over the traditional chemotherapeutic drugs which are usually designed to influence only one signaling pathway within malignant cells. Natural flavonoids can interfere with chemotherapy-induced cell cycle arrest and apoptotic cell death, inhibit cell proliferation, invasion, migration, metastasis and angiogenesis at a number of different steps, through regulation of various molecular mechanisms, dependent on the type and stage of malignancy [12-14]. Furthermore, due to their wide intake as important constituents of plant-based food items or herbal products by human beings already for several centuries, flavonoids have steadily proven their safety profile.

Despite the structural similarity of the main backbone of flavonoids, each of them might act in different ways in diverse malignant systems, requiring separate evaluation for every type of flavonoid-chemotherapeutic drug combination. Based on the current preclinical findings, there are some common natural flavonoids for which only synergistic or additive (or no) interactions with different conventional anticancer agents have been reported, with no antagonistic interactions found so far; including myricetin, isorhamnetin, wogonin or naringenin. However, this observation can be associated with the relatively small amount of studies still performed using combined chemotherapeutic treatment of malignant cells with these flavonoids. Furthermore, each tumor has its own distinct phenotype and consequently, sensitivity of flavonoids to certain chemotherapeutic drugs can vary considerably from one type of malignancy to another. Combinations that are synergistic in one type of tumor may be antagonistic in another type of tumor; moreover, malignant tissues are usually of heterogenous nature. Therefore, each type of cancer cells should be considered individually concerning possible interactions between conventional chemotherapeutic drugs and natural dietary flavonoids. From clinical point of view, it means that careful consideration should be given to individual characteristics of each patient to decide about the most beneficial adjuvant agent for chemotherapy with certain cytotoxic drugs [15-19]. This is probably one of the most feasible areas where the principles of personal medicine should be applied in the clinical oncology in the near future. With no doubt, individualized counseling of cancer patients concerning recommended and unrecommended plant-based food items during the active treatment phase with certain cytotoxic drugs is almost imperative for achievement of the best therapeutic outcome, besides improvement of quality of life of patients. Based on the preclinical findings presented in the Chapter 6 of this book, there are some cancer sites for which only synergistic or additive (or no) interactions between dietary flavonoids and traditional antineoplastic agents have been described so far, with no antagonistic data still reported; including tumors in the head and neck region, i.e., oral cavity, tongue, larynx, hypopharynx and nasopharynx (Table 7.1), liver (Table 7.2), pancreas (Table 7.3), esophagus and endometrium. However, lack of antagonistic interactions in these cancer sites can be associated with the relatively small number of studies performed to date by combining conventional chemotherapeutic drugs with different natural flavonoids. In any case, the prospect of using a safe dietary supplement containing plant flavonoids to enhance the efficacy of chemotherapeutic treatment, reduce its adverse side effects and improve clinical outcome is exciting and certainly deserves further investigations.

Table 7.1. Chemosensitization of head and neck cancers by flavonoids (composed by preclinical findings)*

Cytotoxic drug	Chemosensitizers
Cisplatin	Apigenin, chrysin, EGCG, isoliquiritigenin, quercetin, wogonin
Doxorubicin	DMC, ECG, EGCG, myricetin, quercetin, rutin, tamarixetin
5-Fluorouracil	Apigenin, EGCG
Vincristine	Quercetin
Paclitaxel	EGCG, luteolin

* Neoplasms in tongue, larynx, hypopharynx, nasopharynx and oral cavity are included in this group of cancers. DMC, 2`,4`-Dihydroxy-6`-methoxy-3`,5`-dimethylchalcone.

Table 7.2. Chemosensitization of liver cancers by flavonoids (composed by preclinical findings)

Cytotoxic drug	Chemosensitizers
Mitomycin C	Quercetin
Cisplatin	Alpinetin, chrysin, genistein, luteolin, quercetin, wogonin
Carboplatin	Quercetin
Nedaplatin	Ampelopsin
Hydrocamptothecin	Baicalein, wogonin
Etoposide	Rhamnetin, wogonin
Doxorubicin	Apigenin, chrysin, DMC, ECG, EGCG, ethylated EGCG (Y6), icaritin, quercetin, rhamnetin, silibinin
Daunorubicin	ECG, EGCG
Epirubicin	Baicalein
Mitoxantrone	Malvidin
5-Fluorouracil	Apigenin, baicalein, DMC, EGCG, luteolin, oroxylin A, quercetin, wogonin
Paclitaxel	Apigenin, phloretin, quercetin, rhamnetin

DMC, 2`,4`-Dihydroxy-6`-methoxy-3`,5`-dimethylchalcone.

Table 7.3. Chemosensitization of pancreatic cancers by flavonoids (composed by preclinical findings)

Cytotoxic drug	Chemosensitizers
Cisplatin	Apigenin, genistein, luteolin
Oxaliplatin	Apigenin, luteolin
Doxorubicin	Deguelin
5-Fluorouracil	Apigenin, genistein, luteolin
Gemcitabine	Apigenin, baicalein, EGCG, fisetin, genistein, luteolin, quercetin
Docetaxel	Baicalein, genistein

The synergistic interactions between dietary flavonoids and chemotherapeutic drugs in diverse malignant cells, presented in this book, set the basis for further in-depth and more complex studies, including additional *in vitro* tests using a larger number of cancer cell lines with distinct molecular characteristics, *in vivo* assays in different animal models to confirm the *in vitro* results, but also human clinical trials to validate the clinical potential and benefit and develop the best therapeutic protocols for clinical application of the combinations in the future. It is well known that *in vitro* data may not completely represent the *in vivo* results. As metabolic differences between cellular cultures and rodents can change the synergistic relationships of two agents, the results observed *in vitro* may not be always verified in animals [20, 21]. In general, nude mice tumor xenografts are widely accepted models to further evaluate anticancer efficacy of test compounds, assess their toxicity and bioavailability. Although the use of orthotopic injection of malignant cells to experimental animals is considered ideal and preferred to subcutaneous injection in modelling the soft tissue growth, even this process can be sometimes challenging. For example, mice have four biologically different and anatomically separated prostatic lobes and it is still not certainly clear how well any of them corresponds to the human prostate [22]. Therefore, appropriate clinical trials with cancer patients, especially patients with advanced tumors resistant to conventional cytotoxic drugs, are required to initiate to obtain the most reliable data about the usefulness of flavonoids as adjuvant agents for chemotherapeutic regimens and to support the combined strategy for the treatment of various types of human cancers.

Despite hundreds of preclinical studies performed to date about the effects of flavonoids on chemotherapeutic efficacy of antineoplastic drugs in various cancer cells, our current knowledge on combinations is still rather scarce; especially considering the large chemodiversity of flavonoids in the nature (more than 8000 structurally different compounds described so far). In this way, several commonly occurring flavonoids in the human diet have received only very little, if any, attention at all. Therefore, screenings *in vitro* level should also be continued and expanded in the next few years to investigate a wide variety of flavonoids as potential agents with therapy-enhancing effects. In addition, this structural diversity of natural flavonoids might hopefully inspire scientists in terms of synthetic modifications to design semisynthetic derivatives with stronger chemosensitizing properties. Moreover, as flavonoids usually exist in the form of different mixtures in plant-based foods and herbal products, the combined effects of multiple flavonoids instead of a single flavonoid on the therapeutic efficacy of anticancer drugs would also be interesting and attractive to establish. In different mixtures, flavonoids can potentiate beneficial effects of each other, leading to even higher potency to sensitize malignant cells towards chemotherapeutic drugs and block diverse survival and metastatic mechanisms of tumoral cells. On the other hand, interactions of different flavonoids with some new-generation cytotoxic agents are also needed to examine in the near future. Last but not least, further mechanistic studies might help to fully understand the alterations in cellular physiology and molecular events regulated by combined treatments with flavonoids and anticancer drugs in diverse cancer cells. Molecular targets and cellular signaling pathways modulated by flavonoids in interfering with drug-induced antitumor responses are needed to be clarified in further investigations. Therefore, the research field to find the best combinations of flavonoids and chemotherapeutic drugs to bring them into clinical practice is very broad, multipronged and multilevel.

In conclusion, numerous findings on interactions with natural dietary flavonoids and traditional antineoplastic agents set an attractive scientific basis for development of non-toxic adjuvant agents for current chemotherapeutic regimens against different types of human cancers allowing to maximize clinical outcome, while simultaneously improving quality of life and survival of patients. In the meantime, and from the practical perspective of cancer patients, the incredibly strong potential of plant secondary metabolites, which constitute an essential but still modifiable part of the everyday diet of human beings, to modulate the therapeutic efficacy of traditional anticancer drugs should not be ignored, but rather consciously utilized for the best therapeutic responses. In particular, it is important to bear in mind that certain flavonoids can work antagonistically with specific chemotherapeutic drugs, resulting in decrease or even abolishing the treatment efficacy. Therefore, personal counseling of patients about the recommended and contraindicated flavonoids-containing plant-based food products and dietary supplements during the active treatment phase with traditional cytotoxic antineoplastic agents is highly important.

REFERENCES

[1] Ma W, Feng S, Yao X, Yuan Z, Liu L, Xie Y. Nobiletin enhances the efficacy of chemotherapeutic agents in ABCB1 overexpression cancer cells. *Sci Rep* 2015; 5: 18789.

[2] Davenport A, Frezza M, Shen M, Ge Y, Huo C, Chan TH, Dou QP. Celastrol and an EGCG pro-drug exhibit potent chemosensitizing activity in human leukemia cells. *Int J Mol Med* 2010; 25: 465-70.

[3] Mihaila M, Bostan M, Hotnog D, Ferdes M, Brasoveanu LL. Real-time analysis of quercetin, resveratrol and/or doxorubicin effects in MCF-7 cells. *Rom Biotechnol Lett* 2013; 18: 8106-14.

[4] Raina K, Agarwal R. Combinatorial strategies for cancer eradication by silibinin and cytotoxic agents: Efficacy and mechanisms. *Acta Pharmacol Sin* 2007; 28: 1466-75.

[5] Iriti M, Kubina R, Cochis A, Sorrentino R, Varoni EM, Kabala-Dzik A, Azzimonti B, Dziedzic A, Rimondini L, Wojtyczka RD. Rutin, a quercetin glycoside, restores chemosensitivity in human breast cancer cells. *Phytother Res* 2017; 31: 1529-38.

[6] Ho BY, Lin CH, Apaya MK, Chao WW, Shyur LF. Silibinin and paclitaxel cotreatment significantly suppress the activity and lung metastasis of triple negative 4T1 mammary tumor cell in mice. *J Tradit Complement Med* 2011; 2: 301-11.

[7] Khoshyomn S, Nathan D, Manske GC, Osler TM, Penar PL. Synergistic effect of genistein and BCNU on growth inhibition and cytotoxicity of glioblastoma cells. *J Neurooncol* 2002; 57: 193-200.

[8] Bieg D, Sypniewski D, Nowak E, Bednarek I. Morin decreases galectin-3 expression and sensitizes ovarian cancer cells to cisplatin. *Arch Gynecol Obstet* 2018; 298: 1181-94.

[9] Li Y, Ahmed F, Ali S, Philip PA, Kucuk O, Sarkar FH. Inactivation of nuclear factor kappaB by soy isoflavone genistein contributes to increased apoptosis induced by chemotherapeutic agents in human cancer cells. *Cancer Res* 2005; 65: 6934-42.

[10] Wang P, Henning SM, Heber D, Vadgama JV. Sensitization of docetaxel in prostate cancer cells by green tea and quercetin. *J Nutr Biochem* 2015; 26: 408-15.

[11] Maciejczyk A, Surowiak P. Quercetin inhibits proliferation and increases sensitivity of ovarian cancer cells to cisplatin and paclitaxel. *Ginekol Pol* 2013; 84: 590-5.

[12] de Oliveira Junior RG, Christiane Adrielly AF, da Silva Almeida JRG, Grougnet R, Thiery V, Picot L. Sensitization of tumor cells to chemotherapy by natural products: A systematic review of preclinical data and molecular mechanisms. *Fitoterapia* 2018; 129: 383-400.

[13] Kuo CY, Zupko I, Chang FR, Hunyadi A, Wu CC, Weng TS, Wang HC. Dietary flavonoid derivatives enhance chemotherapeutic effect by inhibiting the DNA damage response pathway. *Toxicol Appl Pharmacol* 2016; 311: 99-105.

[14] Lecumberri E, Dupertuis YM, Miralbell R, Pichard C. Green tea polyphenol epigallocatechin-3-gallate (EGCG) as adjuvant in cancer therapy. *Clin Nutr* 2013; 32: 894-903.

[15] Budak-Alpdogan T, Chen B, Warrier A, Medina DJ, Moore D, Bertino JR. Retinoblastoma tumor suppressor gene expression determines the response to

sequential flavopiridol and doxorubicin treatment in small-cell lung carcinoma. *Clin Cancer Res* 2009; 15: 1232-40.

[16] Borska S, Chmielewska M, Wysocka T, Drag-Zalesinska M, Zabel M, Dziegiel P. In vitro effect of quercetin on human gastric carcinoma: targeting cancer cells death and MDR. *Food Chem Toxicol* 2012; 50: 3375-83.

[17] Gomez LA, de Las Pozas A, Perez-Stable C. Sequential combination of flavopiridol and docetaxel reduces the levels of X-linked inhibitor of apoptosis and AKT proteins and stimulates apoptosis in human LNCaP prostate cancer cells. *Mol Cancer Ther* 2006; 5: 1216-26.

[18] Klimaszewska-Wisniewska A, Halas-Wisniewska M, Tadrowski T, Gagat M, Grzanka D, Grzanka A. Paclitaxel and the dietary flavonoid fisetin: a synergistic combination that induces mitotic catastrophe and autophagic cell death in A549 non-small cell lung cancer cells. *Cancer Cell Int* 2016; 16: 10.

[19] Abaza MS, Orabi KY, Al-Quattan E, Al-Attiyah RJ. Growth inhibitory and chemo-sensitization effects of naringenin, a natural flavanone purified from Thymus vulgaris, on human breast and colorectal cancer. *Cancer Cell Int* 2015; 15: 46.

[20] Zhang J, Luo Y, Zhao X, Li X, Li K, Chen D, Qiao M, Hu H, Zhao X. Co-delivery of doxorubicin and the traditional Chinese medicine quercetin using biotin-PEG2000-DSPE modified liposomes for the treatment of multidrug resistant breast cancer. *RSC Adv* 2016; 6: 113173.

[21] Wang T, Gao J, Yu J, Shen L. Synergistic inhibitory effect of wogonin and low-dose paclitaxel on gastric cancer cells and tumor xenografts. *Chin J Cancer Res* 2013; 25: 505-13.

[22] Mukhtar E, Adhami VM, Siddiqui IA, Verma AK, Mukhtar H. Fisetin enhances chemotherapeutic effect of cabazitaxel against human prostate cancer cells. *Mol Cancer Ther* 2016; 15: 2863-74.

ABOUT THE AUTHOR

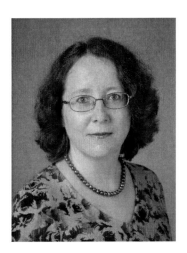

Dr. *Katrin Sak*, was born in Viljandi, Estonia, in 1975, the daughter of schoolteachers Aita Sak and Toivo Sak. After studies in the University of Tartu, she received a bachelor degree (BSc) in chemistry in 1996 and a master degree (MSc) in bioorganic chemistry in 1997. In 2001, Katrin Sak graduated with doctorate degree (PhD) in bioorganic chemistry. During 2001-2004, Dr. Sak did postdoctoral research at the Free University of Brussels, Belgium. In 2011-2012, she completed a special training in nutritional oncology and acquired diploma in cancer nutrition in the Health Schools Australia. Katrin Sak has improved her knowledge at the top universities in Sweden, Finland, Spain, Germany, Israel, Austria, Czech Republic, Italy, etc. Her work has been honored by several awards.

Dr. Sak is the author of international monography *Flavonoids in the Fight against Upper Gastrointestinal Tract Cancers* (Nova Science Publishers, Inc., New York, 2018). She has published more than 75 articles in international peer-reviewed journals; most of them dealing anticancer activities of various flavonoids in the cellular models of different cancer types. She is also the author of three chapters of books, including *Nutraceuticals Nanotechnology in the Agri-Food Industry, Vol. 4* (Academic Press, 2016) and *Food*

Bioconversion Handbook of Food Bioengineering, Vol. 2 (Academic Press, 2017). In addition, Dr. Sak is the author of the book *Food and Cancer* (in Estonian, 2013) and numerous popular-scientific articles published in the Estonian health journals.

The major research topics of Katrin Sak involve different anticancer actions of plant-derived flavonoids in diverse malignant systems, engaged cellular signaling pathways and molecular mechanisms; besides the metabolic bioconversion of these food polyphenols in the human body and bioactivities of various metabolites. In addition, scientific activity of Dr. Sak is also focused on the interactions between dietary flavonoids and conventional anticancer treatment modalities, including chemotherapy and radiotherapy.

Katrin Sak is the head of the NGO Praeventio.

INDEX OF DRUGS

#

4-Hydroxycyclophosphamide (4HO-CY), **137-140**

5-Fluorouracil (5-FU), 4, 5, 6, 53, 56, 58, 60, 62, 63, 65, 201, 225, **271-288**, 304, 389, 390

A

Asparaginase (ASP), 343, **345**

B

Bleomycin (BLM), 63, **343**, **344**

Busulfan, 150, **151**

C

Cabazitaxel (CBZ), 10, 305, **340-342**

Camptothecin (CPT), 60, 63, 89, **206**, 207, 211, 213, 214, 386

Capecitabine (CAPE), 281, **288**, **289**

Carboplatin (CBP), 58, 65, 153, **198-200**, 389

Carmustine (BCNU), 150, **151**

Chlorambucil (CMB), xxi, 39, **149-151**

Cisplatin (CDDP), 3, 9, 11, 12, 35, 53, 54, 56, 58, 60, 63, 64, 136, **153-198**, 201, 202, 203, 205, 267, 272, 278, 291, 292, 322, 326, 335, 338, 389, 390

Cyclophosphamide (CY), 13, 15, 16, 35, 39, **137-141**

Cytarabine (ARA-C), 14, 282, **295-298**, 300, 304

D

Dacarbazine (DTIC), 13, 142, **148**, **149**, 150

Dactinomycin (ACT), 10, 53, 54, **270**

Daunorubicin (DNR), 14, 53, 54, 60, 63, 206, 238, 240, **259-263**, 312, 313, 389

Decitabine (AZA), 282, **299**, **300**

Docetaxel (DOC), 10, 53, 54, 58, 60, 66, 305, **334-340**, 341, 342, 390

Doxorubicin (DOX), 6, 8, 12, 16, 53, 54, 58, 60, 63, 64, 66, 136, 155, 171, 194, 206, 217, **220-258**, 261, 270, 301, 310, 311, 312, 313, 316, 322, 323, 334, 343, 389, 390

E

Epirubicin (EPI), 7, 63, 206, 238, 240, **263-266**, 270, 389

Etoposide (VP-16), 13, 53, 54, 60, 63, 66, 171, **214-220**, 236, 386, 389

F

Fludarabine (FLU), 15, 62, 282, **302**, **303**

G

Gemcitabine (GEM), 6, 8, 53, 60, 63, 66, 281, 282, **289-295**, 304, 390

Index of Drugs

H

Hydrocamptothecin (HCPT), **206**, 207, 210, **211**, 214, 389

I

Idarubicin, 14
Irinotecan (CPT-11), 5, 54, 207, 210, **211**, **212**, 214
Irinotecan active metabolite (SN-38), 53, 54, 207, 208, 209, **211**, **212**, 214

M

Methotrexate (MTX), 10, 13, 14, 53, 54, **300-302**
Mitomycin C (MMC), 53, 54, 150, **151**, **152**, 389
Mitoxantrone (MX), 53, 54, 63, **267-270**, 389

N

Nedaplatin (NDP), 153, **200**, **201**, 202, 205, 389

O

Oxaliplatin (OXA), 5, 53, 54, 153, 166, 189, **201-205**, 230, 246, 390

P

Paclitaxel (PTX), 9, 35, 53, 54, 60, 62, 63, 66, 89, 136, 231, 248, 260, 262, 277, 285, 305, **315-333**, 334, 335, 336, 342, 386, 389
Photofrin or Porfimer sodium (DHE), 343, **344**, **345**
Pirarubicin (THP), 206, **267**

T

Temozolomide (TMZ), 11, **142-148**
Tiazofurin (TCAR), **303**, **304**
Topotecan (TPT), 53, 54, 209, **213**, **214**

V

Vinblastine (VBL), 53, 54, 60, 89, 259, 260, 262, **305-308**, 318, 320, 321, 323, 386
Vincristine (VCR), 14, 16, 53, 54, 60, 89, 305, **309-315**, 342, 386, 389

INDEX OF FLAVONOIDS

#

2`,4`-Dihydroxy-6`-methoxy-3`,5`-dimethylchalcone (DMC), 93, 225, 237, 238, 240, 255, 258, 274, 279, 280, 282, 286, 287, 389

2`,5`-Dihydroxychalcone (2`,5`-DHC), 155, 197

2`-Hydroxychalcone, 149, 150

3`,4`,5`,5,7- Pentamethoxyflavone (3`,4`,5`,5,7-PMF), 94, 155, 192, 196

4`,7- Dimethoxyflavone (4`,7-DMF), 259, 262, 306, 307, 308

4`,7-Dimethoxyisoflavone, 259, 262, 263, 306, 307

4-Methoxychalcone (4-MC), 155, 195, 196

5,7,4`-Trihydroxy-8-methoxyflavanone, 194

5,7-Dimethoxyflavone (5,7-DMF), 139, 140, 267, 268, 296, 297, 298, 310, 313, 315, 343, 345

6-Methoxynaringenin or 5,7,4`-trihydroxy-6-methoxyflavanone, 155, 194

8-Hydroxydaidzein, 95, 263, 265, 266

8-Methylflavone, 267, 268

A

Acacetin or 4`-methylapigenin, 94, 207, 212, 214, 222, 247, 258, 268

Afrormosin, 264, 265

Alopecurone B, 95, 155, 222, 257, 258, 301, 310, 313, 334, 339, 343, 344

Alpinetin, 93, 155, 174, 194, 389

Amorphigenin, 264, 265

Ampelopsin or dihydromyricetin, 93, 198, 199, 200, 202, 204, 205, 225, 238, 256, 258, 318, 331, 333, 389

Apigenin, 91, 94, 96, 102, 155, 156, 174, 188, 189, 196, 198, 202, 204, 208, 212, 214, 215, 216, 218, 222, 223, 238, 245, 246, 249, 257, 258, 267, 268, 274, 280, 281, 283, 287, 290, 292, 293, 294, 295, 304, 310, 313, 314, 315, 318, 328, 333, 389, 390

Astragalin or kaempferol 3-O-glucoside, 208

Avicularin or quercetin 3-O-arabinofuranoside, 156, 174, 182, 196, 273, 274

B

Baicalein, 92, 94, 156, 174, 190, 191, 193, 196, 198, 207, 210, 211, 214, 223, 238, 247, 264, 265, 266, 274, 284, 287, 290, 293, 295, 301, 302, 310, 313, 314, 318, 325, 329, 330, 332, 333, 334, 336, 339, 340, 342, 389, 390

Baicalin or baicalein 7-O-glucuronide, 92, 94, 157, 192, 193, 196, 198, 223, 248, 258, 334, 336, 337

Baptigenin Ψ, 259, 262, 263, 306, 307, 308

Barbigerone, 223, 238, 253, 258

Biochanin A or 4`-methylgenistein, 223, 253, 258, 259, 262, 263, 268, 306, 307

Butein, 149, 150, 157, 174, 195, 196

Index of Flavonoids

C

Calycosin, 95, 157, 188, 196, 223, 253, 274, 286
Catechin, xix, 92, 93, 155, 185, 207, 223, 224, 237, 251, 258,
Chrysin, 94, 157, 158, 174, 190, 196, 198, 208, 209, 212, 213, 214, 224, 246, 247, 249, 257, 258, 259, 262, 263, 264, 265, 267, 268, 306, 307, 334, 336, 337, 339, 340, 389
CJY, 224, 253, 258

D

Daidzein, 92, 95, 102, 158, 188, 196, 198, 263, 306, 307, 308, 318, 326
Deguelin, 95, 216, 218, 219, 220, 224, 225, 238, 256, 257, 258, 282, 296, 297, 298, 302, 303, 390
Diosmetin, 208, 212, 214
Diosmin or diosmetin 7-O-rutinoside, 208

E

Epicatechin (EC), 92, 93, 161, 185, 196, 219, 227, 251, 260, 261
Epicatechin 3-gallate (ECG), 92, 93, 225, 226, 250, 258, 259, 261, 263, 389
Epigallocatechin (EGC), 92, 93, 150, 151, 226, 251, 259, 261, 264, 265, 275, 283, 290, 294
Epigallocatechin 3-gallate (EGCG), 92, 93, 96, 97, 102, 103, 142, 143, 145, 147, 148, 149, 150, 151, 152, 158, 159, 160, 161, 174, 175, 182, 183, 184, 185, 186, 196, 197, 198, 201, 202, 204, 216, 218, 219, 226, 227, 238, 240, 249, 250, 251, 258, 259, 260, 261, 263, 270, 273, 275, 281, 283, 287, 288, 290, 293, 294, 295, 296, 297, 298, 299, 300, 301, 304, 306, 307, 308, 310, 311, 313, 314, 318, 319, 325, 327, 328, 332, 333, 334, 337, 338, 339, 340, 342, 343, 344, 345, 389, 390
Equol, 155, 188, 196, 198
Eriodictyol, 208
Ethylated EGCG (Y6), 227, 250, 389
Eupatorin, 94, 227, 228, 248, 258

F

Fisetin, 91, 94, 137, 138, 140, 141, 161, 162, 175, 180, 196, 208, 215, 216, 218, 228, 244, 245, 257, 267, 269, 273, 275, 290, 293, 294, 295, 301, 316, 317, 319, 320, 332, 333, 340, 341, 342, 390
Flavokawain B, 93, 260, 262
Flavone, 260, 262, 263, 306, 307, 308
Formononetin or 4`-methyldaidzein, 95, 162, 188, 228, 253, 264, 265, 266

G

Galangin, 94, 162, 175, 180, 181, 196, 198, 208, 212, 214, 228, 244, 245, 257, 258
Genistein, 92, 95, 96, 101, 102, 139, 141, 150, 151, 163, 164, 165, 175, 186, 187, 188, 196, 197, 198, 207, 208, 209, 210, 211, 212, 213, 214, 216, 217, 218, 219, 228, 229, 239, 252, 253, 254, 257, 258, 260, 262, 263, 268, 269, 275, 280, 281, 282, 285, 286, 287, 289, 290, 291, 292, 294, 295, 296, 297, 299, 300, 301, 302, 303, 304, 306, 307, 308, 311, 312, 320, 325, 326, 333, 334, 335, 337, 338, 339, 340, 341, 342, 343, 344, 345, 389, 390
Genistin or genistein 7-O-glucoside, 95, 306, 308, 320, 326

H

Heptamethoxyflavone, 311, 313, 314
Hesperetin, 93, 96, 102, 138, 208, 210, 212, 214, 217, 218, 219, 229, 252, 257, 258, 268, 269
Hesperidin or hesperetin 7-O-rutinoside, 93, 96, 138, 139, 141, 165, 194, 229, 239, 252, 258, 296, 297
Hispidulin or 6-methylscutellarein, 94, 144, 145, 148, 276, 285, 287, 291, 293, 294
Hydnocarpin, 95, 310, 313
Hyperoside or quercetin 3-O-galactoside, 94, 165, 181, 196

I

Icariin, 95, 144, 145, 148, 229, 256, 258, 276, 280, 282, 286, 287, 291, 294

Index of Flavonoids

Icariside II, 95, 229, 256, 320, 332, 333

Icaritin, 95, 229, 256, 258, 264, 265, 266, 389

Intricatinol, 95, 165, 196, 197

Isoliquiritigenin, 93, 96, 139, 140, 141, 165, 195, 196, 198, 239, 240, 256, 264, 265, 266, 276, 286, 320, 331, 389

Isorhamnetin or 3`-methylquercetin, 165, 180, 196, 198, 199, 229, 245, 273, 276, 281, 288, 289, 295, 297, 298, 388

Isoxanthohumol, 95, 165, 197, 198, 229, 256, 257, 320, 325, 332

K

Kaempferide or 4`-methylkaempferol, 208, 212, 214, 268, 269

Kaempferol, 91, 94, 166, 181, 196, 198, 208, 212, 214, 229, 230, 244, 245, 257, 258, 264, 266, 268, 269, 295, 297, 298, 306, 308, 317, 321, 333

Kaempferol 7-O-neohesperidoside, 208

L

Licochalcone A, 93, 96, 175, 197, 276, 286, 287

Liquiritigenin, 93, 96, 166, 176, 193, 196, 291, 293

Luteolin, 91, 94, 166, 167, 176, 189, 190, 193, 196, 197, 201, 202, 203, 204, 208, 212, 214, 230, 246, 249, 257, 258, 276, 277, 282, 284, 287, 291, 293, 294, 295, 321, 325, 328, 329, 332, 333, 343, 344, 389, 390

Luteolin 4`-O-glucoside, 208, 212, 214

M

Malvidin, 93, 267, 269, 389

Morin, 94, 149, 150, 151, 167, 181, 196, 197, 230, 244, 258, 317, 321, 325, 333

Myricetin, 91, 94, 167, 180, 196, 209, 230, 231, 244, 245, 258, 273, 277, 280, 287, 295, 297, 298, 317, 321, 333, 388, 389

N

Naringenin, 93, 96, 138, 140, 167, 193, 199, 200, 206, 207, 209, 212, 214, 217, 219, 231, 239, 251, 252, 258, 268, 269, 277, 286, 311, 312, 388

Naringin or naringenin 7-O-neohesperidoside, 93, 96, 210, 212, 296, 298

Nobiletin or hexamethoxyflavone, 94, 96, 167, 192, 198, 199, 200, 203, 204, 231, 248, 258, 260, 262, 263, 277, 285, 287, 311, 313, 314, 321, 330, 332, 333, 335, 336, 340

O

Orobol, 95, 167, 188, 196, 322, 326, 333

Oroxylin A or 6-methylbaicalein, 92, 94, 231, 239, 247, 248, 258, 277, 280, 284, 287, 306, 308, 322, 330, 333, 389

P

Pelargonidin, 93, 267, 269

Peltatoside or quercetin 3-O-arabinoglucoside, 209

Phloretin, 93, 167, 168, 195, 196, 231, 255, 322, 325, 332, 333, 389

Prenylated chalcone (PC2), 322, 332

Pro-EGCG, 259, 261, 297

Protoapigenone, 168, 176, 193

Prunin or naringenin 7-O-glucoside, 209, 212, 214, 268, 269

Puerarin or daidzein 8-C-glucoside, 95, 277, 280, 286, 287

Q

Quercetin , 91, 92, 94, 96, 101, 138, 143, 144, 145, 146, 148, 149, 150, 151, 152, 154, 168, 169, 170, 176, 177, 178, 179, 180, 196, 197, 198, 199, 201, 203, 209, 210, 212, 213, 214, 215, 217, 218, 232, 233, 234, 235, 239, 241, 242, 243, 244, 257, 258, 260, 262, 263, 267, 272, 273, 277, 278, 281, 287, 288, 291, 293, 294, 295, 298, 302, 303, 304, 306, 308, 309, 310, 311, 312, 314, 316, 322, 323, 333, 335, 339, 340, 342, 389, 390

R

Rhamnetin or 7-methylquercetin, 215, 217, 218, 235, 244, 317, 323, 333, 389

Rhoifolin, 209

Robinin, 264, 266
Rotenone, 264, 266
Rubone, 323, 325, 331, 332, 333
Rutin or quercetin 3-O-rutinoside, 94, 138, 140, 144, 146, 147, 148, 170, 182, 209, 235, 245, 273, 295, 296, 298, 301, 317, 323, 333, 389

S

Salvigenin, 94, 235, 248, 258
Scutellarein, 170, 191, 285
Scutellarin or scutellarein 7-O-glucoside, 94, 171, 193, 278, 285, 287
Silibinin, xxiii, 92, 95, 96, 144, 146, 148, 150, 152, 171, 177, 194, 195, 196, 197, 198, 199, 200, 207, 209, 212, 217, 219, 236, 239, 240, 254, 255, 258, 267, 269, 278, 281, 286, 296, 298, 299, 300, 301, 323, 324, 325, 330, 331, 333, 335, 339, 340, 389
Sinensetin, 312, 313, 314
Spiraeoside or quercetin 4`-O-glucoside, 171, 182

T

Tangeretin, 94, 96, 172, 192, 196, 312, 313, 314
Taxifolin, 237, 256, 258, 312, 313, 314, 324, 331, 333
Tectorigenin, 324, 326, 333
Tricin, 335, 336
Troxerutin, 94, 273, 278, 281, 287

V

Vicenin-2, 94, 335, 336, 337, 340

W

Wogonin, 92, 94, 172, 173, 177, 191, 192, 196, 203, 204, 206, 207, 211, 214, 215, 217, 218, 219, 237, 240, 247, 258, 279, 281, 284, 285, 287, 306, 308, 324, 325, 330, 333, 388, 389

Related Nova Publications

Food for Huntington's Disease

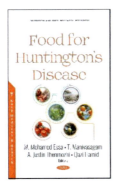

AUTHORS: Musthafa Mohamed Essa, Ph.D., Thamilarasan Manivasagam, Arokiasamy Justin Thenmozhi, and Qazi Hamid

SERIES: Nutrition and Diet Research Progress

BOOK DESCRIPTION: *Food and Huntington's Disease* is another book in a series of books related to the benefits of food on brain function. This book designates the possible beneficial effects of edible natural products and their active materials on Huntington's disease.

HARDCOVER ISBN: 978-1-53613-854-2
RETAIL PRICE: $195

Flour: Production, Varieties and Nutrition

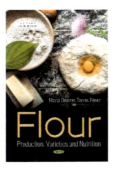

EDITOR: María Dolores Torres Pérez

SERIES: Nutrition and Diet Research Progress

BOOK DESCRIPTION: *Flour: Production, Varieties and Nutrition* is divided into fifteen chapters. The prestigious authors of this book discuss traditional and alternative flours for different application fields, covering a broad range of gluten and novel gluten-free flours.

HARDCOVER ISBN: 978-1-53613-761-3
RETAIL PRICE: $230

To see a complete list of Nova publications, please visit our website at www.novapublishers.com

Related Nova Publications

SCIENCE, TECHNOLOGY AND APPLICATION OF FOLIC ACID ENCAPSULATION

AUTHORS: Honest Sindile Madziva and Kasipathy Kailasapathy

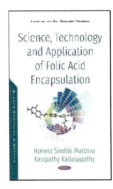

SERIES: Nutrition and Diet Research Progress

BOOK DESCRIPTION: This book elaborates an alternative approach to protect and stabilise the bio-functionality of folic acid through a novel and robust microencapsulation technique. It contains comprehensive science and technology information on folic acid that describes how to protect it from natural plant sources during processing through novel encapsulation techniques and to produce innovative and smart foods and supplements.

HARDCOVER ISBN: 978-1-53614-007-1
RETAIL PRICE: $160

FLAVONOIDS IN THE FIGHT AGAINST UPPER GASTROINTESTINAL TRACT CANCERS

AUTHOR: Katrin Sak

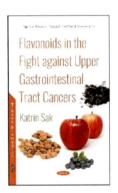

SERIES: Nutrition and Diet Research Progress

BOOK DESCRIPTION: This book gives a comprehensive and contemporary survey about the different anticancer actions of various natural and semisynthetic flavonoids in experimental models of oral, pharyngeal, esophageal and gastric cancers, involving the data obtained from studies of both cell lines as well as laboratorial animals.

HARDCOVER ISBN: 978-1-53613-570-1
RETAIL PRICE: $230

To see a complete list of Nova publications, please visit our website at www.novapublishers.com